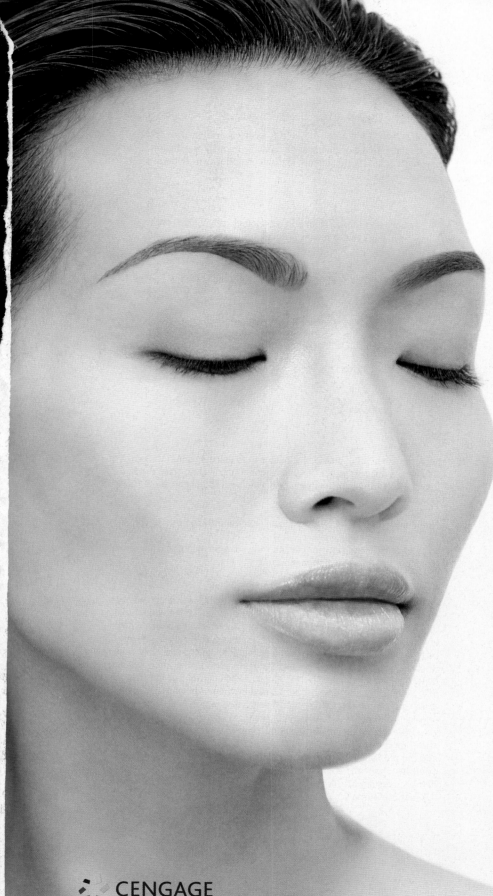

CONTRIBUTING AUTHORS:

Linda Amato

Helen Bickmore

Jeanna Doyle

Mary Nielsen

Lydia Sarfati

Jean Schlaiss

Laura Todd

SERIES EDITOR:

Sallie Deitz

STANDARD ESTHETICS

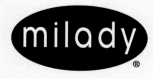

milady®

CENGAGE

Australia • Brazil • Canada • Mexico • Singapore • United Kingdom • United States

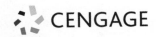

Milady Standard Esthetics: Fundamentals,
Twelfth Edition
Linda Amato, Helen Bickmore, Jeanna Doyle, Mary Nielsen, Lydia Sarfati, Jean Schlaiss, Laura Todd

Vice President and General Manager, Milady: Sandra Bruce

Product Director: Kara Melillo

Product Manager: David Santillan

Learning Design Manager: Jessica Mahoney

Senior Content Manager: Nina Tucciarelli

Content Manager: Sarah Koumourdas

Learning Designer: Beth Williams

Marketing Manager: Kim Berube

Marketing Director: Slavik Volinsky

Design Director, Creative Studio: Jack Pendleton

Cover Designer: Joe Devine

Cover Image:

Makeup by: JP Ramirez

Photography: Julie Stahl

For product information and technology assistance, contact us at
**Cengage Customer & Sales Support, 1-800-354-9706
or support.cengage.com.**

For permission to use material from this text or product, submit all requests online at **www.cengage.com/permissions.**

Library of Congress Control Number: 2019932668

ISBN: 978-1-337-09502-0

Cengage
200 Pier 4 Boulevard
Boston, MA 02210
USA

Cengage is a leading provider of customized learning solutions with employees residing in nearly 40 different countries and sales in more than 125 countries around the world. Find your local representative at **www.cengage.com/global**.

For your lifelong learning solutions, visit **www.milady.com**

To register or access your online learning solution or purchase materials for your course, visit **www.cengage.com**.

Notice to the Reader
Publisher does not warrant or guarantee any of the products described herein or perform any independent analysis in connection with any of the product information contained herein. Publisher does not assume, and expressly disclaims, any obligation to obtain and include information other than that provided to it by the manufacturer. The reader is expressly warned to consider and adopt all safety precautions that might be indicated by the activities described herein and to avoid all potential hazards. By following the instructions contained herein, the reader willingly assumes all risks in connection with such instructions. The publisher makes no representations or warranties of any kind, including but not limited to, the warranties of fitness for particular purpose or merchantability, nor are any such representations implied with respect to the material set forth herein, and the publisher takes no responsibility with respect to such material. The publisher shall not be liable for any special, consequential, or exemplary damages resulting, in whole or part, from the readers' use of, or reliance upon, this material.

Printed in the United States of America
Print Number: 10   Print Year: 2022

Brief Contents

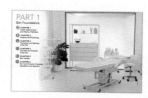

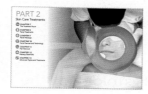

Contents

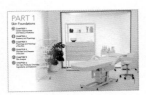

5 Skin Analysis   162

6 Skin Care Products: Chemistry, Ingredients, and Selection   196

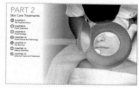

PART 2
Skin Care Treatments   /260

7 The Treatment Room   262

8 Facial Treatments   296

Procedures at a Glance

Preface

A Letter to You: Our Fabulous Student

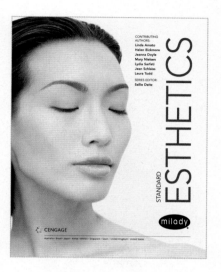

Well done! You have made a terrific decision to study esthetics. Career opportunities for estheticians will continue to surprise and excite you every day. As with many choices, it will be important to follow that which you are drawn to, rather than feeling pushed in any one direction. Naturally, there are subjects and components of study that you may find more interesting than others; however, you will find new ways to learn and grow beyond any of those limitations, and most of all you will surprise yourself.

Your Milady Team

Within the many decades of writing, research, and knowledge within this text, your Milady mentors, reviewers, authors, and educators have preceded you, and know what you need to learn. They have spent many dedicated years in preparing to teach you all that they know and are here to help you not only in preparation in obtaining your license but can support you to become your best…as an esthetician.

Your Classmates

One note of observance about your colleagues. Your classmates will become important in your study of esthetics, as you will learn quickly that you need each other. For some of you, this experience in school may be your first career. For others it may be a fourth or fifth career, and one that you have always dreamed about. Have patience with them, and mostly, with yourself. You will serve as models for each other in practicing techniques, role playing to learn how to present ingredients and products to future clients. You may find that you become best friends.

You Will Learn About

In the 12th Edition of *Milady Standard Esthetics: Fundamentals* the team has curated the most current information on the sciences, facial treatments, skin types, product knowledge, and makeup. You will learn about advanced topics such as peels, microdermabrasion, lasers, and light therapies. Additionally, you will be introduced to client intake forms and documentation, which are among some of the most important maintenance details of your practice.

The Future

On the matter of your practice, once you've graduated and have license in hand there is reason to be optimistic about growth in our industry. According to the Bureau of Labor Statistics in the United States, the projected growth for estheticians is 14% from 2017 to 2026. This is higher than other industries, a situation that has been consistently in our favor for over two decades.

Your future is bright! Study hard, use your creativity, don't give up, and allow yourself to grow.

"The world is waiting for you...Believe it!"

—Sallie Deitz. LME
Esteemed Milady Author and Master Esthetician

The Industry Standard

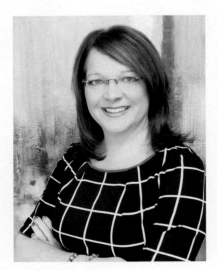

Sandra Bruce

Since 1927, Milady has been committed to quality education for beauty professionals. Over the years, tens of millions of licensed professionals have begun their careers studying from Milady's industry-leading textbooks.

We at Milady are dedicated to providing the most comprehensive learning solutions in the widest variety of formats to serve you, today's learner. The newest edition of *Milady Standard Esthetics: Fundamentals* is available to you in multiple formats, including the traditional print version, an eBook version, and MindTap, which provides an interactive learning experience complete with activities, learning tools, and brand-new video content.

Milady would like to thank the educators and professionals who participated in surveys and reviews to best determine the changes that needed to be made for this edition. We would also like to thank learners, past and present, for being vocal about your needs and giving Milady the opportunity to provide you with the very best in esthetics education.

Thank you for trusting Milady to provide the valuable information you need to build the foundation for your career. Our content combined with your passion, creativity, and devotion to your craft and your customers will set you on the path to a lifetime of success. Congratulations for taking the first step toward your future as an esthetician and a beauty professional!

Sandra Bruce
Vice President and General Manager, Milady

The Benchmark for Esthetics Education

Milady's Standard Textbook for Professional Estheticians was first published in 1978 and was the creation of Joel Gerson. It soon became the textbook choice of esthetics educators and has seen 12 revisions. Throughout this period, it has consistently been the most widely used esthetics textbook in the world. As the science and business of skin care evolve, new editions of the text are needed periodically, and Milady is committed to producing the best in esthetics education. We have thoroughly updated the content and design of this textbook to bring you the most valuable, effective educational resource available. To get the most out of the time you will spend studying, take a few minutes now to learn about the text and how to use it before you begin.

This 12th Edition of *Milady Standard Esthetics: Fundamentals* combined with *Milady Standard Foundations* provides you with the basic information you need in an esthetics training course up to 600 hours. While *Milady Standard Foundations* focuses on interpersonal skills and keeping you and your clients safe, *Milady Standard Esthetics: Fundamentals* contains comprehensive information to prepare you with the technical skills you will need as an esthetician to prepare you for employability.

Milady Standard Esthetics: Fundamentals, 12th Edition, contains comprehensive information on many subjects, including preparing your treatment room, facial treatments, devices, and more. As a part of your esthetics education, this book provides you with a valuable guide for learning the techniques you will be performing. No matter which career path you choose in the esthetics field, you will refer to this text again and again as the foundation upon which to build your success.

In Memoriam

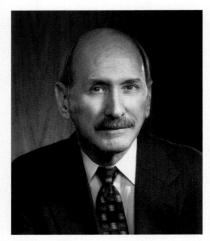

Joel Gerson

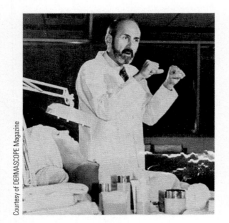

Courtesy of DERMASCOPE Magazine

Joel Gerson, PhD, was an icon in the esthetics educational industry, setting the path for us to develop an esthetics industry in the United States. With a PhD in health science from New York University, Dr. Gerson's professional credits also include Resident Makeup Artist for the House of Revlon; Spokesman for Lever Brothers; Vice President of Education for Christine Valmy, Inc.; and Technical Director for the International School for Estheticians and Makeup Specialists. Dr. Gerson was a licensed cosmetologist, holding a teaching license for Esthetics, Scientific Facial Treatments, and Makeup from the University of the State of New York. He also served as Esthetic Examiner with the New York Department of State.

Brief history

When Joel Gerson graduated from high school in Detroit, he had no career plans in place. Early on he pursued truck driving and served in the U.S. Army for two years. Upon his return he continued to feel unsure about his occupation.

A friend of the family owned a beauty salon and suggested that Joel attend cosmetology school. When he began the program, he did not know the difference between a hair pin and a bobby pin. Three months later, he told his father that hairdressing was not for him and he was going to drop out of school. While reminiscing he thought, "One day I was holding an M-1 rifle, and the next a Lady Ellen hair clip." It was then that his father gave him the following advice: "Finish school, and get a license, and no matter where you go, you will always be able to find work." His father was correct, and the world may have missed the great spirit, love, and the many gifts and talents of Dr. Gerson had he not listened to the wise advice of his dear father.

Our first meeting and awards

I first met Dr. Gerson in 1974 when he championed the first skin care show with Robert Opennheim and Ann Kean. He was named a Legend by *Dermascope* magazine and received the Crystal Award from Les Nouveau Esthétiques. In 2016, Dr. Gerson received his most cherished award, a certificate of merit from CIDESCO (Comité International d'Esthétique et de Cosmétology) USA. (Recently, it was my privilege to travel to Dublin with Paul Dysktra, CEO of CIDESCO USA to accept the honor for him.)

One of Joel's greatest achievements was one that would impact the esthetics community for all time. It was the development and writing of the *Standard Textbook for Professional Estheticians* by Milady. Joel came to understand skin care and esthetics through cosmetology, and thus was able to set a high bar for esthetics standards. Erica Miller, friend and fellow esthetician, and Diplomat of CIDESCO International, said, "In a sentence, this book is an answer to an esthetician's prayer, and sets America on its own in the field of esthetics. Whether a prospective student of esthetics or the veteran cosmetologist, it is a must read for the study of esthetics." From the many concepts and original needs for esthetician education as recognized by Dr. Gerson, Milady continues to lead and develop education materials in esthetics, cosmetology, and manicuring programs in schools today.

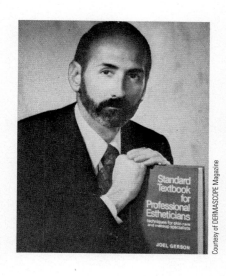
_{Courtesy of DERMASCOPE Magazine}

Dr. Gerson was humble about his contributions and had a tremendous sense of humor. To me, he was Joel; my friend, my champion, and a member of my family. One of my favorite memories is how he was so proud when at the ABA Beauty Ball in NYC he was asked to perform a facial massage in front of more than 800 people and did so with beautiful movements to the strum of a harpist. It was so gorgeous, I cried.

Joel always called me "kiddo" and said, "You are my family." And indeed, over the decades, he was part of my family. He was there for me in happiness and sorrow, at my daughter's bat mitzvahs, graduations, weddings, and all holidays, even Thanksgiving dinner.

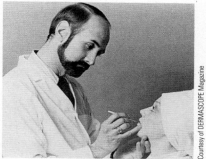
_{Courtesy of DERMASCOPE Magazine}

I loved him and he will be in my heart forever. We all must remember that it was Joel who created our beautiful and thriving skin care community where every esthetician can enjoy success and flourish. We also all need to remember his personal motto for success: **"Love what you do and care to be different."**

—Lydia Sarfati
CEO and Founder, Repêchage
Honorary Chairwoman, CIDESCO, USA

Meet the Contributors

Message to the Authors

Milady recognizes the many gifts and talents of its authors worldwide. It is with our gratitude that we thank these very special authors of the 12th edition of *Milady Standard Fundamentals: Esthetics* for their dedication to writing this volume and without whom it would not be the great educational resource that it has become. We are pleased to share their biographies, which no doubt, provide just a glimpse of all that they have accomplished. Well done!

Sallie Deitz, Series Editor

Sallie Deitz, BA, LME, author, speaker, and consultant, has been an esthetics practitioner and Learning Leader in a variety of settings. Her background and experience include medical esthetics; product

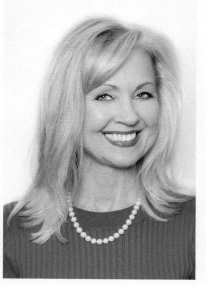
Sallie Deitz

development (both products and devices); and business and education management for medical spas, sole proprietors, manufacturers, and esthetics schools.

Sallie has also served with the National Interstate Council of State Boards in test development for basic and master estheticians, and in manicuring. She has served on numerous boards; has been a contributing author with Milady, a division of Cengage, since 2002; and is the author of *Skin Care Practices and Clinical Protocols* (Milady, 2013), *The Clinical Esthetician* (Milady, 2005), and *Amazing Skin for Girls* (Drummond Publishing, 2005).

A special worldwide focus of Sallie's is in the coaching of women skin care entrepreneurs, to help them become self-sufficient through education, self-esteem and confidence building, and practical business applications.

Mary Nielsen, Author

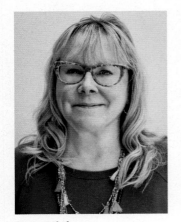

Mary Nielsen

A technician, educator, mentor, and business owner, Mary Nielsen has been at the forefront in medical esthetics since its infancy in the early 1990s. She is a Certified Advanced Esthetician in the state of Oregon and a Master Esthetician in Washington. She is a licensed esthetics instructor. She is also a licensed nurse. She is currently vice chair and industry expert on the Oregon Board of Certified Advanced Estheticians. She is the author of *A Compendium for Advanced Aesthetics: A Guide for the Master Esthetician* (FriesenPress, 2017) and writes regularly for MiladyPro. She is also a diplomate with the American Board of Laser Surgery in Cosmetic Laser Procedures.

She is the executive director of Spectrum Advanced Aesthetics, the founder of the Cascade Aesthetic Alliance, as well as the creator of Skintelligent Resources.

Linda Amato, Author

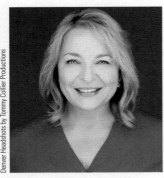

Linda Amato

Linda Amato started her career in esthetics over 20 years ago practicing as an esthetician and laser technician at day spas and medical clinics. Throughout the years she has gained valuable experience in many aspects of the esthetics industry, including marketing, sales, and medical spa management. Linda found her true passion in esthetics training and education 15 years ago, and has helped develop advanced training programs for estheticians, beauty therapists, and medical professionals throughout the world.

Linda is currently the Midwest US Regional Manager and international educator for Lira Clinical SkinCare. She enjoys presenting seminars on ingredient technology and providing hands-on workshops for advanced techniques in chemical peeling. Through training and education, Linda truly believes in helping fellow skin care professionals become successful while enjoying an amazing career in esthetics.

Helen Bickmore, Author

Helen Bickmore, an esthetics industry veteran of more than 40 years, received her diplomas in beauty therapy (esthetics), body treatments, massage, and electrolysis in 1979 through both the London College of Fashion and the City and Guilds of London Institute (CGLI). She is a New York State licensed esthetician and massage therapist (LMT) and has been a certified professional electrologist (CPE) with the American Electrology Association (AEA) and a certified clinical medical electrologist (CME) with the Society of Clinical and Medical Hair Removal (SCMHR).

Helen has taught esthetics at the former Scarborough Technical College, now called the Yorkshire Coast College, in England, and over the years she has worked in salons providing services and as a spa director. In addition, she has owned her own businesses in both England and the United States. Moving toward retirement she still continues to provide services to a large clientele. In addition, Helen has reviewed manuscripts, written articles, and worked on esthetics video projects with Milady. She has also appeared on television news programs, given workshops, and served on a number of panels and professional association boards, including the Board of the New York Electrolysis Association (NYEA).

Since 2004 she has been a contributing author to a number of Milady's textbooks, including *Milady Standard Cosmetology* (2016) and *Milady Standard Esthetics: Advanced* (2012), and now *Milady Standard Esthetics: Fundamentals* (2020). Helen is the author of *Milady's Hair Removal Techniques: A Comprehensive Manual* and its companion *Course Management Guide* as well as coauthor of *Milady Aesthetician Series: Advanced Hair Removal* (2007).

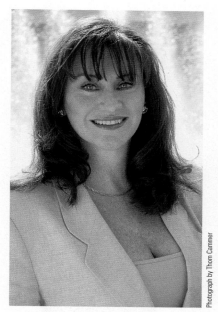

Helen Bickmore

Jeanna Doyle, Author

Jeanna Doyle is a licensed cosmetologist and Medical Aesthetic Provider with special training in oncology esthetics and corrective makeup. Her innovative work in corrective makeup has been part of two scientific studies, both at UT Southwestern one was in plastic surgery, and one was in oncology esthetics and was presented as a best new practice at the AOSW (Association of Oncology Social Workers) National Conference in 2015.

Jeanna has worked in medical and media settings. Her work in the medical community has taken her from private practices to hospitals, cancer centers, and children's hospitals working directly with plastic and reconstructive surgeons, dermatologists, oncologists, psychologists, and social workers. In media settings Jeanna has worked on print, television, and film projects with A-list actors, athletes, models, musicians, politicians, and even a former president and first lady of the United States.

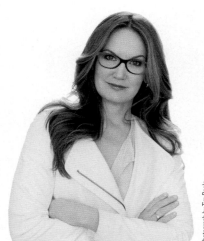

Jeanna Doyle

Jeanna founded the 501(c)(3) nonprofit Suite HOPE (Helping Oncology Patients Esthetically). She is also the developer of a corrective makeup curriculum, The HOPE Method, designed to teach other esthetics professionals corrective makeup. Additionally, Jeanna is the author of *Wig ED* (Books-Ruhl, 2017), the first beauty book on wig selection.

Jeanna writes articles and delivers keynote speeches for medical and beauty industry giants like MD Anderson, the Cancer Knowledge Network, the Cancer Support Community, and the Mary Kay Foundation.

Lydia Sarfati, Author

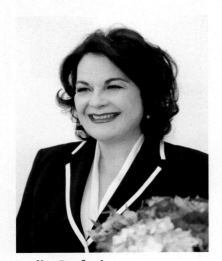

Lydia Sarfati

Lydia Sarfati, an educational leader in esthetics for over 40 years, is a licensed Master Esthetician and the founder and CEO of Repêchage Skin Care. Throughout her career, Ms. Sarfati has made major contributions to the elevation of esthetics, serving as the chairperson of CIDESCO Section U.S.A, an international organization promoting the world standard for beauty and spa therapy, since 2005. She is also the recipient of the Independent Cosmetic Manufacturers and Distributors (ICMAD) Cosmetic Entrepreneur Award for Leadership, the National Cosmetology Association (NCA) Pillar Award for Education Leadership, the *Les Nouvelles Esthétiques (LNE)* magazine Crystal award, and the *Dermascope* magazine Legend award.

Sarfati was born in Legnica, Poland. After receiving her esthetics license, she opened Klisar, the first day spa in Manhattan, in 1977. In 1980, she launched Repêchage, the first company to bring seaweed-based skin care treatments and cosmetics to the U.S market. With the launch of the world-renowned Repêchage Four-Layer Facial, Sarfati garnered a reputation as a leading esthetics educator, spa owner, manufacturer, and consultant. She has been featured as an expert in *Vogue, InStyle, Glamour, Elle, Allure,* and the *New York Times* as well as on CNN, CBS, and FOX. Her prominence as a leading promoter of excellence in education led to the establishment of the Lydia Sarfati Post Graduate Skincare Academy, now located at the Repêchage headquarters in Secaucus, New Jersey.

Sarfati appears nationally and internationally at esthetics trade shows, and attends and conducts overseas conferences in Asia, Europe, the Middle East, Central and South America, and South and West Africa. Sarfati is the author of *Success at Your Fingertips: How to Succeed in the Skin Care Business* (L.S. Publications, Inc., 2013); has produced 17 step-by-step instructional videos, including a comprehensive facial massage video; and has written and published *Repêchage: The Book, Skincare Science & Protocols* (L.S. Publications, Inc., 2018), a comprehensive review of skin conditions, skin care, body treatments, and esthetics. In 2014, Sarfati was named honorary ambassador to her home city of Legnica, Poland.

Jean Schlaiss, Author

Jean Schlaiss has been working in the beauty industry since 1991. Throughout her career, she has worn many hats, including nail technician; esthetician; medical aesthetician; cosmetologist; cosmetology, esthetics, and nail technology teacher; salon manager, author; makeup artist; and permanent makeup artist. She is also a certified personal trainer and a certified group fitness instructor.

As a freelance makeup artist, Jean has been performing makeup services since 1996. Working with organizations such as *Spri, Maybelline, Teen People, Nexxus,* and *Diamond Jack's Casino,* she has been published in various media formats, including magazines, books, and online. Jean continues to pursue the creativity that makeup artistry brings by working with models and photographers.

Jean has served on the Illinois Board of Barber, Cosmetology, Esthetics, Hair Braiding, and Nail Technology and is involved in other related organizations as a subject matter expert. She has also completed her bachelor's in science to further expand her knowledge base as she continually strives for self-improvement.

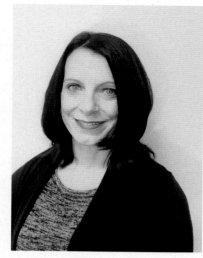

Jean Schlaiss

Laura Todd, Author

Laura Todd has over 20 years of experience in the industry, including as owner of a medical spa and the Institute of Advanced Medical Esthetics, an accredited esthetics school in the state of Virginia.

Laura participates in legislative issues, and previously served as the co-chair of the Virginia Panel for Esthetics Licensure, where she helped to establish two-tier esthetics (Basic and Master) licensure. Appointed by the governor, Laura was Virginia's first appointed full-term esthetician in 2005, serving on the board as the main contributor to the development of Virginia's esthetics regulations. She then served as a subject matter expert to help create the licensure examinations for NIC.

Laura was then appointed by the American Association of Cosmetology Schools as Virginia's State Relations Committee representative and also participated in policy development for the medical board concerning the use of esthetics lasers in Virginia.

She is also director of the Virginia State Association of Skin Care Professionals, where she continues to work toward advancements and the protection of Virginia's esthetics industry.

As a result of her dedication to Virginia's esthetics industry, the State Board staff issued her license #1 for her school as well as license #1 as a Master Instructor in Virginia. She was later recognized by the State Board as well as her fellow board members with an appreciation of service award.

Laura's academic focus was pre-med, and she holds several university degrees, including a bachelor's of science, and she continued on with coursework for a master's degree in education.

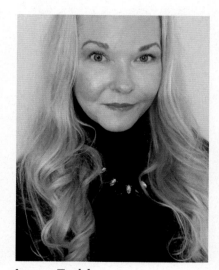

Laura Todd

Contributing Authors for Previous Editions of *Milady Standard Esthetics: Fundamentals*

We want to sincerely thank the following individuals who have contributed their skin care expertise and business knowledge to students and educators in past editions.

Janet M. D'Angelo

Catherine M. Frangie

Sallie Deitz

John Halal

Shelley Lotz

Jean Schlaiss

New Organization Of Chapters

By learning about and using the tools in this text together with your teachers' instruction, you will develop the abilities needed to build a loyal and satisfied clientele. To help you locate information more easily, the chapters are now grouped into two main parts:

Part 1: Skin Foundations

"Skin Foundations" includes six chapters that cover the past, present, and future of the field of esthetics. Chapter 1, "Career Opportunities and History of Esthetics," outlines the exciting career options available to estheticians as well as the origin of esthetics, tracing its evolution through the twenty-first century and speculating on where it will go in the future. Chapter 2, "Anatomy and Physiology," provides essential information that will help guide your work with clients and enable you to make decisions about treatments. Chapter 3, "Physiology and Histology of the Skin," includes skin anatomy and skin function; Chapter 4, "Disorders and Diseases of the Skin," explores the many maladies of the skin, including acne, sensitive skin, and the danger of sun exposure. Chapter 5, "Skin Analysis," addresses skin types and conditions, stressing the necessity of a thorough client consultation. The foundation on which almost every retail sale is built is covered in Chapter 6, "Skin Care Products: Chemistry, Ingredients, and Selection."

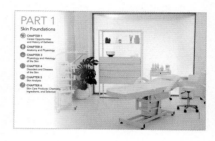

Part 2: Skin Care Treatments

"Skin Treatments" focuses on actual practices performed by the esthetician. Setting up the treatment room and creating the correct atmosphere for both the client and the esthetician are covered in Chapter 7, "The Treatment Room." Chapter 8, "Facial Treatments," instructs in the methods used during several types of facials and their benefits and contraindications, as well as the unique considerations and techniques of the men's facial. Chapter 9, "Facial Massage," covers the benefits of massage along with contraindications and basic massage movements. Chapter 10, "Facial Devices and Technology," is devoted to machines used in esthetic treatments and provides instruction on the use of the steamer, galvanic machine, diamond tip microdermabrasion, and more. Chapter 11, "Hair Removal," covers the critical information you'll need for these increasingly requested services from head to toe. Color theory, face shapes, and advice about selecting a product line are some of the topics addressed in Chapter 12, "Makeup Essentials." In closing, Chapter 13, "Advanced Topics and Treatments," provides an overview of the body and clinical procedures used with cosmetic surgery and also covers the increasingly popular spa body treatments.

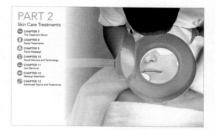

Features of this Edition

In response to advances in learning science and the growing importance of competency-based education, several changes have been made to the *Esthetics: Fundamentals* text you may be familiar with. Features have been added or tweaked with the hope of making your learning experience more intuitive, more effective, and above all more relevant.

Photography and Art

Milady conducted a photo shoot and video shoot to capture the hundreds of new four-color photographs that appear throughout the book, in both chapter content and step-by-step procedures. As Joel Gerson stated, "Love what you do and care to be different." Each model featured in the chapter openers could be a client who will walk into your salon or spa, and you need to be ready to serve them. As estheticians, it is our job to adapt our treatment plans to each client and embrace the differences in everyone's skin. Your clientele will rely on you to help them relax and relieve their skin challenges, and you need to provide services that cater to their individual needs.

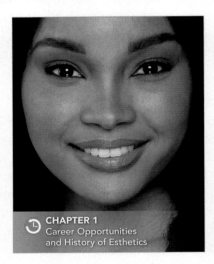

CHAPTER 1
Career Opportunities
and History of Esthetics

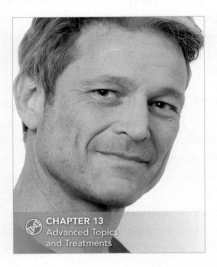

CHAPTER 13
Advanced Topics
and Treatments

Table of Contents

Whether you're getting started, reviewing for your exams, or just feeling lost, the table of contents at the beginning of this text will be your learning roadmap through the content. The Contents section shows you the structure of the text as a whole, making it easier to find the section you're looking for. In addition, because the section headers double as learning objectives, this table of contents also shows you at a glance all the objectives you will need to achieve in order to master each chapter.

Chapter Icons

Each chapter of *Esthetics: Fundamentals* has its own icon, which connects it across all of the supplements. Think of these icons as badges—once you've achieved all of a chapter's learning objectives, you've successfully earned a chapter icon!

Learning Objectives

At the beginning of each chapter is a list of learning objectives that tell you what important information you will be expected to know after studying the chapter. Throughout the chapter, these learning objectives are also used as the titles of the major sections themselves. This is done for ease of reference and to reinforce the main competencies that are critical to learn in each chapter to prepare for licensure. In addition, learning objectives have been written to focus on measurable results, helping you know what it is you should be able to do after mastering each section.

Learning Objectives

After completing this chapter, you will be able to:

1. Explain how career opportunities and the history of the profession are critical to esthetics.
2. Describe the career options available to licensed estheticians.
3. List types of existing esthetics practices to help chart your career path.
4. Outline skin care practices from earlier cultures to today.
5. Summarize the current and future states of the esthetics industry as described in this chapter.

The First Learning Objective

Milady knows, understands, and appreciates how excited students are to delve into the newest and most exciting products and equipment, and we recognize that students can sometimes feel restless spending time learning the basics of the profession. The first objective in every chapter is to help you understand why you are learning each chapter's material and to help you see the role it will play in your future career as an esthetician. The section includes bullet points that tell you why the material is important and how you will use the material in your professional career.

Explain How Career Opportunities and the History of the Profession are Critical to Esthetics

Esthetics is a career in which you can continuously learn new skills and make a difference in the lives of others every day (Figure 1–1). Whether you are coming to esthetics as your first, second, or third career path, it holds the promise of independence, pride, and community. Being a professional esthetician opens many doors that are not available in other industries. Once you become proficient and master the basics, the only limits that you will experience are those that you allow to define you.

Estheticians should study and have a thorough understanding of the career opportunities and history of esthetics because:

- You can learn about the many and diverse career opportunities to begin planning for your career.
- It is good to have a historical perspective on where we have been to know how far we have come.
- Materials used in early beauty preparations may have been instrumental in determining how materials are used today, such as in color formulations and cosmetics.
- You will have a better understanding of how culture can shape product development and how it can bring about the necessity for change.

Check-In Questions

Instead of placing review questions at the end of each chapter, check-in questions have been added to the end of the relevant section. In this way you can check your understanding as you progress through a chapter, as opposed to waiting until the chapter is over to check your memory. Check-in questions also make it easier to find any answers you need help with. The answers to the check-in questions are provided to your instructor.

 CHECK IN

1. Draw and label the basic structures of a cell.
2. Summarize cell metabolism and its purpose.

Competency Progress

The list of learning objectives is repeated at the end of each chapter, with added checkboxes. At this point you'll be invited to review your progress through the content you have just covered, including checking off the learning objectives you feel you have mastered. Anything not checked off will stand out as a clear reminder of work you still need to do to complete that chapter.

COMPETENCY PROGRESS

How are you doing with Anatomy and Physiology? **Check off the Chapter 2 Learning Objectives below that you feel you have mastered; leave unchecked those objectives you will need to return to:**

☐ Explain why estheticians need knowledge of anatomy and physiology.
☐ Describe the basic structure and function of a cell.
☐ Describe the four types of tissue found in the body.

Procedures

All step-by-step procedures offer clear, easy-to-understand directions and multiple photographs to help you learn the techniques. At the beginning of each procedure, you will find a list of the needed implements and materials, along with any preparation that must be completed before beginning the procedure.

In order to avoid interrupting the flow of the main content, all of the procedures have been moved to a **Procedures** section at the end of each chapter.

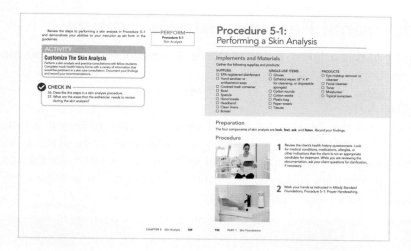

Pre- and Post-Service Procedures

To drive home the point that pre-service cleaning, disinfecting, and preparing for the client are important, you will find that a unique *pre-service procedure* has been created in Chapter 7, "*The Treatment Room,*" to specifically address setting up your facial room before a client arrives. Protocols related to meeting, greeting, and escorting your client to your service area now appear in Chapter 8, "Facial Treatments." Additionally, a *post-service procedure* has been created to address cleaning, disinfecting, and organizing after servicing a client and at the end of the day. Look for the Perform icons that appear in every chapter with procedures as a reminder and call to action to perform and practice the steps until they become natural to you.

Perform Icons

Some students may want to review a procedure at the time it is mentioned in the main content. To make it easy for you to find the procedure you are looking for at these times, Milady has added Perform icons. These icons appear where each procedure is mentioned within the main content of the chapter, and they direct you to the procedure number located at the end of the chapter.

---PERFORM---
Procedure 8-2
Remove Eye Makeup
and Lipstick

Procedure 8-3
Applying a Cleansing Product

Procedure 8-4
Removing Products

Additional Features of this Edition

As part of this edition, many features are available to help you master key concepts and techniques.

Focus On

Throughout the text, short boxed sections draw attention to various skills and concepts that will help you reach your goal. The Focus On pieces target sharpening technical skills, new research, further explanation of complex subjects, and interesting facts. These topics are key to your success as a student and as a professional.

> **FOCUS ON**
>
> ### Scientific Research
>
> When researching topics, keep an open mind and determine the reliability of the source providing the information. What is found to be true one year may change with new evidence and discoveries.

Did You Know?

These features provide interesting information that will enhance your understanding of the material in the text and call attention to special points.

> **DID YOU KNOW?**
>
> Hormones are actually chemicals. There are over 30 hormones telling your body what it should do every day.

Caution!

Some information is so critical for your safety and the safety of your clients that it deserves special attention. The text directs you to this information in the CAUTION! boxes.

> **CAUTION!**
>
> Each regulatory agency is different, so check your local laws to see what is acceptable related to performing exfoliation services under your esthetics license.

> **CAUTION!**
>
> To avoid overstimulation and damage to capillaries, do not use steam or hot towels on rosacea-prone or couperose skin. Use an additional facial mask instead.

Activity

The Activity boxes describe hands-on classroom exercises that will help you understand the concepts explained in the text.

ACTIVITY

Create flashcards for the nerves of the head, face, and neck.

Web Resources

The Web Resources features provide you with web addresses where you can find more information on a topic and references to additional sites for more information.

Web Resources

Here are some great websites for more information:
American Society of Plastic Surgeons: www.plasticsurgery.org
eMedicine: www.emedicine.com
Mayo Clinic: www.mayoclinic.com
The medical journal for skin care professionals: www.pcijournal.com

Glossary List

A complete list of key terms appears in the glossary at the end of each chapter. In addition to the key terms, you will find the *page reference* for where the key terms are defined and discussed in the chapter material. *Phonetic spellings* for all terms are included along with the glossary definition. The combined key term and chapter glossary is a way to learn important terms that are used in the beauty and wellness industry and to prepare for licensure. This list is a one-stop resource to help you create flash cards or study for quizzes on a particular chapter.

All key terms are included in the Chapter Glossary, as well as in the Glossary/Index at the end of the text.

CHAPTER GLOSSARY

acne AK-nee	p. 131	chronic inflammatory skin disorder of the sebaceous glands that is characterized by comedones and blemishes; commonly known as *acne simplex* or *acne vulgaris*
actinic keratosis ak-TIN-ik Kara-toe-sis	p. 129	pink or flesh-colored precancerous lesions that feel sharp or rough; results from sun damage

Acknowledgments

Milady recognizes, with gratitude and respect, the many professionals who have offered their time to contribute to this edition of *Milady Standard Esthetics: Fundamentals* and wishes to extend enormous thanks to the following people who have played a part in this edition:

- Becky Kuehn, LME, COS, founder, president, and leading U.S. educator of Oncology Spa Solutions, for introducing oncology esthetics as a career for estheticians in the new edition. www.OncologySpaSolutions.com.

- Mary Scully MacLean, writer extraordinaire, for all your support and editing of Chapter 7, "The Treatment Room"; Chapter 8, "Facial Treatments"; and Chapter 9, "Facial Massage."

- Matthew England, Licensed Master Esthetician Instructor, for his research assistance on chapters 10 and 13.

- Many thanks to Annette Hanson, founder of Atelier Esthétique Institute (www.aeinstitute.net), a New York State licensing esthetics school, and her staff and students for their assistance and collaboration in the creation of many of the photos and videos that appear in this new edition. Annette allowed us to focus on creating the perfect content by opening up her school to the Milady staff and models to perform practice runs and test equipment. This act of kindness shows her dedication to the project and her commitment to quality education.

- A special thanks to educator Janette Van Zyl and professional esthetician Raechel Lowe for their support and participation in the video shoot planning and execution by performing services on camera. We appreciate the knowledge and energy that they brought to the set every day.

- Michael Gallitelli, Tiago M. Mello, and Tom Stock, professional photographers, whose photographic expertise helped bring many of these pages to life.

- Odalisa (Lisa) Dominguez and Natalie Fedorchenko for impeccable professionalism and talent behind the scenes and on camera providing instruction and performing waxing and facial services for the photos and videos.

- Michelle D'Allaird-Brenner, owner of Aesthetic Science Institute in Latham, New York, who, along with her instructors and students, welcomed the Milady team to their beautiful school in order to conduct a photo shoot, and who were supportive and hospitable to our entire team.

- Andrea Gregaydis (lead instructor) at Aesthetics Science Institute, for generously performing soft and hard wax services at the photo shoot as well as overseeing students and the shoot details.

- Thank you, Blonde + Co, for your overall support in capturing our new procedures. We appreciate your expertise and contributions including your photographers, videographers, set designers, and SMEs (JP Ramirez).

Reviewers of Milady Standard Esthetics: Fundamentals, 12th Edition

- Selisha Abbas, Regional Director, Northwest College School of Beauty, OR
- Jocelyn Ash L.E., L.E.I., Esthetics Director of Education, Atlanta Institute of Aesthetics, GA
- Peggy Braswell, Southeastern Technical College, GA
- Dannette Corirossi, Director of Education, Bellus Academy, CA
- Dina Costello, Benes Career Academy, New Port Richey, FL
- Alayne Curtiss, Owner of Make Me Fabulous, Saratoga Springs, NY
- Kimberly Cutter-Williams, Savannah Technical College, Savannah, GA
- Meagan Delange, Education Director, Acaydia Spa and School of Aesthetics, UT
- Cindy Heidemann, ABC School of Cosmetology, Esthetics & Nail Technology Inc., Lake in the Hills, IL
- Sarah Herb, Evergreen Beauty College, Everett, WA
- Shelley M. Hess, Beauty & Wellness Author and Lecturer, CA
- Cassandra Hutchison, LME & Skincare Educator, Shear Excellence Academy, FL
- Donna L. Joy, Spa Consultant, NY
- Beth Ann Maloney, Lead/Head Instructor for Skin Care/Paramedical Program, Boca Beauty Academy, FL
- Suzette Christian Marchetti, Vice President, Industry Relations, Advance Beauty College, CA
- Erika Luckert McGrath, LE, Lead Instructor, New York Institute of Beauty, NY
- Malinda A. McHenry, Owner and Education Director, Academy of Advanced Aesthetic Arts, KS
- Angela Frazier McTair, Owner, Harlem Zen Med Spa Treatment Lounge, NY and GA
- Suzanne Mulroy, Consultant in Market Development, Business Development, and Product Development, CA
- Elizabeth Myron, General Manager and Educational Instructor, Imperial Salon and Spa and The Salon Professional Academy, FL
- Jessica Olsen, Master Esthetics Instructor, Chrysm Institute of Esthetics, VA
- Aliesh D. Pierce, Makeup Artist and Esthetician, Ask Aliesh, CA
- Kathy Davis Rees, Education Director, National Institute of Medical Aesthetics, UT
- Leslie Roste, RN, National Director of Education & Market Development, King Research/Barbicide, WI

- Ashley Smith, Educator, Atlanta Institute of Aesthetics, GA
- Maggie Staszcuk, Director of Education for the College of International Esthetics, Inc., CO
- Elaine Sterling, Founder and CEO, The Elaine Sterling Institute, GA
- Kitra Tailor, Paul Mitchell the School, Dallas, TX
- Roseann Terrill, Director of Education, Boca Beauty Academy, FL
- Marina Valmy de Haydu, Owner of Christine Valmy Company and Schools, NY
- Sharicka Washington, Owner and Director, Institute of Skin Science, NH
- Madison Weinrich, Instructor at Continental School of Beauty, NYS Practical Exam Supervisor, NY
- Patrice Wilson, Bennett Career Institute, Washington, DC
- Chamagne Williams Sr. Lead Instructor, Ann Webb Skin Institute, Austin, TX

PART 1
Skin Foundations

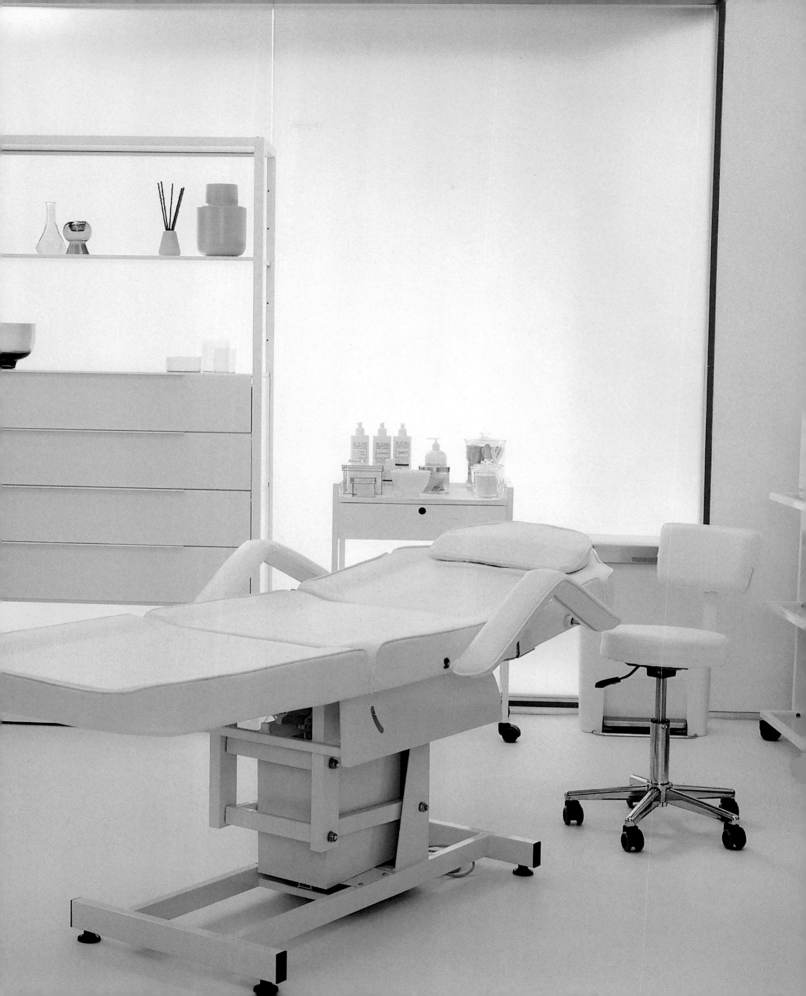

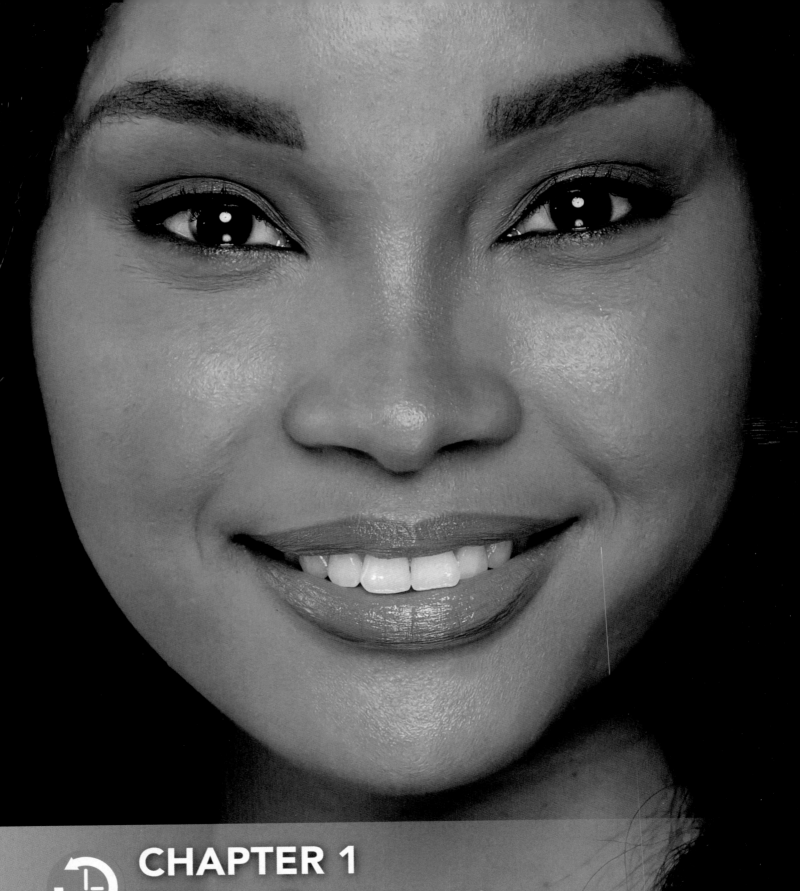

CHAPTER 1
Career Opportunities
and History of Esthetics

"Let the beauty of what you love be what you do."

–Rumi

Learning Objectives

After completing this chapter, you will be able to:

1. Explain how career opportunities and the history of the profession are critical to esthetics.
2. Describe the career options available to licensed estheticians.
3. List types of existing esthetics practices to help chart your career path.
4. Outline skin care practices from early cultures.
5. Summarize the current and future states of the esthetics industry as described in this chapter.

Explain How Career Opportunities and the History of the Profession are Critical to Esthetics

Esthetics is a career in which you can continuously learn new skills and make a difference in the lives of others every day (**Figure 1–1**). Whether you are coming to esthetics as your first, second, or third career path, it holds the promise of independence, pride, and community. Being a professional esthetician opens many doors that are not available in other industries. Once you become proficient and master the basics, the only limits that you will experience are those that you allow to define you.

Estheticians should study and have a thorough understanding of the career opportunities and history of esthetics because:

- You can learn about the many and diverse career opportunities to begin planning for your career.

- It is good to have a historical perspective on where we have been to know how far we have come.

- Materials used in early beauty preparations may have been instrumental in determining how materials are used today, such as in color formulations and cosmetics.

- You will have a better understanding of how culture can shape product development and how it can bring about the necessity for change.

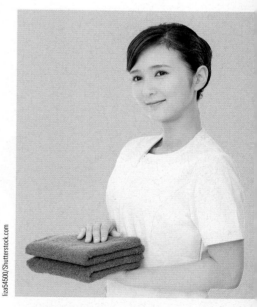

liza54500/Shutterstock.com

▲ **FIGURE 1–1** Esthetics is a rewarding field that allows for a variety of career options.

Describe the Career Options Available to Licensed Estheticians

Esthetics *(es-THET-iks)*, also known as **aesthetics**, from the Greek word *aesthetikos* (meaning "perceptible to the senses"), is a branch of anatomical science that deals with the overall health and well-being of the skin, the largest organ of the human body.

An **esthetician** *(es-thuh-TISH-un)* is a specialist in the cleansing, beautification, and preservation of the health of skin on the entire body, including the face and neck. Some establishments may also call this specialist an *aesthetician*, which is more common in medical settings.

Estheticians provide preventive care for the skin and offer treatments to keep the skin healthy and attractive. They may also manufacture, sell, or apply cosmetics. They are trained to detect skin problems that may require medical attention. However, unless an esthetician is also a licensed dermatologist, physician, or physician's assistant, they cannot make a diagnosis, prescribe medication, or give medical treatments.

Esthetics is an exciting, ever-expanding field. Over the past few decades, it has evolved from a minor part of the beauty industry into an array of specialized services offered in elegant, full-service salons, day spas, and wellness centers. As a licensed esthetician, you can choose from a wide range of career options. The information in this chapter highlights only a few opportunities to consider when starting to plot a path that is right for you to launch your career. Almost everything you do is a stepping stone to the next level of advancement in your career, so while still in school start dreaming early, stay open-minded, and consider your future as an esthetician.

Salon or Day Spa Esthetician

Description: Estheticians in a salon or day spa are skin care specialists and consultants.

Place of Employment: Estheticians work at full-service salons, skin care salons, or day spas. These may be independent businesses or national chains, and they may operate within hotels or department stores.

Preferred Skills/Common Duties: Performing facials and facial massage; waxing; and providing body treatments, applied both manually and with the aid of machines (**Figure 1–2**); and providing makeup services. Other job duties may include doing laundry, confirming appointments, and making follow-up calls to clients that have come in for a treatment; keeping records of the services provided and the products clients use; behaving pleasantly toward clients; and being skillful at selling products and services.

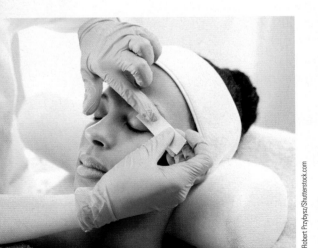

Robert Przybysz/Shutterstock.com

▲ **FIGURE 1–2** Being a salon or day spa esthetician allows you to offer a variety of services.

Growth Opportunities: You can work your way up to management and supervisory positions. With experience, you may decide to open your own salon or buy an established business or franchise. Most private salon or franchise owners have multiple responsibilities. Besides running the business, you may perform some or all of the services your business offers; or you may choose to limit your services to the areas of skin care and makeup.

Clinical Esthetician

Description: Clinical esthetics (clin-i-kuhl es-THET-iks), previously known as medical esthetics, involves the integration of surgical procedures and esthetic treatments. In this setting, the physician concentrates on surgical work while the esthetician assists with esthetic treatments. Contact your state board to find out the rules and regulations for estheticians working in a medical setting.

Place of Employment: In medical settings, estheticians perform services ranging from working with pre- and postoperative patients to managing a skin care department in a medical spa. The settings may include outpatient clinics, dermatology clinics, medical spas, laser clinics, dental offices, or research and teaching hospitals.

Preferred Skills/Common Duties: Providing patient education; marketing, buying, and selling products; applying camouflage makeup; and—with a physician's supervision—performing advanced treatments, including laser and light therapies (depending on state licensing rules) (Figure 1–3). In addition, an experienced esthetician may manage the cosmetic surgery office or act as a patient care coordinator. Some estheticians are certified nursing assistants (CNAs), licensed practical nurses (LPNs), or registered nurses (RNs).

Growth Opportunities: This type of work is very demanding, and it is important to be adaptable. Many rules and regulations must be understood and followed in a medical setting, and there is much at stake. You must be a good leader but also be able to follow instructions explicitly. Teamwork is the number one priority in a medical organization.

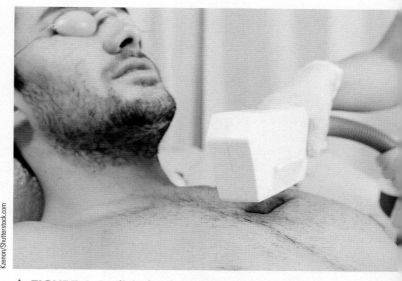

Kzenon/Shutterstock.com

▲ **FIGURE 1–3** Clinical estheticians work alongside medical professionals to offer a range of advanced services.

Waxing Specialist/Brow Specialist

Description: Waxing specialists remove hair from the face and/or body mainly by using hard or soft wax but also by threading, sugaring, and

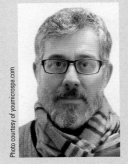

Owner of You, MicroSpa, a skin health and wellness retreat based in Reno, Nevada, Leeder is a Reiki master, is the former president of the Nevada State Board of Cosmetology, and has worked as an art director, a visual merchandiser, a makeup artist, and an editor at Skin Sense.

What inspired you to make a career in esthetics?

When I was young I suffered from acne—cystic, painful, scarring acne. I tried every available treatment, prescription, and other advice people gave me. But then I decided to learn about skin care by attending beauty school and becoming a licensed esthetician.

What has been the most defining moment in your esthetics career?

Serving Nevadans and the cosmetology industry as a 10-year member and three-term president of the Board of Cosmetology and being credited for including education in its mission certainly define my career in professional esthetics.

What would you tell someone considering an esthetics career?

No matter how large or small your skin care center or spa, the client experience requires that we exceed their expectations. Your career as an esthetician depends on your ability to care for yourself and to provide superior care for each client who is on your schedule.

How do you give back to the industry?

I enjoy sharing my knowledge and experience, including "tips and tricks," treatment protocols, and regulatory changes that affect our profession. I make every effort to mentor and am humbled when asked for advice. Frequently I have received a message or bumped into a colleague who tells me, "That one piece of advice you gave has really helped me." Giving a helping hand to someone is a gift that you witness being opened.

How do you grow yourself as a professional?

A licensed esthetician cares for themselves in the constant pursuit of education. I give myself the gift of routine, daily health and wellness, and focusing my energy on the client in front of me. I also enroll in classes such as mathematics at the university, which expand my current knowledge base and encourage my interest in diverse topics.

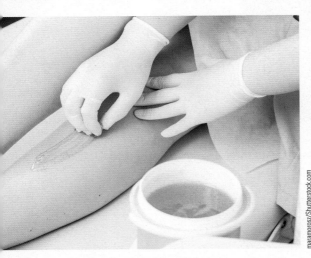

▲ **FIGURE 1–4** Sugaring is one extraction method used by waxing specialists in addition to threading, waxing, and tweezing.

tweezing. Brow specialists specialize in brow shaping by waxing, tweezing, and other extraction methods (**Figure 1–4**).

Place of Employment: There are corporate-owned waxing salons along with privately owned ones. Brow specialists are hired by salons and makeup companies.

Preferred Skills/Common Duties: Being capable and skilled in removing all face and body hair by tweezing and waxing as well as being willing to help out around the salon by answering phones and performing infection control duties. A minimum of one year of retail sales may be required in some situations.

Growth Opportunities: Between 2011 and 2015, the waxing business grew by 7.6 percent annually, according to IBISWorld's Industry Market Report.[1] With the rise of waxing salons and a

[1] Le, Vanna. (February 12, 2016). Why the Multibillion-Dollar Hair-Removal Business Is About to Get Even Bigger. Accessed October 19, 2017. https://www.inc.com/vanna-le/why-the-billion-dollar-hair-removal-industry-is-about-to-see-an-even-bigger-boom.html

continued consumer focus on physical appearance, more and more estheticians are taking jobs as waxing specialists.

Makeup Artistry

Description: Makeup artists must develop a keen eye for color and color coordination so they can select the most flattering cosmetics for each client. They may offer facials and facial massage as part of their services, or they may concentrate only on applying makeup (**Figure 1–5**).

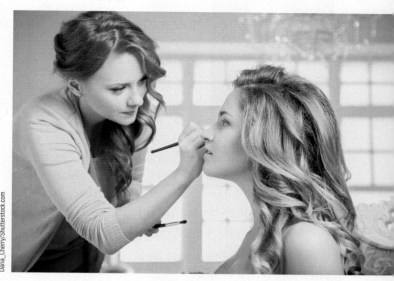

Place of Employment: Makeup artists in salons, spas, and department stores work for an hourly wage, commission, salary, or various combinations of all three.

Preferred Skills/Common Duties: Being skilled in makeup techniques and application, having retail skills to recommend makeup products and colors for home use, staying informed on the latest trends in color, and being efficient and creative.

▲ **FIGURE 1–5** Makeup artistry offers an exciting and creative career with many different work environments.

Growth Opportunities: Job opportunities for a makeup artist are vast, and only a few are listed here. Makeup artists can work in a salon setting or can freelance. They can also work with commercial photographers, television, theater, fashion, camouflage makeup, or mortuary science, which is preparing and applying cosmetics for the deceased under the direction of a mortician. A more detailed explanation of makeup artist roles appears in Chapter 12, Makeup Essentials.

Manufacturer's Representative

Description: Manufacturer's representatives are responsible for selling products and training estheticians and other staff members on how to properly use those products as well as how to retail and merchandise.

Place of Employment: Product companies hire knowledgeable estheticians to represent their company and their products.

Preferred Skills/Common Duties: Calling on spas, salons, drugstores, department stores, and specialty businesses to help build clientele and increase product sales. Traveling a great deal and exhibiting products at trade shows and conventions. Upon selling a product, being well versed in the product line in order to educate the customer as to why it is beneficial and how to use it.

Growth Opportunities: Product companies offer the opportunity to advance within the company. One could be a regional manager or move up within other divisions of the company.

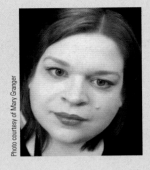

Photo courtesy of Mary Granger

Licensed esthetician, accomplished educator, and curriculum writer Granger has over 18 years' experience in the beauty Industry. In her career, Granger has been a sales rep and trainer for many well-known International skin care and spa lines, the director of operations for two large spa chains, a franchise spa trainer, a regional waxing trainer, and a district manager for a major waxing franchise.

What inspired you to make a career in esthetics?

My whole life, I was very self-conscious and had low self-esteem. For me, the ability to make someone feel beautiful and more self-confident is an amazing thing that I can do for others. When a woman feels beautiful and confident, she expands and can conquer the world!

What has been the most defining moment in your esthetics career?

Having the opportunity to meet and attend a three-day train the trainer workshop with Carol Phillips. She not only gave me the tools I needed to be an amazing trainer/teacher, but she also believed in me and told me I was amazing. To hear such powerful words from such a remarkable trainer gave me the confidence I needed to really own my place in the esthetics industry.

What has been your most challenging moment, and how did you deal with the adversity?

When I was 21, I was the national trainer for a very large spa company known for catering to an older clientele. I knew people would challenge my knowledge base due to the age difference between my clients and me, so I made sure I stepped into each training knowing everything to perfection. I always won over my class by lunchtime and became the most requested trainer in this major company.

What would you tell someone considering an esthetics career?

Don't ever let anyone tell you, "Oh, you just do facials." No! You help men and women feel beautiful and confident. You touch lives!

How do you give back to the industry?

I am a guest speaker at local beauty schools on a variety of advanced topics. I also have an "open door" policy with the students I meet, helping them with study sessions for state board exams and even providing complimentary training on services postgrad to help them get a head start in the industry.

Salesperson or Sales Manager

Description: A salesperson or sales manager is responsible for the sales of the product(s) sold within the salon or store (**Figure 1–6**).

Place of Employment: Salespeople and sales managers work at salons, spas, department stores, boutiques and specialty businesses.

Preferred Skills/Common Duties: Keeping records of sales and stock on hand, demonstrating products, selling to clients, cashiering, thoroughly understanding the products and being able to explain the benefits to customers, and cross-selling services and treatments.

Growth Opportunities: Starting in this position allows you to work your way to top management positions and possibly ownership.

Cosmetics Buyer

Description: Cosmetics buyers purchase the products that are sold within a retail setting.

Place of Employment: Cosmetics buyers work at department stores, salons, and specialty businesses.

Preferred Skills/Common Duties: Keeping up with the latest products; being able to recognize and anticipate trends in skin care; being willing to travel frequently to visit markets, trade shows, and manufacturers' showrooms to learn more about potential products that could be brought into the retail area; keeping records of purchases and sales; and estimating the amount of stock an operation will need over a particular period.

Growth Opportunities: There is always room for growth in a retail setting. Moving up to store manager or regional manager is one option.

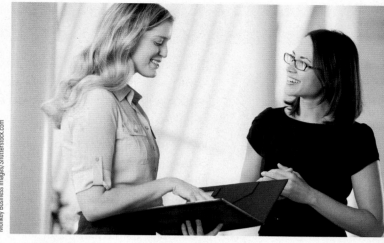

▲ **FIGURE 1–6** A salesperson or sales manager spends their day showcasing the products that they represent.

Esthetics Writer or Beauty Editor

Description: Esthetics writers and beauty editors write articles, blogs, or posts for magazines, newspapers, online magazines, or publishing companies (**Figure 1–7**).

Place of Employment: Esthetics writers and beauty editors can be freelance contributors, or they may hold permanent positions at newspapers, magazines, education and technology companies, or publishers.

Preferred Skills/Common Duties: Writing intriguing articles/posts that are of interest and value to the esthetics community; proofreading and verifying references; having strong communication, research, and writing skills; having a social media presence; and being well immersed in industry trends, skin care topics, and beauty-related research.

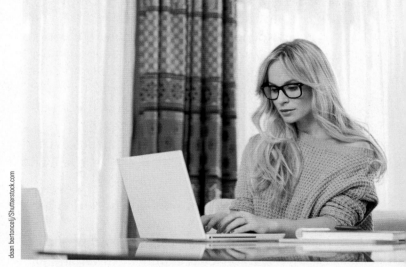

▲ **FIGURE 1–7** A writer with a background in esthetics can write for magazines, newspapers, television, or publishers.

Growth Opportunities: Esthetics writers and beauty editors can manage a team of contributors and content creators or become permanent writers for a marketing firm or publisher. Some writers even move into the role of editor.

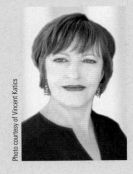

Photo courtesy of Vincent Katics

Farmer-Katics currently works part-time at Alexander's Aesthetics in Burlingame, California, as an independent skin care educator. Her focus is teaching various facial massage techniques to licensed estheticians, including lymphatic drainage massage, facial acupressure, and facial aromatherapy.

What inspired you to pursue a career in esthetics?

Honestly, my esthetics career happened by accident. Driven by my ambition to work for the BBC television company as a makeup artist, I studied cosmetology and esthetics for three years in the UK. After two unsuccessful interviews with the BBC, I decided to use all of my esthetics training and began a home visiting practice offering facials, electrolysis, waxing, and body massage, to name a few. All of these services were in my scope of practice in the UK.

What has been the most defining moment in your esthetics career?

The most thrilling moment was my first day of work at Dermalogica, where I was employed as a skin care instructor. I had been inspired by Jane Wurwand, founder of Dermalogica and the International Dermal Institute, 10 years previously when I first heard her lecture at the Olympia trade show. I had very little confidence back then and couldn't imagine myself standing up in front of a class of fellow estheticians and teaching. Yet, here I was. Standing in front of the head office in Leatherhead, Surrey, I could hardly believe it was happening to me.

What would you tell someone considering an esthetics career?

Whilst building your own clientele and providing a professional service is extremely rewarding in itself, there are numerous opportunities in this industry outside of the treatment room. My personal career has included running my own businesses, both a home visiting practice and a brick and mortar establishment; travelling the world working aboard luxury cruise ships; teaching nationally and internationally for skin care companies in the UK and U.S.; training skin therapists at the original Dermalogica Flagship store in Santa Monica, California; managing Dermalogica in Montana; creating my own independent esthetic education company; being education manager for Eve Taylor Aromatherapy Skincare; and writing articles for trade magazines.

How do you give back to the industry?

Teaching allows me to pass on the skills and knowledge I've accumulated over the years so estheticians may share with their clients, thus touching a greater number of people. When we hold ourselves to a high standard of work ethics, we maintain the bar for fellow estheticians and reflect to our clients that we are professional service providers, raising the reputation of our industry.

How do you grow yourself as a professional?

I feel very fortunate to have received an incredibly rich and comprehensive initial training back in the early 1980s. However, if I hadn't updated my skills and knowledge since then, I would be ignorant of all the amazing discoveries we have made about skin physiology, skin care ingredients, and advances in equipment technology. I choose to stay flexible, open minded, and receptive. In nature, stagnation and withering occurs without growth and change.

Travel Industry Professional

Description: Travel industry professionals perform esthetic services within the travel industry (**Figure 1–8**).

Place of Employment: Travel industry professionals can work on cruise ships, at airports, for private airline companies, or at destination spas.

Preferred Skills/Common Duties: Performing all esthetic services in order to meet traveling clients' needs.

Growth Opportunities: Travel industry professionals can advance into a skin care or cosmetic store manager, general manager, or regional manager positions.

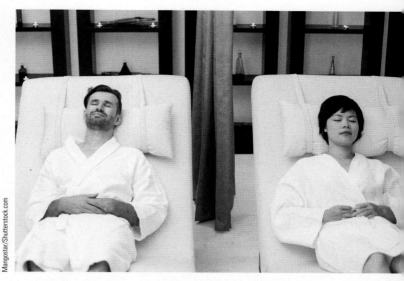

▲ **FIGURE 1–8** Travel industry professionals can offer a work environment on land or water.

Educator

Description: Educators teach the theory and technical application of esthetics (**Figure 1–9**).

Place of Employment: Educators can teach esthetics in a public, vocational, industrial, or technical high school. With the necessary certification, private cosmetology and esthetics schools are also a viable option.

Preferred Skills/Common Duties: Taking some basic teacher-training courses; developing lesson plans, curriculum, worksheets, tests, and any other supplements to assist in teaching others; executing the topics in a clear and concise manner; and being able to demonstrate the practical tasks that an esthetician will have to perform.

Growth Opportunities: Teachers can become a part of many associations that will help develop their career. They can also advance within the school where they teach by becoming a team leader, department director, or school director.

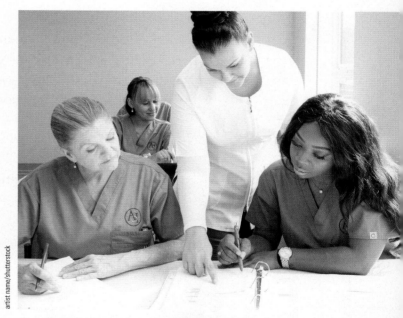

▲ **FIGURE 1–9** Educators have the ability to share their knowledge and provide quality learning for future estheticians.

Cosmetic Chemist and Product Developer

Description: Cosmetic chemists and product developers should be interested in cosmetic chemistry and ingredients. They create new products and develop new technologies (**Figure 1–10**).

Place of Employment: Cosmetic chemists and product developers work at skin care product companies.

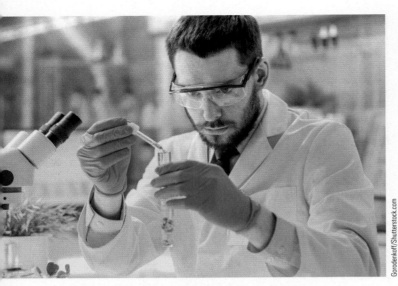

▲ FIGURE 1–10 Cosmetic chemistry and product development are for estheticians who enjoy creating skin care products.

Preferred Skills/Common Duties: Being involved in all phases of development from ideation to a final new product, having a full understanding of the industry and business, and attending trade shows to keep up to date on new ingredients; thoroughly understanding cosmetic chemistry along with what is beneficial and how different ingredients would work together.

Growth Opportunities: Estheticians can take classes on cosmetic chemistry offered through universities and other community and vocational colleges in order to advance their careers.

State Licensing Inspector or Examiner

Description: A licensed, experienced cosmetologist and/or esthetician may become a state inspector or examiner.

Place of Employment: Licensed, experienced cosmetologists and estheticians work in government buildings and state board offices.

Preferred Skills/Common Duties: Inspectors—conducting regular salon and spa inspections to ensure that managers and employees are following state rules and regulations and meeting ethical standards. State examiners—preparing and conducting examinations, enforcing rules and regulations, investigating complaints, and conducting hearings.

Growth Opportunities: Most states have laws governing cosmetology and other personal services and give examinations for cosmetology and related licenses. The experience required for this role varies from state to state, but staying current on the latest laws, regulations, and trends is important for job development. Inspectors could extend their job outreach by obtaining dual licenses.

State Board Member

Description: State board members are highly qualified and experienced estheticians that support and help to develop content for the laws and rules for licensed professionals. The laws are enforced by the state (**Figure 1–11**).

Place of Employment: State board members work in government buildings and state board offices.

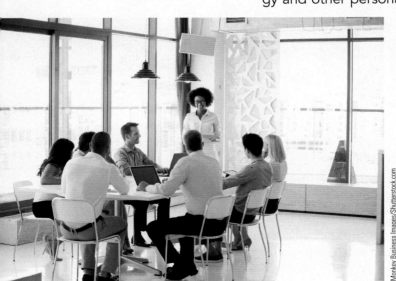

▲ FIGURE 1–11 Board members create, assess, and enforce rules and regulations.

Preferred Skills/Common Duties: Assisting in the development of laws that will protect the public; listening to and ruling over issues of a licensed professional or a license applicant; being prepared to conduct examinations, grant licenses, and inspect schools to ensure that certain physical standards, such as those for space and equipment, are maintained; and making sure that educational materials meet certain specifications.

Growth Opportunities: State board members can become state inspectors or work for the state government.

Oncology-Trained Esthetician

Description: Oncology-trained esthetics is a specialized field that helps clients who have cancer. Physicians often treat cancer with chemotherapy or radiation, and each of these has skin-related side effects. Oncology-trained estheticians can ease the discomfort of the damaged skin while enhancing clients' quality of life (**Figure 1–12**).

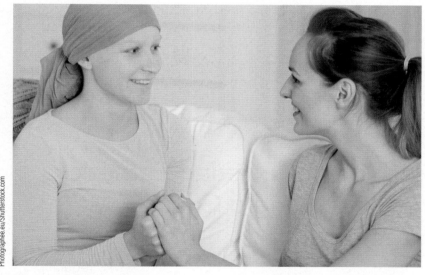

Photographee.eu/Shutterstock.com

▲ **FIGURE 1–12** Oncology-trained esthetics is a specialized field that helps clients who have cancer.

Place of Employment: Oncology training creates many opportunities for estheticians in spa and medical settings. Oncology-trained estheticians can become valued assets in the circle of care by working alongside or receiving referrals from oncologists, radiologists, hospitals, wellness centers, and cancer centers.

Preferred Skills/Common Duties: Knowing how and when to modify spa services for clients' safety, which is critical during all phases—before, during, and after—of cancer treatments.

---

2 "Oncology." Merriam-Webster.com. Accessed October 19, 2017. https://www.merriam-webster.com/dictionary/oncology

> **"Believe you can and you're halfway there."**
>
> **—Theodore Roosevelt**

DID YOU KNOW?

Oncology (ong-kol-uh-jee) is "the study and treatment of cancer and tumors."[2]

DID YOU KNOW?

Look Good Feel Better (LGFB) is a free public service program that teaches beauty techniques to people with cancer, helping them boost their self-image and camouflage their hair loss. The program is open to all people who have cancer and are actively undergoing treatment.

Look Good Feel Better
www.lookgoodfeelbetter.org

Growth Opportunities: Oncology-trained esthetician is a relatively new position that has expanded quickly based on need. The cancer survivor count in the U.S. in January 2016 was estimated to be 15.5 million and is expected to be 20.3 million by 2026.[3] With this growing number of survivors, there will be spa clients with specific skin care needs now and possibly for the rest of their life. Anyone interested in pursuing this career path must add oncology training to their basic esthetic skills. The best preparation for this line of work is training with an experienced instructor who offers hands-on work with real patients who have cancer. Volunteering with the American Cancer Society's Look Good Feel Better program is another viable option.

 CHECK IN

1. What career options are available to estheticians at salons and day spas?
2. What is clinical esthetics? In what ways can estheticians practice their skills in a medical setting?
3. List the different environments in which makeup artists can be employed.
4. What are the duties of a manufacturer's representative?
5. Discuss employment options open to an esthetics educator.

List Types of Existing Esthetics Practices to Help Chart Your Career Path

Start to create your own plan of action early on. You may enter the field of esthetics with the dream of working in a particular setting. Some might want to work at a chic urban day spa or a health and wellness center, while others crave a more intimate atmosphere. Understanding more about the qualitative differences in salon and spa environments will help you to narrow your search and find the best fit for your personality and style.

Skin care salons and spas range from basic to glamorous, and prices vary according to location and clientele. These options exist in urban, suburban, and rural settings. Salons and spas may be franchised, independent, or corporately owned. They can be full service, specialized,

---

[3] National Institutes of Health, National Cancer Institute. (2016). Statistics. Accessed October 19, 2017. https://cancercontrol.cancer.gov/ocs/statistics/statistics.html

or health oriented, and they may be categorized as skin care clinics, salons, day spas, destination spas, or medical spas (**Figure 1–13**).

Franchised salon or spa	• Owned by individuals who pay a certain fee to use the company name • Part of a larger organization or chain of salons • Operates according to a specified business plan and set protocols • Offer certain corporate advantages, such as national marketing campaigns and employee benefits packages • Important decisions such as the size, location, décor, and menu of services are dictated by the parent company.
Independently owned skin care clinics and day spas	• Owner has greater freedom and control in decision making • Benefits may be fewer; however, this does not necessarily mean that income is inadequate. • A good fit for practitioners who prefer a more intimate setting and like to work closely with a smaller group of practitioners • Greater opportunity to build long-lasting relationships with clientele
Full-service salon or day spa	• Fast-paced hub of activity • Appealing to those who appreciate the full spectrum of beauty • Opportunity to become part of a larger team or network
Resort or destination spa	• Associated with a hotel facility • Just the right fit for the esthetician who likes to work with a constantly changing clientele • May include more corporate-style benefits and educational opportunities
Medical spa or wellness center	• For those estheticians who are more focused on the health benefits or age-management aspect of skin care

▲ **FIGURE 1–13** Business options for the esthetician.

Before you decide on the setting that is best for you, take time to research and visit a variety of operations. If you do not find the type of spa or salon you are looking for in your locale, there are many trade publications, consumer magazines, and websites that can provide you with more in-depth information to help you make your decision.

Getting Started as an Esthetician

As an esthetician, you are part of an exciting, rewarding, and well-respected profession that will only grow in importance and earning power in the years ahead. If you can dream of your ideal career, you can make it happen. This is a time of revolutionary changes in what we know about skin and the ways we care for it. With this said, it is important to learn about the origin of esthetics and where we have been to know how far we have come on this skin care journey.

Web Resources

For more information about the esthetics profession, visit these websites:
www.lookgoodfeelbetter.org
www.ncea.tv
www.dol.gov
www.cosmeticplasticsurgerystatistics.com
www.themakeupgallery.info
www.beauty.about.com

Outline Skin Care Practices from
EARLY CULTURES

Much of today's skin and body care therapies are rooted in the practices and attempts of earlier civilizations to ward off disease in order to live healthier, longer lives. The brief history outlined in this section will acquaint you with some of the ways men and women have improved upon skin health and nature by changing and enhancing their appearance. Learn the history of your profession to understand how far the industry has advanced and help you predict and understand the origins of skin care ingredients and techniques.

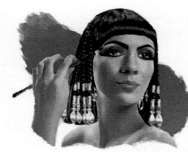

Ancient Egypt

- The Egyptians used cosmetics as part of their personal beautification habits, for religious ceremonies, and in preparing the deceased for burial.
- One of the earliest uses of **henna** (hen-uh), a dye obtained from the mignonette tree, was as a reddish hair dye and as a temporary tattoo, as well as for body art and on fingernails.

Ancient Greece

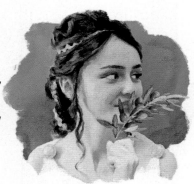

- The words cosmetics and cosmetology come from the Greek word **kosmetikos** (kos-MET-i-kos), meaning "skilled in the use of cosmetics."
- The Greeks viewed the body as a temple, and they frequently bathed in olive oil and then dusted their bodies in fine sand to regulate their body temperature and to protect themselves from the sun.
- Honey and olive oil were also used for elemental protection.

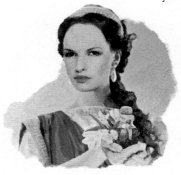

Ancient Rome

- The ancient Romans are famous for their bathhouses, which were magnificent public buildings with separate sections for men and women.
- Steam therapy, body scrubs, massage, and other physical therapies were all available at bathhouses.
- Bathing and grooming rituals included applying rich oils and fragrances made from flowers, saffron, almonds, and other ingredients.

Asia: China and Japan

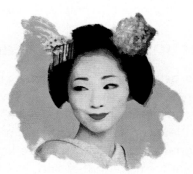

- Geishas removed their body hair using a technique similar to today's threading—they wrapped a thread around and extracted each hair.
- Japanese women used a type of paper called *aburatorigami* to blot oil from the skin and reduce shine.
- Chinese women mixed rice with water as a toner and used turmeric as a main ingredient in their facial masks to prevent wrinkles and skin discoloration. Recipes for masks and creams using crushed pearls, ginger, ginseng based on plants date back to thousands of years. More recently recipes from the Ming Dynasty (1300) are being rediscovered today.[4]

---

[4] 10 Chinese Beauty Secrets. *Beauty and Tips*. Accessed October 19, 2017. https://www.beautyandtips.com/beauty-2/10-chinese-beauty-secrets/

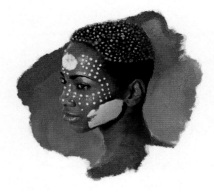

Africa

- Since ancient times, Africans have created remedies and grooming aids from the materials found in their natural environment such as roots, berries, and clay.
- Ancient Africans often adorned themselves with a variety of colors to blend into their environment for hunting.

The Middle Ages

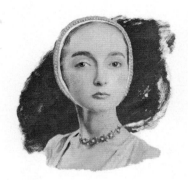

- Healing, particularly with herbs, was largely in the hands of the church.
- Pale skin was a sign of wealth and status.
- Women wore colored makeup on their cheeks and lips but not on their eyes.
- Bathing was not a daily ritual, but those who could afford them used fragrant oils.

The Renaissance Era

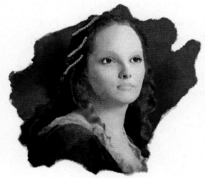

- Women shaved their eyebrows and hairline to show a greater expanse of forehead for a look of greater intelligence.
- Fragrances and cosmetics were used, although highly colored preparations for lips, cheeks, and eyes were discouraged.
- During the mid-1500s reign of Elizabeth I, men and women actually used lead and arsenic face powder to adorn themselves.

Age of Extravagance

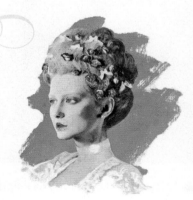

- Marie Antoinette was queen of France during the Age of Extravagance from 1755 to 1793.
- Women of status bathed in strawberries and milk and used extravagant cosmetic preparations, such as scented face powder made from pulverized starch.
- Lips and cheeks were often brightly colored in pink and orange shades by crushed geranium petals.
- Small silk patches were used to decorate the face and conceal blemishes.

The Victorian Age

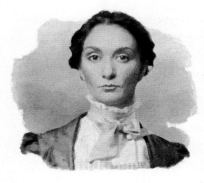

- Modesty was greatly valued, and makeup and showy clothing were discouraged except in the theater.
- To preserve skin health and beauty, women used beauty masks and packs made from honey, eggs, milk, oatmeal, fruits, vegetables, and other natural ingredients.
- Victorian women pinched their cheeks and bit their lips to induce natural color rather than using cosmetics such as lipstick and rouge.

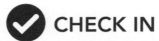

CHECK IN

6. Which Greek word does the word *cosmetics* come from? What does the Greek word mean?
7. In ancient Rome, what body therapies were provided for bathhouse patrons?
8. Describe the facial masks women used during the Victorian age.

Summarize the Current and Future States of the Esthetics Industry

Each decade of the twentieth and twenty-first centuries has seemed to have an inherently different look, whereas in earlier history it may have taken a century to bring about change. Today changes occur much more rapidly. For example, the first women's razor was offered in 1915, laser hair removal services were offered in the 1990s, and today the use of personal, at-home hair reduction devices is on the rise (**Figure 1–14**).

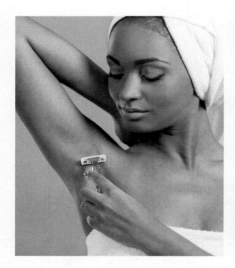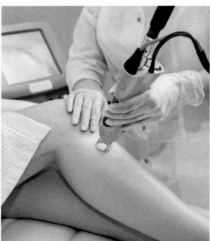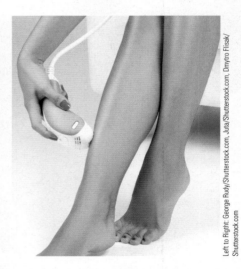

Left to Right: George Rudy/Shutterstock.com, Juta/Shutterstock.com, Dmytro Flisak/Shutterstock.com

▲ **FIGURE 1–14** Hair removal options have evolved over time from razors to laser hair removal to personal at-home devices.

Since life has become more fast-paced and stressful, environmental assaults on the skin have increased. This enhances the value of an esthetician's services, particularly to consumers who are more knowledgeable and more affluent than those in previous generations. Skin care options today are more *science based,* and the results are more dramatic. Consumers view these personal services and products as necessary to their health and sense of well-being, and consider them more as a routine than a luxury.

With information on facial services, treatments, and product ingredients readily available, consumers are making more informed, discerning

EXPERT Q&A: PAMELA SPRINGER

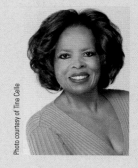

Photo courtesy of Tina Celle

Founder of Global Skin Solutions, a corrective skin care line; and a professional speaker and former national training director for major skin care companies, Springer's passion is to educate other skin care professionals on the unique nuances of pigmented skin.

What inspired you to make a career in esthetics?

In the early 1990s, a recession affected major retailers throughout the country. I was a fashion show producer, but the need for large promotions decreased. During this time, I was recruited to become a national training director for an ethnic skin care product line. This is when I finally found my passion.

What has been the most defining moment in your esthetics career?

The hallmark of my career was in 2000 when I became the first esthetician in the state of Arizona to own a freestanding esthetics school.

What would you tell someone considering an esthetics career?

This can be a very lucrative career if:

- You are self-motivated, have a passion for skin health and beauty regimens.

- After graduating, you continue postgraduate technical training and find a mentor; a mentor helped to catapult my career within two years of graduation and open an esthetics school within five years of graduation.

How do you give back to the industry?

Doing research for a chapter in a book highlighting oncology esthetics, I was so surprised at the scarcity of information on the skin of individuals of color, as well as those with skin and breast cancer. My goal is to give informational workshops on cancer awareness focused on external manifestations of chemotherapy and radiation along with ingredients to avoid.

How do you grow yourself as a professional?

I constantly take classes and read the latest advancements in technology and ingredients.

---

decisions about cosmetics in general. The birth of the medical spa has created growth in a segment of the skin care industry and with that, new procedures and products are continuing to increase at a rapid pace.

The future for esthetics is promising! The U.S. Bureau of Labor Statistics predicts job opportunities for estheticians will increase by 12 percent from 2014 to 2024.[5]

Consider the following facts about the recent past, current, and future states of the industry.

Consumers

- Anti-aging will continue to be a top priority.
- Men's skin care will continue to grow.

---

[5] Esthetician: Career Outlook and Job Profile. Study.com. Accessed December 3, 2017. http://study.com/articles/Esthetician_Career_Outlook_and_Job_Profile.html

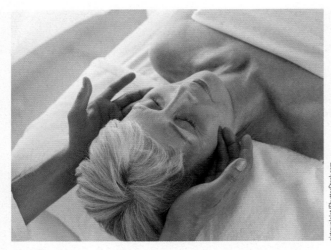

▲ **FIGURE 1–15** Baby boomers are a large customer base and can be made aware of the value of wellness, ingredients and treatments for anti-aging.

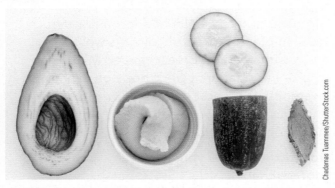

▲ **FIGURE 1–16** Natural ingredients are popular in skin care.

DID YOU KNOW?

Remember that it is against the law for an esthetician to inject Botox® (or similar substances) or fillers of any kind. It is legal in some states for estheticians to perform laser hair reduction or other types of laser treatments; however, your state laws should always be referenced. When it comes to other treatments such as chemical peels or microdermabrasion, laws should also be referenced, but these services can be performed in most states.

- According to the Google Beauty Trends 2017 report, U.S. consumers have an increased interest in vegan skin care and facial masks (especially charcoal and clay).
- Development of gluten-free skin care and makeup products are on the rise with the increased awareness of gluten intolerance.

BABY BOOMERS
- The baby boomers—Americans born between 1946 and 1964—constitute the largest generation in U.S. history.
- They are also the largest single market for skin care products and services. Baby boomers and their children enjoy the benefits the skin care market offers.
- There will be plenty of opportunities for estheticians in newer settings such as lifestyle and retirement centers (**Figure 1–15**).

Ingredients
- Organic cosmetics grew in popularity in the twentieth century, following the overall trend of other types of organic products.
- New ingredients and therapies for wrinkles, skin cancer, and general skin health will continue to be developed.
- Cell and tissue protectants will be sought by consumers—nurture over nature takes the lead role when defining anti-aging methodologies.
- Technologically advanced ingredients that are effective for various skin problems include plant stem cells and different types of peptides that improve the health of the skin and truly have anti-aging properties.
- Antioxidants and other vitamins are being used for the many different ways they affect the skin (**Figure 1–16**).

Technology
- The twentieth century brought about Tretinoin (Retin-A®), Botox®, alpha hydroxy acid, and oxygen facials; the use of galvanic current, radio frequency, lasers, high-frequency machines; and a myriad of sought-after cosmetic surgery procedures.
- The interest in less invasive technology is here to stay.

- Device manufacturers will continue to innovate and improve on existing technologies and create new ones, for example, ultrasound and ultrasonic machines continue to be reinvented and improved upon.

Facilities/Services

- The U.S. Department of Labor predicts the rapid growth of full-service day spas and a growing demand for practitioners licensed to provide a broad range of services (Figure 1–17).
- Subspecialties such as esthetics, massage, wellness, and women's fitness centers may be partnered with medical facilities. For example, cosmetic dentists are partnering with cosmetic surgeons, and plastic surgeons are partnering with gynecologists.
- Teaching hospitals that run clinical studies in human potential also have medical spas and fitness centers to enhance the benefits of these studies.
- We may see more estheticians as independent practitioners who make home, office, and hotel visits.

Table 1–1 provides a summary of the procedures, advancements, ingredients, and technologies transforming the esthetics industry.

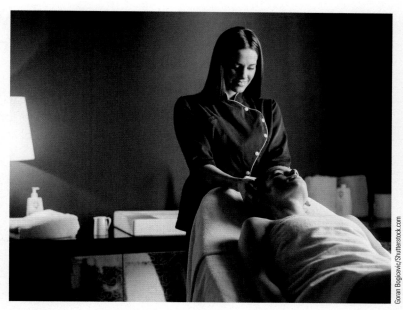

▲ FIGURE 1–17 Estheticians are equipped to work in any environment such as wellness centers, hotels, offices, home visits, plastic surgeon's offices, and more.

Goran Bogicevic/Shutterstock.com

ACTIVITY

Skin Care Advancements

Learn about a new trend or technique that is on the rise. Search online for trend reports, skin care articles, or tradeshows/conferences that you can attend.

▼ TABLE 1–1 Advancements in the Esthetics Industry, 2000s

Popular procedures in medical spas	Laser hair reduction, chemical peels, microdermabrasion, and injectables (e.g., Botox®)
Advancements in esthetic procedures	Light therapies, lasers, microcurrent, ultrasound, microneedling, dermaplaning, chemical peels, microcurrent, and ultrasonic cavitation
Product ingredient delivery systems	Microencapsulation and microsponge
Device treatments to allow for better ingredient delivery	Dermal rolling, dermaplaning, microneedling, ultrasound, and ultrasonic machines
Anti-aging ingredients	Antioxidants, peptides, sodium PCA, sodium hyaluronate, polyphenols, and retinols

Apply Your Knowledge of Career Opportunities and the History of Esthetics

Use your time in school to learn everything you can to craft your skills and consider your career options. Work hard to represent your best every day as you get involved in this dynamic, innovative, and rewarding profession.

 CHECK IN

9. Which important cosmetic products and procedures were introduced in the late twentieth century?
10. What are some of the newer esthetic procedures that are offered?

COMPETENCY PROGRESS

How are you doing with career opportunities and the history of esthetics? **Check the Chapter 1 Learning Objectives below that you feel you have mastered; leave unchecked those concepts you will need to return to.**

☐ Explain how career opportunities and the history of the profession are critical to esthetics.

☐ Describe the career options available to licensed estheticians.

☐ List types of existing esthetics practices to chart your career path.

☐ Outline skin care practices from early cultures.

☐ Summarize the current and future states of the esthetics industry as described in this chapter.

CHAPTER GLOSSARY

clinical esthetics clin-i-kuhl es-THET-iks	p. 7	Previously known as *medical esthetics*; the integration of surgical procedures and esthetic treatments.
esthetician es-thuh-TISH-un	p. 6	Also known as *aesthetician*; a specialist in the cleansing, beautification, and preservation of the health of skin on the entire body, including the face and neck.
esthetics es-THET-iks	p. 6	Also known as *aesthetics*; from the Greek word *aesthetikos* (meaning "perceptible to the senses"); a branch of anatomical science that deals with the overall health and well-being of the skin, the largest organ of the human body.

henna hen-uh	p. 18	A dye obtained from the powdered leaves and shoots of the mignonette tree; used as a reddish hair dye and in temporary design tattooing.
kosmetikos kos-MET-i-kos	p. 18	Greek word meaning skilled in the use of cosmetics.
oncology ong-kol-uh-jee	p. 15	The study and treatment of cancer and tumors.

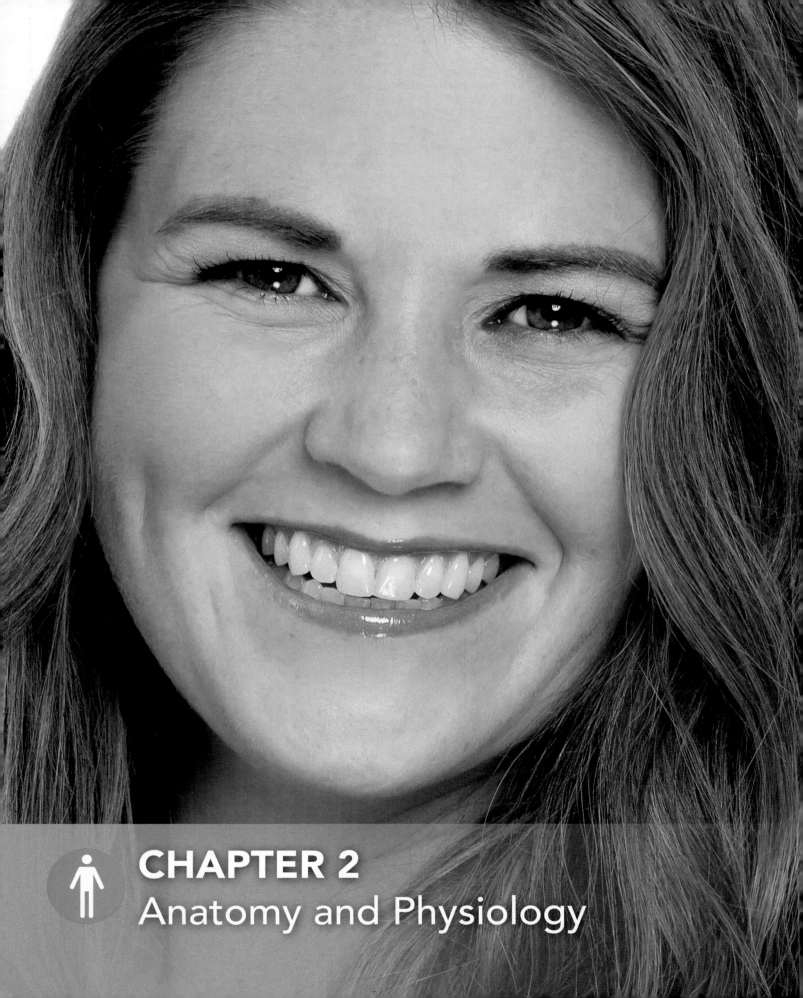

CHAPTER 2
Anatomy and Physiology

"Impossible is not a scientific term."

–Vanna Bonta

Learning Objectives

After completing this chapter, you will be able to:

1. Explain why estheticians need knowledge of anatomy and physiology.
2. Describe the basic structure and function of a cell.
3. Describe the four types of tissue found in the body.
4. Define the functions of major organs and systems of the body that intersect with the integumentary system and esthetics.
5. List the five accessory organs to the skin.
6. Identify the five functions of the skeletal system.
7. Recognize the muscles involved in esthetic massage.
8. Describe the three nerve branches of the head, neck, and face essential for performing facial treatments.
9. Outline how the circulatory system influences the health of the skin.
10. Explain the interdependence of the lymphatic, circulatory, and immune systems.
11. Identify the glands that make up the endocrine system.
12. List how hormonal changes in the reproductive system can affect the skin.
13. Describe what occurs during inhalation and exhalation.
14. Explain the five steps in digestion.
15. List the five organs that comprise the excretory system.

Explain Why Estheticians Need Knowledge of Anatomy and Physiology

Did your heart start beating faster when you opened this chapter? Correct, you are not expected to be a medical assistant, but this chapter will guide you through all of the body systems that need to work together to achieve healthy-looking skin. Estheticians focus primarily on the muscles, bones, nerves, and circulation of the head, face, neck, arms, and hands. Whether applying product, giving a treatment, or doing a skin care analysis, as licensed estheticians, we touch people as part of our profession. This is true of very few other occupations, and it is an honor to be able to aid others in a greater sense of well-being.

Estheticians should study and have a thorough understanding of anatomy and physiology because:

- Estheticians need to understand how the human body functions as an integrated whole. Body systems are interdependent on each other and if one system is not functioning optimally, it affects the entire body and can be evident on the skin.
- As a service provider, you must be able to recognize skin changes from earlier visits, and you may need to change a treatment plan or refer the client to a medical provider for evaluation.
- Estheticians must understand the effect that services will have on tissues, organs, and body systems.
- Recommendations for treatment plans and protocols for a client are based on the decisions made during a skin analysis and consultation and review of the client intake form.
- Understanding the complexity of the human body and how body systems are interrelated will help you take the information into consideration when advising a treatment plan, recommending skin care products, or performing a service.

Define Anatomy, Physiology, and Histology

As an esthetic professional, an overview of human anatomy and physiology will enable you to perform your services knowledgeably, effectively, and safely on a consistent basis.

Anatomy (ah-NAT-ah-mee) is the study of the structures of the human body and the substances these structures are made of. It is the science of the interconnected detail of organisms, or of their parts.

Physiology (fiz-ee-AHL-uh-jee) is the study of the functions and activities performed by the body structures, including physical and chemical processes.

Histology (his-TAHL-uh-jee), also known as *microscopic anatomy*, is the study of the structure and composition of tissue.

Describe the Basic Structure and Function of a Cell

Cells (SELLZ) are the basic unit of all living things—from bacteria to plants to animals to human beings. Without cells, life does not exist. As a basic functional unit, the cell is responsible for carrying on all life processes. There are trillions of cells in the human body, and they vary widely in size, shape, and purpose.

Basic Structure of the Cell

The cells of all living things are composed of a substance called **protoplasm** (PROH-toh-plaz-um), a colorless, jellylike substance in which nutrients such as proteins, fats, carbohydrates, mineral salts, and water are present. These nutrient materials are necessary for cell growth, reproduction, and self-repair. You can visualize the protoplasm of a cell as being similar to the clear gel of a raw egg. In addition to protoplasm, most cells also include a nucleus, **organelles** (or-guh-NELZ) (small organs), and the cell membrane (**Figure 2–1**).

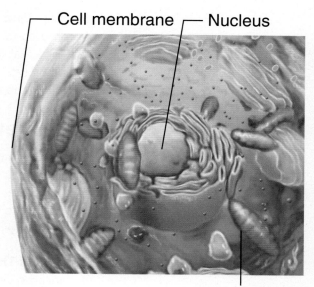

▲ **FIGURE 2–1** The cell is responsible for carrying on all life processes.

- The **nucleus** (NOO-klee-us) is the dense, active protoplasm found in the center of the cell. It plays an important part in cell reproduction and metabolism. You can visualize the nucleus as the yolk of a raw egg. Within the nucleus of the cell is the **nucleoplasm** (NEW-clee-oh-plasm), which is a fluid that contains proteins, and a very important acid known as **deoxyribonucleic acid (DNA)** (DEE-ox-ee-RYE-boh-NEW-clayic ASUD). DNA is what determines our genetic makeup, including the color of our eyes, skin, and hair.

- Protoplasm is a watery gel-like fluid containing the nutrient material necessary for cell growth, reproduction, and self-repair.

- **Mitochondria** (mahy-tuh-KON-dree-uh) take in nutrients, break them down, and create energy for the cell. Mitochondria work to keep the cell full of energy. This chemical energy used within cells for metabolism is called **ATP** (adenosine triphosphate) (uh-DEN-uh-seen try-FAHS-fayt). Mitochondria are small organelles floating freely throughout the cell. Some cells have several thousand mitochondria, such as muscle cells, while others have none, like red blood cells. Muscle cells need a lot of energy, so they have many mitochondria. **Neurons** (NOO-rahn) or nerve cells (cells that transmit nerve impulses) don't need as many.

- The **cell membrane** (SELL mem-brain) is the part of the cell that encloses the protoplasm and permits **soluble** (SAHL-yuh-bul) substances to enter and leave. It is selectively permeable, controlling the introduction of beneficial substances into the cell and the removal of waste and other substances that do not benefit the life of the cell. The cell membrane protects the cell from its surroundings. It also communicates with other cells, linking like cells together to form tissues.

Cell Reproduction and Division

Cells have the ability to reproduce, thus providing new cells for the growth and replacement of worn or injured ones. **Mitosis** (my-TOH-sus) is the normal process of cell reproduction in human tissues that occurs when the cell divides into two identical cells called daughter cells. As long as conditions are favorable, the cell will grow and reproduce. Favorable conditions include an adequate supply of nutrients, oxygen, and water; suitable temperatures; and the ability to eliminate waste products. Unfavorable conditions include toxins (poisons), disease, and injury, where the cell will become impaired or may be destroyed.

Cell Metabolism

Metabolism (muh-TAB-uh-liz-um) is a chemical process that takes place in living organisms. Metabolism converts nutrients to energy so the cell can function. Metabolism also eliminates waste. These functions allow organisms to grow and reproduce, respond to their environments, and maintain their structures.

How Is This Important? Aging influences the cell's metabolism and the cell begins to function less efficiently. As an esthetician, cell metabolism is something you will consider when working with your clients. Clients' response to treatment and response to the active ingredients in skin care products will be influenced by the efficiency and speed of their metabolism.

According to Jeffrey Utz, MD, from the Department of Neuroscience at Allegheny University:

- Men's bodies contain more water than women's bodies do.
- Water content differs throughout various tissues in the body
- Blood is made up of 83 percent water, and muscle is 75 percent water.
- The human brain is 73 percent water.
- Even bones are about 31 percent water.

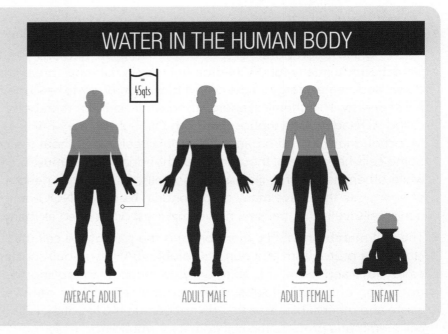

WATER IN THE HUMAN BODY

AVERAGE ADULT   ADULT MALE   ADULT FEMALE   INFANT

 CHECK IN

1. Draw and label the basic structures of a cell.
2. Summarize cell metabolism and its purpose.

Describe the Four Types of Tissue Found in the Body

Tissue (TISH-oo) is a collection of similar cells that perform a particular function. Each tissue has a specific function and can be recognized by its characteristic appearance. There are four types of tissue in the body.

1. **Connective tissue** (Kun-neck-tiv TISH-oo) supports, protects, and binds together other tissues of the body. Examples of connective tissue are bone, cartilage, ligaments, tendons, fascia (which separates muscles), blood, and fat, which is also called **adipose tissue** (AD-uh-pohs TISH-oo) (**Figure 2–2**). Adipose stores energy and gives smoothness and contour to the body. Collagen and elastin are protein fibers, and also a part of connective tissue.

2. **Epithelial tissue** (ep-ih-THEE-lee-ul TISH-oo) is a protective lining on cavities of the body and surfaces of organs. Examples are skin, mucous membranes, the lining of the heart, digestive and respiratory organs, and the glands (**Figure 2–3**).

3. **Muscle tissue** (MUS-uhl TISH-oo) contracts and moves the various parts of the body (**Figure 2–4**).

4. **Nerve tissue** (NURV TISH-oo) carries messages through the central nervous system to control and coordinate all bodily functions. Nerve tissue is composed of special cells known as neurons, which make up the nerves, brain, and spinal cord (**Figure 2—5**).

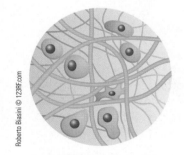

▲ **FIGURE 2–2**
Connective tissue

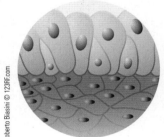

▲ **FIGURE 2–3**
Epithelial tissue

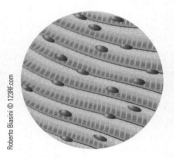

▲ **FIGURE 2–4**
Muscle tissue

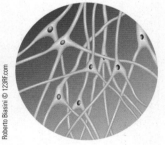

▲ **FIGURE 2–5**
Nerve tissue

✓ CHECK IN

3. List and describe the functions of the four types of tissue found in the human body.

Define the Functions of Major Organs and Systems of the Body that Intersect with the Integumentary System and Esthetics

Functions in the body are carried out by organs. **Organs** (OR-gunz) are a collection of tissues that have an identifiable structure and that perform specific functions . For example, the heart has muscle tissue that pumps blood, fibrous tissue that comprise the heart valves, and special tissue that maintains the rhythm of the heart beating.

Body systems (BAHD-ee SYS-tumz) are groups of organs acting together for one or more functions.

Table 2–1 lists the body systems as well as some of the most important organs of the body whose functioning affects the integrity of the skin.

▼ **TABLE 2–1 Body systems**

System	Function	Organs	Why know this?
Integumentary	Largest organ of the body, first line of defense against infection and water loss; regulates temperature, perceives sensation, produces vitamin D; and has absorption capabilities	Skin and accessory organs such as oil and sweat glands, sensory receptors, hair, and nails	As skin is the largest organ in the body, learning its functions and the work of the accessory organs is a critical component in a skin care therapist's success
Skeletal	Forms the physical foundation of the body; consists of the bones and movable and immovable joints	Bones	Important for protecting your own body mechanics when working, as well as knowing physical landmarks when providing treatments, including makeup applications
Muscular	Covers, shapes, and supports the skeletal tissue; also contracts and moves various parts of the body; consists of muscles	Muscles	Important when doing massage and performing electrical treatments such as microcurrent; also important to understand muscle movement to prevent repetitive motion fatigue when you are performing treatments
Nervous	Carries messages through the central nervous system, controlling and coordinating all bodily functions	Brain, spinal cord, nerves	Need to know the location of the facial nerves and their actions when performing treatments; nerves control the muscle movements of the face
Circulatory	Controls the steady delivery of the blood through the body; works with the lymphatic channels	Heart with blood vessels	Health of the circulatory system affects skin tissue health; circulatory issues are often contraindications and precautions to treatments; when performing body wraps, for example, understanding which direction to wrap is essential for a good outcome, or an adverse event can occur

(Continues)

(Continued)

Immune/ Lymphatic	Protects the body from disease by developing resistances and destroying disease-causing toxins, foreign material, and bacteria	Spleen, lymph	Many treatments require action from the lymphatic system, including performing lymphatic massage
Endocrine 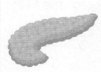	Affects growth, development, sexual activities, and normal regulatory processes of the body; consists of specialized glands	Adrenal gland, pituitary gland, pancreas	Hormones excreted by the endocrine system have a significant effect on the skin, and an understanding of that functioning will help when recognizing the need to refer a client for a medical evaluation; acne breakouts, hair growth, and skin oiliness or dryness are a few
Reproductive 	Performs the function of producing children and passing on our genetics from one generation to another; differentiates between the sexes	Uterus, ovaries, penis, testes	The reproductive system and hormonal influences accompanying puberty, pregnancy, perimenopause, and menopause make significant demands on the skin that require knowledge in order to provide a skin-care treatment
Respiratory 	Enables breathing, supplies the body with oxygen, and eliminates carbon dioxide as a waste product	Lungs, trachea, bronchi	Adequate oxygenation of the tissue allows optimum cell functioning; possibility of the respiratory spread of infection affects safety and cleanliness
Digestive 	Breaks down food into smaller and smaller particles to absorb nutrients or for excretion	Esophagus, stomach, gall bladder, liver, small and large intestines	Good nutrition allows optimum functioning of all body systems
Excretory 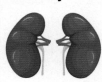	Refers to elimination of waste matter	Kidneys, bladder	Functions to eliminate toxic substances that can affect other body system functions

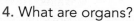

✓ CHECK IN

4. What are organs?
5. Name the body systems and their main functions.
6. Explain why knowledge of each body system is important to esthetics.

List the Five Accessory Organs to the Skin

The **integumentary system** (in-TEG-yuh-ment-uh-ree SIS-tum) is made up of the skin and its various accessory organs, such as sensory receptors, hair, nails, and the oil and sweat glands, also called **exocrine glands** (EK-suh-krin GLANDZ) **(Figure 2–6)**. Skin anatomy and physiology are discussed in detail in Chapter 3, Physiology and Histology of the Skin.

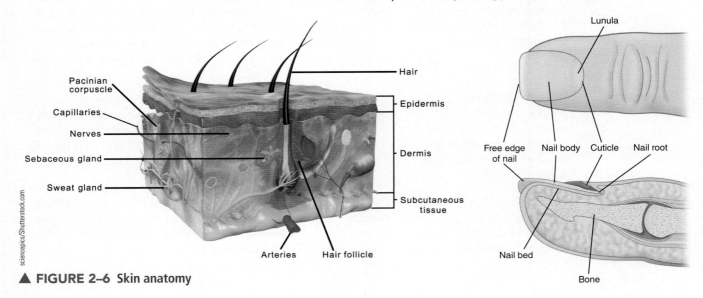

Pacinian corpuscle

Capillaries

Nerves

Sebaceous gland

Sweat gland

Hair

Epidermis

Dermis

Subcutaneous tissue

Arteries

Hair follicle

Lunula

Free edge of nail

Nail body

Cuticle

Nail root

Nail bed

Bone

sciencepics/Shutterstock.com

▲ **FIGURE 2–6 Skin anatomy**

The word *integument* means a natural covering. So, you can think of the **skin** as a protective overcoat for your body against the outside elements that you encounter every day such as germs, chemicals, and sun exposure.

 CHECK IN

7. Name five accessory organs to the skin.

Identify the Five Functions of the Skeletal System

The **skeletal system** (SKEL-uh-tul SIS-tum) forms the physical foundation of the body.

How Is This Important? As an esthetician, an understanding of the skeletal system is important when you are performing makeup applications. Certain treatments may require you treat the ocular ridge. It is essential that you know that location on the anatomy. Some states do not allow estheticians to perform treatments beyond the seventh cervical vertebrae, for example. Additionally, to understand how to protect your own body by using proper body mechanics when you work.

The Number of Bones and Composition

The adult skeleton has 206 bones that form a rigid framework to which the softer tissues and organs of the body are encased and acts as anchor points for muscles and ligaments to provide support for movement.

Muscles are connected to bones by tendons. Bones are connected to each other by ligaments (**Figure 2–7**).

The bone tissue is composed of several types of bone cells embedded in a web of inorganic salts (mostly calcium and phosphorus) and collagenous fibers. The web gives the bone strength, and the fibers give the bone flexibility.

The place where bones meet one another is typically called a joint. A **joint** (JOYNT) is the connection between two or more bones of the skeleton. There are two types of joints: movable, such as elbows, knees, and hips; and immovable, such as the pelvis and skull, which allow little or no movement.

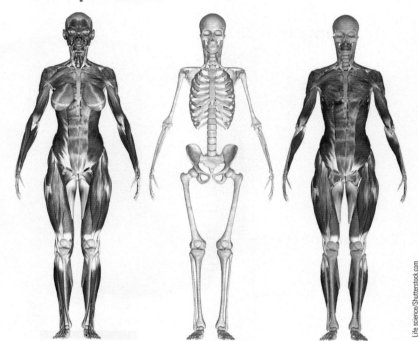

▲ **FIGURE 2–7** Muscles and tendons

Life science/Shutterstock.com

Functions

The primary functions of the skeletal system are to:

- Give shape and support to the body
- Protect various internal structures and organs
- Serve as attachments for muscles and act as levers to produce body movement
- Help produce both white and red blood cells (one of the functions of bone marrow)
- Store most of the body's calcium supply as well as phosphorus, magnesium, and sodium.

DID YOU KNOW?

People often complain of joint pain; however, the pain is usually caused by inflammation of the tissue surrounding the joint and not by the joint itself.

You have over 230 moveable and semi-moveable joints in your body.

Bones of the Skull

The human head contains 22 bones divided into two groups: the cranium and the facial bones. The **cranium** (KRAY-nee-um) is an oval, bony case that protects the brain, and it is formed by eight bones. The face consists of 14 bones, including the maxilla (upper jaw) and mandible (lower jaw). Small openings in the skull allow the cranial nerves to extend to various locations on the head.

BONES OF THE CRANIUM

The cranium is made up of eight bones (**Figure 2–8a**):

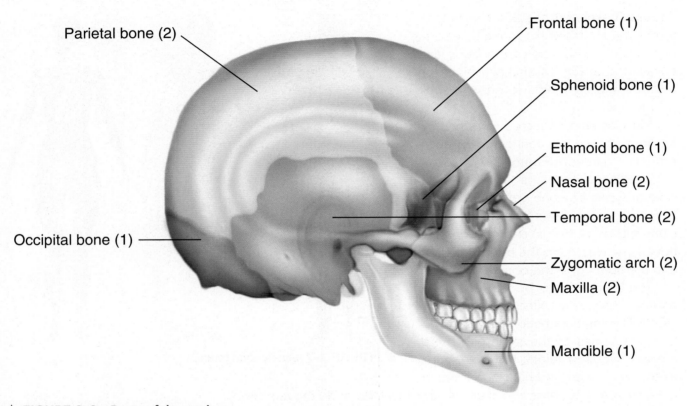

▲ **FIGURE 2–8a Bones of the cranium**

- The **occipital bone** (ahk-SIP-ut-ul BOHN) forms the back of the skull above the **nape** (NAYP).
- The two **parietal bones** (puh-RY-ate-ul BONZ) form the sides and crown (top) of the cranium.
- The **frontal bone** (FRUNT-ul BOHN) forms the forehead.
- The two **temporal bones** (TEM-puh-rul BONZ) form the sides of the head in the ear region.
- The **ethmoid bone** (ETH-moyd BOHN) is the light, spongy bone between the eye sockets that forms part of the nasal cavities.
- The **sphenoid bone** (SFEE-noyd BOHN) forms the sides of the eye socket.

The ethmoid and sphenoid bones are not affected when performing services or giving a massage.

BONES OF THE FACE

The bones of the face that estheticians need to know include (**Figure 2–8b**):

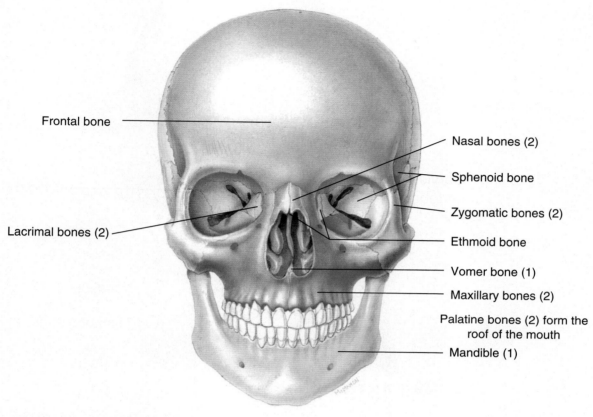

Frontal bone

Nasal bones (2)

Sphenoid bone

Zygomatic bones (2)

Ethmoid bone

Lacrimal bones (2)

Vomer bone (1)

Maxillary bones (2)

Palatine bones (2) form the roof of the mouth

Mandible (1)

▲ **FIGURE 2–8b Bones of the Face**

- Two **nasal bones** (NAY-zul BONZ) form the bridge of the nose.
- Two **lacrimal bones**, (LAK-ruh-mul BONZ) the smallest and most fragile bones of the face, are situated at the front inside part of the eye socket.
- Two **zygomatic bones**, (zy-goh-MAT-ik BONZ) also known as **malar bones** (mey-ler BONZ) or **cheekbones** (CHEEK-bonz), form the prominence of the cheeks.
- Two **maxillae bones** (mak-SIL-uh BONZ) form the upper jaw.
- The **mandible** (MAN-duh-bul) forms the lower jawbone, the largest and strongest bone of the face.

Bones of the Neck

The main bones of the neck are the following (**Figure 2–9**):

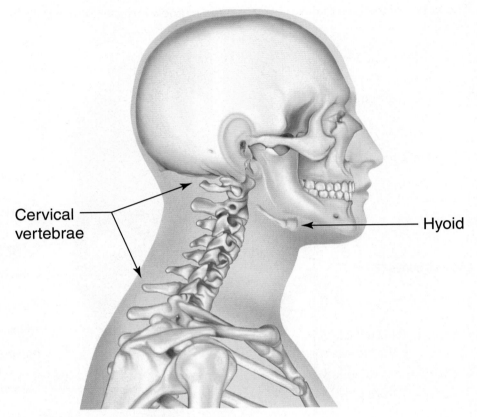

Cervical vertebrae

Hyoid

▲ **FIGURE 2–9** Bones of the neck

- **Hyoid bone**, (HY-oyd BOHN) a U-shaped bone at the base of the tongue that supports the tongue and its muscles
- **Cervical vertebrae** (SUR-vih-kul VURT-uh-bray), the seven bones of the top part of the vertebral column located in the neck region

Bones of the Chest

Bones of the chest are important when performing full-body treatments, such as body wraps (**Figure 2–10**), as well as for massage that will include touching the sternum, scapula, and clavicle as body reference landmarks. The bones of the trunk or torso include:

- **Thorax** (THOR-aks): the chest or pulmonary trunk consisting of the sternum, ribs, and thoracic vertebrae; it is an elastic, bony cage that serves as a protective framework for the heart, lungs, and other internal organs
- **Ribs** (RIBZ): twelve pairs of bones forming the wall of the thorax
- **Scapula** (SKAP-yuh-luh) also known as **shoulder blade** (SHOHL-dur blayd): the large, flat, triangular bone of the shoulder; there are two scapulae

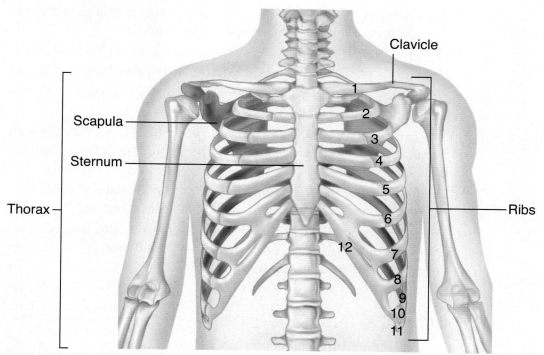

▲ FIGURE 2–10 Bones of the chest

- **Sternum** (STUR-num), also known as **breastbone** (BREST-bohn): the flat bone that forms the ventral (front) support of the ribs
- **Clavicle** (KLAV-ih-kul), also known as **collarbone** (KAHL-ur-BOHN): the bone that joins the sternum and scapula

Bones of the Arms and Hands

The important bones of the arms and hands are as follows (**Figure 2–11**):

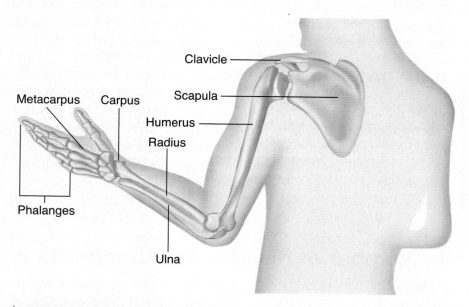

▲ FIGURE 2–11 Bones of the arm and hands

- The **humerus** (HYOO-muh-rus) is the uppermost and largest bone of the arm, extending from the elbow to the shoulder.
- The **ulna** (UL-nuh) is the inner and larger bone of the forearm (lower arm), attached to the wrist and located on the side of the little finger.
- The **radius** (RAY-dee-us) is the smaller bone in the forearm on the same side as the thumb.
- The **carpus** (KAR-pus), also known as **wrist** (RIST), is a flexible joint composed of eight small, irregular bones (carpals) held together by ligaments.
- The **metacarpus** (met-uh-KAR-pus), also known as **palm** (PAHM), consists of five long, slender bones called metacarpal bones.
- The **phalanges** (FA-lanj-eez) (singular: phalanx, FAY-langks), also known as **digits** (DIJ-utz), are the bones in the fingers, three in each finger and two in each thumb, totaling 14 bones.

 CHECK IN

8. List the primary functions of the skeletal system.
9. Identify the bones in the skull, cranium, face, neck, chest, and arms and hands and their location.

Recognize the Muscles Involved in Esthetic Massage

The **muscular system** (MUS-kyuh-lur SIS-tum) covers, shapes, and supports the skeletal tissue. Muscles are fibrous tissues with the ability to stretch and contract according to the demands of the body's movements. This system can contract and move various parts of the body.

How Is This Important? An esthetician will need familiarity with muscles for a number of reasons. Esthetic massage involves manipulating the muscles of the face, neck, shoulders, arms, and hands. Many treatments using electrical modalities involve an understanding of the muscle's movements in order to achieve the desired result. Your posture and positioning during treatments will require you to demonstrate good body mechanics in order to prevent muscle fatigue.

The Number of Muscles and Composition

The human body has over 630 muscles, which are responsible for approximately 40 percent of the body's weight. Out of the over 630 muscles, 30 are facial muscles.

There are three types of muscle tissue:

1. Skeletal, or voluntary muscles contract with conscious thought.
2. Smooth, or involuntary muscles are not under conscious control.
3. Cardiac muscles are specific to heart function and are not under conscious control.

Estheticians work with skeletal, or voluntary, muscles. These are the muscles attached to bones and are controlled by thought processes. Nerve impulses trigger a reaction from the muscle, which contracts, moving the bone or joint it is associated with.

A skeletal or voluntary muscle has three parts (**Figure 2–12**):

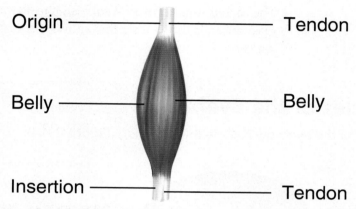

▲ FIGURE 2–12 Parts of skeletal muscle

1. The **origin** (OR-ih-jin) is the more fixed part of the muscle closest to the skeleton, which flexes but remains stationary (does not move).
2. The **belly** (BELL-ee) is the middle part of the muscle.
3. The **insertion** (in-SUR-shun) is the part of the muscle that is the movable attachment and farthest from the skeleton.

Pressure in massage is usually directed from the insertion to the origin. Muscle tissue can be positively influenced during an esthetic treatment by:

- Massage (hand or mechanical vibrations)
- Electrical therapy current (See Chapter 10, Facial Devices and Technology, for additional information on high-frequency current, galvanic current, or microcurrent.)
- Light rays (infrared light, light-emitting diode [LED])
- Dry heat (heating lamps or heating caps)
- Moist heat (steamers or moderately warm steam towels).

Muscles of the Scalp

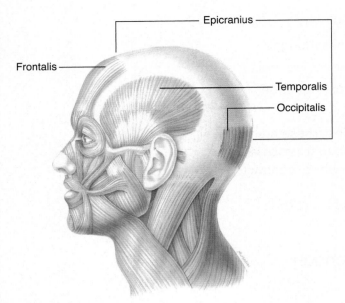

- There are four muscles of the scalp: frontalis, occipitalis, and two temporalis on the sides.
- The esthetician is most concerned about the **frontalis** (frun-TAY-lus), the scalp muscle that raises the eyebrows, draws the scalp forward, and causes wrinkles in the forehead.
- The **epicranius** (ep-ih-KRA-nee-us), also known as the **occipitofrontalis** (ahk-SIP-ihtoh-frun-TAY-lus) is a broad muscle that covers the top of the skull. It has two parts, occipitalis and frontalis.
- The **occipitalis** (ahk-SIP-i-tahl-is), the back of the epicranius, is the muscle that draws the scalp backward.

▲ **FIGURE 2–13a** Muscles of the scalp.

Muscles of the Eyebrow

Muscles of the eyebrow include the following (**Figure 2–13**):

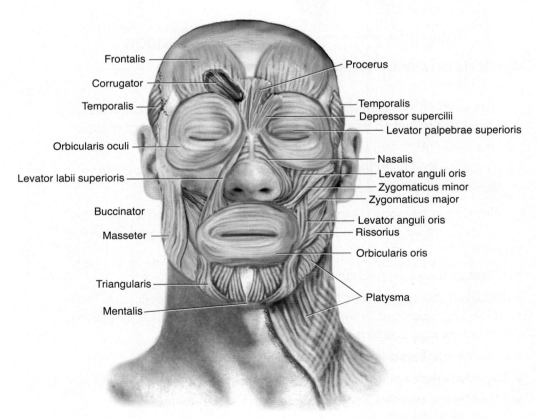

▲ **FIGURE 2–13b** Muscles of the scalp, eyebrow, nose, mouth, and mastication

- The **corrugator** (KOR-uh-gayt-or) is the muscle located beneath the frontalis and orbicularis oculi. It draws the eyebrow down and wrinkles the forehead vertically.
- The **orbicularis oculi** (or-bik-yuh-LAIR-is AHK-yuh-lye) is the ring muscle of the eye socket; it closes the eyes.
- The **levator palpebrae superioris muscle** (lih-VAYT-ur PAL-puh-bree soo-peer-ee-OR-is MUS-uhl) controls the eyelid and can be easily damaged during makeup application.

Muscles of the Nose

Figure 2–13 also shows the two primary muscles of the nose.

- The **procerus** (proh-SEE-rus) lowers the eyebrows and causes wrinkles across the bridge of the nose.
- The **nasalis** (nay-ZAY-lis) is a two-part muscle that covers the nose and includes the *transverse part* and the *alar part*, which flair the nostrils.

Muscles of the Mouth

The following are important muscles of the mouth (see **Figure 2–13**):

- The **buccinator** (BUK-sih-nay-tur) is the thin, flat muscle of the cheek between the upper and lower jaw that compresses the cheeks and expels air between the lips, as in when blowing a whistle.
- The **triangularis** (try-ang-gyuh-LAY-rus), also known as the **depressor anguli oris** (dee-PRES-ur ANG-yoo-lye OH-ris), is the muscle extending alongside the chin that pulls down the corners of the mouth.
- The **mentalis** (men-TAY-lis) is the muscle that elevates the lower lip and raises and wrinkles the skin of the chin.
- The **orbicularis oris** (or-bik-yuh-LAIR-is OH-ris) is the flat band around the upper and lower lips that compresses, contracts, puckers, and wrinkles the lips.
- **Levator anguli oris** (lih-VAYT-ur ANG-yoo-ly OH-ris) is a muscle associated with smiling.
- The **risorius** (rih-ZOR-ee-us) is the muscle that draws the corners of the mouth out and back when grinning.
- **Levator labii superioris** (lih-VAYT-ur LAY-bee-eye soopeer-ee-OR-is) is a muscle associated with lifting the wings of the nose and upper lip. It is sometimes called the **quadratus labii superioris** (kwah-DRA-tus LAY-bee-eye soo-eeree-OR-is).
- **Zygomaticus** (zy-goh-MAT-ih-kus) major and minor are muscles extending from the zygomatic bone to the angle of the mouth that elevates the lip, as in laughing.

Muscles of Mastication (Chewing)

The main muscles of mastication coordinate to open and close the mouth and bring the jaw forward or backward. These muscles are sometimes referred to as the *chewing muscles.* The esthetician needs to know the location of these muscles when performing facial massage and electrical modality treatments.

- **Masseter** (muh-SEET-ur)
- **Temporalis** (tem-poh-RAY-lis)

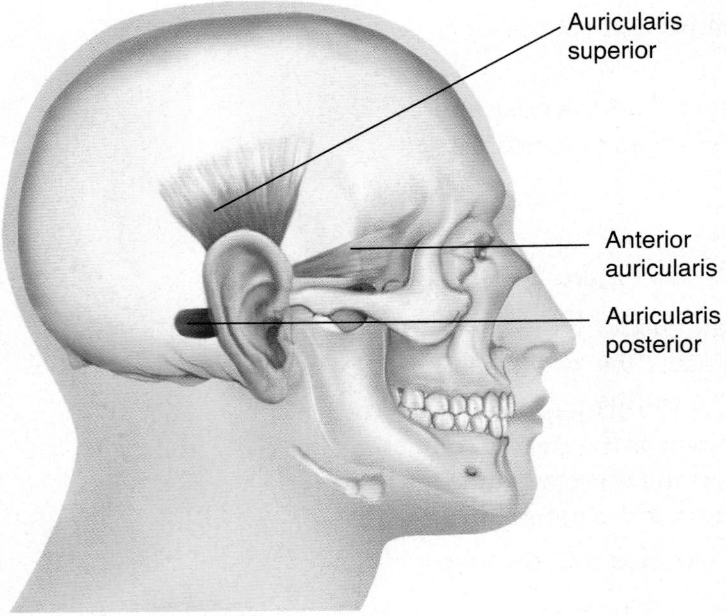

Auricularis superior

Anterior auricularis

Auricularis posterior

▲ FIGURE 2–14 Muscles of the ear

Muscles of the Ear

- The three muscles of the ear are called the **auricularis muscles** (aw-rik-yuh-LAIR-is MUS-uhlz). They work together to move the ear upward, forward or backward (**Figure 2–14**).

Muscles of the Neck

Muscles of the neck include the following (**Figure 2–15**):

- The **platysma** (plah-TIZ-muh) is a broad muscle extending from the chest and shoulder muscles to the side of the chin. It is responsible for lowering the lower jaw and lip.
- The **sternocleidomastoid (SCM)** (STUR-noh-KLY-doh-MAS-toyd) is the muscle extending alongside of the neck from the ear to the collarbone. It acts to rotate the head from side to side and up and down.

Muscles That Attach the Arms to the Body

Muscles attaching the arms to the body include the following:

- The **latissimus dorsi** (lah-TIS-ih-mus DOR-see) is a large, flat, triangular muscle that covers the lower back. It comes up from the lower half of the vertebral column and iliac crest (hip bone) and narrows to a rounded tendon attached to the front of the upper part of the humerus (**Figure 2–16**).
- The **pectoralis major** (pek-tor-AL-is MAY-jor) and **pectoralis minor** (pek-tor-AL-is MY-nur) are muscles of the chest that assist the swinging movements of the arm.

ACTIVITY

Muscles Flashcards

Make flashcards for the muscles of the scalp, eyebrow, ear, nose, mouth, chewing, neck, shoulder, and arm.

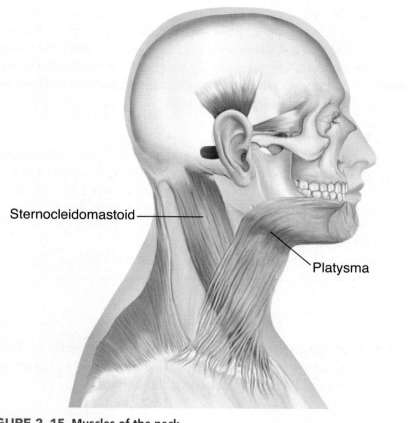

Sternocleidomastoid

Platysma

▲ FIGURE 2–15 Muscles of the neck

Muscles of the Shoulder and Arm

Here are the principal muscles of the shoulders and upper arms (**Figure 2–16**):

- The **trapezius** (truh-PEE-zee-us) muscle covers the back of the neck, shoulders, and upper and middle region of the back; shrugs shoulders; and stabilizes the scapula.

- The **biceps** (BY-seps) muscles produce the contour of the front and inner side of the upper arm; they lift the forearm, flex the elbow, and turn the palms outward.

- The **deltoid** (DEL-toyd) is a large, triangular muscle covering the shoulder joint that allows the arm to extend outward and to the side of the body.

- The **triceps** (TRY-seps) is a large muscle that covers the entire back of the upper arm and extends the forearm.

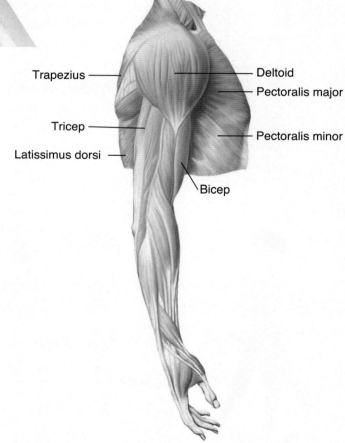

Trapezius

Tricep

Latissimus dorsi

Deltoid

Pectoralis major

Pectoralis minor

Bicep

▲ FIGURE 2–16 Muscles of the shoulders and upper arms

MUSCLES OF THE FOREARM

The forearm is made up of a series of muscles and strong tendons. As an esthetician, you will be concerned with the muscles of the forearm so you can ensure you use good body mechanics when performing treatments. In addition, you may also be performing some hand and forearm massage during a relaxing facial session.

MUSCLES OF THE HAND

The hand is one of the most complex parts of the body, with many small muscles that overlap from joint to joint, providing flexibility and strength to open and close the hand and fingers. Massage can help relax and maintain the pliability of these muscles.

MUSCLE MOVEMENTS

Important muscle movements to know include the following (**Figure 2–17**):

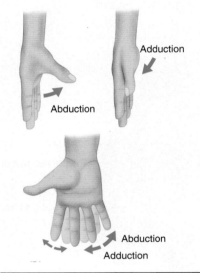

- **Abduction** (ab-DUK-shun): muscles that draw a body part, such as a finger, arm, or toe, away from the midline of the body or of an extremity. In the hand, abduction separates the fingers.

- **Adduction** (ah-DUK-shun): muscles that draw a body part, such as a finger, arm, or toe, inward toward the median axis of the body or of an extremity. In the hand, adduction draws the fingers together.

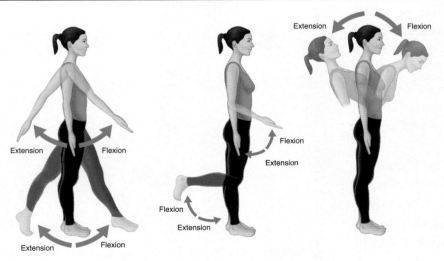

- **Flexion** (FLEK-shun) is when muscles move to pull the body part toward the core of the body, such as when the biceps of the arm are activated toward the body.

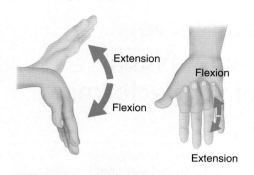
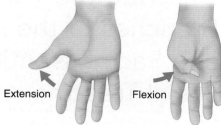

Extension
Flexion
Flexion
Extension
Extension
Flexion

- **Extension** (ik-STEN-shun) is when muscles straighten. When the wrist, hand, and fingers form a straight line, for example.

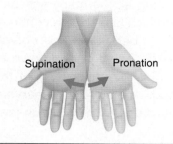

Supination   Pronation

- **Pronate** (proh-NAYT) is when muscles turn inward. For example, when the palm faces downward.

- **Supinate** (SOO-puh-nayt) is when muscles rotate. For example, in the forearm, the radius turns outward and the palm upward.

▲ **FIGURE 2–17** Important muscle movements

 CHECK IN

10. List the primary functions of the muscular system.
11. Name the three parts of a voluntary muscle.
12. Identify how muscle tissue can be positively influenced in an esthetic treatment.
13. Identify and explain the muscles of each of these areas of anatomy:
    a. Scalp
    b. Eyebrow
    c. Ear
    d. Nose
    e. Mouth
    f. Chewing
    g. Neck
14. Identify and explain the muscles of each of these areas:
    a. Muscles that attach the arms to the body
    b. Muscles of the shoulder and arm
15. What do the muscles of the hand do?
16. Identify and explain the functions of:
    a. Abduction
    b. Adduction
    c. Flexion
    d. Extension
    e. Supination
    f. Pronation

Describe the Three Nerve Branches of the Head, Neck, and Face Essential for Performing Facial Treatments

The **nervous system** (NUR-vus SIS-tum) is an exceptionally well-organized system that is responsible for coordinating all the many activities that are performed by the body. Every square inch (2.5 square centimeters) of the human body is supplied with fine fibers known as *nerves*; there are over 100 billion nerve cells, known as *neurons*, in the body. The scientific study of the structure, function, and pathology of the nervous system is known as **neurology** (nuh-RAHL-uh-jee).

> **How Is This Important?** Understanding the sensory nerve functions of the skin and the power of touch will enhance your career. An understanding of how nerves work will help you perform massage more proficiently and understand the effects of treatments on the body as a whole.

Divisions of the Nervous System

The nervous system is divided into three main subdivisions (**Figure 2–18**).

1. The **central nervous system (CNS)** (SEN-trul NUR-vus SIS-tum) consists of the brain, spinal cord, spinal nerves, and cranial nerves. It controls consciousness and many mental activities, involuntary functions of the five senses (seeing, hearing, feeling, smelling, and tasting), and voluntary muscle actions, including all body movements and facial expressions.

2. The **peripheral nervous system (PNS)** (puh-RIF-uh-rul NUR-vus SIS-tum) is a system of nerves that connects the peripheral (outer) parts of the body to the central nervous system; it has both sensory and motor nerves. Its function is to carry impulses,

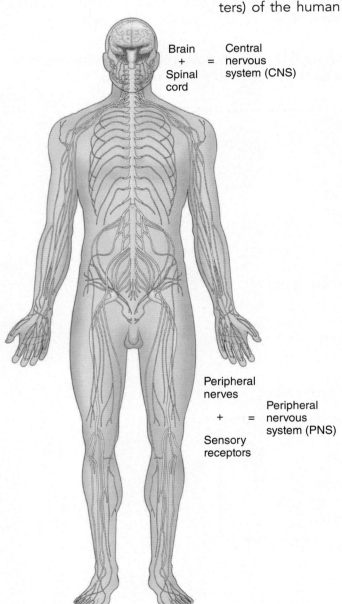

Brain + Spinal cord = Central nervous system (CNS)

Peripheral nerves + Sensory receptors = Peripheral nervous system (PNS)

▲ **FIGURE 2–18** Divisions of the Nervous System

or messages, to and from the central nervous system.

3. The **autonomic nervous system (ANS)** (aw-toh-NAHM-ik NUR-vus SIS-tum) is the part of the nervous system that controls the involuntary muscles; it regulates the action of the smooth muscles, glands, blood vessels, heart, and breathing.

The Brain and Spinal Cord

The **brain** (BRAYN) is the largest and most complex mass of nerve tissue in the body. The brain is contained in the cranium and controls sensation, muscles, and glandular activity It sends and receives messages through 12 pairs of cranial nerves that reach various parts of the head, face, and neck (**Figure 2–19**).

- The **brain stem** (BRAYN stem) connects the spinal cord to the brain. The brain stem is involved in regulating such vital functions as breathing, heartbeat, and blood pressure.
- The **spinal cord** (SPY-nal KORD) is a continuation of the brain stem and originates in the brain, extends down to the lower extremity of the trunk, and is protected by the spinal column. Thirty-one pairs of spinal nerves extending from the spinal cord are distributed to the muscles and skin of the trunk and limbs.

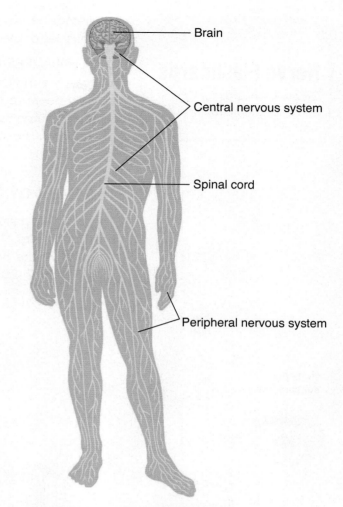

▲ **FIGURE 2–19** The Brain and Spinal Cord

Nerve Cell Structure and Function

Nerves (NURVZ) are whitish cords, made up of bundles of nerve fibers held together by connective tissue, through which impulses are transmitted. Nerves originate in the brain and spinal cord, and their branches extend to all parts of the body.

TYPES OF NERVES

There are two types of nerves:

1. **Sensory nerves** (SEN-soh-ree NURVZ) carry impulses or messages from the sense organs to the brain, where sensations such as touch, cold, heat, sight, hearing, taste, smell, pain, and pressure are experienced. Sensory nerve endings called **receptors** (ree-SEP-turz) are located close to the surface of the skin. As impulses pass from the sensory nerves to the brain and back through the motor nerves to the muscles, a complete circuit is established, resulting in movement of the muscles.

2. **Motor nerves** (MOH-tur NURVZ) carry impulses from the brain to the muscles or glands. These transmitted impulses produce movement.

A **reflex** (REE-fleks) is an automatic nerve reaction to a stimulus that involves the movement of an impulse from a sensory receptor along the sensory nerve to the spinal cord and a responsive impulse back along a motor neuron to a muscle, causing a reaction (e.g., the quick removal of the hand from a hot object). Reflexes do not have to be learned; they are automatic.

Nerves of the Head, Face, and Neck

There are 12 pairs of cranial nerves arising at the base of the brain and the brain stem. The cranial nerves activate the muscles and sensory structure of the head and neck, including skin, membranes, eyes, and ears (**Figure 2–20**).

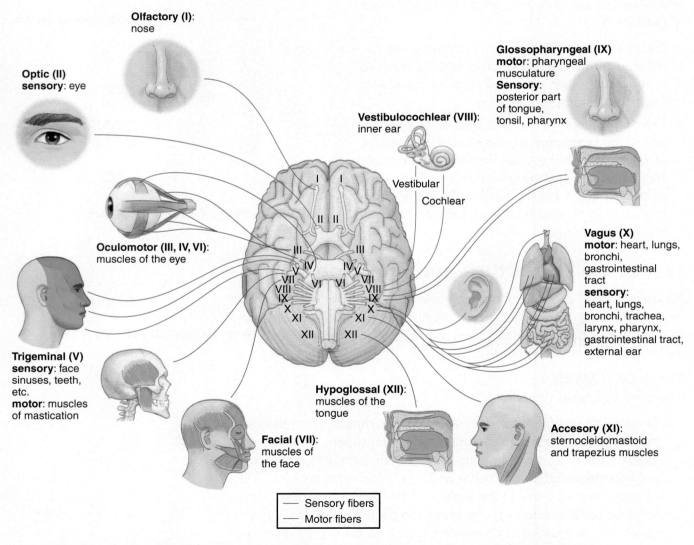

Olfactory (I): nose

Optic (II) sensory: eye

Oculomotor (III, IV, VI): muscles of the eye

Trigeminal (V) sensory: face sinuses, teeth, etc. **motor**: muscles of mastication

Facial (VII): muscles of the face

Hypoglossal (XII): muscles of the tongue

Vestibulocochlear (VIII): inner ear

Vestibular

Cochlear

Glossopharyngeal (IX) motor: pharyngeal musculature **Sensory**: posterior part of tongue, tonsil, pharynx

Vagus (X) motor: heart, lungs, bronchi, gastrointestinal tract **sensory**: heart, lungs, bronchi, trachea, larynx, pharynx, gastrointestinal tract, external ear

Accesory (XI): sternocleidomastoid and trapezius muscles

— Sensory fibers
— Motor fibers

▲ **FIGURE 2–20** The cranial nerves activate the muscles and sensory structures of the head, neck, and face

Estheticians are primarily concerned with nerves V, VII, and XI, and each one has several branches (**Figure 2–21**).

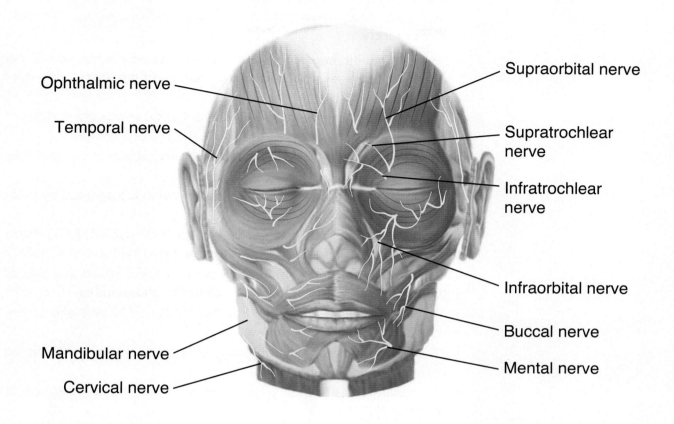

Ophthalmic nerve

Temporal nerve

Mandibular nerve

Cervical nerve

Supraorbital nerve

Supratrochlear nerve

Infratrochlear nerve

Infraorbital nerve

Buccal nerve

Mental nerve

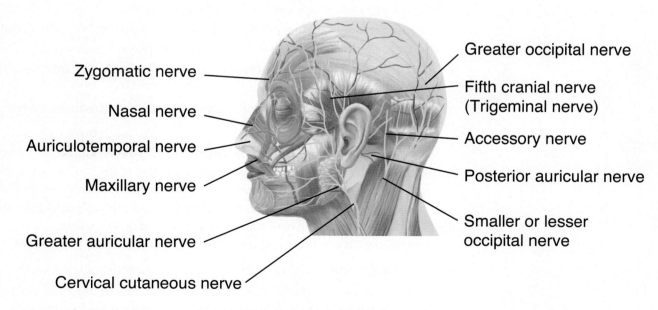

Zygomatic nerve

Nasal nerve

Auriculotemporal nerve

Maxillary nerve

Greater auricular nerve

Cervical cutaneous nerve

Greater occipital nerve

Fifth cranial nerve (Trigeminal nerve)

Accessory nerve

Posterior auricular nerve

Smaller or lesser occipital nerve

▲ **FIGURE 2–21** Nerves V, VII, and XI and their branches

The largest of the cranial nerves is the **fifth cranial nerve** (FIFTH KRAY-nee-ul NURV), also known as the **trifacial** (try-FAY-shul) or **trigeminal** (try-JEM-un-ul) nerve. It is the chief sensory nerve of the face, and it serves as the motor nerve of the muscles that control chewing. It consists of three branches:

- The **ophthalmic nerve** (ahf-THAL-mik NURV) affects the skin of the forehead, upper eyelids, and interior portion of the scalp, orbit, eyeball, and nasal passage.
- The **mandibular nerve** (man-DIB-yuh-lur NURV) affects the muscles of the chin and lower lip.
- The **maxillary nerve** (MAK-suh-lair-ee NURV) affects the upper part of the face.

The following branches of the fifth cranial nerve are affected by facial or lymphatic massage.

- The **auriculotemporal nerve** (aw-RIK-yuh-loh-TEM-puh-rul NURV) affects the external ear and skin above the temple, up to the top of the skull.
- The **infraorbital nerve** (in-fruh-OR-bih-tul NURV) affects the skin of the lower eyelid, side of the nose, upper lip, and mouth.
- The **infratrochlear nerve** (in-frah-TRAHK-lee-ur NURV) affects the membrane and skin of the nose.
- The **mental nerve** (MEN-tul NURV) affects the skin of the lower lip and chin.
- The **nasal nerve** (NAY-zul NURV) affects the point and lower side of the nose.
- The **supraorbital nerve** (soo-pruh-OR-bih-tul NURV) affects the skin of the forehead, scalp, eyebrow, and upper eyelid.
- The **supratrochlear nerve** (soo-pruh-TRAHK-lee-ur NURV) affects the skin between the eyes and upper side of the nose.
- The **zygomatic nerve** (zy-goh-MAT-ik NURV) affects the muscles of the upper part of the cheek.

The branches of the fifth cranial nerve are affected by facial or lymphatic massage.

The **seventh cranial nerve** (SEV-AHNTH CRAN-ee-ahl NURV) also known as the **facial nerve** (FAY-shul NURV), is the chief motor nerve of the face. It emerges near the lower part of the ear and extends to the muscles of the neck. Its divisions and their branches supply and control all the muscles of facial expression and the secretions of saliva.

The following are the most important branches of the facial nerve.

- The **buccal nerve** (BUK-ul NURV) affects the muscles of the mouth.
- The **cervical nerves** (SUR-vih-kul NURVZ) (branches of the facial nerve) affect the side of the neck and the platysma muscle.
- The mandibular nerve affects the muscles of the chin and lower lip.
- The **posterior auricular nerve** (poh-STEER-ee-ur aw-rik-yuh-LAYR NURV) affects the muscles behind the ear at the base of the skull.

- The **temporal nerve** (TEM-puh-rul NURV) affects the muscles of the temple, side of the forehead, eyebrow, eyelid, and upper part of the cheek.
- The zygomatic nerve (upper and lower) affects the muscles of the upper part of the cheek.

The **eleventh cranial nerve** (ee-LEV-unth CRAY-nee-ul NURV), also known as **accessory nerve** (ak-SESS-uh-ree NURV), is a type of motor nerve that controls the motion of the neck and shoulder muscles. This nerve is important to estheticians because it is affected during facials, primarily with massage.

Cervical nerves originate at the spinal cord, and their branches supply the muscles and scalp at the back of the head and neck as follows:

- The **cervical cutaneous nerve** (SUR-vih-kul kyoo-TAY-nee-us NURV), located at the side of the neck, affects the front and sides of the neck as far down as the breastbone.
- The **greater auricular nerve** (GRAY-tur aw-RIK-yuh-lur NURV), located at the side of the neck, affects the face, ears, neck, and parotid gland.
- The **greater occipital nerve** (GRAY-tur ahk-SIP-ut-ul NURV), located in the back of the head, affects the scalp as far up as the top of the head.
- The **smaller occipital nerve** (SMAWL-ur ahk-SIP-ut-ul NURV), also known as the **lesser occipital nerve** (LES-ur ahk-SIP-ut-ul NURV), located at the base of the skull, affects the scalp and muscles behind the ear.

Nerves of the Arm and Hand

The principal nerves supplying the superficial parts of the arm and hand include (**Figure 2–22**):

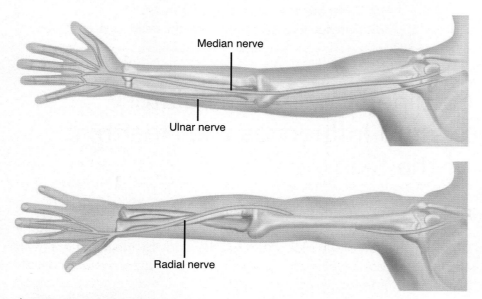

▲ **FIGURE 2–22 Nerves of the Arm**

DID YOU KNOW?

The ulnar nerve runs along the bottom of the elbow. This explains why leaning on one's elbows for long periods can cause the little fingers to go numb. This is due to localized inflammation (irritation and swelling) around the nerve.

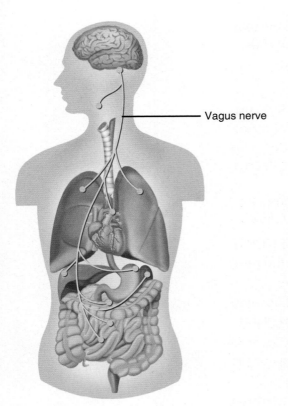

Vagus nerve

▲ **FIGURE 2–23** The vagus nerve

- The **digital nerve** (DIJ-ut-tul NURV) is a sensory-motor nerve that, with its branches, supplies the fingers.
- The **radial nerve** (RAY-dee-ul NURV) is a sensory-motor nerve that, with its branches, supplies the thumb side of the arm and back of the hand.
- The **median nerve** (MEE-dee-un NURV) is a smaller sensory-motor nerve than the ulnar and radial nerves; with its branches, it supplies the arm and hand.
- The **ulnar nerve** (UL-nur NURV) is a sensory-motor nerve that, with its branches, affects the little-finger side of the arm and palm of the hand.

VAGUS NERVE

The **vagus nerve** (VAY-gus NURV) is located in the abdominal cavity, but its function can impact the esthetician in a surprising way, so knowledge of its function is important (**Figure 2–23**). The vagus nerve is a nerve of the autonomic nervous system. When it overreacts to a trigger, it can cause a sudden drop in blood pressure, and the result is fainting. It is the most common cause of fainting. Some triggers are standing up too quickly, the sight of blood, stress, pain, and even pressing on certain areas of the throat, sinus cavities, and eyes.

 CHECK IN

17. Compare and contrast the three divisions of the nervous system.
18. What are the functions of the brain, brain stem, and spinal cord?
19. What are the two types of nerves?
20. Describe the nerves that affect the head, face, and neck.

Outline How the Circulatory System Influences the Health of the Skin

The **circulatory system** (SUR-kyoo-lah-tohr-ee SIS-tum), also known as **cardiovascular system** (kahr-dee-oh-VAS-kyoo-ler SIS-tum), controls the steady circulation of the blood through the body by means of the heart and blood vessels (veins and arteries). The circulatory system consists of the heart, arteries, veins, and capillaries for the distribution of blood throughout the body.

How Is This Important? The circulatory system and the role it plays in nourishing and oxygenating the cells is important to the esthetician's ability to interpret skin reactions to treatments. Impaired circulatory function can create a sallowness in the skin, as the tissue is not being oxygenated. Impaired circulatory function can also delay healing times. Recognizing the fragility of couperose skin (redness; distended capillaries from weakening of the capillary walls) and revising a treatment plan to benefit the client is a skill that comes from a knowledge of the circulatory system. Impaired circulatory conditions are often a contraindication to treatment.

The Heart

The **heart** (HART) is often referred to as the body's pump (**Figure 2–24**); it is a muscular, cone-shaped organ that keeps the blood moving within

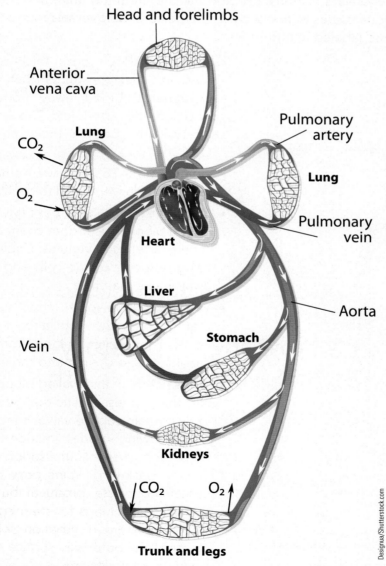

▲ **FIGURE 2–24** The human circulatory system

the circulatory system. The heartbeat is regulated by the vagus (tenth cranial) nerve and other nerves in the autonomic nervous system. In a normal resting state, the heart beats 72 to 80 times per minute.

The blood is in constant and continuous circulation. Two systems ensure this circulation is intact:

1. **Pulmonary circulation** (PUL-muh-nayr-ee sur-kyoo-LAY-shun) carries the blood from the heart to the lungs to be oxygenated.

2. **Systemic circulation** (sis-TEM-ik sir-KYU-lay-shun), also known as general circulation, carries the oxygenated blood from the heart throughout the body and back to the heart again.

Blood Vessels

The **blood vessels** (BLUD VES-ulz) are tubelike structures that include the arteries, arterioles, capillaries, venules, and veins. The function of these vessels is to transport blood to and from the heart and then on to various tissues of the body. The types of blood vessels found in the body are labeled in **Figure 2–25**.

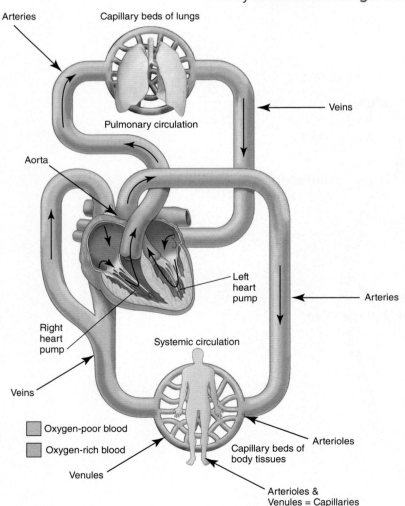

▲ FIGURE 2–25 Types of blood vessels found in the body

- **Arteries** (AR-tuh-reez): thick-walled, muscular, flexible tubes that carry oxygenated blood away from the heart to the arterioles. The largest artery in the body is the **aorta** (ay-ORT-uh).

- **Arterioles** (ar-TEER-ee-ohlz): small arteries that deliver blood to capillaries.

- **Capillaries** (KAP-ih-lair-eez): tiny, thin-walled blood vessels that connect the smaller arteries to venules. Capillaries bring nutrients to the cells and carry away waste materials.

- **Venules** (VEEN-yoolz): small vessels that connect the capillaries to the veins. They collect blood from the capillaries and drain it into the veins.

- **Veins** (VAYNS): thin-walled blood vessels that are less elastic than arteries. They contain cuplike valves that keep blood flowing in one direction to the heart and prevent the blood from flowing backward. Veins carry blood containing waste products back to the heart and lungs for cleaning and to pick up oxygen. Veins are located closer to the outer skin surface of the body than arteries are.

The Blood

Blood (BLUD) is a nutritive fluid circulating through the circulatory system and is considered connective tissue because it connects body systems together, bringing oxygen, nutrients, and hormones and removing waste products.

Quick Facts

✓ There are 8 to 10 pints (3.8 to 4.7 liters) of blood in the human body

✓ Sticky and salty

✓ Normally 98.6 degrees Fahrenheit (36 degrees Celsius)

FUNCTIONS OF THE BLOOD

Blood performs the following critical functions:

- Carries water, oxygen, nutrition, and minerals to all cells and tissues of the body

- Carries away carbon dioxide and waste products to be eliminated through the lungs, skin, and kidneys

- Helps to equalize the body's temperature, thus protecting the body from extreme heat and cold

- Aids in protecting the body from harmful bacteria and infections through the action of the white blood cells

- Closes injured tiny blood vessels by forming clots, thus preventing blood loss.

COMPOSITION OF THE BLOOD

Blood is composed of red blood cells, white blood cells, platelets, and plasma. **Red blood cells** (RED BLUD SELLS) carry oxygen to the body cells. **White blood cells** (WHYT BLUD SELLS) perform the function of destroying disease-causing microorganisms. **Platelets** (PLAYT-lets) contribute to the blood-clotting process, which stops bleeding. **Plasma** (PLAZ-muh) is the fluid part of the blood. It is about 90 percent water and contains proteins, sugars, and minerals. The main function of plasma is to act as a delivery system, carrying vital components, including nutrients, hormones, and minerals, to the cells and to take waste away from the cells.

Arteries of the Head, Face, and Neck

The **common carotid arteries** (KAHM-un kuh-RAHT-ud ART-uh-reez) are the main source of blood supply to the head, face, and neck (**Figure 2–26**). They are located on either side of the neck, and each one is divided into an internal and external branch.

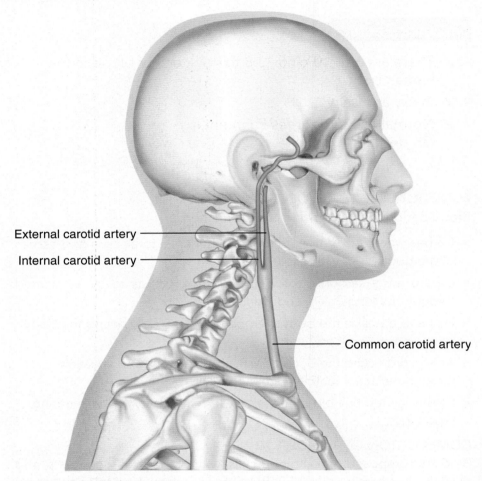

External carotid artery

Internal carotid artery

Common carotid artery

▲ **FIGURE 2–26** The common carotid arteries

Veins of the Head, Face, and Neck

The blood returning to the heart from the head, face, and neck flows on each side of the neck in two principal veins: the **internal jugular vein** (in-TUR-nul JUG-yuh-lur VAYN) and **external jugular vein** (eks-TUR-nul JUG-yuh-lur VAYN) (**Figure 2–27**). These veins run parallel to the carotid arteries.

- The external carotid artery branches off supplying blood to the face. The facial artery is the fourth branch of the external carotid artery. It is very flexible and strong. It can tolerate head movements, swallowing, and facial movements of the cheeks, lips and jaws. The facial artery branches off into smaller arteries that specifically supply the cheeks, chin, ocular area, forehead, lips and even the teeth.

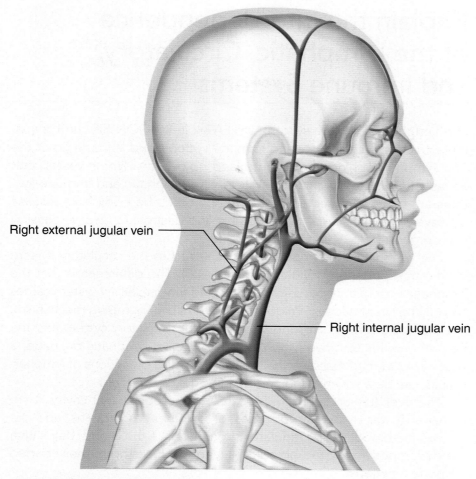

Right external jugular vein

Right internal jugular vein

▲ **FIGURE 2–27 The veins of the head**

- Facial vein branches return the blood to the external jugular, similarly from the same facial locations as the arteries.

- The facial vessels can be intimidating because they are so numerous, but they are very important for the esthetician to know. Understanding vessel locations can help you avoid bruising during a treatment or even the possible adverse event of a vessel occlusion during a dermal filler session.

 CHECK IN

21. What is the body's pump?
22. What two forms of circulation keep blood flowing to all parts of the body, and how do they work?
23. List the types of blood vessels and their functions.
24. List the components in blood and their functions.
25. Describe the location of the arteries and veins that supply blood to the head, face, and neck and their functions.

Explain the Interdependence of the Lymphatic, Circulatory, and Immune Systems

The **lymphatic/immune system** (lim-FAT-ik ih-MYOON SIS-tum) is a vital factor to the circulatory and immune systems and is made up of the liver, lymph, lymph nodes, thymus gland, spleen, and lymph vessels that act as an aid to the circulatory system. The lymphatic and immune systems are closely connected in that they protect the body from disease by developing resistance to pathogens and destroying disease-causing microorganisms.

The lymphatic system is closely connected to the circulatory system for the transportation of fluids (**Figure 2–28**). The difference is that the lymphatic system transports lymph fluid, and the circulatory system carries blood. The lymphatic system does not have its own pumping mechanism, like the heart. It relies on some actions in the circulatory system and the help of muscles to move lymphatic fluid. Manual lymphatic drainage, a specialized form of massage that assists in moving collections of lymphatic fluid, can be a very healing part of an esthetician's work.

The **liver** (LIV-ur) is a gland located in the abdominal cavity. It secretes enzymes necessary for digestion, synthesizes proteins, and detoxifies the blood. It also regulates sugar levels in the blood, helps with the decomposition of red blood cells, and produces hormones needed for body functions.

The spleen is a large **lymph node** (LIMF NOHD) (gland-like structures found inside lymphatic vessels) that fights infection and detoxifies the blood.

Lymph (LIMF) is a liquid composed of changing components in the interstitial fluid as the fluid is circulating throughout the body, dispersing white blood cells and cell nutrients, such as sugars, fats, and salts, as well as absorbing toxins and waste.

Functions

The primary functions of the lymphatic system are to:

- Act as a defense against disease and invading bacteria and toxins by developing resistance
- Drain tissue spaces of excess **interstitial fluid** (INTER-stih-shall FLU-id) in the blood. Interstitial fluid is a solution that bathes and surrounds the cells and provides the cells with nutrients and a method of removing cell waste. The fluid contains components that are involved in blood clotting and wound healing

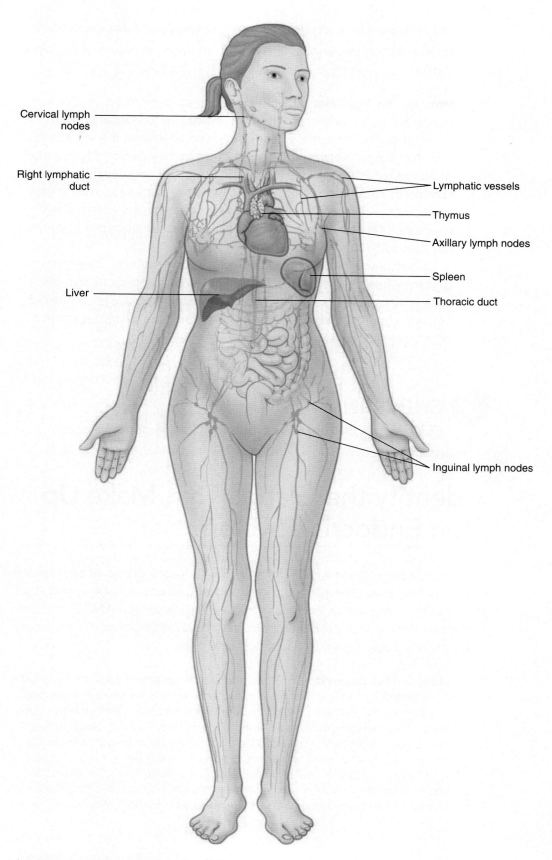

Cervical lymph nodes

Right lymphatic duct

Lymphatic vessels

Thymus

Axillary lymph nodes

Spleen

Liver

Thoracic duct

Inguinal lymph nodes

▲ FIGURE 2–28 The lymphatic system

- Carry the excess fluid, waste, and impurities away from the cells
- Aid in reducing swelling, inflammation, and accumulations in the blood vessels.

How Is This Important? Many treatments performed on the skin create a mild wounding of the skin. Inflammation occurs due to the wounding. The immune system is alerted to relieve the inflammation and repair the wounding. Estheticians may perform lymphatic drainage, which improves lymphatic flow, reduces swelling, and stimulates circulation. Additionally, lymphatic drainage may create a sense of well-being and provide relaxation for the client. Body wraps must be performed with a technique that does not impede the flow of lymph.

Understanding the lymphatic and immune systems is very important when treating the skin. A client with an autoimmune disease may require special consideration when you are recommending skin care regimens; a compromised immune system is often a contraindication for treatments.

 CHECK IN

26. Describe the functions of the lymphatic/immune system.

Identify the Glands That Make Up the Endocrine System

The **endocrine system** (EN-duh-krin SIS-tum) is a group of specialized glands that affect the growth, development, sexual activities, and state of health in the entire body (**Figure 2–29**). **Glands** (GLANDZ) are specialized organs that produce chemicals, including hormones, necessary for various body systems to function optimally.

How Is This Important? The esthetician's treatment plan can be greatly impacted by the functioning of the client's endocrine system. Hormonal imbalances can cause hair growth, affect oil production, and increase acne breakouts, melanin production, and skin sensitivity. Uncontrolled diabetes, which is a disease influenced by the production of insulin, affects the nerves, vision, and immune system to name a few. A person with diabetes may have neuropathy and sensation loss in the extremities, for example. If you were to do a paraffin wax treatment and the wax was too hot, the client with diabetes may be unable to sense the burn and alert you.

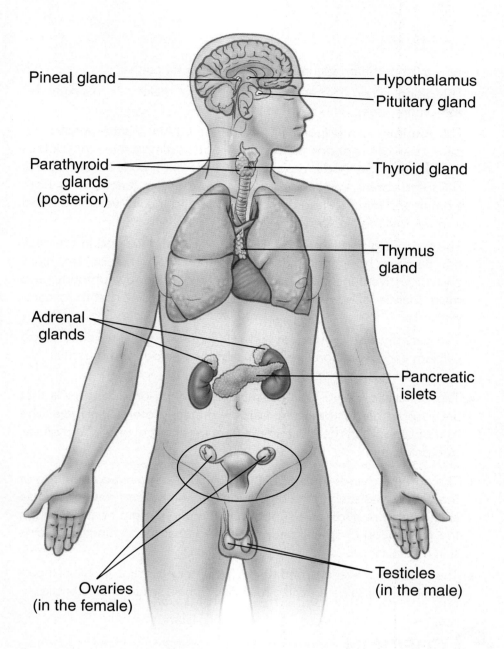

Pineal gland

Hypothalamus

Pituitary gland

Parathyroid glands (posterior)

Thyroid gland

Thymus gland

Adrenal glands

Pancreatic islets

Ovaries (in the female)

Testicles (in the male)

▲ **FIGURE 2–29** The endocrine system

Endocrine glands (EN-duh-krin GLANDZ), also known as **ductless glands** (DUKT-lis GLANDZ), release secretions called *hormones* directly into the bloodstream, which in turn influences the welfare of the entire body. **Hormones** (HOR-mohnz) such as insulin, adrenaline, and estrogen stimulate functional activity or secretion in other parts of the body.

ACTIVITY

Research & Report

Research and write about an endocrine gland disorder. Report to the rest of the class.

Functions

Here is a list of the endocrine glands and their functions:

- The **pineal gland** (PY-nee-ul GLAND) plays a major role in sexual development, sleep, and metabolism.
- The **pituitary gland** (puh-TOO-uh-tair-ee GLAND) is the most complex organ of the endocrine system. It affects almost every physiologic process of the body: growth, blood pressure, contractions during childbirth, breast-milk production, sexual organ functions in both women and men, thyroid gland function, and the conversion of food into energy (metabolism).
- The **thyroid gland** (THY-royd GLAND) is a gland located in the neck that secretes hormones that regulate the body's metabolism, heart and digestive functions, muscle control, brain development, and maintenance of bone mass. It needs iodine from the diet to function properly.
- The **parathyroid glands** (payr-uh THY-royd GLANDZ) regulate blood calcium and phosphorus levels so that the nervous and muscular systems can function properly.
- The **pancreas** (PANG-kree-us) secretes enzyme-producing cells that are responsible for digesting carbohydrates, proteins, and fats. The islet of Langerhans cells within the pancreas control insulin and glucagon production.
- The **adrenal glands** (uh-DREEN-ul GLANDZ) are located at the top of the kidneys assisting in the regulation of metabolism, stress response and blood pressure, and support of immune system health through the generation of specific hormones. Adrenal gland function affects skin melanization.
- The **ovaries** (OH-var-eez) and **testes** (TESS-teez) function in sexual reproduction as well as determining male and female sexual characteristics.

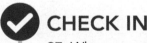 **CHECK IN**

27. What are seven endocrine glands and their functions?

List How Hormonal Changes in the Reproductive System Can Affect the Skin

The **reproductive system** (ree-proh-DUK-tiv SIS-tum) includes the ovaries, fallopian tubes, uterus, and vagina in the female and the testes, prostate gland, penis, and the urethra in the male (**Figure 2–30**).

MALE

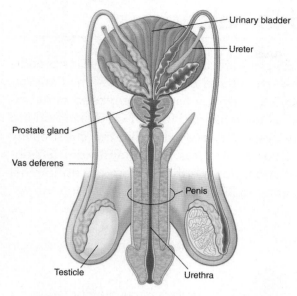

- Urinary bladder
- Ureter
- Prostate gland
- Vas deferens
- Penis
- Testicle
- Urethra

FEMALE

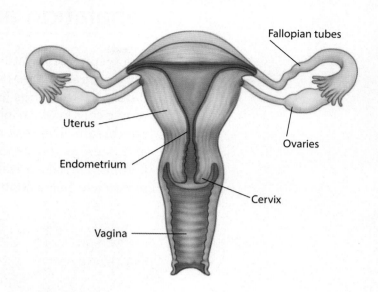

- Fallopian tubes
- Uterus
- Ovaries
- Endometrium
- Cervix
- Vagina

▲ **FIGURE 2–30 The reproductive system**

It performs the function of producing children and passing on our genetics from one generation to another.

How Is This Important? The hormonal changes that occur with the reproductive system affect the skin in many ways. Understanding that you cannot cure acne because of the hormonal changes of puberty or perimenopause will help you create skin care options that will help your clients treat the symptoms. Loss of collagen and elastin related to hormonal changes with aging, assisting your client with hair removal options due to fluctuations in hormones, or spending time treating your client's melasma will be rewarding because you have a solid understanding of the cycles of the reproductive system.

The reproductive system produces the hormones estrogen, progesterone, and testosterone. Estrogen is dominant in females, and testosterone is dominant in males. Hormone balance, or lack thereof, affect the skin in several ways. Acne, loss of collagen and elastin, loss of scalp hair, facial hair growth and color, and changes in skin pigmentation such as **melasma** (mel-AZ-muh) (pregnancy mask) are some of the results of changing, or fluctuating, hormones.

 CHECK IN

28. What is the function of the reproductive system?
29. What are the reproductive hormones?

Describe What Occurs During Inhalation and Exhalation

The **respiratory system** (RES-puh-rah-tor-ee SIS-tum) enables breathing (**respiration** [res-puh-RAY-shun]) and consists of the lungs and air passages. The **lungs** (LUNGZ) are spongy tissues composed of microscopic cells in which inhaled air is exchanged for carbon dioxide during one breath. The respiratory system is located within the chest cavity and is protected on both sides by the ribs. The **diaphragm** (DY-uh-fram) is a muscular wall that separates the thorax from the abdominal region and helps control breathing (**Figure 2–31**).

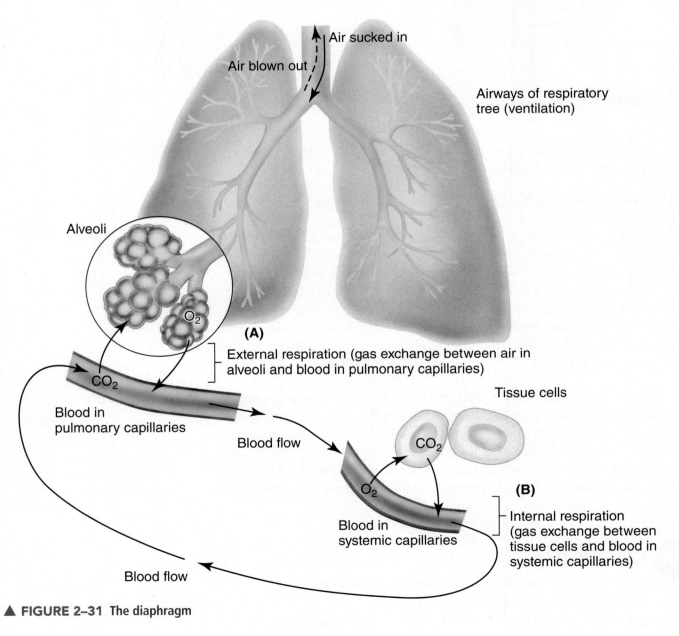

Air sucked in

Air blown out

Airways of respiratory tree (ventilation)

Alveoli

O_2

(A)

CO_2

External respiration (gas exchange between air in alveoli and blood in pulmonary capillaries)

Blood in pulmonary capillaries

Blood flow

Tissue cells

CO_2

O_2

(B)

Blood in systemic capillaries

Internal respiration (gas exchange between tissue cells and blood in systemic capillaries)

Blood flow

▲ FIGURE 2–31 The diaphragm

With each breathing cycle, an exchange of gases takes place. During **inhalation** (in-huh-LAY-shun), or breathing in, oxygen is absorbed into the blood. During **exhalation** (eks-huh-LAY-shun), or breathing out, carbon dioxide is expelled from the lungs.

How Is This Important? Healthy skin needs oxygen. A strong respiratory system will help keep the skin oxygenated for maximum benefits. Skin that is poorly oxygenated will be sallow and gray. It will take longer to respond to treatments or may not respond at all.

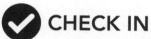 CHECK IN

30. What happens with each breath?
31. Based on the response to the previous question, why is respiration important to the esthetician?

Explain the Five Steps in Digestion

The **digestive system** (dy-JES-tiv SIS-tum), also called the **gastrointestinal system** (gas-troh-in-TES-tun-ul SIS-tum), is responsible for changing food into nutrients and waste (**Figure 2–32**). **Digestive enzymes** (dy-JES-tiv EN-zymz) are chemicals that break down food into a form that can be used by the body. The food, now in soluble form, is transported by the bloodstream and used by the body's cells and tissues.

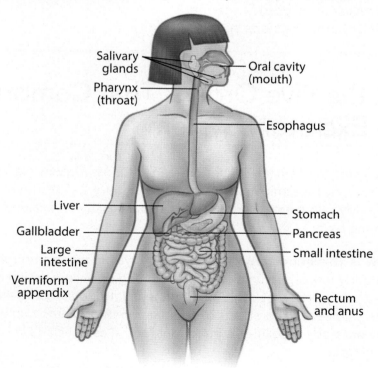

▲ **FIGURE 2–32 The digestive system**

How Is This Important? A thorough knowledge of the processes of the digestive system helps the esthetician perform better because what we eat affects the condition of the skin. An unbalanced diet leaves cells without the nutrients they need to function well. For example, the thyroid gland requires a dietary intake of iodine to function properly. Our bodies do not make iodine and rely on a diet with iodine-rich foods.

Functions

The digestive system prepares nutrients for use by the cells through five basic activities:

- Eating, or **ingestion** (in-JES-chun)—taking food into the body
- Moving food along the digestive tract—known as **peristalsis** (payr-ih-STAWL-sis)
- Breakdown of food by mechanical and chemical means, with the use of **enzymes** (EN-zymz)—known as **digestion** (dy-JES-chun)
- **Absorption** (ub-SORP-shun) of the digested food into the circulatory systems for transportation to the tissues and cells
- Elimination of solid waste from the body—known as **defecation** (def-ih-cay-shun)

 CHECK IN

32. What are digestive enzymes?
33. Describe the steps in digestion.

List the Five Organs That Comprise the Excretory System

The **excretory system** (EKS-kruh-toh-ree SIS-tum) is responsible for purifying the body by eliminating waste matter (**Figure 2–33**). The metabolism of body cells creates various toxic substances that, if retained, could poison the body.

How Is This Important? The excretory system works throughout the body to keep it functioning, preventing an accumulation of toxic substances that could be detrimental. Understanding the process, particularly the effects of perspiration through the skin and how our body detoxifies is important for the esthetician's knowledge base.

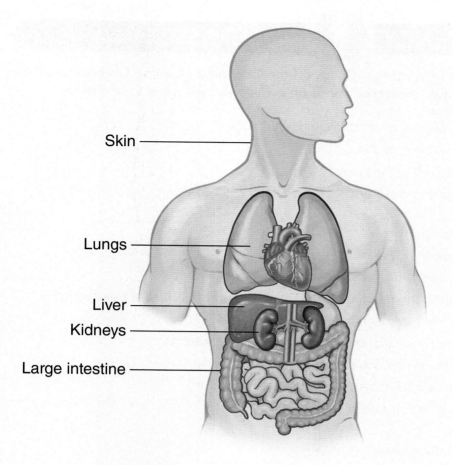

Skin

Lungs

Liver

Kidneys

Large intestine

▲ FIGURE 2–33 The excretory system

Functions

The organs work in other body systems, but each of the following organs plays a crucial role in the excretory system.

- The **kidneys** (KID-neez) excrete urine; eliminating water and waste products.
- The liver discharges bile, which breaks down digestive fat.
- The skin eliminates salts and minerals through perspiration.
- The large intestine eliminates decomposed and undigested food.
- The lungs exhale carbon dioxide.

Web Resources

For more information about systems in the body and how they work, visit these websites:
www.innerbody.com
www.getbodysmart.com

 CHECK IN

34. What body organs work to contribute to the excretory system? What do they do?

COMPETENCY ⬤ PROGRESS

How are you doing with Anatomy and Physiology? **Check off the Chapter 2 Learning Objectives below that you feel you have mastered; leave unchecked those objectives you will need to return to:**

☐ Explain why estheticians need knowledge of anatomy and physiology.

☐ Describe the basic structure and function of a cell.

☐ Describe the four types of tissue found in the body.

☐ Define the functions of major organs and systems of the body that intersect with the integumentary system and esthetics.

☐ List the five accessory organs to the skin.

☐ Identify the five functions of the skeletal system.

☐ Recognize the muscles involved in esthetic massage.

☐ Describe the three nerve branches of the head, neck essential for performing facial treatments.

☐ Outline how the circulatory system influences the health of the skin.

☐ Explain the interdependence of the lymphatic, circulatory, and immune systems.

☐ Identify the glands that make up the endocrine system.

☐ List how hormonal changes in the reproductive system can affect the skin.

☐ Describe what occurs during inhalation and exhalation.

☐ Explain the five steps in digestion.

☐ List the five organs that comprise the excretory system.

GLOSSARY

abduction ab-DUK-shun	pg. 46	muscles that draw a body part, such as a finger, arm, or toe, away from the midline of the body or of an extremity. In the hand, abduction separates the fingers
absorption ub-SORP-shun	pg. 68	the transport of fully digested food into the circulatory system to feed the tissues and cells
accessory nerve ak-SESS-uh-ree NURV	pg. 53	also known as *eleventh cranial nerve*; a type of motor nerve that controls the motion of the neck and shoulder muscles
adduction ah-DUK-shun	pg. 46	muscles that draw a body part, such as a finger, arm, or toe, inward toward the median axis of the body or of an extremity. In the hand, adduction draw the fingers together
adenosine triphosphate (ATP) uh-DEN-uh-seen try-FAHS-fayt	pg. 29	transports chemical energy within cells for metabolism
adipose tissue AD-uh-pohs TISH-oo	pg. 31	a specialized connective tissue considered fat, which gives smoothness and contour to the body and cushions and insulates the body
adrenal glands uh-DREEN-ul GLANDZ	pg. 64	glands that are located at the top of the kidneys assisting in the regulation of metabolism, stress response and blood pressure, and support of immune system health through the generation of specific hormones

anatomy ah-NAT-ah-mee	pg. 28	the study of human body structure, how the body parts are organized, and the science of the structure of organisms or of their parts
aorta ay-ORT-uh	pg. 56	the body's largest artery, the arterial trunk that carries blood from the heart to be distributed by branch arteries through the body
arteries AR-tuh-reez	pg. 56	thick-walled muscular, flexible tubes that carry oxygenated blood from the heart to the capillaries throughout the body
arterioles ar-TEER-ee-ohlz	pg. 56	small arteries that deliver blood to capillaries
auricularis muscles aw-rik-yuh-LAIR-is MUS-uhlz	pg. 44	the three muscles of the ear that work together to move the ear upward, forward, or backward
auriculotemporal nerve aw-RIK-yuh-loh-TEM-puh-rul NURV	pg. 52	affects the external ear and skin above the temple, up to the top of the skull
autonomic nervous system aw-toh-NAHM-ik NUR-vus SIS-tum	pg. 49	abbreviated ANS; the part of the nervous system that controls the involuntary muscles; regulates the action of the smooth muscles, glands, blood vessels, and heart.
belly BELL-ee	pg. 41	the middle part of the muscle
biceps BY-seps	pg. 45	muscle producing the contour of the front and inner side of the upper arm
blood BLUD	pg. 57	nutritive fluid circulating through the cardiovascular system (heart, veins, arteries, and capillaries) to supply oxygen and nutrients to cells and tissues and to remove carbon dioxide and waste from them
blood vessels BLUD VES-ulz	pg. 56	tubelike structures that transport blood to and from the heart, and to various tissues of the body; include arteries, arterioles, capillaries, venules, and veins
body systems BAHD-ee SYS-tumz	pg. 32	groups of body organs acting together to perform one or more functions. The human body is composed of 11 major systems
brain BRAYN	pg. 49	part of the central nervous system contained in the cranium; largest and most complex nerve tissue; controls sensation, muscles, glandular activity
brain stem BRAYN stem	pg. 49	structure that connects the spinal cord to the brain
buccal nerve BUK-ul NURV	pg. 52	affects the muscles of the mouth
buccinator BUK-sih-nay-tur	pg. 43	the thin, flat muscle of the cheek between the upper and lower jaw that compresses the cheeks and expels air between the lips, as in when blowing a whistle
capillaries KAP-ih-lair-eez	pg. 56	tiny, thin-walled blood vessels that connect the smaller arteries to the veins. Capillaries bring nutrients to the cells and carry away waste materials
cardiovascular system kahr-dee-oh-VAS-kyoo-ler SIS-tum	pg. 54	body system consisting of the heart, arteries, veins, and capillaries for the distribution of blood throughout the body
carpus KAR-pus	pg. 40	also known as *wrist*; a flexible joint composed of eight small, irregular bones (carpals) held together by ligaments

cell membrane SELL mem-brain	pg. 29	part of the cell that encloses the protoplasm and permits soluble substances to enter and leave the cell
cells SELLZ	pg. 28	basic unit of all living things; capable of performing all the fundamental functions of life
central nervous system SEN-trul NUR-vus SIS-tum	pg. 48	abbreviated CNS; cerebrospinal nervous system; consists of the brain, spinal cord, spinal nerves, and cranial nerves
cervical nerves SUR-vih-kul NURVZ	pg. 52	a branch of the facial nerve that affects the side of the neck and the platysma muscle
cervical cutaneous nerve SUR-vih-kul kyoo-TAY-nee-us NURV	pg. 53	located at the side of the neck, affects the front and sides of the neck as far down as the breastbone
cervical vertebrae SUR-vih-kul VURT-uh-bray	pg. 38	the seven bones of the top part of the vertebral column located in the neck region
circulatory system SUR-kyoo-lah-tohr-ee SIS-tum	pg. 54	also known as *cardiovascular system*; system that controls the steady circulation of the blood through the body by means of the heart and blood vessels
clavicle KLAV-ih-kul	pg. 39	also known as *collarbone*; bone joining the sternum and scapula
common carotid arteries KAHM-un kuh-RAHT-ud ART-uh-reez	pg. 58	arteries that supply blood to the face, head, and neck, located on either side of the neck, having an internal and external branch
connective tissue Kun-neck-tiv TISH-oo	pg. 31	fibrous tissue that binds together, protects, and supports the various parts of the body such as bone, cartilage, and tendons. Examples of connective tissue are bone, cartilage, ligaments, tendons, blood, lymph, and fat
corrugator muscle KOR-uh-gayt-or MUS-uhl	pg. 43	facial muscle that draws eyebrows down and wrinkles the forehead vertically
cranium KRAY-nee-um	pg. 36	oval, bony case that protects the brain
defecation def-ih-cay-shun	pg. 68	elimination of feces from the body
deltoid DEL-toyd	pg. 45	large, triangular muscle covering the shoulder joint that allows the arm to extend outward and to the side of the body
deoxyribonucleic acid DEE-ox-ee-RYE-boh-NEW-clayic ASUD	pg. 29	abbreviated DNA; the blueprint material of genetic information; contains all the information that controls the function of every living cell
depressor anguli oris dee-PRES-ur ANG-yoo-lye OH-ris	pg. 43	also known as *triangularis muscle*; muscle extending alongside the chin that pulls down the corner of the mouth
diaphragm DY-uh-fram	pg. 66	muscular wall that separates the thorax from the abdominal region and helps control breathing
digestion dy-JES-chun	pg. 68	breakdown of food by mechanical and chemical means
digestive enzymes dy-JES-tiv EN-zymz	pg. 67	chemicals that change certain kinds of food into a form that can be used by the body

digestive system dy-JES-tiv SIS-tum	pg. 67	also called the *gastrointestinal system*; responsible for changing food into nutrients and wastes; consists of the mouth, stomach, intestines, salivary and gastric glands, and other organs
digital nerve DIJ-ut-tul NURV	pg. 54	sensory-motor nerve that, with its branches, supplies impulses to the fingers
digits DIJ-utz	pg. 40	also known as *phalanges*; the bones in the fingers, three in each finger and two in each thumb, totaling 14 bones
ductless glands DUKT-lis GLANDZ	pg. 63	also known as *endocrine glands*; glands that release secretions called hormones directly into the bloodstream
eleventh cranial nerve ee-LEV-unth CRAY-nee-ul NURV	pg. 53	also known as *accessory nerve*; a motor nerve that controls the motion of the neck and shoulder muscles
endocrine glands EN-duh-krin GLANDZ	pg. 63	also known as *ductless glands*; release secretions called hormones directly into the bloodstream which in turn influence the welfare of the entire body
endocrine system EN-duh-krin SIS-tum	pg. 62	group of specialized glands that affect the growth development, sexual activities, and health of the entire body
enzymes EN-zymz	pg. 68	a group of complex proteins produced by living cells that act as catalysts in specific chemical reactions in the body, such as digestion
epicranius ep-ih-KRA-nee-us	pg. 42	also known as *the occipitofrontalis*; a broad muscle that covers the top of the skull and includes the occipitalis and frontalis
epithelial tissue ep-ih-THEE-lee-ul TISH-oo	pg. 31	protective covering on body surfaces, such as the skin, mucous membranes, and lining of the heart; digestive and respiratory organs; and glands
ethmoid bone ETH-moyd BOHN	pg. 36	light, spongy bone between the eye sockets that forms part of the nasal cavities
excretory system EKS-kruh-toh-ree SIS-tum	pg. 68	group of organs—including the kidneys, liver, skin, large intestine, and lungs—that purify the body by elimination of waste matter
exhalation eks-huh-LAY-shun	pg. 67	breathing outward; expelling carbon dioxide from the lungs
exocrine glands EK-suh-krin GLANDZ	pg. 34	also known as *duct glands*; produce a substance that travels through small, tubelike ducts. sweat and oil glands of the skin belong to this group
extension ik-STEN-shun	pg. 47	when muscles straighten. when the wrist, hand, and fingers form a straight line, for example
external jugular vein eks-TUR-nul JUG-yuh-lur VAYN	pg. 58	vein located on the side of the neck that carries blood returning to the heart from the head, face, and neck
facial nerve FAY-shul NURV	pg. 52	it is the chief motor nerve of the face. It emerges near the lower part of the ear and extends to the muscles of the neck
fifth cranial nerve FIFTH KRAY-nee-ul NURV	pg. 52	also known as *trifacial* or *trigeminal nerve*; it is the chief sensory nerve of the face, and it serves as the motor nerve of the muscles that control chewing. It has three branches

flexion FLEK-shun	pg. 46	when muscles move to pull the body part toward the core of the body, such as when the biceps of the arm are activated toward the body
frontal bone FRUNT-ul BOHN	pg. 36	bone forming the forehead
frontalis frun-TAY-lus	pg. 42	front (anterior) portion of the epicranius; muscle of the scalp that raises the eyebrows, draws the scalp forward, and causes wrinkles across the forehead
gastrointestinal system gas-troh-in-TES-tun-ul SIS-tum	pg. 67	responsible for changing food into nutrients and waste, also called the digestive system
glabella gluh-BEL-uh	pg. 43	the corregator and procerus muscles; considered an area or region such as between eyebrows, and or on the frontal bone. Not specifically a muscle or a bone
glands GLANDZ	pg. 62	an organ that contributes to keeping the body in homeostasis by producing chemicals, including hormones, that are passed directly into the bloodstream because the glands have no duct system to travel through
greater auricular nerve GRAY-tur aw-RIK-yuh-lur NURV	pg. 53	located at the side of the neck, affects the face, ears, neck, and parotid gland
greater occipital nerve GRAY-tur ahk-SIP-ut-ul NURV	pg. 53	located in the back of the head, affects the scalp as far up as the top of the head
heart HART	pg. 55	muscular cone-shaped organ that keeps the blood moving within the circulatory system
histology his-TAHL-uh-jee	pg. 28	also known as *microscopic anatomy*; the study of the structure and composition of tissue
hormones HOR-mohnz	pg. 63	secretions produced by one of the endocrine glands and carried by the bloodstream or body fluid to another part of the body, or a body organ, to stimulate functional activity or secretion, such as insulin, adrenaline, and estrogen
humerus HYOO-muh-rus	pg. 40	uppermost and largest bone in the arm, extending from the elbow to the shoulder
hyoid bone HY-oyd BOHN	pg. 38	U-shaped bone at the base of the tongue that supports the tongue and its muscle
infraorbital nerve in-fruh-OR-bih-tul NURV	pg. 52	affects the skin of the lower eyelid, side of the nose, upper lip, and mouth
infratrochlear nerve in-frah-TRAHK-lee-ur NURV	pg. 52	affects the membrane and skin of the nose
ingestion in-JES-chun	pg. 68	eating or taking food into the body
inhalation in-huh-LAY-shun	pg. 67	breathing in through the nose or mouth; oxygen is absorbed by the blood
insertion in-SUR-shun	pg. 41	point where the skeletal muscle is attached to a bone or other more movable body part
integumentary system in-TEG-yuh-MEN-tuh-ree SIS-tum	pg. 34	the skin and its accessory organs, such as the oil and sweat glands, sensory receptors, hair, and nails

internal jugular vein in-TUR-nul JUG-yuh-lur VAYN	pg. 58	vein located at the side of the neck to collect blood from the brain and parts of the face and neck
interstitial fluid INTER-stih-shall FLU-id	pg. 60	a solution that bathes and surrounds the cells and provides the cells with nutrients and a method of removing cell waste; the fluid contains components that are involved in blood clotting and wound healing
joint JOYNT	pg. 35	connection between two or more bones of the skeleton
kidneys KID-neez	pg. 69	one of the organs which supports the excretory system by eliminating water and waste products
lacrimal bones LAK-ruh-mul BONZ	pg. 37	smallest, most fragile, thin bones located in the front inside wall of the orbits (eye sockets)
latissimus dorsi lah-TIS-ih-mus DOR-see	pg. 44	large, flat, triangular muscle covering the lower back
lesser occipital nerve LES-ur ahk-SIP-ut-ul NURV	pg. 53	also known as *smaller occipital nerve*; located at the base of the skull, affects the scalp and muscles behind the ear
levator anguli oris lih-VAYT-ur ANG-yoo-ly OH-ris	pg. 43	a muscle associated with smiling
levator palpebrae superioris muscle lih-VAYT-ur PAL-puh-bree soo-peer-ee-OR-is MUS-uhl	pg. 43	thin muscle that controls the eyelid and can be easily damaged during makeup application
levator labii superioris lih-VAYT-ur LAY-bee-eye soopeer-ee-OR-is	pg. 43	a muscle associated with lifting the wings of the nose and upper lip. It is sometimes called the quadratus labii superioris
liver LIV-ur	pg. 60	a gland in the abdominal cavity that secretes enzymes necessary for digestion, synthesizes proteins, and detoxifies the blood. It regulates sugar levels in the blood and helps with decomposition of red blood cells and produces hormones necessary for body functions
lungs LUNGZ	pg. 66	main organs of the respiratory system. Two of them, located on either side of the heart, take oxygen from the environment and transfer it to the bloodstream. They also exchange oxygen for carbon dioxide during a breath.
lymph LIMF	pg. 60	a liquid composed of changing components in the interstitial fluid as the fluid is circulating throughout the body, dispersing white blood cells and cell nutrients, such as sugars, fats, and salts, as well as absorbing toxins and waste
lymph node LIMF NOHD	pg. 60	gland-like structure found inside lymphatic vessels; filters the lymphatic vessels and helps fight infection
lymphatic/immune system lim-FAT-ik ih-MYOON SIS-tum	pg. 60	vital to the circulatory and immune systems; made up of lymph, lymph nodes, thymus gland, spleen, and lymph vessels that act as an aid to the blood system; the lymphatic and immune systems are closely connected in that they protect the body from disease by developing resistances and destroying disease-causing microorganisms
mandible MAN-duh-bul	pg. 37	lower jawbone; largest and strongest bone of the face

mandibular nerve man-DIB-yuh-lur NURV	pg. 52	affects the muscles of the chin and lower lip
masseter muh-SEET-ur	pg. 44	one of the muscles that coordinate with the temporalis, medial pterygoid, and lateral pterygoid muscles to open and close the mouth and bring the jaw forward; sometimes referred to as chewing muscles
maxillae bones MAK-suh-lair-ee BONZ	pg. 37	form the upper jaw
maxillary nerve MAK-suh-lair-ee NURV	pg. 52	affects the upper part of the face
median nerve MEE-dee-un NURV	pg. 54	nerve, smaller than the ulnar and radial nerves, that supplies the arm and hand
melasma mel-AZ-muh	pg. 65	also referred to as pregnancy mask; a form of hyperpigmentation that is characterized by bilateral patches of brown pigmentation on the cheeks, jawline, forehead, and upper lip due to hormonal imbalances, such as pregnancy, birth control pills, or hormone replacement therapy
mental nerve MEN-tul NURV	pg. 52	affects the skin of the lower lip and chin
mentalis men-TAY-lis	pg. 43	muscle that elevates the lower lip and raises and wrinkles the skin of the chin
metabolism muh-TAB-uh-liz-um	pg. 30	(1) chemical process taking place in living organisms whereby the cells are nourished and carry out their activities. (2) the process of changing food into forms the body can use as energy
metacarpus met-uh-KAR-pus	pg. 40	also known as *palm*; consists of five long, slender bones called metacarpal bones
mitochondria mahy-tuh-KON-dree-uh	pg. 29	a cell structure that takes in nutrients, breaks them down, and creates energy for the cell, called ATP, adenosine triphosphate
mitosis my-TOH-sus	pg. 29	cells dividing into two new identical cells (daughter cells); the normal process of cell reproduction of human tissues
motor nerves MOH-tur NURVZ	pg. 50	carry impulses from the brain to the muscles or glands. These transmitted impulses produce movement
muscle tissue MUS-uhl TISH-oo	pg. 31	tissue that contracts and moves various parts of the body
muscular system MUS-kyuh-lur SIS-tum	pg. 40	body system that covers, shapes, and supports the skeletal tissue; contracts and moves various parts of the body
nape NAYP	pg. 36	back of the neck
nasal bones NAY-zul BONZ	pg. 37	bones that form the bridge of the nose
nasal nerve NAY-zul NURV	pg. 52	affects the point and lower side of the nose
nasalis muscle nay-ZAY-lis MUS-uhl	pg. 43	two-part muscle that covers the nose
nerve tissue NURV TISH-oo	pg. 31	tissue that controls and coordinates all body functions

nerves NURVZ	pg. 49	whitish cords made up of bundles of nerve fibers held together by connective tissue, through which impulses are transmitted
nervous system NUR-vus SIS-tum	pg. 48	body system composed of the brain, spinal cord, and nerves; controls and coordinates all other systems and makes them work efficiently, in sync with each other
neurology nuh-RAHL-uh-jee	pg. 48	the scientific study of the structure, function, and pathology of the nervous system
neuron NOO-rahn	pg. 29	also known as *nerve cell*; cells that make up the nerves, brain, and spinal cord and transmit nerve impulses
nucleoplasm NEW-clee-oh-plasm	pg. 29	fluid within the nucleus of the cell that contains proteins and DNA; determines our genetic makeup
nucleus NOO-klee-us	pg. 29	the central part, core. In anatomy and histology, the dense, active protoplasm found in the center of a cell that acts as the genetic control center; it plays an important role in cell reproduction and metabolism
occipital bone ahk-SIP-ut-ul BOHN	pg. 36	hindmost bone of the skull, below the parietal bones; forms the back of the skull above the nape
occipitalis ahk-SIP-i-tahl-is	pg. 42	back of the epicranius; muscle that draws the scalp backward
ophthalmic nerve ahf-THAL-mik NURV	pg. 52	affects the skin of the forehead, upper eyelids, and interior portion of the scalp, orbit, eyeball, and nasal passage
orbicularis oculi or-bik-yuh-LAIR-is AHK-yuh-lye	pg. 43	ring muscle of the eye socket; closes the eyelid
orbicularis oris or-bik-yuh-LAIR-is OH-ris	pg. 43	flat band around the upper and lower lips that compresses, contracts, puckers, and wrinkles the lips
organelles or-guh-NELZ	pg. 29	small structures or miniature organs within a cell that have their own function
organs OR-gunz	pg. 32	structures composed of specialized tissues; perform specific functions in plants and animals
origin OR-ih-jin	pg. 41	part of the muscle that does not move; it is attached to the skeleton and is usually part of a skeletal muscle
ovaries OH-var-eez	pg. 64	function in sexual reproduction as well as determining male and female sexual characteristics
pancreas PANG-kree-us	pg. 64	secretes enzyme-producing cells that are responsible for digesting carbohydrates, proteins, and fats. the islet of Langerhans cells within the pancreas control insulin and glucagon production
parathyroid glands payr-uh THY-royd GLANDZ	pg. 64	regulate blood calcium and phosphorus levels so that the nervous and muscular systems can function properly
parietal bones puh-RY-ate-ul BONZ	pg. 36	bones that form the sides and top of the cranium
pectoralis major and minor pek-tor-AL-is MAY-jor / MY-nur	pg. 44	muscles of the chest that assist the swinging movements of the arm
peripheral nervous system puh-RIF-uh-rul NURV-vus SIS-tum	pg. 48	abbreviated PNS; system of nerves and ganglia that connects the peripheral parts of the body to the central nervous system; has both sensory and motor nerves

peristalsis payr-ih-STAWL-sis	pg. 68	moves food along the digestive tract
phalanges (singular: phalanx, FAY-langks**)** FA-lanj-eez	pg. 40	also known as *digits*; the bones in the fingers, three in each finger and two in each thumb, totaling 14 bones
physiology fiz-ee-AHL-uh-jee	pg. 28	study of the functions or activities performed by the body's structures.
pineal gland PY-nee-ul GLAND	pg. 64	a gland located in the brain; plays a major role in sexual development, sleep, and metabolism
pituitary gland puh-TOO-uh-tair-ee GLAND	pg. 64	a gland found in the center of the head; the most complex organ of the endocrine system; affects almost every physiologic process of the body: growth, blood pressure, contractions during childbirth, breast-milk production, sexual organ functions in both women and men, thyroid gland function, and the conversion of food into energy (metabolism)
plasma PLAZ-muh	pg. 57	fluid part of the blood and lymph that carries food and secretions to the cells and carbon dioxide from the cells
platelets PLAYT-lets	pg. 57	also known as *thrombocytes*; much smaller than red blood cells; contribute to the blood-clotting process, which stops bleeding
platysma plah-TIZ-muh	pg. 44	broad muscle extending from the chest and shoulder muscles to the side of the chin; responsible for depressing the lower jaw and lip
posterior auricular nerve poh-STEER-ee-ur aw-rik-yuh-LAYR NURV	pg. 52	affects the muscles behind the ear at the base of the skull
procerus proh-SEE-rus	pg. 43	muscle that covers the bridge of the nose, depresses the eyebrows, and causes wrinkles across the bridge of the nose
pronate proh-NAYT	pg. 47	when muscles turn inward. for example, when the palm faces downward
protoplasm PROH-toh-plaz-um	pg. 29	colorless, jellylike substance in cells; contains nutrients such as protein, fats, carbohydrates, mineral salts, and water
pulmonary circulation PUL-muh-nayr-ee sur-kyoo-LAY-shun	pg. 56	sends the blood from the heart to the lungs to be purified, then back to the heart again
quadratus labii superioris kwah-DRA-tus LAY-bee-eye soo-eeree- OR-is	pg. 43	a muscle associated with lifting the wings of the nose and upper lip. It is sometimes called the levator labii superioris
radial nerve RAY-dee-ul NURV	pg. 54	a sensory-motor nerve that, with its branches, supplies the thumb side of the arm and back of the hand
radius RAY-dee-us	pg. 40	smaller bone in the forearm on the same side as the thumb
receptors ree-SEP-turz	pg. 49	sensory nerve endings located close to the surface of the skin
red blood cells RED BLUD SELLS	pg. 57	blood cells that carry oxygen from the lungs to the body cells and transport carbon dioxide from the cells back to the lungs

reflex REE-fleks	pg. 50	automatic reaction to a stimulus that involves the movement of an impulse from a sensory receptor along the sensory nerve to the spinal cord. A responsive impulse is sent along a motor neuron to a muscle, causing a reaction (e.g., the quick removal of the hand from a hot object). Reflexes do not have to be learned; they are automatic
reproductive system ree-proh-DUK-tiv SIS-tum	pg. 64	body system that includes the ovaries, uterine tubes, uterus, and vagina in the female and the testes, prostate gland, penis, and urethra in the male. This system performs the function of procreation and passing on the genetic code from one generation to another
respiration res-puh-RAY-shun	pg. 66	process of inhaling and exhaling; the act of breathing; the exchange of carbon dioxide and oxygen in the lungs and within each cell
respiratory system RES-puh-rah-tor-ee SIS-tum	pg. 66	body system consisting of the lungs and air passages; enables breathing, which supplies the body with oxygen and eliminates carbon dioxide as a waste product
ribs RIBZ	pg. 38	twelve pairs of bones forming the wall of the thorax
risorius rih-ZOR-ee-us	pg. 43	muscle that draws the corners of the mouth out and back when grinning
scapula SKAP-yuh-luh	pg. 38	also known as *shoulder blade*; one of a pair of large, flat triangular bones of the shoulder
sensory nerves SEN-soh-ree NURVZ	pg. 49	carry impulses or messages from the sense organs to the brain, where sensations such as touch, cold, heat, sight, hearing, taste, smell, pain, and pressure are experienced; sensory nerve endings called receptors are located close to the surface of the skin
seventh cranial nerve SEV-AHNTH CRAN-ee-ahl NURV	pg. 52	also known as *facial nerve*; the chief motor nerve of the face; emerges near the lower part of the ear and extends to the muscles of the neck
skeletal system SKEL-uh-tul SIS-tum	pg. 34	physical foundation of the body, composed of the bones and movable and immovable joints
skin skin	pg. 34	external protective coating that covers the body; the body's largest organ; acts as a barrier to protect body systems from the outside elements; part of the integumentary system
smaller occipital nerve SMAWL-ur ahk-SIP-ut-ul NURV	pg. 53	also known as *lesser occipital nerve*; located at the base of the skull, affects the scalp and muscles behind the ear
soluble SAHL-yuh-bul	pg. 29	capable of being dissolved or liquefied
sphenoid bone SFEE-noyd BOHN	pg. 36	forms the sides of the eye socket
spinal cord SPY-nal KORD	pg. 49	portion of the central nervous system that originates in the brain, extends down to the lower extremity of the trunk, and is protected by the spinal column
sternum STUR-num	pg. 39	also known as *breastbone*; the flat bone that forms the ventral support of the ribs
sternocleidomastoid STUR-noh-KLY-doh-MAS-toyd	pg. 44	the muscle extending alongside of the neck from the ear to the collarbone; acts to rotate the head from side to side and up and down

supinate SOO-puh-nayt	pg. 47	when muscles rotate, for example, in the forearm, the radius turns outward and the palm upward
supraorbital nerve soo-pruh-OR-bih-tul NURV	pg. 52	affects the skin of the forehead, scalp, eyebrow, and upper eyelid
supratrochlear nerve soo-pruh-TRAHK-lee-ur NURV	pg. 52	affects the skin between the eyes and upper side of the nose
systemic circulation sis-TEM-ik sir-KYU-lay-shun	pg. 56	also known as *general circulation*; circulation of blood from the heart throughout the body and back again to the heart
temporal bones TEM-puh-rul BONZ	pg. 36	bones forming the sides of the head in the ear region
temporal nerve TEM-puh-rul NURV	pg. 53	affects the muscles of the temple, side of the forehead, eyebrow, eyelid, and upper part of the cheek
temporalis muscle tem-poh-RAY-lis MUS-uhl	pg. 43	temporal muscle; one of the muscles involved in mastication (chewing)
testes TESS-teez	pg. 64	male organs that produce the male hormone testosterone
thorax THOR-aks	pg. 38	also known as *chest*; consists of the sternum, ribs, and thoracic vertebrae; elastic, bony cage that serves as a protective framework for the heart, lungs, and other internal organs
thyroid gland THY-royd GLAND	pg. 64	a gland located in the neck that secretes hormones that regulate the body's metabolism, heart and digestive functions, muscle control, brain development, and maintenance of bone mass; needs iodine from the diet to function properly
tissue TISH-oo	pg. 31	collection of similar cells that perform a particular function
trapezius truh-PEE-zee-us	pg. 45	muscle that covers the back of the neck and upper and middle region of the back; stabilizes the scapula and shrugs the shoulders
triangularis try-ang-gyuh-LAY-rus	pg. 43	also known as the *depressor anguli oris*; is the muscle extending alongside the chin that pulls down the corners of the mouth
triceps TRY-seps	pg. 45	large muscle that covers the entire back of the upper arm and extends the forearm
trifacial (trigeminal) nerve try-FAY-shul (try-JEM-un-ul) NURV	pg. 52	chief sensory nerve of the face; serves as the motor nerve of the muscles that control chewing; consists of three branches: ophthalmic nerve, mandibular nerve, and the maxillary nerve
ulna UL-nuh	pg. 40	inner and larger bone of the forearm, attached to the wrist on the side of the little finger
ulnar nerve UL-nur NURV	pg. 54	a sensory-motor nerve that, with its branches, affects the little-finger side of the arm and palm of the hand
vagus nerve VAY-gus NURV	pg. 54	located in the abdominal cavity, a nerve of the autonomic nervous system
veins VAYNS	pg. 56	thin-walled blood vessels that are less elastic than arteries; they contain cuplike valves to prevent backflow and carry impure blood from the various capillaries back to the heart and lungs

venules VEEN-yoolz	pg. 56	small vessels that connect the capillaries to the veins; they collect blood from the capillaries and drain it into veins
white blood cells WHYT BLUD SELLS	pg. 57	perform the function of destroying disease-causing germs
zygomatic bones zy-goh-MAT-ik BONZ	pg. 37	also known as *malar bones* or *cheekbones*; bones that form the prominence of the cheeks; the cheekbones
zygomatic nerve zy-goh-MAT-ik NURV	pg. 52	affects the muscles of the upper part of the cheek
zygomaticus zy-goh-MAT-ih-kus	pg. 43	consists of major and minor muscles extending from the zygomatic bone to the angle of the mouth that elevates the lip, as in laughing

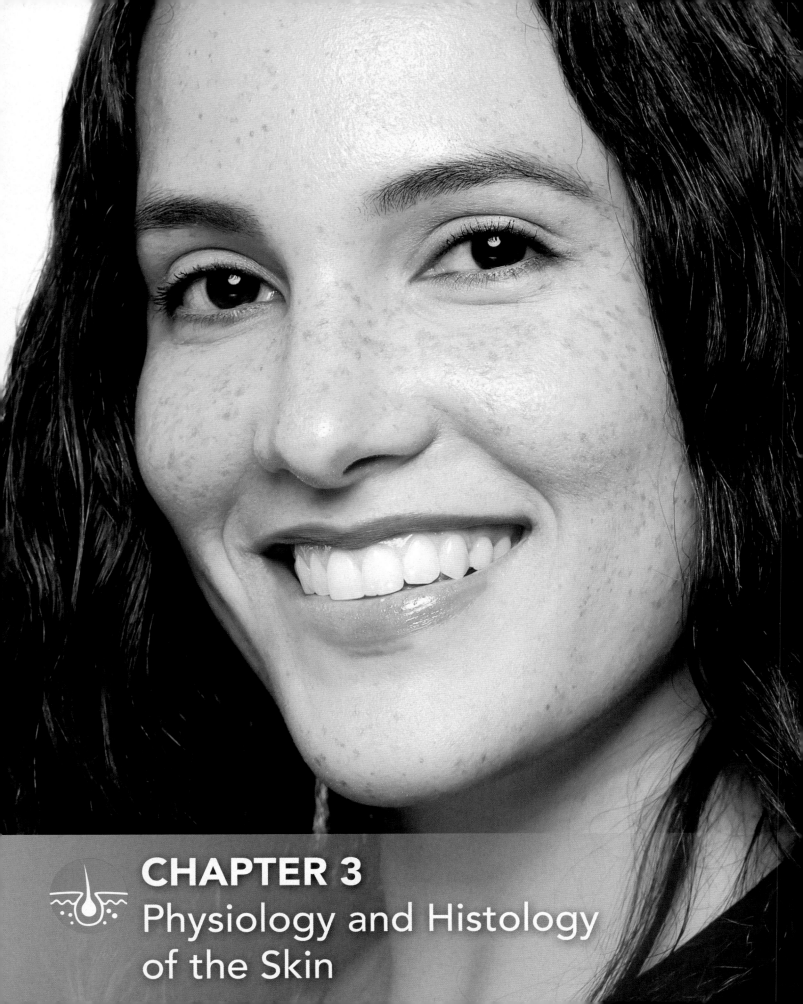

CHAPTER 3
Physiology and Histology
of the Skin

"Though we travel the world over to find the beautiful, we must carry it with us or we find it not."

–Ralph Waldo Emerson

Learning Objectives

After completing this chapter, you will be able to:

1. Describe why learning the physiology and histology of the skin makes you a better esthetician.
2. Describe the attributes of healthy skin.
3. Distinguish the six primary functions of the skin.
4. Explain the function of each layer of the skin, from the deepest to the surface.
5. Identify a hair follicle as an appendage of the skin.
6. Identify nails as an appendage of the skin.
7. Describe the functions of the two types of nerves.
8. Explain what is produced by the two types of glands of the skin.
9. Distinguish the factors influencing skin health.

Describe Why Learning the Physiology and Histology of the Skin Makes You a Better Esthetician

Estheticians have an opportunity to study a most fascinating science. Skin *histology* and *physiology* involves the study of the anatomy, layers, and functions of the skin. Recall that Chapter 2 defined physiology as the study of the functions and activities performed by the body structures, including physical and chemical processes. Histology is also known as *microscopic anatomy*, the study of the structure and composition of tissue. So, skin physiology and histology involves the study of the structure and composition of the skin tissue. These are the foundational sciences estheticians need to have a solid grasp of before caring for the skin.

Estheticians who specialize in the health and beauty of skin are sometimes referred to as *technicians*, *skin therapists*, or *specialists*. There is much more to being an esthetician than simply performing facials and selling products (**Figure 3–1**). As scientific research in the industry changes and advances constantly, new understandings of how

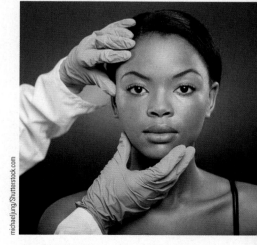

michaeljung/Shutterstock.com

▲ **FIGURE 3–1** Consulting with a client.

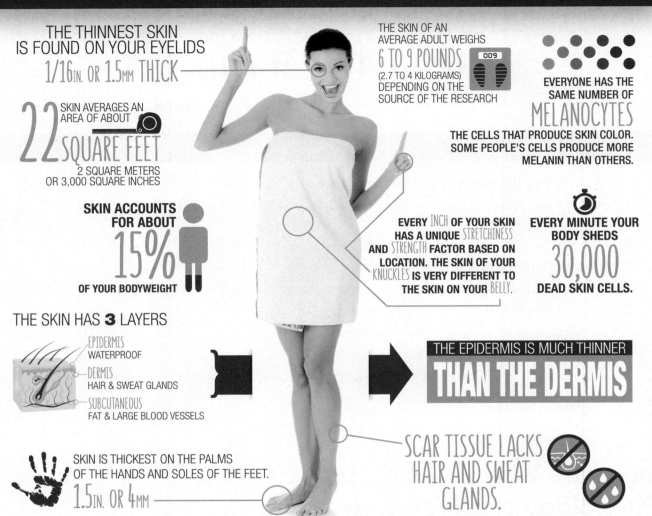

THE THINNEST SKIN IS FOUND ON YOUR EYELIDS
1/16IN. OR 1.5MM THICK

22 SKIN AVERAGES AN AREA OF ABOUT SQUARE FEET
2 SQUARE METERS OR 3,000 SQUARE INCHES

SKIN ACCOUNTS FOR ABOUT 15% OF YOUR BODYWEIGHT

THE SKIN HAS **3** LAYERS
EPIDERMIS WATERPROOF
DERMIS HAIR & SWEAT GLANDS
SUBCUTANEOUS FAT & LARGE BLOOD VESSELS

SKIN IS THICKEST ON THE PALMS OF THE HANDS AND SOLES OF THE FEET.
1.5IN. OR 4MM

THE SKIN OF AN AVERAGE ADULT WEIGHS
6 TO 9 POUNDS
(2.7 TO 4 KILOGRAMS) DEPENDING ON THE SOURCE OF THE RESEARCH

EVERYONE HAS THE SAME NUMBER OF MELANOCYTES
THE CELLS THAT PRODUCE SKIN COLOR. SOME PEOPLE'S CELLS PRODUCE MORE MELANIN THAN OTHERS.

EVERY INCH OF YOUR SKIN HAS A UNIQUE STRETCHINESS AND STRENGTH FACTOR BASED ON LOCATION. THE SKIN OF YOUR KNUCKLES IS VERY DIFFERENT TO THE SKIN ON YOUR BELLY.

EVERY MINUTE YOUR BODY SHEDS
30,000 DEAD SKIN CELLS.

THE EPIDERMIS IS MUCH THINNER **THAN THE DERMIS**

SCAR TISSUE LACKS HAIR AND SWEAT GLANDS.

B-D-S Piotr Marcinski/Shutterstock.com

the skin functions and interacts with new technologies are emerging. How other body systems are integrally linked with the integumentary system are being revealed as researchers look for new ways to treat chronic diseases and disorders, work on anti-aging efforts, and battle cancer. Estheticians must commit to being lifelong learners. Clients value an esthetician's comprehensive understanding of the skin in general. Committing to becoming a skin expert means you develop an understanding of your client's unique skin characteristics and responses. You can make personalized treatment recommendations and prescribe a home care regimen that will help keep the skin healthy and vibrant. By educating clients, estheticians are sharing their knowledge and expertise. An esthetician's primary focus is on preserving, protecting, and nourishing the skin.

Estheticians should study and have a thorough understanding of the physiology and histology of the skin because:

- The complexity of the skin is astonishing. The layers, components, and functions all work with other body systems to protect and regulate the skin and other parts of the body.

- The study of skin physiology and histology includes learning about the aging process as well as interpreting the effects of ultraviolet (UV) damage, hormonal influences, and nutrition on skin health. Each of these factors affect the skin's health and appearance.

- There is much to study about the body's largest organ and how to best maintain its optimum health and with a deeper understanding, the skin therapist can confidently treat this sophisticated system.

Describe the Attributes of Healthy Skin

Skin, or the *integumentary system*, is the largest organ in the body. It is a strong barrier designed to protect us from the outside elements. Skin layers, nerves, cellular functions, hair follicles, and glands all work together harmoniously to regulate and protect the body. Hormones, growth factors, and other biochemicals control the skin's intricate functions (**Figure 3–2**).

The basic material and building blocks for our body's tissues are proteins. Amino acids are the building blocks of proteins. Amino acids form peptides, and peptides form proteins. Proteins have many roles in maintaining skin health.

Our skin is an industrious manufacturer, with miles (kilometers) of blood vessels, millions of sweat glands, and an array of nerves within a network of fibers. Appendages of the skin include hair, nails, sweat glands, and oil glands. Healthy skin is slightly moist, soft, smooth, and somewhat acidic.

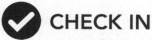 **CHECK IN**

1. List five interesting facts about healthy skin.

ACTIVITY

Skin Factoids

Use a photo collage app on your phone, tablet, or computer to create a collage showing fun facts about the skin. Share the collage with your instructor.

Factoid example: Over 50% of the dust in your house is really dead skin cells.

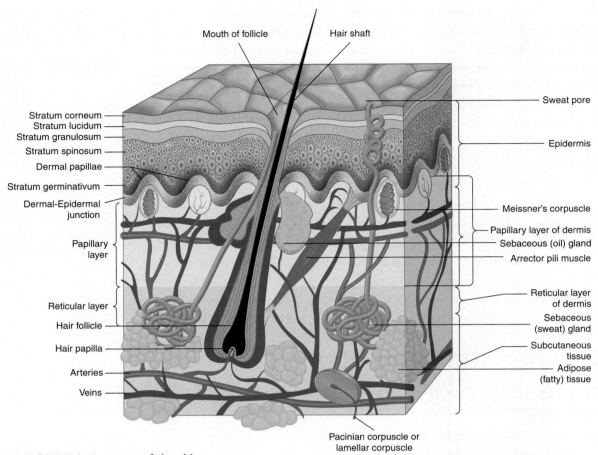

Mouth of follicle

Hair shaft

Stratum corneum
Stratum lucidum
Stratum granulosum
Stratum spinosum
Dermal papillae
Stratum germinativum
Dermal-Epidermal junction
Papillary layer
Reticular layer
Hair follicle
Hair papilla
Arteries
Veins

Sweat pore
Epidermis
Meissner's corpuscle
Papillary layer of dermis
Sebaceous (oil) gland
Arrector pili muscle
Reticular layer of dermis
Sebaceous (sweat) gland
Subcutaneous tissue
Adipose (fatty) tissue

Pacinian corpuscle or lamellar corpuscle

▲ **FIGURE 3–2** Layers of the skin.

Distinguish the Six Primary Functions of the Skin

The skin is similar to a multifunction tool. It acts as a shield for the body. It is waterproof, and an insulator that protects the body against extreme heat, cold, and damaging UV rays. Skin is a barrier that protects against harmful chemicals and bacteria, preventing infection. Skin plays an important role in bone health by producing vitamin D. In addition, our skin is a huge sensory storehouse that keeps our brain in touch with the world around us. Skin does all of this while being flexible enough for the body to engage in motion while maintaining a healthy exterior to allow us to look good and feel comfortable. For these reasons, the six primary functions of the skin are sensation, protection, heat regulation, excretion, secretion, and absorption.

Sensation

Touch is one of the first senses to develop. Nerve fibers in the skin sense when we are touched. Depending on the type of stimulation, sensations felt on our skin cause us to feel, react, or move. Different nerve sensors help us to detect different sensations and perceive changes in our environment, such as heat, cold, touch, pain, and pressure (**Figure 3–3**). Nerve sensors send messages to the brain and motor nerves send messages back to relay to the body how to respond. The sensation of heat will cause us to pull away from a hot stove burner. A massage sends messages to the brain through nerve stimulation and lowers stress in the body as well as promotes circulation. Studies have shown stress reduction in babies and older adults when they experience more touch and interaction with others. Sensory nerve fibers are most abundant in the fingertips and are designed to be one of the most sensitive parts of the body.

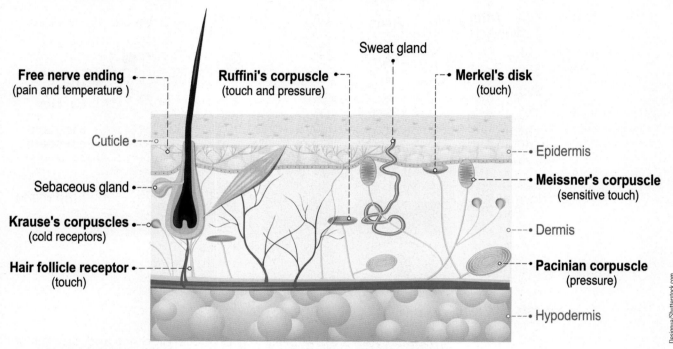

Free nerve ending (pain and temperature)
Cuticle
Sebaceous gland
Krause's corpuscles (cold receptors)
Hair follicle receptor (touch)
Ruffini's corpuscle (touch and pressure)
Sweat gland
Merkel's disk (touch)
Epidermis
Meissner's corpuscle (sensitive touch)
Dermis
Pacinian corpuscle (pressure)
Hypodermis

Designua/Shutterstock.com

▲ **FIGURE 3–3** Pressure, vibration, temperature, pain and itching are transmitted via special receptory organs and nerves.

Protection

The skin is a thin, yet strong, protective barrier to outside elements and microorganisms. It has many defense mechanisms to protect the body from injury and invasion. Sebum (oil) on the epidermis gives protection from external factors such as invasion by certain bacteria. The acid mantle is the protective barrier made up of sebum, lipids, sweat, and water. These components form a **hydrolipidic** (hy-droh-li-PID-ic) film to protect the skin from drying out and from exposure to external factors that could damage it. *Hydro* means "water". *Lipidic* means "oil". A *hydrolipidic film* provides an oil–water balance on the skin's surface.

The acid mantle has an average pH of 5.5. The balanced pH of the skin is important to protect the body from pathogens and to regulate enzymatic functions.

The acid mantle is part of the skin's natural barrier function. The **barrier function** (BEAR-ee-ore FUNK-shun) is the skin's mechanism that protects us from irritation and intercellular **transepidermal water loss** (TEWL; TRANS-ep-uh-der-muhl WAH-tur LOSS), the water loss caused by evaporation on the skin's surface. Lipids are substances that contribute to the barrier function of the epidermis. Lipids are protective oils and are part of the **intercellular matrix** (in-tur-SEL-yuh-lur MAY-tricks) (fluid) between epidermal cells. Damage to the barrier layer is the cause of many skin problems, including sensitivities, aging, and dehydration (**Figure 3–4**).

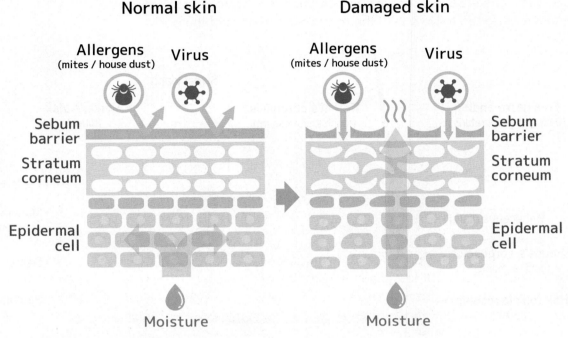

▲ **FIGURE 3–4** Barrier function.

Melanocytes are the cells that produce pigment and protect our bodies from harmful ionizing UV rays. Melanocytes produce pigment granules called melanosomes. Melanosomes produce a protein called melanin. Melanin travels from the deeper basal cell layer of the stratum germinativum to the surface through fingerlike projections called dendrites, acting as an umbrella to shield the skin from the negative effects of the sun and indoor tanning. UV rays can damage the DNA in melanocytes and cause skin cancer. The three types of skin cancer are discussed in Chapter 4, "Disorders and Diseases of the Skin".

The skin's most amazing feature is the ability to heal itself. Skin can repair itself when injured, thus protecting the body from infection and damage from injury. Through a hyperproduction of cells and blood clotting, injured skin can restore itself to its normal thickness. Hormones such as **epidermal growth factor** (EGF; ep-ih-DUR-mul GROWTH FAK-tor) stimulate skin cells to reproduce and heal. Proteins and peptides trigger **fibroblasts** (fy-BROH-blasts) (cell stimulators) and cells to rejuvenate. Skin cells are activated to quickly repair the skin. Other protective components of the skin include cells active in the immune system. These processes are discussed later in this chapter.

DID YOU KNOW?

The microscopic view of the structure of the epidermis resembles a brick wall—the cells are the bricks, and the intercellular matrix is the cement mortar between the bricks that holds everything together.

Heat Regulation

The body's average internal thermostat is set at 98.6 degrees Fahrenheit (37 degrees Celsius). When the outside temperature changes, the skin automatically adjusts to warm or cool the body as necessary.

The body maintains thermoregulation through evaporation, perspiration, radiation, and insulation. Millions of sweat glands release heat from the body through perspiration to keep us from overheating. We then cool ourselves through evaporation on the skin's surface. Blood flow and blood vessel dilation also assist in cooling the body.

We protect ourselves from the cold by constriction of the blood vessels and decreased blood flow. Additionally, the body's fat layers help to insulate and warm the body.

Hair follicles also help regulate body temperature and protect from heat loss. When we are cold, the **arrector pili muscles** (ah-REK-tohr-PY-leh MUS-uhls) attached to the hair follicles contract and cause goosebumps. This reaction is thought to warm the skin by the air pockets that are created under the hairs that stand up when the muscle contracts. Shivering is also an automatic response to cold and a way to warm up the body.

Excretion

The **sudoriferous glands** (sood-uh-RIF-uh-rus GLANZ), also known as *sweat glands*, excrete perspiration. Many people believe that sweat detoxifies the body but less than one percent of the body's detoxification comes through perspiration. Sudoriferous glands serve to prevent the body from overheating. The liver and kidneys do the detox work. Heavy sweating can cause a loss of fluids, dehydration, and the loss of the mineral balance needed to keep the body functioning optimally. Sweat, just like sebum, is also part of the acid mantle. The functions of these glands are discussed later in the chapter.

Secretion

Sebum (SEEB-um) is an oily substance that protects the surface of the skin and lubricates both the skin and hair. **Sebaceous glands** (sih-BAY-shus GLANZ), also known as *oil glands*, are appendages attached to follicles that produce sebum. These oils help keep the skin soft and protected from outside elements. The skin is approximately 50 to 70 percent water. Sebum coating the surface of the skin slows down the evaporation of water, also known as transepidermal water loss (TEWL), and helps maintain appropriate water levels in the cells. Emotional stress and hormone imbalances can stimulate oil glands to increase the flow of sebum, which can lead to skin problems such as acneic breakouts.

Absorption

Absorption of chemicals, hormones, moisture, and oxygen is necessary for our skin's health. Vitamin D is also synthesized and produced in the skin upon exposure to the sun. The skin selectively absorbs topical products, serums and creams, through the cells, hair follicles, and sebaceous glands. While absorption is limited, some ingredients with a smaller molecular size can penetrate the skin. The penetration ability of the ingredient is determined by the size of the molecule and other characteristics of the product. Lipid-soluble products penetrate better.

The routes of penetration are through the follicle walls, sebaceous glands, intercellular, or transcellular (**Figure 3–5**). Small molecules with permeable cell walls can penetrate the cells. Larger cells with nonpermeable cell walls can be temporarily absorbed by the glands in the skin and can travel through the intercellular spaces.

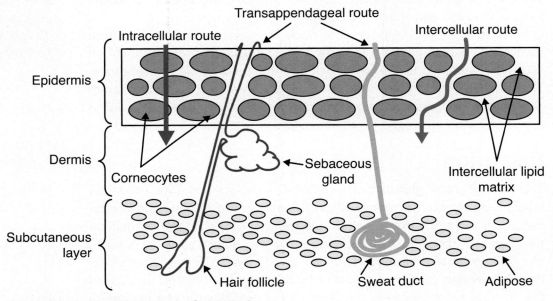

▲ **FIGURE 3–5 Primary routes of penetration.**

Absorption of select topical products helps keep skin moisturized, nourished, and protected. Scientific advances continually result in the creation of new products that are more readily absorbed by the skin, thus making them more effective. New nanotechnology transforms skin care products, micronizing the particles, so they are able to penetrate further into the skin. Many skin care ingredients, including prescription creams, can penetrate the skin's deeper layers. This effect can be either harmful or beneficial, depending on the elements in the topical application.

DID YOU KNOW?

Intercellular means "between" the cells and *transcellular* is "across" or through the cells.

✓ CHECK IN

2. What are the six main functions of the skin?
3. What is the barrier function?
4. How does sebum protect the skin?
5. What is the function of the sudoriferous glands?
6. What routes does the skin have for absorption?

Explain the Function of Each Layer of the Skin, from the Deepest to the Surface

The skin comprises three main components: (1) the hypodermis or subcutaneous layer, (2) the dermis, and (3) the epidermis. We are going to start at the deepest layer and work our way toward the surface. (**Figure 3–6**).

Subcutaneous Tissue

The **subcutaneous layer** (sub-kyoo-TAY-nee-us LAY-ur), also known as *hypodermis* or *superficial fascia*, is composed of loose connective tissue or **subcutis tissue** (sub-KYOO-tis TISH-oo), also known as *adipose tissue*. This layer is 80 percent fat. This tissue creates a protective cushion that gives contour and smoothness to the body, and it is also

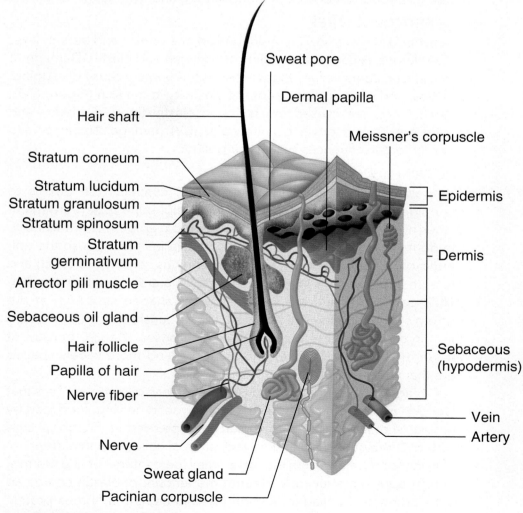

Sweat pore

Dermal papilla

Meissner's corpuscle

Hair shaft

Stratum corneum

Stratum lucidum
Stratum granulosum
Stratum spinosum
Stratum germinativum

Epidermis

Arrector pili muscle

Dermis

Sebaceous oil gland

Hair follicle

Papilla of hair

Sebaceous (hypodermis)

Nerve fiber

Nerve

Vein
Artery

Sweat gland

Pacinian corpuscle

▲ **FIGURE 3–6** Structure of the skin.

a source of energy for the body. Vessels, nerves, fibers, adipose cells, and fibroblasts are just some of the components of the hypodermis. This layer decreases and thins with age. A client with a thick subcutaneous layer may have an underlying hormonal disorder and will deserve further exploration when you perform your skin care consultation. Fat storage in the body is also influenced by hormones and may be reflected, for example, by acneic breakouts, hair growth, excessive oiliness or dryness.

The Dermis

The **dermis** (DUR-mis), also called the *derma*, **corium** (KOH-ree-um), **cutis** (KYOO-tis), or *true skin*, is the support layer of connective tissues above the hypodermis.

The dermis, which is about 25 times thicker than the epidermis, consists of two layers: the reticular layer below and the papillary layer above. The dermis primarily comprises of connective tissues made of collagen protein and elastin fibers. The dermis supplies the skin with oxygen and nutrients through a network of blood vessels and lymphatic channels.

THE RETICULAR LAYER

The **reticular layer** (ruh-TIKyuh-lur LAY-ur), the denser and deeper layer of the dermis, is comprised mainly of collagen and elastin. Damage to these elastin fibers as they break down is the primary cause of sagging, wrinkles, and intrinsic aging—loss of elasticity in the skin (**Figure 3–7**). Stretch marks are caused by damaged elastin fibers. Collagen and elastin are broken down by ultraviolet (UV) damage, smoking, and environmental influences such as air pollution.

THE PAPILLARY LAYER

The **papillary layer** (PAP-uh-lair-ee LAY-ur) connects the dermis to the epidermis. The **dermal papillae** (DUR-mul puh-PILL-ay) are membranes of ridges and grooves that attach to the epidermis. Attached to the dermal papillae are either looped capillaries that nourish the epidermis or tactile corpuscles, the nerve endings sensitive to touch and pressure. Note that papillae in the hair follicle are called **hair papillae** (HAYR pah-PIL-ay) and are the small, cone-shaped structures at the bottom of hair follicles. The blood supplies nourishment within the skin through capillaries. The papillary layer comprises 10 to 20 percent of the dermis. Collagen and elastin are loose and more widely spaced here than in the reticular layer.

Collagen (KAHL-uh-jen) is a protein substance of complex fibers that gives skin its strength and is necessary for wound healing. Produced by fibroblasts, collagen makes up 70 percent of the dermis. Fibroblast cells produce proteins and aid in the production of collagen and elastin.

In contrast, elastin makes up a small percentage of the dermis. There is approximately one-fifteenth the amount of elastin compared to the amount of collagen. **Elastin** (ee-LAS-tin) is the fibrous protein that forms elastic tissue and gives skin its elasticity.

DID YOU KNOW?

Collagen is the most abundant protein in the body and is derived from the Greek words *kolla* for "glue" and *gennan* for "to produce".

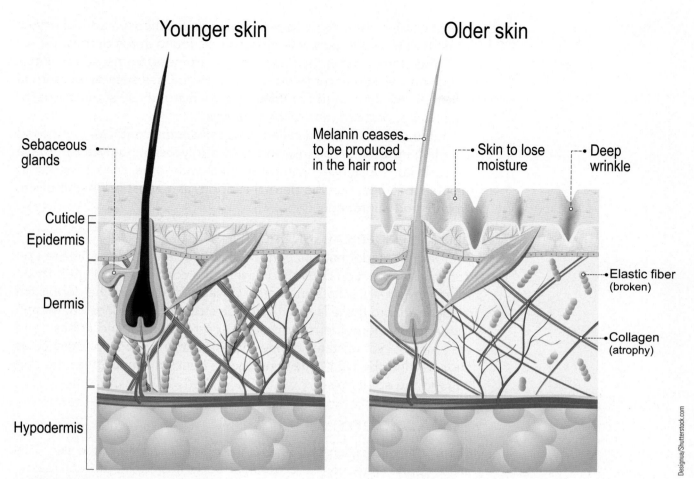

Younger skin

Older skin

Sebaceous glands

Cuticle
Epidermis

Dermis

Hypodermis

Melanin ceases to be produced in the hair root

Skin to lose moisture

Deep wrinkle

Elastic fiber (broken)

Collagen (atrophy)

Designua/Shutterstock.com

▲ **FIGURE 3–7** A comparison of younger and older skin showing the decrease in collagen fibers, atrophy and broken elastin, formed wrinkles, and hair becoming gray in the aging process.

Glycosaminoglycans (GAGs; gly-kose-ah-mee-no-GLY-cans) are large protein molecules and water-binding substances found between the fibers of the dermis. GAGs are polysaccharides, that is, protein and sugar complexes. Glycosaminoglycans work to maintain and support collagen and elastin in the cellular spaces, keeping protein fibers in balance. They also help collagen and elastin retain moisture. They interact with copper peptides in our system for cellular repair. A healthy fluid intake is essential to keep the GAGs functioning properly. Beneficial hydrating fluids such as **hyaluronic acid** (HY-uh-luhr-ahn-ik A-sid) are part of this dermal substance. Hyaluronic acid is a GAG. Ingredients that duplicate these natural intercellular fluids are important in esthetics and skin care products and are discussed in other chapters.

Blood and lymph vessels, capillaries, follicles, sebaceous glands, sudoriferous glands, sensory nerves, additional receptors, and the arrector pili muscles are all located in the dermis. **Lymph vessels** (LIMF ves-uhls) remove waste products, bacteria, and excess fluid. Fibroblasts (cell stimulators), lymphocytes (infection fighters), Langerhans cells

DID YOU KNOW?

Collagenase and elastase are enzymes that help protect collagen and elastin; however, when excessive levels are produced in response to UV radiation or other damage, it causes dermal breakdown, hyperpigmentation, rhytides (wrinkles), and premature aging.

(guard cells), mast cells (involved in allergic reactions), and leukocytes (white blood cells to fight infections) are all found in the dermis.

Other components give tautness, or firmness, to the skin by interacting with elastin and hyaluronic acid. Hormones such as epidermal growth factor (EGF) and fibroblast growth factor (FGF) stimulate fibroblasts, cells, proteins, and DNA synthesis.

In the dermis is a fluid called *extracellular matrix* (ECM) composed of collagen, other proteins, and GAGs (glycosaminoglycans). These intercellular substances comprise fluid with other components to maintain balance, provide dermal support, and assist cell metabolism, growth, and migration.

DERMAL/EPIDERMAL JUNCTION

The dermal/epidermal junction (DEJ) connects the dermis to the epidermis. This junction consists of layers of a connective collagen tissue with many small pockets and holes. Collagen fibrils from the dermis are embedded into these layers to provide strength and adhesion. Keratin filaments on the epidermis side also ensure strength and adhesion to the junction. Some states define the esthetician's scope of practice as "not beyond the DEJ", meaning the esthetician cannot treat the skin beyond the epidermis.

The Epidermis

The **epidermis** (ep-uh-DUR-mis) is the outermost layer of the skin. This is the epithelial tissue that covers our body. It is a thin, protective covering with many nerve endings. The epidermis is composed of the five layers called strata (singular: stratum) (**Figure 3–8**):

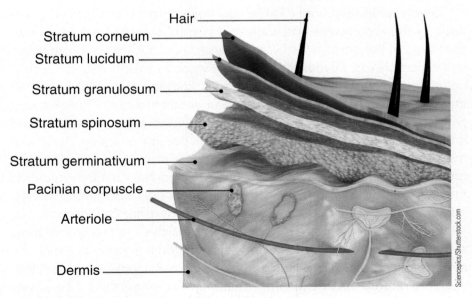

Hair

Stratum corneum

Stratum lucidum

Stratum granulosum

Stratum spinosum

Stratum germinativum

Pacinian corpuscle

Arteriole

Dermis

Sciencepics/Shutterstock.com

▲ **FIGURE 3–8** The five layers of the epidermis.

- Stratum germinativum—"the germination or growth layer"; bottom layer (basal cell layer)
- Stratum spinosum—"the spiny cells"
- Stratum granulosum—"the grainy cells"
- Stratum lucidum—"the clear cells"; present only where the skin is thick, on the soles of the feet and the palms of the hands
- Stratum corneum—"the horny cells"

Understanding how the skin cell layers function is important in choosing ingredients and treatments. Estheticians' scope of practice references working on the epidermis, not the dermis, unless they are working under the direction of a physician or other licensed medical practitioner, such as a nurse practitioner, naturopathic physician, or physician assistant.

KERATINOCYTES

Keratinocytes (kair-uh-TIN-oh-syts), composed of keratin, comprise 95 percent of the epidermis. These cells contain both proteins and lipids. Surrounding the cells in the epidermis are lipids, which protect the cells from water loss and dehydration.

Keratin (KAIR-uh-tin) is a fibrous protein that provides resiliency and protection. Keratin is found in all layers of the epidermis. Hard keratin is the protein found in hair and nails.

Keratinocytes have many different functions and go through changes as they move up through the layers to the top layer of the stratum corneum. Stem cells are the mother cells that divide in the basal layer, or stratum germinativum, forming new daughter cells. These daughter cells move up through the layers before becoming hardened corneocytes of the stratum corneum. Keratinocytes and other cells protect the epidermis. Other cells in the epidermis include melanocytes, immune cells, lamellar granules, and Merkel cells (nerve receptors).

THE STRATUM GERMINATIVUM

The stratum germinativum (STRAT-um jur-min-ah-TIV-um), also known as the *basal cell layer*, is located above the dermis and is composed of a single layer of basal cells laying on a "basement membrane". In this active layer, stem cells undergo continuous cell division (mitosis) to replenish the skin cells that are regularly shed from the surface. Stem cells are basically mother cells that divide to produce daughter cells in a remarkable process.

Mother cells divide to form two daughter cells. Some stem cells and daughter cells always remain undifferentiated and keep dividing for constant self-renewal over a lifetime. These either remain stem cells or are programmed to become something else, such as a keratino-cyte. In the body, some daughter cells go on to become skin cells. Other cells become glands, follicles, tissues, or organs. Daughter cells that are not able to divide anymore have the capability to program themselves to end up as one specific type of cell. This is known as *terminal differentiation*. Cells such as these keratinocytes begin their journey of terminal differentiation as they migrate to the surface and eventually become strong and protective.

Cells in the basal layer produce the necessary lipids that form cell membranes and hold the cells together. Merkel cells (sensory cells) are touch receptors also located in the basal layer. The stratum germinativum also contains **melanocytes** (muh-LAN-uh-syts), which are cells that produce pigment granules in the basal layer (**Figure 3–9**). About 5 to 10 percent of the basal cells are melanocytes. The pigment-carrying granules, called **melanosomes** (MEL-uh-noh-sohms), then produce a complex protein, **melanin** (MEL-uh-nin), which determines skin, eye, and hair color.

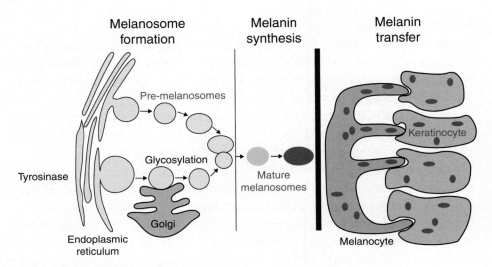

▲ **FIGURE 3–9** Melanin production.

THE STRATUM SPINOSUM

The **stratum spinosum** (STRAT-um spy-NOH-sum), also known as the *spiny layer*, is above the stratum germinativum. Cells continue to divide and change shape here, and enzymes are creating lipids and proteins. Cell appendages, which resemble prickly spines, become desmosomes, the intercellular structures that assist in strengthening and holding cells together. **Desmosomes** (DEZ-moh-somes) are keratin filaments—the protein bonds that create the junctions between the cells. These strengthen the epidermis and assist in intercellular communication.

Also found here are the **Langerhans immune cells** (LAN-ger-han IM-yoon SELLS), which protect the body from infections by identifying foreign material (antigens). The immune cells help destroy these foreign invaders. Keratinocytes and melanocytes work in synergy here, forming the even placement of pigment granules. **Lamellar granules** (la-mel-lar gran-yoolz) are cells that contain lipids to maintain the barrier function. The spinosum is the largest layer of the epidermis.

THE STRATUM GRANULOSUM

The **stratum granulosum** (STRAT-um gran-yoo-LOH-sum), also known as the *granular layer*, is composed of cells that resemble granules and are filled with keratin. The production of keratin and intercellular lipids also takes place here. In this layer, enzymes dissolve the structures (desmosomes) that hold cells together. As these cells become keratinized, they move to the surface and replace the cells shed from the stratum corneum.

Natural moisturizing substances such as triglycerides, ceramides, waxes, fatty acids, and other intercellular lipids are made here and are excreted from cells to form components of the skin's waterproofing barrier function of the top layer. These water-soluble compounds are referred to as natural moisturizing factors (NMFs) and hydrate the lipid layer surrounding cells, absorb water, and prevent water loss.

THE STRATUM LUCIDUM

The **stratum lucidum** (STRAT-um LOO-sih-dum) is a thin, clear layer of dead skin cells under the stratum corneum. It is a translucent layer made of small cells that let light pass through. This layer is thickest on the palms of the hands and soles of the feet. The keratinocytes in this layer contain clear keratin. The cells here release lipids, forming bilayers of oil and water. The thicker skin on the palms and soles is composed of epidermal ridges that provide a better grip while walking and using our hands. This layer also forms our unique fingerprints and footprints.

THE STRATUM CORNEUM

The **stratum corneum** (STRAT-um KOR-nee-um), also known as the *horny layer*, is the top, outermost layer of the epidermis. The esthetician works extensively with this layer. The stratum corneum is very thin, yet it is waterproof and permeable, regenerates itself, detoxifies the body, and responds to stimuli. Keratinocytes on the surface have hardened into **corneocytes** (KOR-nee-oh-sytz), the waterproof protective cells. These "dead" protein cells have dried out and lack nuclei. This layer is referred to as the *horny layer* because of these scale-like cells.

Keratinocytes are continually shed from the skin in a process called **desquamation** (DES-kwuh-MAY-shun). These cells are replaced by new cells coming to the surface from the lower stratums. This process of desquamation and replacement is known as *cell turnover*. The average adult cell turnover rate is every 28 days depending on a person's age, lifestyle, and health. The cell turnover rate slows with age. Average cell turnover when you are a baby is 14 days. In your teens, your cells are replaced every 3 to 4 weeks. By the time you are over 50, your cell turnover has slowed to 42 to 84 days. Understanding the process of cell turnover will help you make better decisions about how to treat aging skin.

Cells and oil combine to form a protective barrier layer on the stratum corneum. Lamellar granules are secreted from keratinocytes, resulting in the formation of an impermeable, lipid-containing membrane that serves as a water barrier and is required for correct skin barrier function. These bodies release components that are required for skin shedding (desquamation) in the stratum corneum. This is the acid mantle. Stratum corneum cells are surrounded by **bilayers** (BY-lay-urz) of oil and water. Lipids of the cell membranes, such as phospholipids and essential fatty acids, determine the health of this protective barrier. To clarify, a bilayer is a thin polar membrane made of two layers of lipid molecules. These membranes are flat sheets that form a continuous barrier around all cells. The cell membranes of almost all living organisms and many viruses are made of a lipid bilayer, as are the membranes surrounding the cell nucleus and other subcellular structures.

In general, the stratum corneum has 15 to 20 layers of cells. The stratum corneum has a thickness between 0.01 and 0.04 mm. The keratinocytes on the surface of the skin are also called *squamous* (flat, scaly) keratinized cells. There are different terms used to describe the same cells, so it is helpful to remember these surface cells are both flat and hardened (squamous and cornified).

SKIN COLOR: MELANIN, MELANOCYTES, AND MELANOSOMES

Melanin is the pigment that protects us from the sun. Every person has the same number of melanocytes, or pigment-producing cells. Both internal and external factors affect melanin activation and production. Differences in genetic skin color are due to the amount of melanin activated in the skin and the way it is distributed. Individuals with darker skin and melanin have more activity in their melanocytes. This is an example of an internal factor. An external factor influencing melanin production is sun exposure.

Melanin production is stimulated by exposure to sunlight and protects the cells below by absorbing and blocking UV radiation. Melanocyte cells make melanosome spheres, which are transferred to keratinocytes (**Figure 3–10**). Melanosomes carry the pigment granules that provide the skin's color. One melanocyte will deposit pigment-carrying melanosomes into about 30 keratinocytes through its dendrites. Dendrites are the arms, or cellular projections, that branch out to interact with other cells in the extracellular matrix between cells. This process is how pigment darkening occurs.

Tyrosinase (TAH-roz-in-ays) is the enzyme that stimulates melanocytes and thus produces melanin. It is estimated that there are over 1,000 melanocytes per square mm (⅛ square inch) of skin.

The body produces two types of melanin: **pheomelanin** (fee-oh-MEL-uh-nin), which is red to yellow in color, and **eumelanin** (yoo-MEL-uh-nin), which is dark brown to black. People with light-colored skin mostly produce pheomelanin, while those with dark-colored skin

FOCUS ON

Melanin

Melanocytes are cells that produce pigment granules, called *melanosomes*. Melanocytes are stimulated to produce melanosomes by the enzyme tyrosinase.

Melanosomes carry and produce the protein called *melanin*.

Melanin is transferred to cells from melanosomes through dendrite branches.

EPIDERMIS

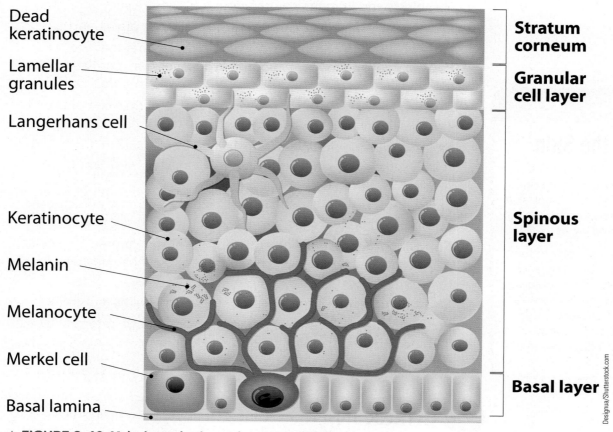

Dead keratinocyte

Lamellar granules

Langerhans cell

Keratinocyte

Melanin

Melanocyte

Merkel cell

Basal lamina

Stratum corneum

Granular cell layer

Spinous layer

Basal layer

Designua/Shutterstock.com

▲ FIGURE 3–10 Melanin production and protection of the skin.

mostly produce eumelanin. Individuals with fair skin have approximately 20 melanosomes per keratinocyte, and people with dark skin have about 200 melanosomes per keratinocyte.

Products that suppress melanin production by interrupting biochemical processes are referred to as *brightening agents*. Some are called *tyrosinase inhibitors*. These products are designed to reduce hyperpigmentation. Pigmentation disorders are discussed in Chapter 4, "Disorders and Diseases of the Skin". Products and treatments for hyperpigmentation are discussed in other chapters.

We have covered a lot of information so far. A summary of the main components of the skin, including their respective layers and functions, is provided here.

Subcutaneous layer—*hypodermis*, or superficial fascia; loose connective tissue, also known as *adipose tissue*; 80 percent fat; creates a protective cushion that gives contour and smoothness to the body; is a source of stored energy

Dermis—divided into two subdivisions, reticular and papillary; fibroblasts and immune cells are found in these layers

Reticular layer—collagen and elastin, glands, blood and lymph vessels, nerve endings, intercellular fluids

Papillary layer—touch receptors, blood vessels, capillaries, dermal papilla

Epidermis—each of the five layers of the epidermis contain keratinocytes, immune cells, and intercellular fluids

Stratum germinativum—single layer of cells, cell mitosis, stem cells, Merkel cells; keratinocytes, melanocytes, and lipids are all produced here

Stratum spinosum—large layer, cell activity, desmosomes created, Langerhans immune cells, melanosome pigment distribution

Stratum granulosum—production of keratin granules in cells, additional lipid production and excretion, desmosomes dissolved by enzymes

Stratum lucidum—clear cells; thickest on the palms and soles

Stratum corneum—hardened corneocytes (also referred to as flattened squamous cells), melanin, barrier layer, acid mantle, desquamation

 CHECK IN

7. Name the two components of the dermis.
8. Name the five layers of the epidermis.
9. What are keratinocytes?
10. Clarify the process of skin melanization.
11. How does the skin repair itself?

Identify a Hair Follicle as an Appendage of the Skin

Hair is an appendage of the skin—it is a slender, threadlike outgrowth of the skin and scalp. An esthetician needs to understand this appendage in order to perform treatments such as body waxing, sugaring, and brow shaping. **Figure 3–11** shows the structure of the hair follicle. There is no sense of feeling in the hair, due to the absence of nerves.

Much of the hair on the body is invisible to the naked eye. Heavier concentrations of hair are on the head, under the arms (in the axillary area), around the genitals, and on the arms and legs. Due to hormonal influences, there are different male and female hair growth patterns. Genetics influence the distribution of each person's hair, along with its

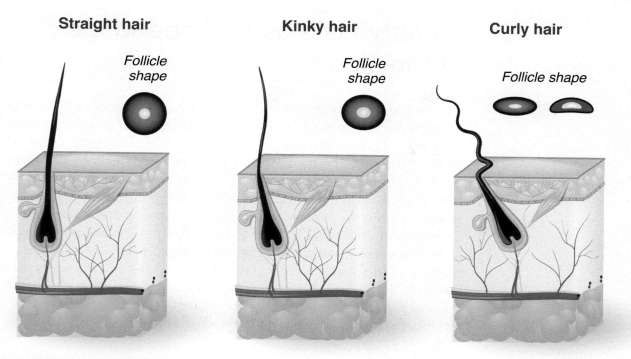

Straight hair

Follicle shape

Kinky hair

Follicle shape

Curly hair

Follicle shape

Designua/Shutterstock.com

▲ **FIGURE 3–11 Shape of a hair follicle**

thickness, quality, color, rate of growth, and whether it is curly or straight. The speed of hair growth is roughly 0.5 inch (1.25 centimeters) per month, which is about 6 inches (15 centimeters) per year. With age, the speed of hair growth might slow down to as little as 0.1 inch (0.25 cm) a month.

There are two types of keratin:

- Alpha (A-keratin) is softer.
- Beta (B-keratin) is harder.

Hair contains 90 percent hard B-keratin. It has lower moisture and fat content than soft A-keratin does, and is a particularly tough, elastic material. Keratin forms continuous sheets (fingernails) or long, endless fibers (hair). Hard keratin does not normally break off or flake away. It remains a continuous structure. Hair also contains melanin, which determines hair color.

Abnormalities such as extremely curly hair and/or rapidly growing bacteria and the inability of the follicle to take in oxygen, along with excessive sebum production, can contribute to ingrown hairs and folliculitis, an inflammation of the follicle. Hair growth is discussed extensively in Chapter 11, "Hair Removal".

 CHECK IN

12. What influences hair growth?
13. What kind of keratin does hair contain?

Identify Nails as an Appendage of the Skin

The nail, an appendage of the skin, is a hard translucent plate that protects fingers and toes. The nail is composed of hard keratin. **Figure 3–12** shows the nail structure. *Onyx* (AHN-iks) is the technical term for the nail. The hard, or horny, nail plate contains no nerves or blood vessels. Fingernails grow faster than toenails and grow faster over the summer than over the winter, lengthen about $\frac{1}{10}$ inch to $\frac{1}{8}$ inch (2.5 mm to 3 mm) per month, which means that it takes a fingernail about four to six months to fully grow out. An esthetician may work in a state where performing nail services is part of the scope of practice. Additionally, some symptoms of diseases and disorders that influence the skin are evident on the nails. A person with a circulatory disorder may have cyanotic nails, for example. Cyanosis is when a person has a purple or bluish tone under their fingernails.

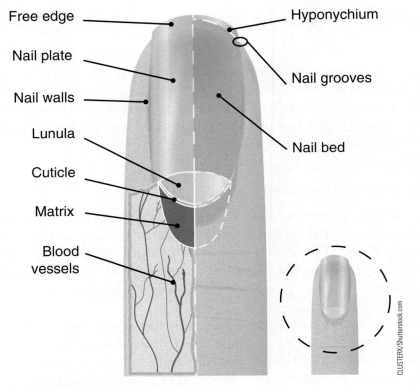

Free edge — Nail plate — Nail walls — Lunula — Cuticle — Matrix — Blood vessels

Hyponychium — Nail grooves — Nail bed

CLUSTERX/Shutterstock.com

▲ **FIGURE 3–12** Nail structure.

✔ **CHECK IN**

14. What kind of keratin do nails contain?

Describe the Functions of the Two Types of Nerves

Nerves are cordlike bundles of fibers made up of neurons through which sensory stimuli and motor impulses pass between the brain or other parts of the central nervous system and the eyes, glands, muscles, and other parts of the body. Nerves form a network of pathways for conducting information throughout the body. There are two types of nerves: motor and sensory.

- *Motor*, or *efferent*, nerve fibers convey impulses from the brain or spinal cord to the muscles or glands. These nerve fibers stimulate muscles, such as the arrector pili muscles, attached to the hair follicles. Arrector pili muscles cause "goosebumps" when you are cold or frightened. *Secretory* nerve fibers are motor nerves attached to sweat and oil glands. They regulate excretion from the sweat glands and control sebum output to the surface of the skin.

- *Sensory*, or *afferent*, nerve fibers send messages to the central nervous system and brain to react to heat, cold, pain, pressure, and touch.

 CHECK IN

> 15. Name the two main types of nerves and describe what they do.

Explain What is Produced by the Two Types of Glands of the Skin

The dermis of the skin contains two types of duct glands, each producing different substances. The sebaceous glands secrete oil, while the sudoriferous glands excrete sweat (**Figure 3–13**).

The Sebaceous (Oil) Glands

Sebaceous glands are connected to the hair follicles and produce oil, which protects the surface of the skin. Glandular sacs open into the follicles through ducts. If the ducts become clogged, open or closed comedones (blackheads or whiteheads) are formed. The oily secretions lubricate both the skin and hair. Sebaceous glands are larger on the face and scalp than on the rest of the body. Other chapters include further discussion on sebaceous glands and acne.

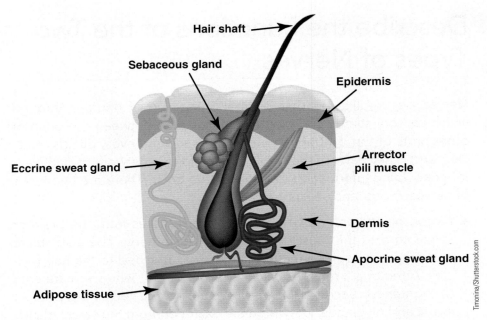

Hair shaft

Sebaceous gland

Epidermis

Arrector
pili muscle

Eccrine sweat gland

Dermis

Apocrine sweat gland

Adipose tissue

Timonina/Shutterstock.com

▲ FIGURE 3–13 Oil and sweat glands.

The Sudoriferous (Sweat) Glands

Sudoriferous glands help to regulate body temperature and eliminate minute amounts of waste products by excreting sweat. They have a coiled base and duct openings at the surface, known as pores. Fluids and minerals are eliminated daily through these pores. Excess fluid loss can result in the loss of electrolytes, which may lead to dehydration in the body. The excretion of sweat is controlled by the nervous system. Normally, 1 to 2 pints (0.5 to 1 liter) of fluids containing trace amounts of minerals such as sodium, potassium, and magnesium are eliminated daily through sweat pores in the skin. There are two kinds of sweat glands—apocrine and eccrine.

The **apocrine glands** (AP-uh-krin GLANZ) are coiled structures attached to the hair follicles found under the arms (in the axillary region) and in the genital area. Their secretions are released through the oil glands. Apocrine function is sensitive to adrenaline, so sweating can occur during times of anxiety, stress, fear, sexual arousal, and pain. Odors associated with these glands are due to the interaction of the secretions and bacteria on the surface of the skin. According to some medical authorities, apocrine glands are not true sweat glands because their openings connect to oil glands instead of pore openings directly on the skin's surface.

The **eccrine glands** (EK-run GLANZ) are found all over the body but are primarily on the forehead, palms of the hands, and soles of the feet. They have a duct and pore through which secretions are released on the skin's surface. These glands are not connected to hair follicles. Eccrine glands are more active when the body is subjected to physical activity and high temperatures. Eccrine sweat does not typically produce an offensive odor.

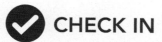

CHECK IN

16. What glands help regulate the body's temperature?
17. What are the two main glands associated with the skin?
18. What are the two types of sweat glands?

Distinguish the Factors Influencing Skin Health

In order to survive, cells need these important elements: nourishment, protection, and the ability to function properly through respiration, circulation, elimination of wastes, and continual replacement or proliferation. Skin health and aging of the skin are both influenced by many different factors, including heredity, sun exposure, the environment, health habits, nutrition, and general lifestyle. This topic is discussed thoroughly in Chapter 5, "Skin Analysis".

The Immune System and the Skin

Our immune system is a complex defense mechanism that protects the body from foreign substances. The immune system is activated when antigens (foreign invaders) are identified. Antibodies are molecules formed to fight and neutralize bacteria, viruses, and antigens. Langerhans cells, T cells, and leukocyte cells are part of the immune system.

Langerhans cells are dendritic in form. They are present predominantly in the stratum spinosum, but also other layers of the skin. They work to absorb, process, and carry antigens to the nearest lymph node for further immune system action.

Another part of the immune system involves **leukocytes** (LOO-koh-syts), the white blood cells that have enzymes to digest and kill bacteria and parasites. These white blood cells also respond to allergies. A **T cell** (TEE SELL) is a type of lymphocyte. T cells play an important role in the immune system by attacking virus-infected cells, foreign cells, and cancer cells. T cells get their name from the thymus gland, where they mature.

There are additional components of the immune system that protect the body from foreign substances, bacteria, and infections. Infections and allergic reactions speed up cell growth and migration rates for faster healing. The skin's capacity to heal, fight infection, and protect itself is truly extraordinary.

Skin Nourishment

Blood and lymph are the fluids that nourish the skin (**Figure 3–14**). Networks of arteries and lymphatics send essential materials for growth and repair throughout the body. Water, vitamins, minerals, and other

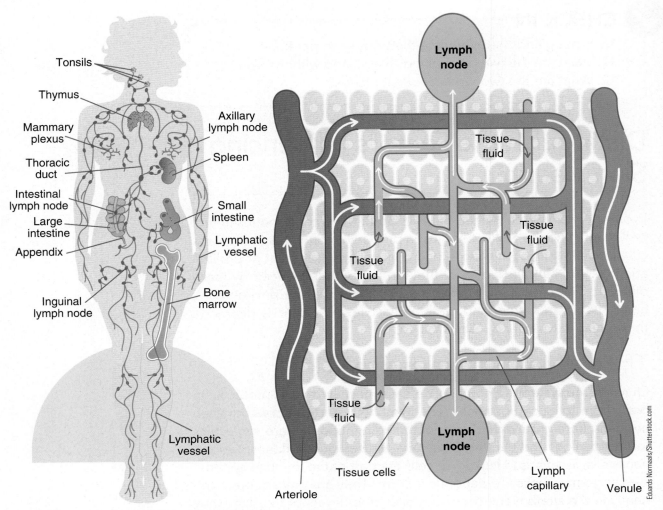

Tonsils

Thymus

Mammary plexus

Thoracic duct

Intestinal lymph node

Large intestine

Appendix

Inguinal lymph node

Axillary lymph node

Spleen

Small intestine

Lymphatic vessel

Bone marrow

Lymphatic vessel

Lymph node

Tissue fluid

Tissue fluid

Tissue fluid

Tissue fluid

Tissue fluid

Lymph node

Tissue cells

Arteriole

Lymph capillary

Venule

Eduards Normaals/Shutterstock.com

▲ FIGURE 3–14 Nourishment through the blood and lymph systems.

nutrients are all important for skin health. Blood supplies nutrients and oxygen to the skin. Nutrients are molecules from food such as protein, carbohydrates, and fats. Topical products with small molecules can nourish the epidermis.

Lymph, the clear fluid of the body that resembles blood plasma but contains only colorless corpuscles, bathes the skin cells, removes toxins and cellular waste, and has immune functions that help protect the skin and body against disease. Networks of arteries and lymph vessels in the subcutaneous tissue send their smaller branches up to dermal papillae, follicles, and skin glands.

Cell Protection

The health of skin cells depends on the cellular membrane and the water-holding capacity of the stratum corneum. Phospholipids, glycolipids, cholesterol, triglycerides, squalene, and waxes are all different types of lipids found in the stratum corneum and cell membranes. Intercellular lipids and proteins surround cells and provide protection, hydration, and nourishment to the cells. **Ceramides** (SARA-mydes) are a group of waxy lipid molecules such as glycolipids that are important to barrier function and water-holding capacity. Fifty percent of the lipids in the stratum corneum are ceramides. Fatty acids are also components of the intercellular substances.

Lipids are reduced if the skin is dry, damaged, or mature. Topical products containing peptides, hyaluronic acid, ceramides, and other lipids benefit skin that is damaged from both intrinsic and extrinsic aging. These products expedite the regenerative processes of the body and promote healing. Exfoliation removes and depletes lipids, so topical product reapplication is necessary to balance what was lost in exfoliation. Cell recovery depends on water to function properly, so drinking water and keeping the skin hydrated is essential to keep cells healthy.

Cell Replacement

The body replaces billions of cells daily. The cells of organs such as the skin, heart, liver, and kidneys are replaced every six to nine months. Cells of the bones are replaced every seven years. Unfortunately, elastin and collagen are not easily replaced by the body, and the skin does not regain its once pliable shape after being stretched or damaged by UV radiation and environmental pollution; however, research shows that certain skin care treatments and ingredients, such as vitamin A, alpha hydroxy acids (AHAs), alpha lipoeic acid, and other growth factors stimulate skin cell turnover and reduce visible signs of aging. Regular cell turnover is necessary to keep skin healthy.

Sun Damage

The sun and ultraviolet (UV) electromagnetic radiation have the greatest impact on how our skin ages. According to the U.S. Department of Health and Human Services, ultraviolet radiation (UVR) is a proven carcinogen. UV exposure alters DNA and can cause skin cancer. Approximately 80 to 85 percent of our aging is caused by sun exposure. As we age, the collagen and elastin fibers of the skin naturally weaken. This weakening is accelerated when the skin is frequently exposed to ultraviolet radiation.

UV reaches the skin in three different forms: UVA, UVB, and UVC. Each of the UV forms affects the skin at different levels (**Figure 3–15**). Cell damage is cumulative, and photodamage (from the sun) causes photoaging. Pigment dysfunction, wrinkles, sagging, collagen and elastin breakdown, and skin cancer result from exposure to UV radiation.

UVA radiation (YOO-VEE-AY ray-DEE-aye-shun), also known as *aging rays*, contributes up to 95 percent of the sun's UVR that reaches the Earth's surface. The longer wavelengths of UVA (320 to 400 nanometers) penetrate deeper into the skin and cause genetic damage

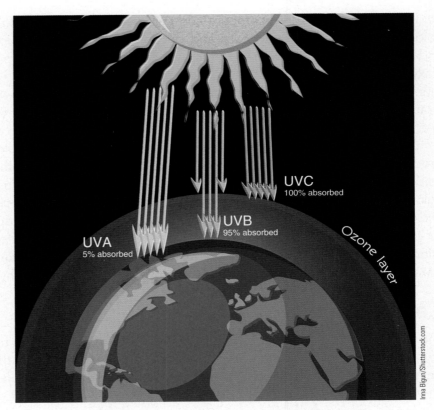

▲ FIGURE 3–15 UV rays penetrate into the skin at different levels.

and cell death. UVA weakens the skin's collagen and elastin fibers, causing wrinkling and sagging in the tissues. UVA can also penetrate glass and clouds. UVA is present all year and more prevalent than UVB.

UVB radiation (YOO-VEE-BEE ray-DEE-aye-shun), also known as *burning rays*, causes burning of the skin as well as tanning, aging, and cancer. UVB wavelengths range between 290 and 320 nanometers. Although UVB penetration is shorter than and not as deep as UVA, these wavelengths are stronger and more damaging to the skin and can damage the eyes as well. On a positive note, UVB radiation contributes to the body's synthesis of vitamin D and other important minerals.

UVC radiation has more energy than UVA or UVB. It reacts with the ozone high in our atmosphere and from humanmade sources, such as welding torches, and UV sanitizing bulbs that kill bacteria and other germs.

The effects of HEV light, or **high-energy visible light** (HAYH-EN-er-jee VIZ-uh-buh-l LAHYT) is a new consideration when working on the skin, and questioning your client's exposure to this light is a valid inquiry during the consultation. Blue light from your TV, computer, and smartphone, that is, HEV light, is said to penetrate the skin more deeply than UV rays and damage collagen, hyaluronic acid, and elastin. There is some evidence that the light may also worsen pigmentation problems such as melasma. Evidence tying it to skin cancers and deep wrinkles is scant, however, in part because the subject is too new for long-term study results to be available.

Melanin is designed to help protect the skin from the sun's UV radiation, but melanin can be altered or destroyed when large, frequent doses of UV are allowed to penetrate the skin. It is important that you advise your clients about the necessary precautions to take when they are exposed to the sun. Sun protection does more than protect the skin; it defends cells from radiation, cell death, tissue breakdown, and premature aging.

In addition to taking sun protection precautions, clients should be advised to see a medical professional specializing in dermatology for regular skin checkups, especially if they detect any changes in the coloration, size, or shape of a mole.

Home self-examinations are an effective way to check for signs of potential skin cancer between scheduled medical visits. When performing a self-care exam, clients should be advised to check for any changes in existing moles and to pay attention to any new visible growths on the skin. Sun damage, skin cancer, and sunscreens are discussed further in Chapter 5, "Skin Analysis", and in other chapters.

Free Radical Damage

All cells in our body like to be in a state of homeostasis, from individual body systems to microscopic cells. Molecules are in balance when electrons are paired. Molecules may lose an electron due to damage from UV rays, the environment, poor nutrition, unhealthy lifestyle, or injuries. Inflammation creates free radicals. Free radicals speed the aging process and creates an unhealthy state. Free radicals have an unbalanced electrical charge. They are unstable and a chain reaction of cellular destruction begins as they steal electrons from other molecules to try to put themselves back into a state of balance. (**Figure 3–16**).

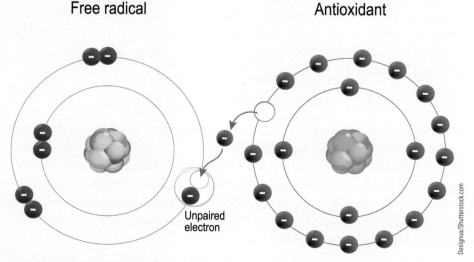

▲ **FIGURE 3–16** Antioxidant donates electron to free radical.

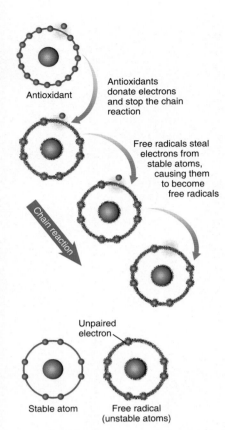

▲ FIGURE 3–17 Free radicals and antioxidants.

These free radicals are reactive oxidants (derived from reactions with oxygen molecules) searching the body for other electrons that will allow them to become stable, neutral molecules again. Free radicals take electrons from compounds in the body such as proteins, lipids, and DNA; this process destabilizes and oxidizes the once healthy molecules and creates more free radicals. (**Figure 3–17**). Free radicals are superoxidizers that not only cause an oxidation reaction but also produce new free radicals in the process.

The prevention of free radical formation is a critical process and a complex task that is necessary for cells to survive. Antioxidants are components that have an extra electron. Antioxidants are vital to neutralize this chain reaction by donating their electrons to stabilize the free radical's electrons. Proteins, enzymes, vitamins, and metabolites are all antioxidants.

Skin cells have built-in antioxidants to protect against sun damage, but their ability to protect cells deteriorates with sun exposure. The melanin pigment produced by tanning darkens the skin and absorbs UV radiation to help keep cells below from being damaged.

Skin Health and the Environment

While the sun may play the predominant role in how the skin ages, changes in our environment also greatly influence this aging process. Pollutants in the air from factories, automobile exhaust, and even secondhand smoke can all influence the appearance and overall health of our skin. While these pollutants affect the surface appearance of the skin, they can also change the health of the underlying cells and tissues, thereby speeding up the aging process.

Climate, humidity levels, and other environmental factors also affect the skin. Routine cleansing at night helps to remove the buildup of pollutants that have settled on the skin's surface throughout the day. Applying daily moisturizers, antioxidants, growth factor serums, peptides, sunscreen, and even foundation products helps to protect the skin from airborne pollutants and the environment.

Skin Health and Lifestyle Choices

What we choose to put into our bodies significantly affects our overall health. The impact of poor choices can be seen most visibly on the skin. Smoking, drinking, drugs, and an unbalanced diet with heavily processed foods all greatly influence the aging process. It is the esthetician's responsibility to be aware of how these habits affect the skin and during consultations to stress the benefits of good nutrition, exercise, balanced lifestyle, and stress reduction.

Smoking and tobacco use not only may cause cancer but are linked to the premature aging and wrinkling of the skin. Nicotine in tobacco causes contraction and weakening of the blood vessels and small capillaries that supply blood to the tissues, causing decreased circulation. Eventually, the tissues are deprived of essential oxygen, and the skin's surface may appear yellowish or gray in color and can look dull (**Figure 3–18**). Lack of oxygen and nutrients accelerates skin aging.

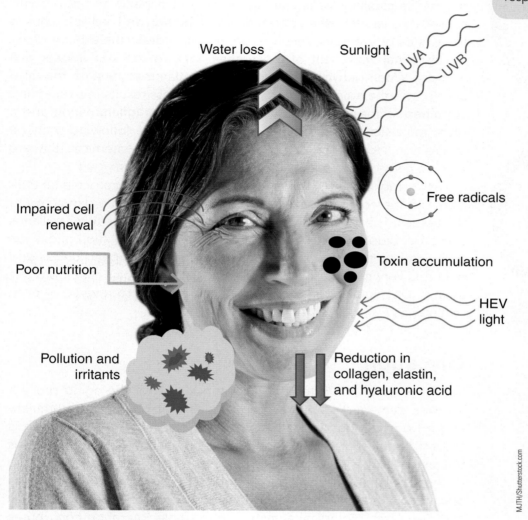

▲ **FIGURE 3–18** Extrinsic aging.

Using some prescription or illegal drugs also affects the skin. Certain drugs have been shown to interfere with the body's intake of oxygen, thus affecting healthy cell growth. Some drugs can even aggravate serious skin conditions, such as acne. Other effects include dryness and allergic reactions on the skin's surface.

As more states move to legalize marijuana, the effects of inhaled cannabis should be a consideration in the skin's aging processes as well.

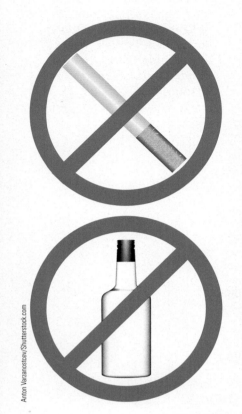

Anton Varzanostaev/Shutterstock.com

There may be documentation about the benefits of skin care containing cannabinoids; however, inhaling marijuana has a detrimental effect on the skin. There is a correlation between marijuana and testosterone that may cause increased acneic breakouts as well as deprive the skin of needed oxygen, further breaking down collagen and elastin.

Similarly, consuming alcohol has a damaging effect on the skin. Heavy or excessive intake of alcohol dilates the capillaries and other blood vessels. Over time, this constant overdilation and weakening of the fragile capillary walls can cause them to expand and burst. This causes a constant flushed appearance of the skin and red splotches in the whites of the eyes. Alcohol can also dehydrate the skin by drawing essential water out of the tissues, making the skin appear dull and dry. When dehydrated, skin is in an inflammatory state that also accelerates the aging process. Alcohol in excess results in a rapid and sustained increase in blood sugar, which causes inflammation and a glycation reaction (see details on glycation in the following section). In addition, alcohol is metabolized by the liver into chemicals that are toxic to cells.

Both smoking and drinking contribute to the aging process on their own, but the combination of the two can be even more damaging to the tissues. The constant dilation and contraction of the tiny capillaries and other blood vessels, as well as the constant deprivation of oxygen and water to the tissues, quickly makes the skin appear lifeless and dull. It is very difficult for the skin to adjust and repair itself from this assault. Damage done by our habits can be hard to reverse or even diminish.

Glycation

Recent research indicates that an intrinsic part of the aging process involves damaged structures and tissues that gradually accumulate in the body through a destructive process called *glycation*, which is caused by an elevation in blood sugar. **Glycation** (GLIE-kay-shun) is the binding of a protein molecule to a glucose molecule, resulting in the formation of damaged, nonfunctioning structures known as *advanced glycation end products*. Glycation alters protein structures and decreases biological activity. For example, glycation contributes to the aging of skin, contributing to wrinkles and hyperpigmentation. Many age-related diseases such as arterial stiffening, cataracts, and neurological impairment are partially attributed to glycation.

Scientists have established that anything that causes a rise in our blood sugar results in inflammation on a cellular level. When blood sugar goes up rapidly and continually, the sugar can actually attach to the collagen in the skin, making it stiff and inflexible. This is glycation. When collagen is cross-linked by sugar, it leads to stiff and sagging skin.

When blood sugar is elevated, we are in an inflammatory state. For example, lack of sleep elevates the hormone cortisol. On days we do not get enough sleep, we tend to crave carbohydrates because cortisol raises blood sugar and insulin levels, setting up this craving. Even though it is an essential hormone in the body, cortisol has many negative side effects in excess quantities. For example, it can break down muscle tissue, thin skin, decalcify bones, and elevate blood sugar. In summary, glycation is an unhealthy biological process for many reasons. A healthy lifestyle and a diet without excess sugar intake can help keep sugar levels balanced in the body.

Aging Skin and Hormones

As we age, our skin changes significantly. This is partially because of shifts in hormone balance. Hormones are the internal messengers for most of the body's systems and are significant internal factors in the skin's appearance, strength, and health. Estrogen (which is present in both men and women, but is predominant in women) is a crucial hormone for good health and the appearance of skin. Estrogen is anti-inflammatory, an antioxidant, and a key factor in tissue repair. The hormone is also responsible for maintaining health in several areas such as coordination, balance, skin moisture, vision, bones, and the nervous system. Estrogen has even been linked to memory and emotions.

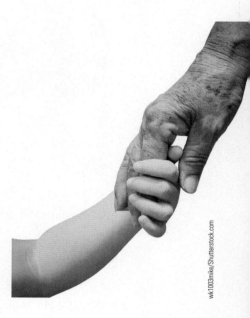

Women's skin is continually in a state of change due to hormonal changes in the reproductive and endocrine systems. From puberty to pregnancy, to the postpartum period, to perimenopause, and to menopause, estrogen levels fluctuate. This affects the skin's protective barrier, epithelial (external covering) tissue, and dermis. As skin ages, capillary and other vascular walls begin to weaken, lipids are reduced, the lymphatic system is less efficient, glands slow down, and there are fewer fibroblasts, thus affecting cells, collagen, and elastin (**Figure 3–19**). The skin thins and collagen has less ability to respond to physical changes from aging and sun damage.

As estrogen is depleted, skin begins to lose its tone. Reduced glycosaminoglycans mean less moisture in the tissues; keratinocytes are reduced (slower cell mitosis); melanocytes are reduced (less protective pigment); and cellular exchanges are reduced. Testosterone levels become dominant as estrogen decreases, which can increase sebum production, pore size, and hair growth on the face. This helps explain why mature women may experience adult onset acne or facial hair growth.

Microcirculation

Microcirculation is the circulation of blood from the heart to arterioles (small arteries), to capillaries, to venules (small veins), and then back to the heart. Hormonal changes are one cause of the microcirculation

Web Resources

www.skincancer.org
www.ncbi.nlm.nih.gov (National Library of Medicine, National Institute of Health)
www.medicinenet.com

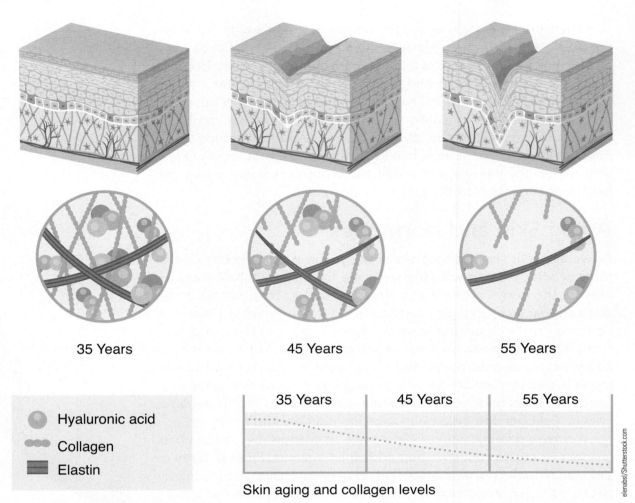

35 Years   45 Years   55 Years

Hyaluronic acid
Collagen
Elastin

| 35 Years | 45 Years | 55 Years |

Skin aging and collagen levels

elenabsl/Shutterstock.com

▲ FIGURE 3–19 Aging of the skin.

problems common in mature skin. One such problem is **couperose** (KOO-per-ohs) skin, or **telangiectasia** (tel-an-jee-ek-TAY-zhuh), the dilation of the capillary walls. As the endothelium (wall of the capillary) atrophies and loses its elasticity, the walls dilate and fill with blood, sometimes bursting.

Other causes of vasodilation are heredity, alimentary (digestive) problems, alcohol, smoking, sun damage, harsh cosmetics, trauma, pregnancy, excess localized heat, topical corticosteroids, inflammation, and heat–cold fluctuations. These could potentially lead to permanent distention of the capillaries.

Rosacea (roh-ZAY-shuh) is a chronic vascular disorder characterized by varying degrees of skin redness and congestion of the skin. Acneic rosacea includes papules and pustules. In some cases, rosacea may be caused by parasitic microorganisms (mites). Skin disorders are discussed in Chapter 4, "Disorders and Diseases of the Skin".

Hormone Replacement Therapy

Hormone replacement therapy (HRT) is often suggested to balance estrogen for women experiencing menopause; however, some HRT may be linked to breast cancer. These therapies may be derived from animal-source estrogens or plant-source estrogens. Estrogens from plants are called *phytoestrogens* (fy-toh-ES-tro-jins); they are about 200 to 400 times weaker than animal estrogens. Plants that provide phytoestrogens include Mexican wild yam, soybeans, red clover, sage, hops, black cohash, flax, Saint John's wort, licorice root, and butcher's broom. Choosing an HRT program should be done with the help of a medical professional. It is not within the scope of practice of an esthetician to make recommendations. In addition to hormone balancing, sustaining good nutrition, the use of good skin care products and treatments, exercise, and a positive outlook can help keep skin looking radiant at any age.

 CHECK IN

19. How do the Langerhans cells, leukocytes, and T cells work to protect the body?
20. Describe the differences between UVA wavelengths, UVB wavelengths, UVC wavelengths, and HEV light and their effect on the skin.
21. How do antioxidants stop free radical damage?
22. What environmental influences affect skin health?
23. What happens to the skin during the aging process?

COMPETENCY PROGRESS

How are you doing with physiology and histology of the skin? **Check off the Chapter 3 Learning Objectives below that you feel you have mastered; leave unchecked those objectives you will need to return to:**

☐ Describe why learning the physiology and histology of the skin makes you a better esthetician.

☐ Describe the attributes of healthy skin.

☐ Distinguish the six primary functions of the skin.

☐ Explain the function of each layer of the skin, from the deepest to the surface.

☐ Identify a hair follicle as an appendage of the skin.

☐ Identify nails as an appendage of the skin.

☐ Describe the functions of the two types of nerves.

☐ Explain what is produced by the two types of glands of the skin.

☐ Distinguish the factors influencing skin health.

CHAPTER GLOSSARY

apocrine glands
AP-uh-krin GLANZ
pg. 104
coiled structures attached to hair follicles found in the underarm (axillary) and genital areas; secrete sweat

arrector pili muscle
ah-REK-tohr-PY-leh MUS-uhls
pg. 89
small, involuntary muscles in the base of the hair follicle that cause goose flesh when the appendage contracts; sometimes called *goosebumps* and *papillae*

barrier function
BEAR-ee-ore FUNK-shun
pg. 87
protective barrier of the epidermis; the corneum and intercellular matrix protect the surface from irritation and dehydration

bilayers
BY-lay-urz
pg. 98
a thin polar membrane made of two layers of lipid molecules; these membranes are flat sheets that form a continuous barrier around all cells

ceramides
SARA-mydes
pg. 107
glycolipid materials that are a natural part of the skin's intercellular matrix and barrier function

collagen
KAHL-uh-jen
pg. 92
fibrous, connective tissue made from protein; found in the reticular layer of the dermis; gives skin its firmness; topically, a large long-chain molecular protein that lies on the top of the skin and binds water; derived from the placentas of cows or other sources

couperose
KOO-per-ohs
pg. 114
redness; capillaries that have been damaged and are now larger, or distended, blood vessels; commonly seen with telangiectasia.

corneocytes
KOR-nee-oh-sytz
pg. 97
another name for a stratum corneum cell; hardened, waterproof, protective keratinocytes; these "dead" protein cells are dried out and lack nuclei

dermal papillae
DUR-mul puh-PILL-ay
pg. 92
membranes of ridges and grooves that attach to the epidermis; contains nerve endings and supplies nourishment through capillaries to skin and follicles

dermis
DUR-mis
pg. 92
also known as the *derma*, *corium*, *cutis*, or *true skin*; support layer of connective tissue, collagen, and elastin below the epidermis

desmosomes
DEZ-moh-somes
pg. 96
the structures that assist in holding cells together; intercellular connections made of proteins

eccrine glands
EK-run GLANZ
pg. 104
sweat glands found all over the body with openings on the skin's surface through pores; not attached to hair follicles; secretions do not produce an offensive odor

elastin
ee-LAS-tin
pg. 92
protein fiber found in the dermis; gives skin its elasticity and firmness

epidermal growth factor
ep-ih-DUR-mul GROWTH FAK-tor
pg. 88
abbreviated EGF; stimulates cells to reproduce and heal

epidermis
ep-uh-DUR-mis
pg. 94
outermost layer of skin; a thin protective layer with many cells, mechanisms, and nerve endings; is made up of five layers: stratum germinativum, stratum spinosum, stratum granulosum, stratum lucidum, and stratum corneum

eumelanin
yoo-MEL-uh-nin
pg. 98
a type of melanin that is dark brown to black in color; people with dark-colored skin produce mostly eumelanin; there are two types of melanin; the other type is pheomelanin

fibroblasts
fy-BROH-blasts
pg. 88
cells that stimulate collagen production and amino acids that form proteins to aid in healing

follicles FAWL-ih-kuls	pg. 89	hair follicles and sebaceous follicles are tubelike openings in the epidermis
glycation GLIE-kay-shun	pg. 112	caused by an elevation in blood sugar, glycation is the binding of a protein molecule to a glucose molecule resulting in the formation of damaged, nonfunctioning structures known as advanced glycation end products (also known as *AGES*); glycation alters protein structures and decreases biological activity
glycosaminoglycans gly-kose-ah-mee-no-GLY-cans	pg. 93	large protein molecules and water-binding substances found between the fibers of the dermis; GAGS are polysaccharide–protein and sugar complexes; they work to maintain and support collagen and elastin in the cellular spaces, keeping protein fibers in balance
hair papillae HAYR pah-PIL-ay	pg. 92	cone-shaped elevations at the base of the follicle that fit into the hair bulb; papillae are filled with tissue that contains the blood vessels and cells necessary for hair growth and follicle nourishment
high-energy visible light HAYH-EN-er-jee VIZ-uh-buh-l LAHYT	pg. 108	abbreviated as *HEV*; light emitting from electronic devices, reported to penetrate the skin more deeply than UV rays; damages collagen, hyaluronic acid, and elastin
hyaluronic acid HY-uh-luhr-ahn-ik A-sid	pg. 93	hydrating fluids found in the skin; hydrophilic agent with water-binding properties
hydrolipidic hy-droh-li-PID-ic	pg. 87	hydrolipidic film is an oil–water balance that protects the skin's surface
intercellular matrix in-tur-SEL-yuh-lur MAY-tricks	pg. 88	lipid substances between corneum cells that protect the cells from water loss and irritation
keratin KAIR-uht-in	pg. 95	fibrous protein of cells that is also the principal component of skin, hair, and nails; provides resiliency and protection
keratinocytes kair-uh-TIN-oh-syts	pg. 95	epidermal cells composed of keratin, lipids, and other proteins
Langerhans immune cells LAN-ger-han IM-yoon SELLS	pg. 96	guard cells of the immune system that sense unrecognized foreign invaders, such as bacteria, and then process these antigens for removal through the lymph system
lamellar granules la-mel-lar gran-yoolz	Pg. 96	Organelles secreted from keratinocytes, resulting in the formation of an impermeable, lipid-containing membrane that serves as a water barrier and required for correct skin barrier function. These bodies release components that are required for skin shedding (desquamation) in the stratum corneum.
leukocytes LOO-koh-syts	pg. 105	white blood cells that have enzymes to digest and kill bacteria and parasites; also respond to allergies
lymph vessels LIMF ves-uhls	pg. 93	located in the dermis; supply nourishment within the skin and remove waste
melanin MEL-uh-nin	pg. 96	tiny grains of pigment (coloring matter) that are produced by melanocytes and deposited into cells in the stratum germinativum layer of the epidermis and in the papillary layers of the dermis; a protein that determines hair, eye, and skin color; produced as a defense mechanism to protect skin from the sun
melanocytes muh-LAN-uh-syts	pg. 96	cells that produce skin pigment granules in the basal layer

melanosomes MEL-uh-noh-sohms	pg. 96	pigment carrying granules that produce melanin, a complex protein
papillary layer PAP-uh-lair-ee LAY-ur	pg. 92	top layer of the dermis; next to the epidermis
pheomelanin fee-oh-MEL-uh-nin	pg. 98	a type of melanin that is red and yellow in color; people with light-colored skin produce mostly pheomelanin; two types of melanin; the other is eumelanin
pores PORZ	pg. 89	tubelike opening for sweat glands on the epidermis
reticular layer ruh-TIKyuh-lur LAY-ur	pg. 92	deeper layer of the dermis that supplies the skin with oxygen and nutrients; contains fat cells, blood vessels, sudoriferous (sweat) glands, hair follicles, lymph vessels, arrector pili muscles, sebaceous (oil) glands, and nerve endings
rosacea roh-ZAY-shuh	pg. 114	chronic condition that appears primarily on the cheeks and nose and is characterized by flushing (redness), telangiectasis (distended or dilated surface blood vessels), and, in some cases, the formation of papules and pustules
sebaceous glands sih-BAY-shus GLANZ	pg. 89	also known as *oil glands*; protect the surface of the skin; appendages connected to follicles
sebum SEEB-um	pg. 89	oil that provides protection for the epidermis from external factors and lubricates both the skin and hair
stratum corneum STRAT-um KOR-nee-um	pg. 97	also known as *horny layer*; outermost layer of the epidermis, composed of corneocytes
stratum germinativum STRAT-um jur-min-ah-TIV-um	pg. 95	also known as *basal cell layer*; active layer of the epidermis above the papillary layer of the dermis; cell mitosis takes place here to produce new epidermal skin cells (responsible for growth)
stratum granulosum STRAT-um gran-yoo-LOH-sum	pg. 97	also known as *granular layer*; layer of the epidermis composed of cells filled with keratin that resemble granules; replaces cells shed from the stratum corneum
stratum lucidum STRAT-um LOO-sih-dum	pg. 97	clear, transparent layer of the epidermis under the stratum corneum; thickest on the palms of hands and soles of feet
stratum spinosum STRAT-um spy-NOH-sum	pg. 96	also known as the *spiny layer*; layer of the epidermis above the stratum germinativum (basal) layer containing desmosomes, the intercellular connections made of proteins
subcutaneous layer sub-kyoo-TAY-nee-us LAY-ur	pg. 91	also known as *hypodermis*; subcutaneous adipose (fat) tissue located beneath the dermis; protective cushion; energy storage for the body
subcutis tissue sub-KYOO-tis TISH-oo	pg. 91	also known as *adipose tissue*; fatty tissue found below the dermis that gives smoothness and contour to the body, contains fat for use as energy, and also acts as a protective cushion for the outer skin
sudoriferous glands sood-uh-RIF-uh-rus GLANZ	pg. 89	also known as *sweat glands*; excrete perspiration, regulate body temperature, and detoxify the body by excreting excess salt and unwanted chemicals
T cells TEE SELL	pg. 105	identify molecules that have foreign peptides; help regulate immune response
telangiectasia tel-an-jee-ek-TAY-zhuh	pg. 114	capillaries that have been damaged and are now larger, or distended, blood vessels; commonly called couperose skin

transepidermal water loss TRANS-ep-uh-der-muhl WAH-tur LOSS	pg. 88	abbreviated *TEWL*; water loss caused by evaporation on the skin's surface
tyrosinase TAH-roz-in-ays	pg. 98	the enzyme that stimulates melanocytes and thus produces melanin
UVA radiation YOO-VEE-AY ray-DEE-aye-shun	pg. 107	also known as *aging rays*; longer wavelengths ranging between 320 and 400 nanometers that penetrate deeper into the skin than UVB; cause genetic damage and cell death; UVA contributes up to 95 percent of the sun's ultraviolet radiation.
UVB radiation YOO-VEE-BEE ray-DEE-aye-shun	pg. 108	also known as *burning rays*; UVB wavelengths range between 290 and 320 nanometers; UVB rays have shorter, burning wavelengths that are stronger and more damaging than UVA rays; UVB causes burning of the skin as well as tanning, skin aging, and cancer

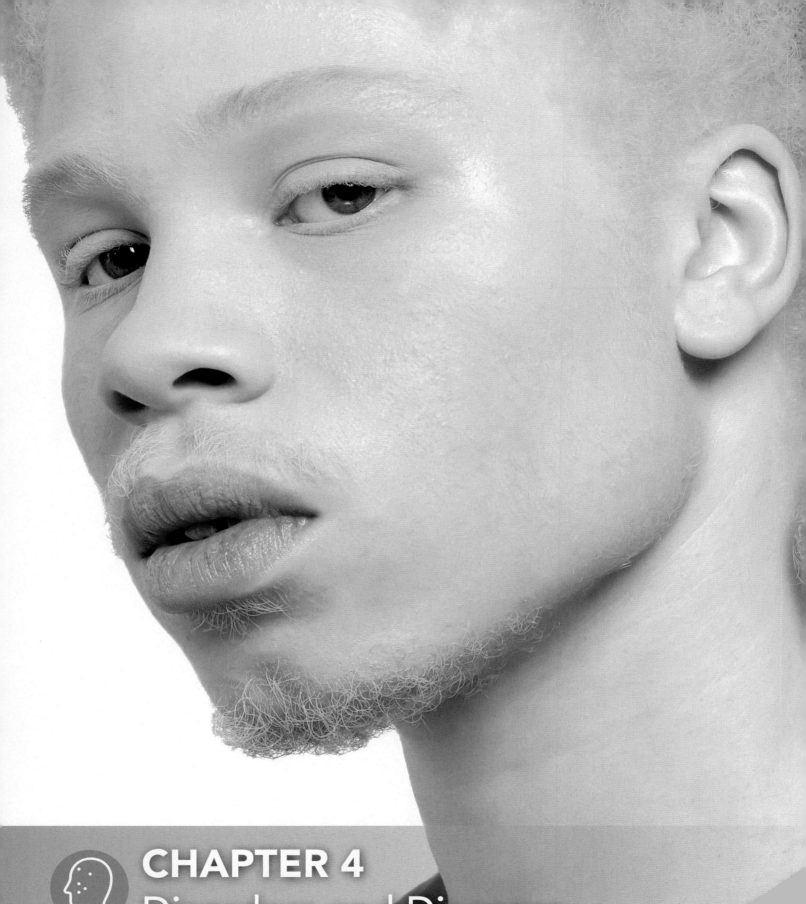

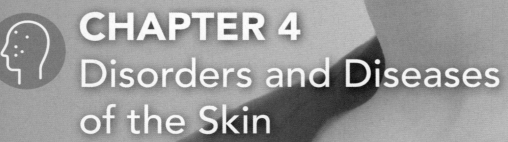

CHAPTER 4
Disorders and Diseases
of the Skin

"Always remember that you are absolutely unique. Just like everyone else."

–Margaret Mead

Learning Objectives

After completing this chapter, you will be able to:

1. Explain why knowledge of diseases and disorders is valuable for an esthetician.
2. Describe how an esthetician and a dermatologist can work collaboratively.
3. Identify the differences between primary, secondary, and tertiary skin lesions.
4. Recognize skin changes that could indicate a type of skin cancer.
5. Describe the types of acne.
6. Describe the symptoms of polycystic ovarian syndrome (PCOS).
7. List common vascular conditions or disorders.
8. Identify pigment disorders.
9. Describe the different types of dermatitis.
10. Identify the types of hypertrophies.
11. Define nine contagious skin and nail diseases.
12. Identify two mental health conditions that may manifest as skin conditions.
13. Recognize common skin conditions related to skin diseases and disorders.
14. Explain five sudoriferous gland disorders.

Explain Why Knowledge of Diseases and Disorders is Valuable for an Esthetician

Skin disorders and diseases are fascinating and complex subjects. Estheticians must be knowledgeable about skin disorders and diseases. As an esthetician, it is not within your scope of practice to diagnose skin diseases, but being savvy enough to recognize common medical conditions can help you work with clients more effectively and safely.

Estheticians can provide client education and help clients with many of their skin concerns. Individuals that have skin problems can be affected emotionally by dealing with such a visible problem. Clients are in a vulnerable position when they bare their skin to you. Sensitivities about visible imperfections can have a lifetime effect on self-esteem. Even in the classroom, permitting our skin to be closely examined by others can be uncomfortable. Use positive words of encouragement and be mindful of how you discuss skin problems tactfully.

Never work on any skin condition you do not recognize. When in doubt, stop the service. Let clients know if you do not recognize a condition or lesion, and they will appreciate your honesty and caution. Posting a photo of your client's skin on social media and asking for advice is not the way to get the right answers on how to treat your client's skin.

Estheticians should study and have a thorough understanding of disorders and diseases of the skin because:

- Recognizing a potentially contagious skin disorder can stop the spread of infection.
- You will help individuals that have skin problems and have been affected emotionally by dealing with such a visible problem.
- Learning when to stop a service and refer a client to a medical professional may save their life.

Describe How an Esthetician and a Dermatologist Can Work Collaboratively

Dermatology (dur-muh-TAHL-uh-jee) is the branch of medical science that studies and treats the skin and its disorders and diseases. A dermatologist (dur-muh-TAHL-uh-jist) is a physician who treats these disorders and diseases. Recognizing skin disorders and diseases is important for the protection of both the technician and the client. Estheticians may not perform services on clients who have contagious or infectious diseases. Dermatologists, physicians, and nurse practitioners are qualified to diagnose skin problems. Estheticians may not diagnose disorders and diseases of the skin. It is outside of their scope of practice. However, once diagnosed, estheticians can help clients with many common disorders and conditions such as rosacea, acne, and hyperpigmentation. Caution and strict infection control practices are imperative when working with skin disorders. Knowledge of skin conditions that *contraindicate* (prohibit) a treatment is also necessary.

Some lesions fit into more than one category and have more than one name or definition. Skin disorders are not easy to categorize, as they can be as diverse as the individuals dealing with the conditions and symptoms.

Estheticians can work as members of a dermatology team to provide skin care treatments that will help to alleviate many of the symptoms of diagnosed diseases and disorders (**Figure 4–1**).

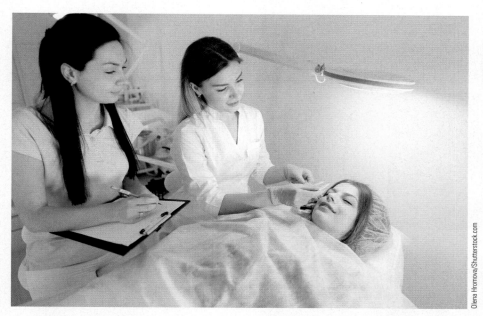

▲ **FIGURE 4–1** Estheticians are valuable members of the dermatology team.

 CHECK IN

1. What is the medical study of the skin called?
2. Why can't an esthetician diagnose disorders or diseases?

Identify the Differences Between Primary, Secondary, and Tertiary Skin Lesions

Lesions (LEE-zhuns) are structural changes in the tissues caused by damage or injury. Any mark, wound, or abnormality is described as a lesion. The three types of lesions are primary, secondary, and tertiary. Some references call tertiary, or third type of lesions, *vascular lesions*. Vascular lesions involve the blood or circulatory system.

Primary Lesions

Primary lesions (PRY-mayr-ee LEE-zhuns) are lesions in the initial stages of development or change. Primary lesions are characterized by flat,

---

CAUTION!

Do not attempt to diagnose or treat medical conditions. Estheticians are not licensed to diagnose skin disorders or diseases. Refer clients to a medical professional if you think they have a disorder or disease that needs medical attention.

ACTIVITY

Research Local Dermatology Offices

Check out the websites of local dermatology offices. Record how many dermatology offices include estheticians as part of their staff. Write down three reasons that a dermatology office should have estheticians on their staff and present to the class.

nonpalpable changes in skin color or by elevations formed by fluid in a cavity, such as vesicles or pustules. Refer to **Table 4–1** for descriptions for primary lesions of the skin and examples of each.

▼ **TABLE 4–1** Primary Lesions

Primary lesions	Pronunciation	Image	Graphic	Description	Examples
Bulla	BULL-uh, (plural: bullae [BULL-ay])			Large blister containing a watery fluid; similar to a vesicle. Requires medical referral.	Contact dermatitis, large second degree burns, bulbous impetigo, pemphigus
Cyst and tubercle	SIST TOO-bur-kul	\n© Courtesy DermNet NZ		Closed, abnormally developed sac that contains pus, semifluid, or morbid matter, above or below the skin. A cyst can be drained of fluid and a tubercle cannot. Requires medical referral.	*Cyst*: Severe acne *Tubercle*: Lipoma, erythema nodosum
Macule	MAK-yool, (plural: maculae [MAK-yuh-ly])	\n© Aneese/Photos.com		Flat spot or discoloration on the skin.	Freckle or 'age spot'
Nodule	NOD-yool	\nSue McDonald /Shutterstock.com		A solid bump larger than 0.4 inches (1 cm) that can be easily felt. Requires medical referral.	Swollen lymph nodes, rheumatoid nodules

(Continues)

(Continued)

Primary lesions	Pronunciation	Image	Graphic	Description	Examples
Papule	PAP-yool			A small elevation on the skin that contains no fluid, but may develop pus.	Acne, warts, elevated nevi
Pustule	PUS-chool			Raised, inflamed, papule with a white or yellow center containing pus in the top of the lesion.	Acne, impetigo, folliculitis
Tumor	TOO-mur			Abnormal mass varying in size, shape, and color. Any type of abnormal mass, not always cancer. Requires medical referral.	Cancer
Vesicle	VES-ih-kel			Small blister or sac containing clear fluid, lying within or just beneath the epidermis. Requires medical referral if cause is unknown or untreatable with over-the-counter products.	Poison ivy, poison oak
Wheal	WHEEL			An itchy, swollen lesion that can be caused by a blow, scratch, bite of an insect, or **urticaria** (ur-tuh-KAYR-ee-ah) (skin allergy), or the sting of a nettle. Typically resolves on its own, but referral to a physician should be considered when the condition lasts more than three days.	Hives, mosquito bites

Image credits: Ocskay Bence/Shutterstock.com; Faiz Zaki/Shutterstock.com; © Courtesy DermNet NZ; Margoe Edwards/Shutterstock.com

Secondary Lesions

Secondary skin lesions (SEK-un-deh-ree SKIN LEE-zhuns) are characterized by piles of material on the skin surface, such as a crust or scab, or by depressions in the skin surface, such as an ulcer. These may require medical referral. Refer to **Table 4–2** for examples and definitions of secondary skin lesions.

▼ **TABLE 4–2** Secondary Lesions

Secondary lesion	Pronunciation	Image	Graphic	Description	Examples
Crust	kruhst	 Pan Xunbin/Shutterstock.com		Dead cells that form over a wound or blemish while healing; accumulation of sebum and pus, sometimes mixed with epidermal cells.	Scab, sore
Excoriation	ek-skor-ee-AY-shun	 R. Baran 'The Nail in Differential Diagnosis" with permission of Informa (London).		Skin sore or abrasion produced by scratching or scraping.	Nail cuticle damage from nail biting
Fissure	FISH-ur	 iibrakv/Shutterstock.com		Crack in the skin that penetrates the dermis.	Severely cracked and/or chapped hands, lips, or feet
Keloid	KEE-loyd			A thick scar resulting from excessive growth of fibrous tissue. Keloids will form along any type of scar for people susceptible to them.	

(Continues)

Secondary lesion	Pronunciation	Image	Graphic	Description	Examples
Scale	skeyl	ibrakv/Shutterstock.com		Thin, dry, or oily plate of epidermal flakes.	Excessive dandruff, psoriasis
Scar or cicatrix	Skahr OR SIK-uh-triks	Geo-grafika/Shutterstock.com		Slightly raised or depressed area of the skin that forms as a result of the healing process related to an injury or lesion.	Post-operative repair
Ulcer	UL-sur	Ilya Andriyanov/Shutterstock.com		Open lesion on the skin or mucous membrane of the body; accompanied by loss of skin depth and possibly weeping of fluids or pus. Requires medical referral, particularly in clients with underlying medical conditions such as diabetes.	Chicken pox, herpes

CHECK IN

3. Name and define the primary lesions.
4. Name and define the secondary lesions.

Recognize Skin Changes that could Indicate a Type of Skin Cancer

Skin cancer risk increases with cumulative ultraviolet (UV) sun exposure and is found in three distinct forms that vary in severity. Each form is named for the type of cells that are affected. Skin cancer is caused by damage to DNA. Skin cancer form when cells begin to divide rapidly and unevenly. See the **Skin Cancer and Sun Exposure** infographic for some facts on skin cancer. If detected early, these abnormal growths can be removed. If not taken care of, they can be deadly.

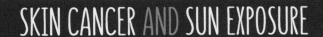

SKIN CANCER AND SUN EXPOSURE

 ABOUT 91,270 NEW MELANOMAS WILL BE DIAGNOSED (ABOUT 55,150 IN MEN AND 36,120 IN WOMEN) **EVERY YEAR**.

SKIN CANCER IS THE MOST COMMON CANCER DIAGNOSIS FOR **MEN OVER AGE 50**.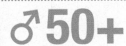

ABOUT **9,320 PEOPLE** ARE EXPECTED TO DIE OF MELANOMA (ABOUT 5,990 MEN AND 3,330 WOMEN) **EVERY YEAR**.

 MORE THAN 90% OF SKIN CANCER IS CAUSED BY SUN EXPOSURE. NON-MELANOMA SKIN CANCER IS CAUSED BY THE **UV RAYS** FROM THE SUN.

 ONE PERSON DIES OF MELANOMA **EVERY HOUR**.

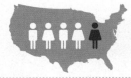 1 IN 5 AMERICANS WILL BE DIAGNOSED IN THEIR LIFETIME WITH SKIN CANCER.

ONE BAD BURN IN CHILDHOOD DOUBLES THE RISK FACTOR FOR MELANOMA LATER IN LIFE. A BLISTERING SUNBURN DURING CHILDHOOD INCREASES THE RISK OF MELANOMA AS AN ADULT. MELANOMA IS **THE DEADLIEST** FORM OF SKIN CANCER.

 SKIN CANCER **KILLS** MORE WOMEN IN THEIR LATE 20s AND EARLY 30s THAN BREAST CANCER DOES.

THERE IS A **75% INCREASE** OF MELANOMA RISK AMONG THOSE WHO USE TANNING BEDS IN THEIR TEENS AND TWENTIES.

Using sensitivity and concern, suggest that the client seek medical advice without diagnosing or speculating about the disorder. For example, you could say, "I'm concerned about this area on your fore-head. Before I do any treatment on it, I need you to see your health care provider for an evaluation. I'll perform your service today and avoid this area." Clients will appreciate your concern and know that you have their best interests at heart. Annual medical skin checks are recommended for everyone to look for changes in the skin.

Actinic keratosis

An **actinic keratosis** (ak-TIN-ik Kara-toe-sis) is a pink or flesh-colored precancerous lesion that feels sharp or rough and is a result of sun damage. It should be checked by a dermatologist.

Types of Skin Cancer

There are three main types of skin cancer. Refer to **Table 4–3** for descriptions of each.

▼ **TABLE 4–3** Types of Skin Cancer

Moles	Description	Image
Normal Mole	Small brownish spot on the skin ranging in color from pale tan to brown or bluish black. *Note:* This is NOT a type of skin cancer.	© D. Kucharski K. Kucharska/Shutterstock.com
Basal Cell Carcinoma (BAY-zul SEL kar-sin-OH-mah)	Most common and least severe type of skin cancer, which often appears as light, pearly nodules; characteristics include sores, reddish patches, or a smooth growth with an elevated border.	
Squamous Cell Carcinoma (SKWAY-mus SEL kar-sin-OH-mah)	More serious than basal cell carcinoma; characterized by scaly, red or pink papules or nodules; also appear as open sores or crusty areas; can grow and spread in the body.	
Malignant Melanoma (muh-LIG-nent mel-uh-NOH-mah)	Most serious form of skin cancer as it can spread quickly (metastasize); black or dark patches on the skin are usually uneven in texture, jagged, or raised; melanomas may have surface crust or bleed. Malignant melanoma is the least common, but is 100 percent fatal if left untreated—early detection and treatment can result in a 94 percent five-year survival rate, but that drops drastically (62 percent) once it reaches local lymph nodes.	

Infrequent, intense UV exposure may increase the risk for melanoma more than chronic continuous exposure does. People with light skin and a tendency to burn with sun exposure are more susceptible to skin cancer.

ONCOLOGY ESTHETICS

A medical niche has emerged for the esthetician certified in *oncology* esthetics. As referenced in chapter 1, oncology is the medical study of cancer, its causes and treatments. Treating skin that has been exposed to radiation and chemotherapy requires a depth of knowledge beyond basic esthetics. The skin can be much more fragile and reactive. Additionally, you don't want to provide any treatment or skin care products that could be contraindicated with their cancer treatment. Clients with cancer still need the healing benefits of touch and can additionally benefit from skin care treatments that are soothing and calming.

ABCDEs of Melanoma Detection

The American Cancer Society recommends using the ABCDE Skin Cancer Checklist to help make potential skin cancer easier to recognize. When checking existing moles, look for changes in any of the following (**Figure 4–2**):

- **A: Asymmetry**—The two sides of the lesion are not identical.
- **B: Border**—The border is irregular on these lesions.
- **C: Color**—Melanomas are usually dark and have more than one color or colors that fade into one another.
- **D: Diameter**—The lesion in a melanoma is usually at least the size of a pencil eraser.
- **E: Evolving**—Melanoma as a lesion often changes appearance.

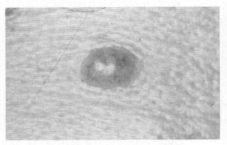
Benign mole—symmetrical

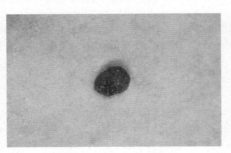
Benign mole—one shade

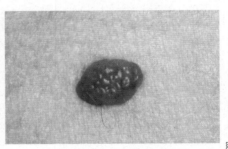
Benign mole—even edges

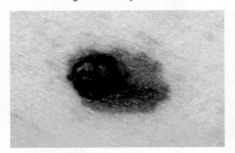
Melanoma—asymmetrical

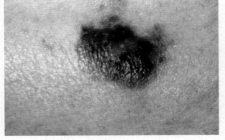
Melanoma—two or more shades

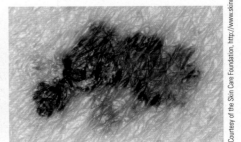
Melanoma—uneven edges

Courtesy of the Skin Care Foundation, http://www.skincancer.org

▲ **FIGURE 4–2** Normal moles compared to cancerous moles that show signs of asymmetry and changes to border, color, and diameter.

Changes to any of these characteristics should be examined by a medical professional. For more information, contact the American Cancer Society at www.cancer.org or (800) ACS-2345.

As estheticians, we may see our clients much more regularly than a client will see their medical provider. We can be key in noting a skin change and referring the client to a dermatologist for diagnosis and treatment.

 CHECK IN

5. Describe the differences between the three types of skin cancer.
6. Explain the checklist system used to identify skin cancers.

Describe the Types of Acne

Acne (AK-nee) is an inflammatory skin disorder of the sebaceous glands, medically known as *acne simplex* or *acne vulgaris*. It is characterized by excess sebum production. This excess oil and dead skin cells can plug pores, creating comedones, papules and pustules, and cysts. This causes a growth of *Propionibacterium acne* (*P. acne*) bacteria. Bacteria in the follicles are anaerobic, that is, the bacteria cannot live in the presence of oxygen. When follicles are blocked with sebum and dead skin buildup, oxygen cannot reach the bottom of the follicle.

Sebum can irritate follicles and cause inflammation. As bacteria and inflammation grow, pressure is exerted on the follicle wall. If the wall ruptures, it becomes infected and debris spills out into the dermis. Redness and inflammation occur when that foreign debris created from the dead white blood cells is detected in the skin, and white blood cells move in to fight the infection.

- *Papules* are red, inflamed lesions caused by this process. Papules may become more infected and pus develops. These infected papules become pustules.

- *Pustules* are filled with fluid from the dead white blood cells that fought the infection.

- *Cysts* are nodules made up of deep pockets of infection. Skin forms hardened tissue around the infection to stop the spread of bacteria, which can lead to both depressed and raised scars from damage to the dermal tissue. Because it is in the dermis, this variety of acne—called *cystic acne*—should be treated by a medical professional.

Causes of Clogged Follicles

Acne is something your clients may have to deal with throughout their lives in various stages. It is important for you to understand the causes of acne and treatments to best serve your client. Your consultation and assessment will be important as you develop a treatment plan that will take the causes of acne into consideration.

Knowledge of the anatomy of the pilosebaceous unit gives you a deeper understanding of how acne behaves. **Pilosebaceous unit** (py-luh-seh-BAY-shus YOO-knit) is the term for the entire follicle that includes the hair shaft, sebaceous gland, and sebaceous duct or canal to the surface. The hairless follicle (with attached sebaceous glands) is the main follicle involved in acne.

Clogged follicles are caused by many factors, including excess oil, retention hyperkeratosis, and **sebaceous filaments** (sih-BAY-shus FILL-ah-mentz). Another reason follicles get clogged is that the opening, or ostium (AHS-tee-um), of the follicle may be too small to let impactions out.

Notable sebaceous gland conditions and disorders are discussed in the following sections.

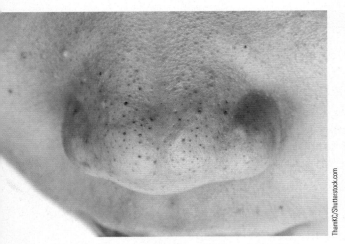

ThamKC/Shutterstock.com

▲ **FIGURE 4–3** An example of a comedo, or comedones.

Types of Clogged Follicles

The types of clogged follicles include the following:

COMEDO

A **comedo** (KAHM-uh-doe) (plural: comedones; KAHM-uh-dohnz) is a noninflamed buildup of cells, sebum, and other debris inside follicles (**Figure 4–3**).

An *open comedo* is a blackhead open at the surface and exposed to air. When the follicle is filled with excess oil a blackhead forms. It is dark because it is exposed to oxygen and oxidation occurs.

A *closed comedo* forms when the openings of the follicles are blocked with debris and white cells. It is also referred to as a *whitehead* but should not be confused with the more hardened white type of papules called milia.

SEBACEOUS FILAMENTS

Sebaceous filaments, similar to open comedones, are mainly small, solidified impactions of oil without the cell matter. These filaments also block the follicle and can cause an acne breakout. They are often found on the nose.

MILIA

Milia (MIL-ee-uh) are small epidermal cysts that appear as firm white papules. Milia are whitish, pearl-like masses of sebum and dead cells under the skin with no visible opening, and are often mistakenly called whiteheads (whiteheads look similar but are soft). Hardened and closed over, milia are more common in dry skin types and may form after skin trauma, such as a laser resurfacing or chronic exposure to UV radiation.

Newborns can sometimes get milia at birth or shortly thereafter. They resemble small sesame seeds and are almost always perfectly round. They are usually found around the eyes, cheeks, and forehead. Milia can also be caused by blocked follicular openings from oil-based moisturizers.

Treatment for milia. Depending on the state, milia can be treated in the salon or spa. Increasing exfoliation and using a retinol product can thin the stratum corneum and gradually eradicate milia. Another treatment option is using an extraction tool to make a tiny opening in the epidermis to expose the milia. With gentle pressure, they usually can be removed from the opening. If they do not pop out, it is best to leave them alone and they will often decompress with regular cleansing, exfoliation, and retinol application.

RETENTION HYPERKERATOSIS

Retention hyperkeratosis (ree-TEN-shun hy-pur-kair-uh-TOH-sis) is a hereditary factor in which dead skin cells build up because they do not shed from the follicles as they do on normal skin. Additionally, excessive sebum production can overtax the sebaceous follicles and cause further cell buildup. Sebum mixed with cells in the follicle become comedones (plugs in the follicles). Consequently, open and closed comedones are formed. While not inflamed, these comedones are the beginning of acne problems if they are not treated with proper skin care to alleviate the impaction.

SEBACEOUS HYPERPLASIA

Sebaceous hyperplasia (sih-BAY-shus hy-pur-PLAY-zhuh) involves benign lesions frequently seen in oilier areas of the face. They are often white, yellow, or flesh-colored. Sebaceous hyperplasia is described as doughnut-shaped with an indentation in the center. Sebaceous material may be found in the center. As cell turnover rate slows with age and androgen levels decline, this causes abnormal cell buildup with very little oil that crowds and enlarges sebaceous glands. Do not mistake these overgrowths of the sebaceous gland for comedones or milia, which may look similar at first. These harmless lesions cannot be removed by extraction. Cryotherapy, surgery, or laser excision are recommended treatment options.

SEBORRHEA

Seborrhea (seb-oh-REE-ah) is a severe oiliness of the skin; an abnormal secretion from the sebaceous glands. When it is in the scalp it is called dandruff or seborrheic dermatitis, but it can occur around the eyebrows, behind the ears, and around the nose or other areas of the face. It is not acne, although the inflammation in the skin from seborrhea can be misidentified as acne. Later in this chapter you will learn more about seborrheic dermatitis.

Grades of Acne

Acne is graded on a scale of 1 to 4 (**Table 4–4**). Grade 1 acne is mild and usually treated with over-the-counter skin care, whereas Grade 4 acne has progressed to consistent breakouts and deep cysts that require medical intervention.

▼ **TABLE 4–4** Grades of Acne

Grades of Acne		
Grade I	Minor breakouts, mostly open comedones, some closed comedones, and a few papules	Kotin/Shutterstock.com
Grade II	Many closed comedones, more open comedones, and occasional papules and pustules	Vladimir Gjorgiev/Shutterstock.com
Grade III	Red and inflamed; many comedones, papules, and pustules	Suzanne Tucker/Shutterstock.com
Grade IV	Cystic acne; cysts with comedones, papules, pustules, and inflammation; scar formation from tissue damage is common	Bangkoker/Shutterstock.com

Acne Triggers

Genetic, hormonal, environmental, lifestyle, certain products, and dietary influences affect acneic breakouts. During the consultation you can ask questions about each of these subjects and learn more to develop a treatment plan to help your client. Educating your client about each of the following factors and getting your client's cooperation in making changes can improve acneic breakouts.

GENETICS

You need to know if your client's parents had acne during puberty or any other time and whether other family members have acne. If acne is a familial disorder, your client's acne will be influenced by that DNA programming.

Treatment for genetic influences. If acne has a genetic component, your client needs to understand that you can help get the breakouts under control but curing the acne will not be possible. With a comprehensive approach that addresses the skin holistically, your clients will experience the best improvements in their skin.

HORMONES

The androgen fluctuations during puberty, monthly menstrual cycle hormone surges, pregnancy, and perimenopause contribute to oil production changes that can bring on comedones, papules, and pustules that usually evidence themselves periodically. Premenstrual water retention can cause slight swelling, enough to influence the epidermis and block pilosebaceous units.

During the consultation, you may have to dig deeper to get a better understanding of hormonally induced acne. You may suggest your client see their medical professional for a change in birth control prescriptions, if the acne developed when the client started on a pill or an intrauterine device (IUD) birth control or following a hormonal injection. If the acne is a result of hormonal changes during pregnancy and perimenopause, you can let your client know that its severity will change as the pregnancy progresses and hormonal fluctuations shift. Your client may be able to influence the breakouts that occur from menstrual cycle hormone surges by limiting sodium intake and increasing water intake.

Treatment for hormonal influences. Treatment options for hormonally induced acne include additional exfoliation to keep the stratum corneum thin so oil can escape to the surface more easily. Commonly this includes chemical peels, enzyme peels, and microdermabrasion options. Home care products can include an antibacterial cleanser, salicylic acid–based products that are lipophilic, and water-based moisturizers.

ENVIRONMENT

Working in an environment with poor air quality, pollutants, or comedogenic exposure can increase the inflammatory response of the sebaceous glands. Dramatic climate changes—including changing seasons, humidity, and temperature—influence oil production.

Understanding your clients' work environment is another aspect of the puzzle you will be solving when helping your clients with acne. Does your client work around oils, chemicals, grease, or ink? Does your client work in an area with poor air quality? Is your client exposed to high levels of carbon dioxide from car exhaust in a city environment?

Treatment for environmental influences. Encouraging your client to cleanse their face at the end of the workday to remove residual pollution, oil, grime, and other pore-clogging factors can improve skin quality. Occlusive products may be too heavy and trap bacteria. Treatments that exfoliate as well as oxygenate the skin can help. The *P. acne* bacteria cannot live in an environment rich with oxygen.

LIFESTYLE

Stress can stimulate the adrenal gland to produce more hormones, which leads to more oil production. Did your client recently start a new job or lose employment? Has your client had a romantic breakup or recently gotten engaged or married? Has there been a death in the family or loss of a close friend? A move to a new home or new town? What about a challenging home situation? A long commute can contribute to stress. Adrenal glands that are constantly excreting adrenalin to keep up with the pace of an overly active lifestyle can create a hormonal imbalance that can affect the skin.

Pressure or friction from cell phones along with wearing hats or scarves and any other device or object that routinely touches the face can transfer bacteria to the face and induce a breakout. Fragrances from dryer sheets, laundry detergents, or shampoos can cause a sensitivity and a breakout.

Treatment for lifestyle influences. Suggesting lifestyle changes to your client can help them find the triggers that stimulate an acne flare-up. Sometimes a simple fix such as more frequent changing of a pillowcase can make a difference.

COSMETICS AND SKIN CARE PRODUCTS

Certain ingredients in products can aggravate acne. Fatty ingredients such as waxes and some oils can clog or irritate follicles. These **comedogenic** (KAHM-uh-doe JEN-ick) ingredients can block follicles, which causes cell buildup, resulting in comedones. Products rich in emollients and occlusive products are too heavy for skin prone to breakouts. Moisturizers and sunscreens should be lighter formulas such as oil-in-water (O/W) emulsions, not water-in-oil (W/O) emulsions. Many makeup products are comedogenic, especially foundations and powders that are made with solids and fatty ingredients. Makeup products become contaminated with unhygienic application techniques. Products for hair and skin can trigger or irritate acne. Products are discussed thoroughly in Chapter 6, Skin Care Products: Chemistry, Ingredients, and Selection.

Treatment for product irritation. Educating your client on routine cleaning of makeup brushes and the use of disposable sponges to apply foundation can help with breakouts.

DIET

An increasing number of studies are linking food allergies or sensitivities to acne. Foods with a higher glucose index, processed foods, foods with heavy iodide content, and dairy are thought to be contributors to acne, although the relationship is not fully understood.

Treatment for dietary influences. You are not a nutritionist or dietician, but you can encourage your clients to eat a healthy diet and drink plenty of water. You can suggest clients see a specialist for dietary changes that may improve the health of their skin.

Medicated Treatment Options for Acne

Regular skin care sessions, with exfoliation and incorporating modalities like high frequency, microdermabrasion, and chemical peels, can help keep the stratum corneum thin, keep oil production under control, add hydration, and oxygenate the skin to eliminate bacteria. Electrical devices and chemical exfoliation are covered in Chapter 10, Facial Devices and Technology, and Chapter 13, Advanced Topics and Treatments. However, treatment options for acne can also include a collaborative approach with medical professionals and the esthetician. They are varied and include the use of topical antibacterial agents to eliminate the *P. acne* bacteria (**Table 4–5**). Antibiotics can be used, both orally and topically. The potential for developing antibiotic resistance is the reason why medical professionals are reducing the use of these drugs to treat chronic acne. If the client acquires a serious infection later in life, antibiotics may not work to fight that infection because of the antibiotic resistance that developed during the long term use to improve the acne.

ACTIVITY

Plan of Care

Develop a plan of care for each grade of acne. Include professional treatment options as well as home care recommendations. Describe your treatment plans to the rest of the class and get feedback on improvements you could make to your plans.

▼ **TABLE 4–5** Common Medications Used in the Treatment of Acne

Drug	Actions	Potential Side Effects
Adapalene (Differin®)	A topical peeling agent similar to retinoic acid; may be less irritating than tretinoin	Drying, redness, and irritation; photosensitivity
Azelaic acid (Azelex®)	A topical acidic agent that flushes out follicles	Drying, redness, and irritation; photosensitivity
Birth control pills	An oral medication used to regulate the androgen hormones that impact oil production	Irregular periods, weight gain, cramps
Clindamycin	Topical antibiotic; kills bacteria	Very drying
Isotretinoin	An oral controlled medication used for severe acne; requires close medical monitoring, including lab work to check liver function, due to its toxicity *Note:* Used as a last resort for severe acne	Severe dryness, birth defects, possible depression, possible suicidal thoughts, and potential for ulcerative colitis; requires participation from both the patient and the medical provider in a mandatory Food and Drug Administration risk management program
Spironolactone	An oral medication used to regulate the androgen hormones that impact oil production; typically prescribed for young women and teens	Irregular menstrual periods, breast tenderness, male pattern facial hair growth, dry mouth
Tazarotene (Tazorac®)	Another retinoid; a topical peeling agent that may be less irritating than tretinoin	Drying, redness, and irritation; photosensitivity
Tretinoin (Retin-A™)	A topical vitamin A acid; a strong peeling agent that is drying and flushes out follicles	Very drying; causes redness and irritation; photosensitivity

CONSIDERATIONS FOR MEDICATED ACNE TREATMENT

You can't "cure" acne, but you can help control the breakouts. The passage of time is often the cure, as a teen moves out of puberty, perimenopause transitions to menopause, or stressful lifestyle habits change. You can help your clients have more confidence in social situations with clearer skin. More information on acne medications available to clients includes the following:

- Home care products should include ingredients with benzoyl peroxide and vitamin A products like tretinoin, retinoids, and adapalene.

- Moisturizers and serums that are low on the comedogenic scale are best. Skin care ingredients are discussed in the chapter on Chapter 6 Skin Care Products: Chemistry, Ingredients, and Selection.

- Benzoyl peroxide products are often combined with topical antibiotics. This combination helps reduce the chances of developing antibiotic resistance. Topical antibiotics alone aren't typically prescribed. These products should be applied in the morning because they can discolor pillowcases.

- Vitamin A products should be applied in the evening because they are photo-sensitizing. Clients should apply a very small pea-sized amount beginning twice a week, increase the application to three times a week, then use the product every other day and finally every day as a tolerance to the product is developed. These products work by thinning the stratum corneum, increasing cell turnover, and preventing hair follicles from becoming clogged with sebum and dead skin cells.

- Salicylic acid and azelaic acid are both antibacterial. Salicylic acid is lipophilic, so it works to digest sebum.

- Oral medications to help with acne in addition to antibiotics are often drugs to counter the effects of androgen hormones. An example is spironolactone.

- Birth control pills are another prescription medication that can influence acne, reducing breakouts from hormonally induced acne.

 CHECK IN

7. Explain the differences between an open and a closed comedone.
8. Describe the four grades of acne.
9. Give examples of three different kinds of medications used to treat acne.

Describe the Symptoms of Polycystic Ovarian Syndrome (PCOS)

Polycystic ovarian syndrome (PCOS) (polee-sistik oh-vair-ee-uh-n sin-druhm), often shortened and pronounced "peecos", is a hormonal condition that affects one in 20 women in their child bearing years, according to the U.S. Department of Health and Human Services (**Figure 4–4**). It is believed to have a genetic component. Symptoms include increased androgen production that causes the development of cysts on the ovaries. The cysts create irregular menstrual cycles and difficulty with fertility. Clients with PCOS are insulin resistant and have challenges with weight loss. Sleep apnea is also a symptom. The esthetician will work with the client who has PCOS because PCOS symptoms include acne, thinning hair in a male hair growth pattern of baldness, which is sparse hair density at the

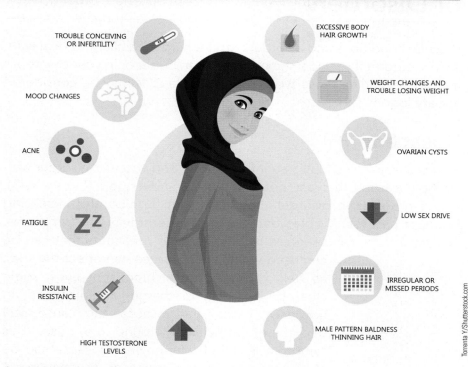

▲ **FIGURE 4–4** Polycystic Ovarian Syndrome (PCOS).

front and top of the scalp. It also causes abnormal hair growth on the face, arms, thighs, neck, and breasts. Clients with PCOS may feel self-conscious about their body image. They may feel they have lost control on many levels.

PCOS is not a condition that is cured, but symptoms can be managed. Birth control pills can help regulate the sex hormones, and androgen-blocking medication can help control hair growth and acne issues. Performing hair removal treatments with waxing or laser services can help keep unwanted hair under better control. Skin care treatments using ingredients that influence the formation of comedones keep the stratum corneum thin. Treatments that influence acne breakouts, like microdermabrasion, high frequency, and an ultrasonic skin scrubber, are helpful. Additionally, providing emotional support can help your client.

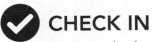 **CHECK IN**

10. Describe how an esthetician could help a client with PCOS.

List Common Vascular Conditions or Disorders

Vascular conditions and disorders can be hard for a client to deal with, so it is important to understand the types to better help your clients. As mentioned earlier, these types of vascular lesions may be considered tertiary lesions.

Rosacea

Rosacea (roh-ZAY-shuh) is an inflammatory and vascular disorder with multiple causes that are not completely understood (**Figure 4–5**). It is a progressive disorder that starts with flushing and increasing bouts of redness. Visible vessels and skin sensitivity are symptoms. The symptoms can progress to pustular-type breakouts that can be confused with acne. Rosacea can affect the eyes as well, causing chronic bloodshot eyes, some clear to yellowish discharge, and irritation. In advanced cases, the rosacea can cause skin thickening, particularly around the nose. This symptom is called *rhinophyma*. Rosacea can be challenging to treat because of its unclear origins. Heredity, bacteria, the dermodex mite, and fungus are possible theories. Certain factors are known to aggravate the condition. **Vasodilation** (vas-oh-dih-LAY-shun) (vascular dilation) of the

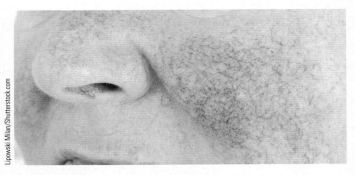

▲ **FIGURE 4–5** An example of rosacea.

blood vessels makes rosacea worse. Spicy foods, alcohol, caffeine, temperature extremes, heat, sun, and stress aggravate rosacea symptoms.

ROSACEA TREATMENTS

Like acne, estheticians can treat the symptoms of rosacea, but cannot cure the disorder. Symptom management is the goal when working with a rosacea client.

Rosacea treatments should include collaboration with medical professionals. Antifungal prescription skin care products may help. Skin calming ingredients and treatments will help decrease the inflammation. Provide soothing facials with gentle massage and light exfoliation. Limit the use of steam. Adding high frequency to oxygenate the skin can help. Some advanced esthetic procedures with lasers, intense pulsed light (IPL), and radio frequency devices can be effective.

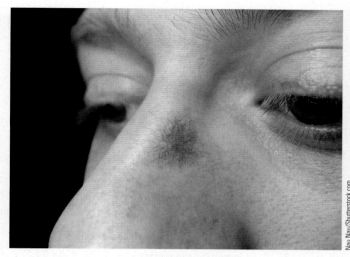

▲ **FIGURE 4–6** An example of telangiectasia.

Telangiectasia

Telangiectasia is visible capillaries, 0.5 to 1.0 mm in diameter, that are commonly found on the face, particularly around the nose, cheeks, and chin (**Figure 4–6**). They can appear due to an injury, heredity, rosacea, hormonal changes, or exposure to extreme cold or heat. A matting of tiny telangiectasia creates a ruddy complexion, called *couperose skin*. Telangiectasia is a cosmetic irregularity and is not a medical condition.

Varicose Veins

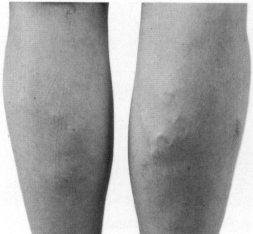

▲ **FIGURE 4–7** An example of varicose veins.

Varicose veins (VAYR-ih-kohs VAYNZ) are visible vascularity that are abnormally dilated and twisted veins that can occur anywhere in the body. They are often on the legs. Pregnancy, extended periods of time standing and sitting, and genetics are contributing factors. Sometimes treatments with *sclerotherapy*, an injection into the vein with a solution that causes the vein to collapse, can cause smaller vessels to disappear (**Figure 4–7**). Varicose veins are a condition that should be treated by a medical professional. Such treatment could include surgery for large twisted vessels.

 CHECK IN

11. Explain the progression of rosacea.
12. List four rosacea triggers.
13. Summarize how to treat rosacea.

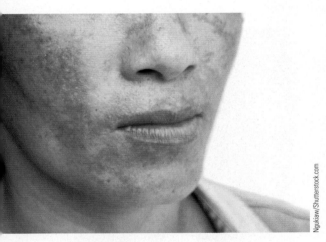

▲ **FIGURE 4–8** Hyperpigmentation.

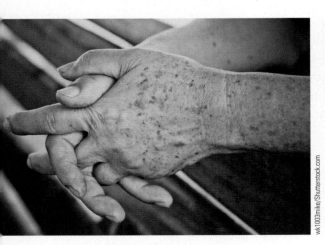

▲ **FIGURE 4–9** Melasma.

Identify Pigment Disorders

The genetic background of a person influences pigmentation disorders. Abnormal pigmentation, referred to as *dyschromia* (diz-KRO-me-ah), can be caused by various internal and external factors. **Hyperpigmentation** (hy-pur-pig-men-TAY-shun), overproduction of pigment, and **hypopigmentation** (hy-poh-pig-men-TAY-shun), lack of pigment, are the two types of pigmentation disorders. Sun exposure is the biggest external cause of pigmentation disorders and can make existing pigmentation disorders worse. Drugs may also cause skin pigmentation abnormalities. Hyperpigmentation is a frequent concern for clients and is discussed in subsequent chapters (**Figure 4–8**).

Hyperpigmentation

Hyperpigmentation appears in the following forms:

MELASMA

Melasma is a type of hormonal hyperpigmentation disorder that first appears during pregnancy or with the use of birth control pills. Melasma has an identifiable pattern of solid fairly symmetrical hyperpigmentation, often on the forehead, cheeks, upper lip, and chin (**Figure 4–9**). Sun exposure can exacerbate the pigmentation of melasma, so a person may have melasma and sun damage.

Addressing the symptoms of melasma can be a challenge for an esthetician. The pigmentation can fade during times of low UV exposure. Hormones returning to normal levels after pregnancy will alleviate the pigmentation. The consistent use of melanocyte-inhibiting skin care products as well as sunscreen application is essential. A series of chemical peels can lighten the pigmentation. Some high-energy laser devices with nanosecond or picosecond technology and fractional radio frequency treatments can offer visible improvements. Melasma is a condition that requires management; there is no cure.

LENTIGO

Lentigo (len-TY-goh) is a flat, pigmented area similar to a freckle; small, yellow-brown spots (**Figure 4–10**). Lentigines (len-tih-JEE-neez) are multiple pigmented lesions. Medical professionals identify lentigenes that result from sunlight exposure as *actinic*, or solar, lentigenes. Your client may call them age spots, as they are associated with aging skin.

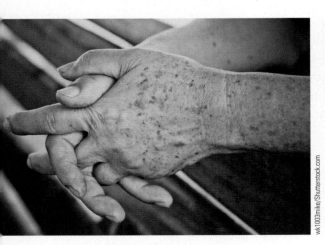

▲ **FIGURE 4–10** Lentigo.

EPHELIDS

Ephelids, also known as freckles, are tiny round or oval pigmented areas of skin on areas exposed to the sun (**Figure 4–11**). Also referred to as *macules*, they are small flat colored spots on the skin.

NEVUS

Nevus (NEE-vus), also known as *birthmark,* is a malformation of the skin from abnormal pigmentation or dilated capillaries that is present at birth or appears shortly after birth. A *port wine stain* is a vascular type of nevus. **Figure 4–12a** is an example of a pigmented nevus. **Figure 4–12b** is an example of a vascular nevus.

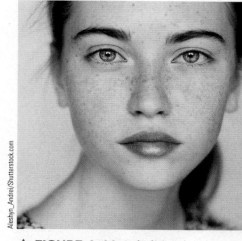

▲ **FIGURE 4–11** Ephelids, also known as freckles.

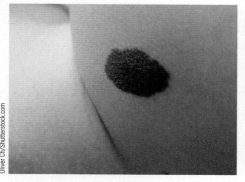

▲ **FIGURE 4–12A** An example of a pigmented nevus.

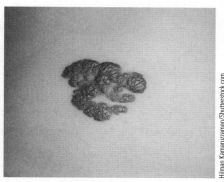

▲ **FIGURE 4–12B** An example of a vascular nevus.

POIKILODERMA OF CIVATTE

Poikiloderma of Civatte (poi-ki-lo-der-ma ov si-vaht) is a skin condition caused by actinic bronzing (chronic sun exposure) to the sides of the face and neck. The skin turns a reddish-brown hue with a distinct white patch under the chin. Poikiloderma is benign, meaning it is not cancerous. Treatment can be a combination of melanocyte-inhibiting skin care, chemical peels, advanced treatments with lasers and IPLs, consistent sunscreen protection, and avoiding irritants, such as heavy fragrances, on the skin.

POSTINFLAMMATORY HYPERPIGMENTATION

Postinflammatory hyperpigmentation (PIH) (POHST-in-flam-uh-tory hy-PER-pig-MEN-tay-shun) is darkened pigmentation due to an injury to the skin or the residual healing after an acne lesion has resolved (**Figure 4–13**). It is often deep red, purple, or brown in appearance.

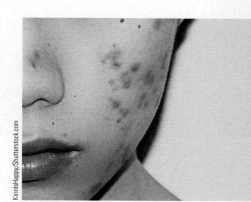

▲ **FIGURE 4–13** Post-inflammatory hyperpigmentation.

TAN

Tan (tan) results from exposure to the sun. Tanning is a change in pigmentation due to melanin production as a defense against UV radiation that damages the skin. A tan is basically visible skin and cell damage.

Hypopigmentation

Hypopigmentation occurs in various forms. It is seen less commonly than hyperpigmentation disorders.

LEUKODERMA

Leukoderma (loo-koh-DUR-ma) is a loss of pigmentation leading to light, abnormal patches of depigmented skin. It is a congenital disorder acquired due to immunological and postinflammatory causes. Vitiligo and albinism are leukodermas.

ALBINISM

Albinism (AL-bi-niz-em) is a rare genetic condition characterized by a lack of melanin pigment in the body, including the skin, hair, and eyes. The person is at risk for skin cancer, is sensitive to light, and ages early without normal melanin protection. The technical term for albinism is *congenital leukoderma or congenital hypopigmentation.*

VITILIGO

Vitiligo (vih-til-EYE-goh) is a pigmentation disease characterized by white irregular patches of skin that are totally lacking pigment (**Figure 4–14**). The condition can worsen with time and sunlight. The disease can occur at any age and is believed to be an autoimmune disorder causing an absence of melanocytes.

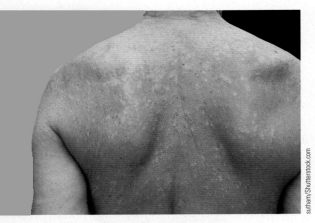

▲ **FIGURE 4–14** White patches of the skin caused by vitiligo.

TINEA VERSICOLOR

Tinea versicolor (TIN-ee-uh VUR-see-kuh-lur), also called *pityriasis versicolor*, is a fungal condition that inhibits melanin production. It is not contagious because it is caused by yeast, a normal part of the human skin. It is characterized by white, brown, or salmon-colored flaky patches (**Figure 4–15**). Sun exposure can stimulate the growth of the fungus. This fungus can be treated with antifungal cream or other medication. Selenium sulfide shampoos can also treat the condition. High humidity and summer heat stimulate the condition. It usually fades in the cold winter season and recurs with warmer weather. To the layperson, tinea versicolor can be misinterpreted as vitiligo, so referral to a medical professional is important.

▲ **FIGURE 4–15** Tinea versicolor.

CHECK IN

14. List three disorders characterized by hyperpigmentation.
15. Describe tinea versicolor and its treatment.

Describe the Different Types of Dermatitis

Dermatitis (derm-a-TIE-tuss) is a generalized term to refer to an inflammatory condition of the skin; various forms include lesions such as eczema, vesicles, or papules (**Figure 4–16**). Dermatitis has many forms, and symptoms of one form can be confused with symptoms of another form. Referral to a medical professional is recommended for appropriate diagnosis.

Types of dermatitis or inflammations of the skin include the following:

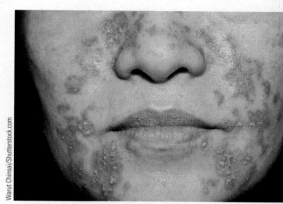

▲ **FIGURE 4–16** An example of dermatitis on the face.

Contact Dermatitis

Occupational disorders from ingredients in cosmetics and chemical solutions can cause **contact dermatitis** (KAHN-takt der-mah-TYT-is), or *dermatitis venenata*. Contact with allergens and caustic chemicals can also cause skin sensitivity or disorders. Allergies and skin eruptions are common. Wearing gloves or protective skin creams while working with chemicals or irritating substances can help prevent contact dermatitis.

Allergic Contact Dermatitis

Allergic contact dermatitis is caused by exposure to and direct skin contact with an allergen. Normally the immune system protects us from pathogens and disease, but with an allergic reaction the immune system causes the problem by trying to do its job too well. An allergic reaction occurs when our immune system mistakes a benign substance for a toxic one and initiates a major defense against it.

Initial exposure to an allergen does not always cause an allergic reaction. The development of hypersensitivity is the result of repeated exposure to an allergen over time. This process is called **sensitization** (SEN-sih-tiz-A-shun), and it may take months or years depending on the allergen and the intensity of exposure. Also remember that different people develop allergies to different allergens. Individual predisposition to allergies may be inherited; sensitivity seems to run in families.

Contact dermatitis and red, itchy skin can be caused by an allergic reaction or contact with an irritant, such as these common allergens:

- Makeup
- Skin care products
- Detergents
- Dyes

CAUTION!

The following reactions from chemicals are commonly seen in the salon:

- On the practitioner's fingers, palms, or on the back of the hand
- On the practitioner's face, especially the cheeks
- On the client's scalp, hairline, forehead, or neckline

If you examine the area where the problem occurs, you can usually determine the cause.

For example, technicians may react to chemicals in disinfectants or strong skin care products. This is both prolonged and repeated contact. Sensitization is an increased or exaggerated sensitivity to products. Wear gloves to avoid potential reactions. Eyes and lungs can also be affected by exposure to strong chemicals or other ingredients.

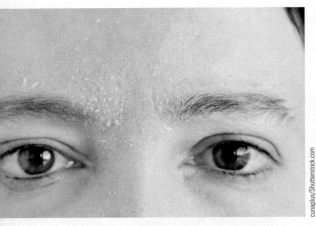

▲ **FIGURE 4–17** Atopic dermatitis caused by allergies.

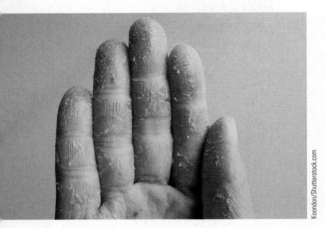

▲ **FIGURE 4–18** Eczema on the hands.

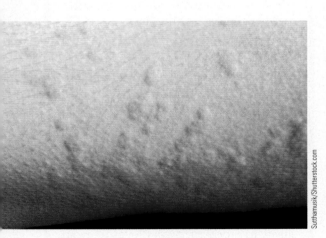

▲ **FIGURE 4–19** Irritant contact dermatitis.

- Fabrics
- Jewelry
- Plants
- Red dyes in products
- Nickel in jewelry

Atopic Dermatitis

Atopic dermatitis (UH-top-ick DERM-uh-tit-is) is a chronic, relapsing form of dermatitis (*atopic* means "excess inflammation from allergies"). Irritants and allergens trigger reactions that include dry, cracked skin (**Figure 4–17**). The redness, itching, and dehydration of the dermatitis make the condition worse. Use of humidifiers and lotion can help keep the skin more hydrated. Topical corticosteroids can relieve the symptoms.

Eczema

Eczema (EG-zuh-muh) is an inflammatory, painful, itching disease of the skin; is acute or chronic in nature; and has dry or moist lesions (**Figure 4–18**). A client with eczema should be referred to a physician. Avoid contact and skin care treatments if a client has eczema.

Irritant Contact Dermatitis

Everyone who comes in contact with an irritant is affected by irritant reactions, although the degree of irritation will vary depending on the individual. In acute cases, symptoms are noticed immediately or within just a few hours. Chronic cases may be delayed reactions that take weeks, months, or years to develop. Symptoms range from redness, swelling, scaling, and itching to serious, painful chemical burns (**Figure 4–19**). Irritating substances temporarily damage the epidermis. Caustic substances are examples of irritants. When the skin is damaged by irritating substances, the immune system springs into action. It floods the tissue with water, trying to dilute the irritant. Therefore, swelling occurs.

The immune system also releases histamines, which enlarge the vessels around the injury. Blood can then rush to the area more quickly and help remove the irritating substance. The extra blood under the skin is easily visible. The entire area becomes red and warm, and it may throb. Histamines cause the itchy feeling that often accompanies contact dermatitis. After everything calms down, the swelling will go away. The surrounding skin is often left damaged, scaly, cracked, and dry. Fortunately, irritations are not permanent.

If you avoid repeated and/or prolonged contact with the irritating substance, the skin will usually quickly repair itself; however, continued or repeated exposure may lead to chronic allergic reactions and skin damage.

You may notice irritant contact dermatitis when a teen client comes in for an acne consultation. You may note a breakout on the client's chin and learn they play football. You must rule out the possibility of irritant contact dermatitis from the football helmet chin strap before beginning a treatment plan for the acne.

Perioral Dermatitis

Perioral dermatitis (pair-ee-OR-ul derm-a-TIE-tuss) is an acne-like condition around the mouth consisting mainly of small clusters of papules. It may be caused by toothpaste or products used on the face (**Figure 4–20**). It is not contagious. Antibiotics can help treat the condition.

Seborrheic Dermatitis

Seborrheic dermatitis (seb-oh-REE-ick derm-a-TIE-tuss) is a form of eczema characterized by inflammation, dry or oily scaling or crusting, and/or itchiness (**Figure 4–21**). The red, flaky skin often appears in the eyebrows, on the scalp and along the hairline, in the middle of the forehead, and along the sides of the nose. One cause is inflammation of the sebaceous glands. This condition is sometimes treated with cortisone creams. Severe cases should be referred to a dermatologist.

Stasis Dermatitis

Stasis dermatitis (stay-sus-dur-muh-TY-tus) is caused by poor circulation in the lower legs that can create a chronic inflammatory state. The legs may sometimes have ulcerations, along with scaly skin, itching, and hyperpigmentation. The hyperpigmentation is caused by hemosiderin staining, a brown-reddish discoloration due to iron deposits in the blood leaking into the tissues (**Figure 4–22**). A client with this type of skin disorder needs a cardiovascular referral. Even when the circulatory issues are resolved, the hemosiderin staining can remain. Advanced esthetic treatments with IPL can help improve the appearance.

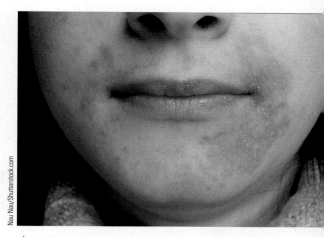
▲ **FIGURE 4–20** Perioral dermatitis around the mouth.

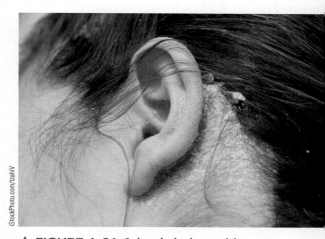
▲ **FIGURE 4–21** Seborrheic dermatitis.

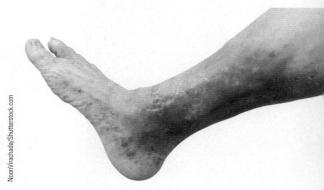
▲ **FIGURE 4–22** Stasis dermatitis caused by poor circulation.

✓ CHECK IN

16. List the inflammations of the skin.

Identify the Types of Hypertrophies

Hypertrophy (hy-PUR-truh-fee) is defined as an abnormal growth; many are *benign*, or harmless; however, some growths are premalignant or malignant and can be dangerous or cancerous. The term *hypertrophic* is used to describe thickening of a tissue. The opposite of hypertrophy is *atrophy*, which means "wasting away or thinning". Keloids are an example of hypertrophies.

Types of hypertrophies include the following:

- **Hyperkeratosis** (hy-pur-kair-uh-TOH-sis)—thickening of the skin caused by a mass of keratinocytes.
- **Keratoma** (kair-uh-TOH-muh)—an acquired thickened patch of epidermis. A callus caused by pressure or friction is a keratoma. If the thickening also grows inward, it becomes a corn.
- **Keratosis** (kair-uh-TOH-sis) (plural: keratoses; kair-uh-TOH-seez)—an abnormally thick buildup of skin cells.
- **Keratosis pilaris** (kair-uh-TOH-sis py-LAIR-us)—redness and bumpiness in the cheeks, upper arms, or thighs; caused by blocked follicles. It has the appearance of "chicken skin" (**Figure 4–23**). It is not well understood but is often genetic and disappears after the age of 30. Many young women feel self-conscious about this condition and will seek an esthetician's help. Topical chemical exfoliants that keep the follicles free of keratin, like alpha hydroxyl acid (AHA) or beta hydroxyl acid (BHA) products, along with light mechanical exfoliation, can help unblock follicles and alleviate the rough feeling. Care must be taken to prevent too aggressive an approach and disturb the acid mantle balance, causing dermatitis or infection.
- **Mole** (MOHL)—a pigmented nevus; a brownish spot ranging in color from tan to bluish black. Some are flat, resembling freckles; others

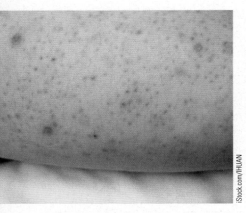

▲ FIGURE 4–23 Keratosis pilaris caused by blocked follicles.

iStock.com/IHUAN

are raised and darker. Most are benign, but changes in mole color or shape should be checked by a physician. Hairs in moles are common. The hair may be tweezed from a mole if the client desires. The belief that hair in moles should not be removed is an old wives' tale. Moles should be observed for changes with the American Cancer Society's ABCDEs of melanoma check.

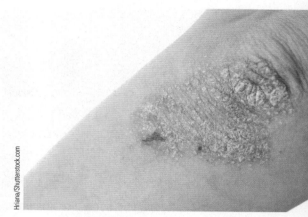

▲ FIGURE 4–24 Psoriasis consisting of red patches.

- **Psoriasis** (suh-RY-uh-sis)—an itchy skin disease characterized by red patches covered with white-silver scales; caused by an overproliferation of skin cells that replicate too fast (**Figure 4–24**). Psoriasis is usually found in patches on the scalp, elbows, knees, chest, and lower back. If patches are irritated, bleeding can occur. Psoriasis is not contagious but can be spread by irritating the affected area. It is thought to be an autoimmune disorder and clients experience flare-ups that can be controlled with oral and topical medications. Light therapy is also thought to be helpful. Clients with psoriasis are often also diagnosed with cardiovascular disease.

- **Skin tag** (skin tag)—small outgrowth or extension of the skin that looks like a flap. They are benign and are common under the arms, on the neck, or breast area caused by friction (**Figure 4–25**).

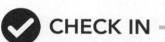 **CHECK IN**

17. What are four hypertrophies of the skin?
18. How is keratosis pilaris treated?

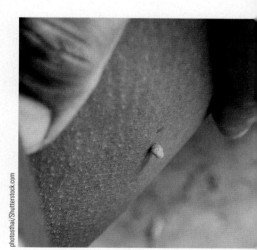

▲ FIGURE 4–25 A skin tag.

Define Nine Contagious Skin and Nail Diseases

The term *contagious disease* is used interchangeably with the terms *infectious* or *communicable disease*. Do not perform services on anyone with a contagious disease because it can spread and infect others. Refer them to a medical professional.

The following are contagious diseases:

- **Conjunctivitis** (kun-junk-tuh-VY-tus), also known as *pinkeye*—inflammation of the mucous membrane (conjunctiva) around the eye due to chemical, bacterial, or viral causes; very contagious (**Figure 4–26**). It can be treated with antibiotics.

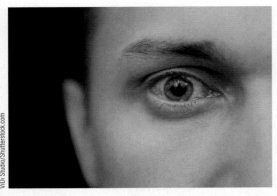

▲ FIGURE 4–26 Conjunctivitis, also known as pinkeye.

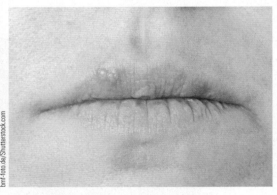

▲ FIGURE 4–27 Herpes simplex virus 1 on the lips.

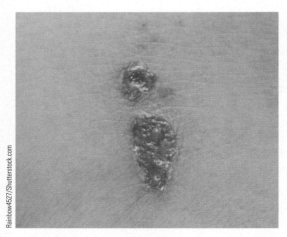

▲ FIGURE 4–28 Never work on a client who has active herpes lesions.

- **Herpes simplex virus 1** (HER-peez SIM-pleks VY-rus ONE)—fever blisters or cold sores; recurring viral infection; a vesicle or group of vesicles on a red, swollen base. The blisters usually appear on the lips or nostrils (**Figure 4–27**). Herpes simplex virus 1 causes cold sores and lesions around the mouth. It is a contagious disease treated with antiviral medication to shorten the outbreak.

- **Herpes simplex virus 2** (HER-peez SIM-pleks VY-rus TOO)—genital herpes; never work on clients with active herpes lesions (**Figure 4–28**). Peels, waxing, or other stimuli may cause a breakout, even if the condition is not currently active. The virus can be spread to other areas on the person that is infected or to other people. This is an example of why reviewing the client intake form is important.

- **Herpes zoster** (HER-peez ZOHS-tur), also known as *shingles*—a painful skin condition due to reactivation of the chickenpox virus; also known as the varicella-zoster virus (VZV). Shingles is a viral infection of the sensory nerves characterized by groups of red blisters that form a rash that occurs in a ring or line (**Figure 4–29**). The rash is typically confined to one side of the body. VZV can cause nerve and organ damage along with severe pain that can last for months or years. Treatment includes antiviral drugs to shorten the length of the outbreak.

- **Impetigo** (im-puh-TEE-go)—a bacterial infection of the skin that often occurs in children; characterized by clusters of small blisters or crusty lesions filled with bacteria (**Figure 4–30**). It is extremely contagious. Oral and topical antibiotics are used in treatment. An untrained eye may misinterpret impetigo and assume herpes, acne, or dermatitis. Professional medical intervention is the correct course of action for your client.

- **Onychomycosis** (ahn-ih-koh-my-KOH-sis)—fungal infection that produces symptoms of thick, brittle, discolored nails (**Figure 4–31**). The fungus lives off the keratin in the nails. Onychomycosis can be challenging to eradicate because fungus likes to grow in dark moist places, and shoes can be the perfect environment. Clients with onychomycosis can feel embarrassed about the appearance of the nails and discouraged during a course of treatment because of slow nail growth. Estheticians could encounter this when doing body wraps, or during hand and foot massages with a facial. If onychomycosis is discovered, the facial service can be continued, but the esthetician should not continue with the hand/foot massage.

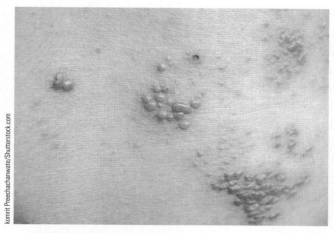

▲ **FIGURE 4–29** Herpes zoster, also known as shingles, is characterized by groups of red blisters that form a rash in a ring or line.

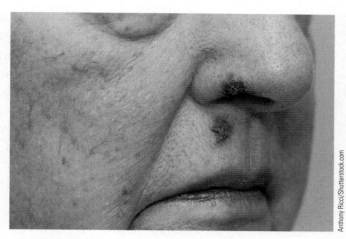

▲ **FIGURE 4–30** Impetigo is characterized by clusters of small blisters or crusty lesions filled with bacteria and is extremely contagious.

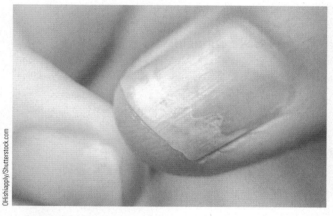

▲ **FIGURE 4–31** Onychomycosis is a fungal infection that produces symptoms of thick, brittle, discolored nails.

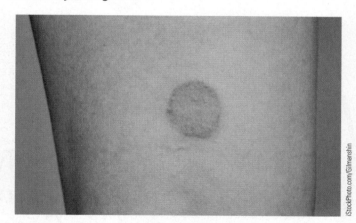

▲ **FIGURE 4–32** Tinea corporis, also known as ringworm, is caused by a fungus that spreads into a red and scaly circular infection.

- **Tinea** (TIN-ee-uh)—fungal infections. Fungi feed on proteins, carbohydrates, and lipids in the skin. Tinea pedis, athlete's foot, is a fungal infection that can be treated with antifungal topical powders, sprays, or creams. Estheticians could encounter this type of infection when doing body wraps, or during hand and foot massages with a facial. If you are reviewing a client intake form and see the word *tinea*, you will know that the client has a fungus and you should determine the location prior to treatment.

- **Tinea corporis** (TIN-ee-uh KOR-pur-is), also known as **ringworm**— caused by a fungus; is not a worm. It looks like a skin irritation that spreads into a circular infection that is red and scaly (**Figure 4–32**). It can be dry or moist. It can be spread by direct contact as well as indirect contact with items that have touched the skin of the infected person. Pets can carry tinea corporis. It is important to use a fungicide to disinfect items that have come in contact with the client who has the infection, including clothing, blankets, and towels. It can be treated with either oral or topical antifungals.

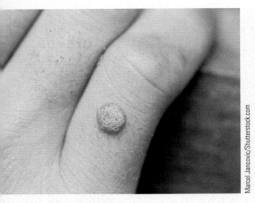

▲ FIGURE 4–33 A wart, or verruca, is typically flesh colored but can be brown or black and may also appear singly or in clusters.

- **Verruca** (vuh-ROO-kuh), also known as *wart*—a hypertrophy of the papillae and epidermis caused by a virus. They are not cancerous, but they are contagious. Verrucas are typically flesh colored but can be brown or black. They can appear singly or in clusters (**Figure 4–33**). Verrucas are not well understood. They can spontaneously disappear but there are several treatment options, including cryotherapy, electric therapy, surgical excision, and chemical exfoliation. Chemical exfoliation involves the application of a strong salicylic acid at home that peels the wart off in layers. When treating a client with warts, it is imperative that you wear gloves to avoid spreading the virus to other locations on the client's body or inadvertently to another client.

CAUTION!

Do not work on clients if you have an open verruca, commonly called a wart, or any other contagious conditions on any area that would contact the client. Do not touch clients' warts or plantar warts on the feet because these are a contagious virus and you could inadvertently spread the virus.

✓ CHECK IN

19. Name and define nine contagious skin and/or nail disorders.
20. Which contagious diseases contraindicate skin care treatments?

Identify Two Mental Health Conditions that May Manifest as Skin Conditions

Dermatillomania (dur-muh-TIL-uh-MAY-nee-uh) is a form of obsessive-compulsive disorder (OCD) in which the person picks at their skin to the point of injury, infection, or scarring. A person with dermatillomania finds the picking stress relieving and not painful. It can often be socially isolating because severe dermatillomania can be disfiguring. Uninformed people may assume the person has a methamphetamine addiction. Treatment includes cognitive behavior therapy, hypnosis, and medication.

Body dysmorphic disorder (BAHD-ee dis-mor-vic dis-OHR-dur) is a psychological disorder in which the client has a preoccupation with their appearance. They do not have a realistic picture of what they look like (**Figure 4–34**). They tend to fixate on minor appearance imperfections and see them as disfiguring. They believe others are viewing them negatively because of their physical appearance. They may check the mirror frequently and need an abnormal amount of reassurance that their appearance is acceptable. They

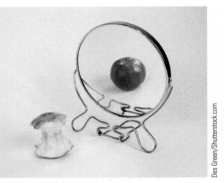

▲ FIGURE 4–34 Body Dysmorphic Disorder is a psychological disorder that causes a client to fixate on imperfections.

may be "spa hoppers" or have a history of many cosmetic surgeries or treatments to fix their perceived flaws. They are dissatisfied with the outcome after treatments. This client will be challenging to manage and will require medical intervention with cognitive behavioral therapy and medication.

CHECK IN

21. Describe dermatillomania and how it is treated.
22. Explain the behavior of a person with body dysmorphic disorder.

Recognize Common Skin Conditions Related to Skin Diseases and Disorders

The skin conditions in **Table 4–6** are often symptoms of more than one skin disease or skin disorder. Several of them look very similar to another. If you encounter these conditions you will need to make an assessment and judgment about treatments. Perhaps a condition is the result of an infection, or is it the appropriate clinical endpoint of an effective treatment? Having confidence in identifying these conditions will give you confidence when determining a treatment plan and also give your client confidence in your skills.

▼ **TABLE 4–6 Common Skin Conditions**

Infection	Definition
Furuncle (FYOO-rung-kul)	Also known as *boil*; a subcutaneous abscess filled with pus; caused by bacteria in glands or hair follicles
Carbuncle (KAHR-bung-kul)	Group of boils
Edema (ih-DEE-muh)	Swelling from a fluid imbalance in the cells or from a response to injury, infection, or medication
Erythema (er-uh-THEE-muh)	Redness caused by inflammation
Folliculitis (fah-lik-yuh-LY-tis)	Hair grows under the surface instead of growing up and out of the follicle, causing a bacterial infection; these ingrown hairs are common in men, usually from shaving (also referred to as *barbae folliculitis, folliculitis barbae, sycosis barbae, or barber's itch*)
Pseudofolliculitis (SOO-doe-fah-lik-yuh-LY-tis)	Also known as *razor bumps*; resembles folliculitis without the pus or infection
Pruritus (proo-RYT-us)	The medical term for itching; persistent itching
Steatoma (stee-ah-TOH-muh)	A sebaceous cyst or subcutaneous tumor filled with sebum; ranges in size from a pea to an orange; usually appears on the scalp, neck, and back; also called a *wen*

 CHECK IN

23. Describe edema, erythema, and pruritis.

Explain Five Sudoriferous Gland Disorders

Disorders of the sudoriferous glands include the following:

- **Anhidrosis** (an-hy-DROH-sis)—a deficiency in perspiration due to failure of the sweat glands; often results from a fever or skin disease. Anhidrosis requires medical treatment.

- **Bromhidrosis** (broh-mih-DROH-sis)—foul-smelling perspiration, usually in the armpits or on the feet. Bromhidrosis is caused by bacteria and yeast that break down the sweat on the surface of the skin.

- **Hyperhidrosis** (hy-pur-hy-DROH-sis)—chronic excessive perspiration caused by heat, genetics, stress, or medications. An FDA-approved treatment for hyperhidrosis includes the use of microwave technology to destroy the underarm sudoriferous glands. One treatment is usually up to 80 percent effective. Neuromodulators, like Botox Cosmetic®, are also used to inhibit the sudoriferous gland production.

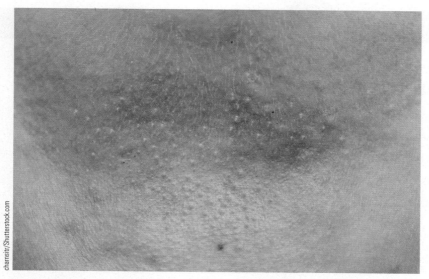

▲ FIGURE 4–35 Miliaria rubra, also known as prickly heat.

- **Diaphoresis** (di-a-fah-re-sis)—excessive perspiration due to an underlying medical condition. Menopause is an example.
- **Miliaria rubra** (mil-ee-AIR-ee-ah ROOB-rah)—also known as *prickly heat*; acute inflammatory disorder of the sweat glands; results in the eruption of red vesicles and burning, itching skin from excessive heat exposure (**Figure 4–35**).

Recognizing a potentially contagious skin disorder can stop the spread of infection. You can formulate a more specific treatment plan and use the appropriate products when you can identify common skin disorders, such as rosacea and acne. Understanding that some skin disorders are contraindications for treatments will help you avoid a negative outcome. The medical field is progressing and the treatment of skin disorders and diseases is becoming easier with advances in technology, ingredients, and medications. Although there are hundreds of disorders and diseases, the majority of the ones you may commonly encounter are discussed in this chapter, along with some that are unique.

Knowledge of skin problems takes years of experience and study, but reference books and credible medical websites are helpful in identifying these disorders and diseases.

Web Resources

www.dermnet.com
www.phil.cdc.gov
www.medicinenet.com
www.rosacea.org
www.skincancer.org
www.pcosaa.org
www.impactmelanoma.org

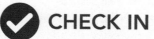 **CHECK IN**

24. Explain five sudoriferous gland disorders.

COMPETENCY PROGRESS

How are you doing with disorders and diseases of the skin? **Check the Chapter 4 Learning Objectives below that you feel you have mastered; leave unchecked those objectives you will need to return to:**

- ☐ Explain why knowledge of diseases and disorders is valuable for an esthetician.
- ☐ Describe how an esthetician and a dermatologist can work collaboratively.
- ☐ Identify the differences between primary, secondary, and tertiary skin lesions.
- ☐ Recognize skin changes that could indicate a type of skin cancer.
- ☐ Describe the types of acne.
- ☐ Describe the symptoms of polycystic ovarian syndrome (PCOS).
- ☐ List common vascular conditions or disorders.
- ☐ Identify pigment disorders.
- ☐ Describe the different types of dermatitis.
- ☐ Identify the types of hypertrophies.
- ☐ Define nine contagious skin diseases.
- ☐ Identify two mental health conditions that may manifest as skin conditions.
- ☐ Recognize common skin conditions related to skin diseases and disorders.
- ☐ Explain five sudoriferous gland disorders.

CHAPTER GLOSSARY

acne AK-nee	p. 131	chronic inflammatory skin disorder of the sebaceous glands that is characterized by comedones and blemishes; commonly known as *acne simplex* or *acne vulgaris*
actinic keratosis ak-TIN-ik Kara-toe-sis	p. 129	pink or flesh-colored precancerous lesions that feel sharp or rough; results from sun damage
albinism AL-bi-niz-em	p. 144	absence of melanin pigment in the body, including skin, hair, and eyes; the technical term for albinism is *congenital leukoderma* or *congenital hypopigmentation*
anhidrosis an-hy-DROH-sis	p. 154	deficiency in perspiration, often a result of a fever or skin disease, that requires medical treatment
atopic dermatitis UH-top-ick DERM-uh-tit-is	p. 146	excess inflammation; dry skin, redness, and itching from allergies and irritants
basal cell carcinoma BAY-zul SEL kar-sin-OH-mah	p. 129	most common and least severe type of skin cancer, which often appears as light, pearly nodules; characteristics include sores, reddish patches, or a smooth growth with an elevated border
body dysmorphic disorder BAHD-ee dis-mor-vic dis-OHR-dur	p. 152	psychological disorder in which the client has a preoccupation with their appearance; they tend to fixate on minor appearance imperfections and see them as disfiguring

bromhidrosis broh-mih-DROH-sis	p. 154	foul-smelling perspiration, usually in the armpits or on the feet
bulla (plural: bullae) BULL-uh	p. 124	large blister containing watery fluid; similar to a vesicle, but larger
carbuncle KAHR-bung-kul	p. 154	cluster of boils; large inflammation of the subcutaneous tissue caused by *Staphylococci* bacterium; similar to a furuncle (boil) but larger
comedo (plural: comedones) KAHM-uh-doe	p. 132	mass of hardened sebum and skin cells in a hair follicle; an open comedo or blackhead when open and exposed to oxygen; closed comedones are whiteheads that are blocked and do not have a follicular opening
comedogenic KAHM-uh-doe JEN-ick	p. 136	tendency for an ingredient to clog follicles and cause a buildup of dead skin cells, resulting in comedones (blackheads)
conjunctivitis kun-junk-tuh-VY-tus	p. 149	also known as *pinkeye*; very contagious infection of the mucous membranes around the eye; chemical, bacterial, or viral causes
contact dermatitis KAHN-takt der-mah-TYT-is	p. 145	also known as *dermatitis venenata*; inflammatory skin condition caused by contact with a substance or chemical; occupational disorders from ingredients in cosmetics and chemical solutions can cause contact dermatitis; allergic contact dermatitis is from exposure to allergens; irritant contact dermatitis is from exposure to irritants
crust kruhst	p. 126	dead cells form over a wound or blemish while it is healing, resulting in an accumulation of sebum and pus, sometimes mixed with epidermal material; an example is the scab on a sore
cyst SIST	p. 124	closed, abnormally developed sac containing fluid, infection, or other matter above or below the skin
dermatillomania dur-muh-**TIL**-uh-**MAY**-nee-uh	p. 152	a form of obsessive-compulsive disorder in which the person picks at their skin to the point of injury, infection, or scarring; a person with dermatillomania finds the picking stress relieving and not painful; it can often be socially isolating because severe dermatillomania can be disfiguring
dermatitis derm-a-TIE-tuss	p. 145	any inflammatory condition of the skin; various forms of lesions such as eczema, vesicles, or papules; the four main categories are atopic, contact, seborrheic dermatitis, and statis dermatitis
dermatologist dur-muh-TAHL-uh-jist	p. 122	physician who specializes in diseases and disorders of the skin, hair, and nails
dermatology dur-muh-TAHL-uh-jee	p. 122	medical branch of science that deals with the study of skin and its nature, structure, functions, diseases, and treatment
diaphoresis di-a-fah-re-sis	p. 155	excessive perspiration due to a medical condition
eczema EG-zuh-muh	p. 146	inflammatory, painful itching disease of the skin, acute or chronic in nature, with dry or moist lesions; clients with this condition should be referred to a physician; *seborrheic dermatitis*, mainly affecting oily areas, is a common form of eczema
edema ih-DEE-muh	p. 154	swelling caused by a fluid imbalance in cells or a response to injury or infection
ephelids EF-ah-lids	p. 143	also known as *freckles*, are tiny round or oval pigmented areas of skin on areas exposed to the sun. Also referred to as *macules*, they are small flat colored spots on the skin.
erythema er-uh-THEE-muh	p. 154	redness caused by inflammation; a red lesion is erythemic

excoriation ek-skor-ee-AY-shun	p. 126	skin sore or abrasion produced by scratching or scraping
fissure FISH-ur	p. 126	crack in the skin that penetrates the dermis; chapped lips or hands are fissures
folliculitis fah-lik-yuh-LY-tis	p. 154	also known as *folliculitis barbae*, *sycosis barbae*, or *barber's itch*; inflammation of the hair follicles caused by a bacterial infection from ingrown hairs; the cause is typically from ingrown hairs due to shaving or other epilation methods
furuncle FYOO-rung-kul	p. 154	also known as *boil*; a subcutaneous abscess filled with pus; furuncles are caused by bacteria in the glands or hair follicles
herpes simplex virus 1 HER-peez SIM-pleks VY-rus ONE	p. 150	strain of the herpes virus that causes fever blisters or cold sores; it is a recurring, contagious viral infection consisting of a vesicle or group of vesicles on a red, swollen base; the blisters usually appear on the lips or nostrils
herpes simplex virus 2 HER-peez SIM-pleks VY-rus TOO	p. 150	strain of the herpes virus that infects the genitals
herpes zoster HER-peez ZOHS-tur	p. 150	also known as *shingles*; a painful viral infection skin condition from the chickenpox virus; characterized by groups of blisters that form a rash in a ring or line
hyperhidrosis hy-pur-hy-DROH-sis	p. 154	excessive perspiration not related to excessive exercise or heat
hyperkeratosis hy-pur-kair-uh-TOH-sis	p. 148	thickening of the skin caused by a mass of keratinized cells (keratinocytes)
hyperpigmentation hy-pur-pig-men-TAY-shun	p. 142	overproduction of pigment
hypertrophy hy-PUR-truh-fee	p. 148	abnormal growth of the skin; many are benign, or harmless
hypopigmentation hy-poh-pig-men-TAY-shun	p. 142	absence of pigment, resulting in light or white splotches
impetigo im-puh-TEE-go	p. 150	a contagious skin infection caused by staphylococcal or streptococcal bacteria, characterized by clusters of small blisters or crusty lesions and often occurring in children
keloid KEE-loyd	p. 126	thick scar resulting from excessive growth of fibrous tissue (collagen)
keratoma kair-uh-TOH-muh	p. 148	acquired, superficial, thickened patch of epidermis; a callus is a keratoma caused by continued, repeated pressure or friction on any part of the skin, especially the hands and feet
keratosis (plural: keratoses) kair-uh-TOH-sis	p. 148	abnormally thick buildup of cells
keratosis pilaris kair-uh-TOH-sis py-LAIR-us	p. 148	redness and bumpiness common on the cheeks or upper arms; it is caused by blocked hair follicles; the patches of irritation are accompanied by a rough texture and small pinpoint white milia
lentigo len-TY-goh	p. 142	freckles; small yellow-brown colored spots; lentigenes that result from sunlight exposure are actinic, or solar; lentigo patches are referred to as *large macules*
lesions LEE-zhuns	p. 123	mark, wound, or abnormality; structural changes in tissues caused by damage or injury

leukoderma loo-koh-DUR-ma	p. 144	skin disorder characterized by light, abnormal patches; causes are congenital, acquired, postinflammation, or other causes that destroy pigment-producing cells; vitiligo and albinism are leukodermas
macule (plural: maculae) MAK-yool	p. 124	flat spot or discoloration on the skin, such as a freckle; macules are neither raised nor sunken
milia MIL-ee-uh	p. 132	epidermal cysts; small, firm papules with no visible opening; whitish, pearl-like masses of sebum and dead cells under the skin; milia are more common in dry skin types and may form after skin trauma, such as a laser resurfacing
miliaria rubra mil-ee-AIR-ee-ah ROOB-rah	p. 155	also known as *prickly heat*; acute inflammatory disorder of the sweat glands resulting in the eruption of red vesicles and burning, itching skin from excessive heat exposure
malignant melanoma muh-LIG-nent mel-uh-NOH-mah	p. 129	most serious form of skin cancer as it can spread quickly (metastasize); black or dark patches on the skin are usually uneven in texture, jagged, or raised; melanomas may have surface crust or bleed
mole MOHL	p. 148	pigmented nevus; a brownish spot ranging in color from tan to bluish black; some are flat, resembling freckles; others are raised and darker
nevus NEE-vus	p. 143	also known as *birthmark*; malformation of the skin due to abnormal pigmentation or dilated capillaries
nodules NOD-yool	p. 124	often referred to as *tumors*, but nodules are smaller bumps caused by conditions such as scar tissue, fatty deposits, or infections
onychomycosis ahn-ih-koh-my-KOH-sis	p. 150	a fungal infection that produces symptoms of thick, brittle, discolored nails; the fungus lives off the keratin in the nails
papule PAP-yool	p. 125	pimple; small elevation on the skin that contains no fluid but may develop pus
perioral dermatitis pair-ee-OR-ul derm-a-TIE-tuss	p. 147	acne-like condition around the mouth; these are mainly small clusters of papules that could be caused by toothpaste or products used on the face
pilosebaceous unit py-luh-seh-BAY-shus YOO-knit	p. 132	the hair unit that contains the hair follicle and appendages: the hair root, hair bulb, dermal papilla, sebaceous appendage, and arrector pili muscle
Poikiloderma of Civatte poi-ki-lo-der-ma ov si-vaht	p. 143	a skin condition caused by actinic bronzing (chronic sun exposure) to the sides of the face and neck. The skin turns a reddish-brown hue with a distinct white patch under the chin. Poikiloderma is benign, meaning it is not cancerous.
Polycystic ovarian syndrome (PCOS) polee-sistik oh-vair-ee-uh-n sin-druhm	p. 139	Often shortened and pronounced "peecos," is a hormonal condition that impacts women in child bearing years believed to have a genetic component. PCOS symptoms include acne, thinning hair in a male hair growth pattern of baldness as in sparse hair density at the front and top of the scalp. It also causes abnormal hair growth on the face, arms, thighs, neck, and breasts.
postinflammatory hyperpigmentation POHST-in-flam-uh-tory hy-PER-pig-MEN-tay-shun	p. 143	abbreviated as *PIH*; darkened pigmentation due to an injury to the skin or the residual healing after an acne lesion has resolved; often deep red, purple, or brown in appearance
primary lesions PRY-mayr-ee LEE-zhuns	p. 123	primary lesions are characterized by flat, nonpalpable changes in skin color such as macules or patches, or an elevation formed by fluid in a cavity, such as vesicles, bullae, or pustules
pruritus proo-RYT-us	p. 154	persistent itching

pseudofolliculitis SOO-doe-fah-lik-yuh-LY-tis	p. 154	also known as *razor bumps*; resembles folliculitis without the pus or infection
psoriasis suh-RY-uh-sis	p. 149	skin disease characterized by red patches covered with white-silver scales; caused by an overproliferation of skin cells that replicate too fast; immune dysfunction could be the cause; usually found in patches on the scalp, elbows, knees, chest, and lower back
pustule PUS-chool	p. 125	raised, inflamed papule with a white or yellow center containing pus in the top of the lesion, referred to as the head of the pimple
retention hyperkeratosis ree-TEN-shun hy-pur-kair-uh-TOH-sis	p. 133	hereditary factor in which dead skin cells build up and do not shed from the follicles as they do on normal skin
scale skeyl	p. 127	flaky skin cells; any thin plate of epidermal flakes, dry or oily; an example is abnormal or excessive dandruff
scar skahr	p. 127	light-colored, slightly raised mark on the skin formed after an injury or lesion of the skin has healed up; the tissue hardens to heal the injury; elevated scars are hypertrophic; a keloid is a hypertrophic (abnormal) scar
sebaceous filaments sih-BAY-shus FILL-ah-mentz	p. 132	similar to open comedones, these are mainly solidified impactions of oil without the cell matter
sebaceous hyperplasia sih-BAY-shus hy-pur-PLAY-zhuh	p. 133	benign lesions frequently seen in oilier areas of the face; an overgrowth of the sebaceous gland, they appear similar to open comedones; often doughnut-shaped, with sebaceous material in the center
seborrhea seb-oh-REE-ah	p. 133	severe oiliness of the skin; an abnormal secretion from the sebaceous glands
seborrheic dermatitis seb-oh-REE-ick derm-a-TIE-tuss	p. 147	common form of eczema; mainly affects oily areas; characterized by inflammation, scaling, and/or itching
secondary lesions SEK-un-deh-ree SKIN LEE-zhuns	p. 126	skin damage, developed in the later stages of disease, that changes the structure of tissues or organs
skin tag skin tag	p. 149	small, benign outgrowth or extension of the skin that looks like a flap; common under the arms or on the neck
squamous cell carcinoma SKWAYmus SEL kar-sin-OHmah	p. 129	type of skin cancer more serious than basal cell carcinoma; characterized by scaly, red or pink papules or nodules; also appear as open sores or crusty areas; can grow and spread in the body
stasis dermatitis stay-sus dur-muh-TY-tus	p. 147	chronic inflammatory state in the legs due to poor circulation; the legs may sometimes have ulcerations, along with scaly skin, itching, and hyperpigmentation
sensitization SEN-sih-tiz-A-shun	p. 145	the development of hypersensitivity due to repeated exposure to an allergen that can take months or years to develop due to the allergen and intensity of exposure.
steatoma stee-ah-TOH-muh	p. 154	sebaceous cyst or subcutaneous tumor filled with sebum; ranges in size from a pea to an orange; usually appears on the scalp, neck, and back; also called a *wen*
tan tan	p. 143	increase in pigmentation due to the melanin production that results from exposure to UV radiation; visible skin damage; melanin is designed to help protect the skin from the sun's UV radiation

tinea TIN-ee-uh	p. 151	contagious condition caused by fungal infection, not a parasite; characterized by itching, scales, and, sometimes, painful lesions
tinea corporis TIN-ee-uh KOR-pur-is	p. 151	also known as *ringworm*; a contagious infection that forms a ringed, red pattern with elevated edges
tinea versicolor TIN-ee-uh VUR-see-kuh-lur	p. 144	also called *pityriasis versicolor*, is a fungal condition that inhibits melanin production. It is not contagious because it is caused by yeast, a normal part of the human skin. It is characterized by white, brown, or salmon-colored flaky patches.
tubercle TOO-bur-kul	p. 124	abnormal rounded, solid lump; larger than a papule
tumor TOO-mur	p. 125	large nodule; an abnormal cell mass resulting from excessive cell multiplication; varies in size, shape, and color
ulcer UL-sur	p. 127	open lesion on the skin or mucous membrane of the body, accompanied by pus and loss of skin depth; a deep erosion; a depression in the skin, normally due to infection or cancer
urticaria ur-tuh-KAYR-ee-ah	p. 125	also known as *hives*; caused by an allergic reaction from the body's histamine production
varicose veins VAYR-ih-kohs VAYNZ	p. 141	vascular lesions; dilated and twisted veins, most commonly in the legs
vasodilation vas-oh-dih-LAY-shun	p. 140	vascular dilation of the blood vessels
verruca vuh-ROO-kuh	p. 152	also known as *wart*; hypertrophy of the papillae and epidermis caused by a virus; infectious and contagious
vesicle VES-ih-kel	p. 125	small blister or sac containing clear fluid; poison ivy and poison oak produce vesicles
vitiligo vih-til-EYE-goh	p. 144	pigmentation disease characterized by white patches on the skin from lack of pigment cells; made worse by sunlight
wheal WHEEL	p. 125	itchy, swollen lesion caused by a blow, insect bite, skin allergy reaction, or stings; hives and mosquito bites are wheals; hives (urticaria) can be caused by exposure to allergens used in products

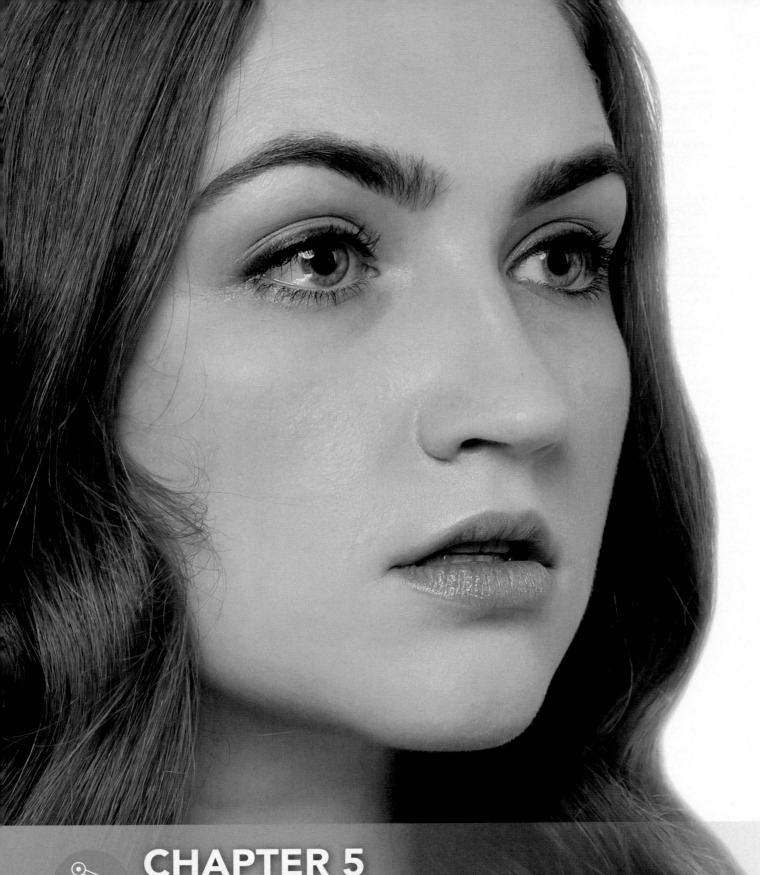

CHAPTER 5
Skin Analysis

"It's not what you look at that matters, it's what you see."

–Henry David Thoreau

Learning Objectives

After completing this chapter, you will be able to:

1. Explain the process of skin analysis.
2. Identify the four genetic skin types through visualization, palpation, and consultation.
3. Differentiate the six Fitzpatrick skin types and accurately identify them.
4. Distinguish the characteristics of sensitive skin.
5. Recognize the intricacies involved with treating skin of color.
6. Identify treatment options for the neck and décolleté.
7. Illustrate examples of skin conditions.
8. Explain the causes of skin conditions.
9. Describe healthy habits for the skin.
10. Determine treatment contraindications through evaluation, analysis, and consultation.
11. Perform a skin analysis.

Explain the Process of Skin Analysis

Being knowledgeable about skin types and conditions is one of the most important competencies for a skin care professional. This interaction with a client sets you up as the skin care expert. Recommendations for the appropriate skin care treatments and products must be uniquely adapted to each person. The skin analysis is the determining factor in deciding what products to use during the service and what products to recommend for home use (**Figure 5–1**). The skin analysis also confirms whether the client is an appropriate candidate for the treatment.

Estheticians should study and have a thorough understanding of skin analysis because:

- Before performing services or selecting products, an individual's skin type and conditions must be analyzed correctly to determine the appropriate treatment and products.

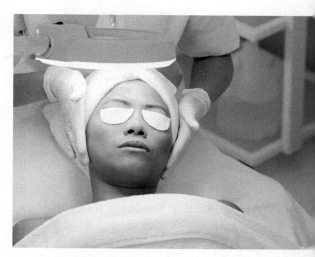

▲ **FIGURE 5–1** Conducting a skin analysis with a magnifying light.

- A thorough skin analysis and client consultation is especially important to determine the causes of skin conditions and any contraindications to treatment or products that the client may have.
- Using a holistic approach, identifying healthy habits and behavior that is detrimental to skin health will give you a better understanding of how to help your clients.

Identify the Four Genetic Skin Types Through Visualization, Palpation, and Consultation

Skin type (SKIN TYPE) is a classification that describes a person's genetic (juh-NET-ik) skin attributes. Skin type is determined by genetics and ethnicity, but like everything else, skin can change over time. Generally, skin becomes drier over time because our cellular metabolism and oil/lipid production slow down as we age. Skin type is based primarily on how much oil is produced in the follicles from the sebaceous glands and on the amount of lipids found between the cells. The T-zone (TEE-ZOHN) is the center area of the face, corresponding to the "T" shape formed by the forehead, nose, and chin (Figure 5–2). Evaluating the pores in the T-zone is the first step in determining skin type.

All skin types need proper cleansing, exfoliating, hydrating, and protecting. Finding the right treatment plan for each individual can be challenging, and this makes the esthetician's role even more interesting. The focus of this chapter is to identify skin types and conditions. Mastering this skill is necessary before learning about which products and treatments to choose for each person. When we perform skin analysis, we are using our visual abilities, often under magnification, to note properties in the skin, such as pore size or irregularities in the skin (e.g., blemishes). We use palpation (pal-PAY-shun) to examine the skin through touch, manipulating it to determine conditions such as oiliness and elasticity. And we use consultation, conversing with our client to determine lifestyle and dietary issues that impact the skin. You will experience more success in your profession as your skills in assessment get stronger.

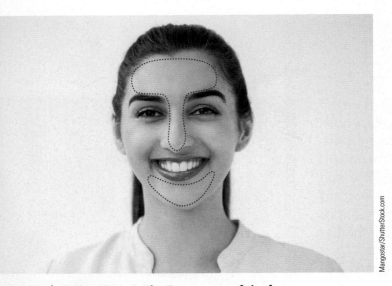

▲ FIGURE 5–2 The T-zone area of the face.

Mangostar/ShutterStock.com

Skin types are categorized as follows (**Table 5–1** and **Figures 5–3 to 5–6**):

- Normal
- Combination
- Oily
- Dry

ACTIVITY

Know Your Skin

Determine your classmates' skin type by utilizing the skills of visualization, palpation, and consultation. Report your findings.

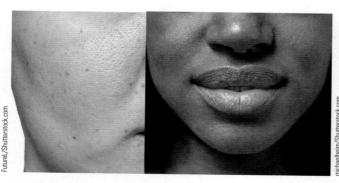

▲ **FIGURE 5–3** Learning to identify skin types will help you formulate the best skin care treatment plan. The oil-hydration balance is easily affected with combination skin.

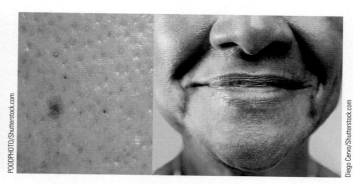

▲ **FIGURE 5–4** Oily skin ages more slowly because the oil acts to protect the skin

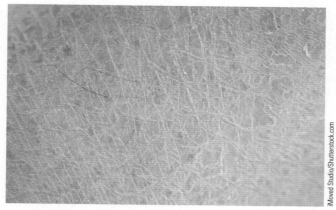

▲ **FIGURE 5–5** Dry skin can have compromised transepidermal water loss (TEWL).

▲ **FIGURE 5–6** Normal skin often changes as we age.

Skin Type	What does it look like, feel like?	How is it treated?	Why?	Expert Tips
Normal	• Oil: balanced • Hydration: balanced • Follicle size: very small • Appearance: uniform luminosity; no or rare blemishes • Feel: soft, smooth texture; good elasticity	• Maintenance and prevention treatments • Use four steps to skin health: • cleanse, exfoliate, nourish, protect	• Body systems functioning **holistically** (hoh-LIS-tik-lee) for balance • Most common in twenties and thirties	• Introduce antiaging products as client matures. • Normal skin will often become drier with age. • Reinforce use of sunscreen.
Combination	• Oil: moderate to high • Hydration: good to dehydrated • Follicle size: larger in T-zone than cheeks and sides of face • Appearance: can have buildup of dead skin and oil in pores around nose but dry or flaking skin outside of T-zone; some blemishes and comedones • Feel: oilier in center T-zone than sides of face	• Cleansing and regular exfoliation • Water-based products • Avoid harsh products and rough exfoliation	• Overproduction of oil in the T-zone • May have normal oil production in the T-zone and dehydrated skin on the sides of the face	• Evaluate often, as oil–hydration balance can be disrupted by hormonal and environmental influences. • Reinforce use of sunscreen.
Oily	• Oil: moderate to high • Hydration: good to dehydrated • Follicle size: moderate to large • Appearance: shiny; comedones and blemishes may be present • Feel: thick and firm, uneven due to congestion	• Regular cleansing and exfoliation and hydrating with water-based products • Treatments to balance oil production	• Overproduction of oil due to genetics, hormonal changes, medication, stress, or environmental factors, such as skin care products or makeup that are comedogenic • Overexfoliation can create oilier skin as sebaceous glands work to increase surface dryness	• Clients with oily skin breakouts and comedones may have them on the neck, back, shoulders, and chest. • Clients with oily skin age more slowly, since the oil acts to protect the skin. • Clients will need to use SPF regularly to avoid post inflammatory hyperpigmentation, a common ailment that accompanies acne.

(Continues)

(Continued)

| Dry | • Oil: minimal production

 • Hydration: minimal production

 • Follicle size: difficult to visualize, fine pores

 • Appearance: dull, lack of luminosity, flaking, blotchy

 • Feel: rough, thin, tight | • Oil-based products to provide protection of the acid mantle and increase the barrier function

 • Dry skin often has compromised **TEWL** (too-wuhl; water loss caused by evaporation on the skin's surface)

 • Treatments to provide nourishment and protection | • Underproduction of oil due to genetics, environmental factors, hormones | • Dry skin may often be dehydrated.

 • Reinforce use of sunscreen. |

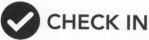 **CHECK IN**

1. Are skin types genetic?
2. List the skin types.
3. What is dry skin lacking?
4. What is skin typing based on?

Differentiate the Six Fitzpatrick Skin Types and Accurately Identify Them

Developed by Dr. Thomas Fitzpatrick, the **Fitzpatrick scale** (FITS-patrick scayl) is used to measure the skin type's ability to tolerate ultraviolet (UV) exposure (**Table 5–2**). Many skin treatment protocols are based on the client's Fitzpatrick skin type. Due to [racially] mixed genetics, there is no true phototype (foh-tuh-tahyp) classification system; therefore, the scale is just a guideline.

When it comes to skin treatments, everyone's level of skin reactivity is different. Lighter skin types are generally more sensitive. Individuals with dark skin have larger melanin deposits in the stratum corneum (SC), which gives more protection from the sun, but dark skin types face other risks. Adverse reaction like hyper- or hypopigmentation and keloid scarring may occur due to aggressive treatments.

ACTIVITY

Skin Deep

Use your cell phone to create a collage of the six Fitzpatrick skin types and send it to your instructor.

▼ **TABLE 5–2** The Fitzpatrick Scale

Fitzpatrick Type	Eyes	Hair	Unexposed Skin	Heritage Heredity	Skin Reaction in UV Exposure
1	Blue, green	Blonde, red	Very white, almost translucent, freckles	English, Irish, Scottish, northern European	Always burns, peels with burn, does not tan
2	Blue, hazel, brown	Red, blonde, brown	Light	Scandinavian and same as Fitzpatrick 1	Burns easily, usually peels, tans minimally
3	Brown	Dark	Fair to olive	Spanish, Greek, Italian	Tans well, burns moderately
4	Dark	Dark	Light brown	Mediterranean, Asian, Hispanic	Tans easily, burns minimally, experiences immediate pigment response
5	Dark	Dark	Dark brown	East Indian, American Indian, Hispanic, Latin American, African American	Rarely burns, tans easily and significantly
6	Dark	Dark	Dark brown, black	African American, Aboriginal	Rarely/never burns, tans easily

Other Skin Classification Systems

There are other classification systems used when evaluating the skin, but Fitzpatrick is the most commonly used. You may want to research other resources for information on the Glogau scale and the Rubin scale.

ACTIVITY

Classification Scales

Research the Rubin skin scale and/or the Glogau scale. Create a poster describing these skin scales.

CHECK IN

5. What is the Fitzpatrick scale?
6. Identify the reaction to UV exposure for each Fitzpatrick skin type.

Distinguish the Characteristics of Sensitive Skin

We are constantly bombarded by environmental stimuli, stress, sun exposure, and other unhealthy elements. Sensitive skin is a condition but can also be genetically predisposed (**Figure 5–7**). Sensitive skin is characterized by fragility, thin skin, and redness. Clients with a heritage that is northern European, Fitzpatrick skin type 1, tend to have fair, light-colored skin that is thinner and more sensitive. It flushes easily and may appear red due to the blood flow being closer to the surface. Individuals with multicultural skin can also be naturally sensitive, without the visible redness.

Sensitive skin is easily irritated by products or by exposure to heat or sun. **Telangiectasia** (tel-an-JEE-ek-tay-juh), visible broken or distended capillaries less than 0.5 mm due to intrinsic or extrinsic causes, may be noticeable on sensitive skin. These conditions are a protective visible reaction to let us know something is irritating the skin.

Fragile or thin skin can also be the result of age or medications. Skin can become reactive and sensitized from exposure to things such as harsh products, heat, or even become dehydrated and chapped from cold weather.

Sensitive or sensitized skin can be difficult to treat because of its low tolerance to products and stimulation. For example, excessive rubbing, heat, exfoliation, or extractions can cause damage and increase redness. Sensitive skin needs to be treated gently with nonirritating, calming products and treatments. It is important to find out what could be causing sensitive conditions by completing a thorough skin analysis.

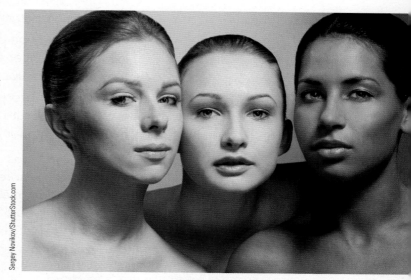

▲ **FIGURE 5–7** Any skin type can be sensitive.

Is it a natural part of their skin condition or is it something the client is exposed to? Primary treatment goals for sensitive skin are to soothe, calm, and protect.

 CHECK IN

7. In addition to a genetic predisposition, what can cause skin to become reactive and sensitized?
8. Why is sensitized skin challenging to treat?
9. What are the goals for treating sensitized skin?

Recognize the Intricacies Involved with Treating Skin of Color

All Fitzpatrick skin types have the same number of melanocytes. Higher Fitzpatrick skin types have melanocytes that produce more melanin. Melanocytes comprise about 5 to 10% of the cells in the basal layer. Most of the differentiation is dependent on the ethnicity of the individual and their geographic location. A person who lives along the equator will have much more active melanocytes than the person who lives at the North Pole. In addition to these considerations, each of these skin types has specific characteristics.

Fitzpatrick skin type 4:

- Considered to be one of the most challenging skin types to treat well
- Has great elasticity and firmness and does not show signs of aging as quickly as Fitzpatrick skin types 1 and 2
- Can become hyperpigmented from treatments or aggressive exfoliating agents; gentler exfoliating products are recommended. May need to add melanin suppressants or other skin lighteners to skin care routine
- Requires sun protection to slow down hyperpigmentation; must avoid sun exposure and use sun protection daily (for anyone prone to hyperpigmentation)

Fitzpatrick skin types 3 and 4 typically have thicker skin that is usually characterized by more oil production and needs more deep-cleansing treatments. Additionally, waxing is more difficult for individuals with any Fitzpatrick skin type that has thicker hair and thicker roots in the follicle. If you want to specialize in skin of color, explore educational resources and advanced classes for this area of study (**Figure 5–8**). No matter what a client's skin type or ethnic background, everyone needs an individualized skin care consultation and treatment plan to maintain healthy skin.

Fitzpatrick skin types 5 and 6:

- Generally have oilier and thicker skin (dermis) but can have the same level of reactivity as lower Fitzpatrick skin types
- Reactions may be more challenging to see on darker skin, but they may be just as intense as those on lighter skin
- Are prone to a form of hyperkeratosis known as *ichthyosis* and dead skin–cell buildup, so those clients need more exfoliation and deep pore cleansing
- May have abnormal hypertrophic scarring (keloids)
- Sun protection still necessary for these skin types

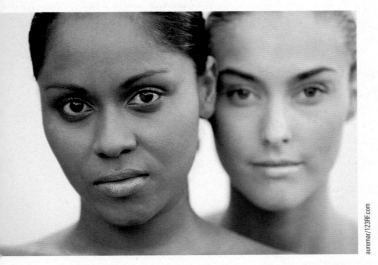

auremar/123RF.com

▲ **FIGURE 5–8** Skin of color is complex and requires advanced knowledge and skill.

CHECK IN

10. Why do clients with higher Fitzpatrick skin types have darker skin?
11. How can you treat the hyperkeratosis that is common in Fitzpatrick skin types 5 and 6?
12. Which Fitzpatrick skin type is often considered the most challenging to treat?
13. What treatment can be difficult for a client of any skin color who has thick hair and thicker roots in the follicle?

Identify Treatment Options for the Neck and Décolleté

The skin on the neck and **décolleté** (dey-kol-TEY) (pertaining to the lower neck and chest) is not the same as the skin on the face. The neck and décolleté have fewer sebaceous glands than the face, so they tend to show aging more quickly (**Figure 5–9**). The neck and décolleté are more susceptible to irritation. Photodamage, broken capillaries, fine lines, and rhytids (wrinkles) develop just as much on the neck and chest as the face. **"Tech neck"** (TEK NEK), a new phenomenon caused by the repeated movement of looking down at a cell phone or other electronic device has created a demand for specialty topical treatments that include antioxidants, growth factor serums, and additional moisture. Be cautious when applying vitamin A or alpha hydroxy acid (AHA) products that may cause excess irritation to the area. A product, such as a retinol, may be fine for the face but may be too aggressive for the neck. Remind your clients that the neck and décolleté need SPF protection as much as the face does.

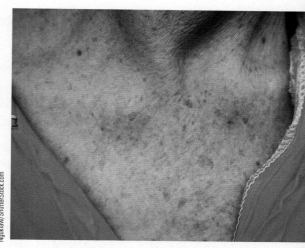

▲ FIGURE 5–9 Often the neck and décolleté can reveal aging more than the face.

CHECK IN

14. Why do the neck and décolleté show aging more quickly than the face does?
15. What is "tech neck"?
16. What kind of products should be used on the neck and décolleté?

ACTIVITY

Quiz Yourself on Skin Conditions

Create flash cards to help you learn about skin conditions.

Illustrate Examples of Skin Conditions

Many internal and external factors affect the condition of a person's skin. Skin conditions are more than our genetic makeup. These conditions are what the esthetician is most concerned about, and they are the focus of skin treatments. Some of the most common skin conditions estheticians see today are adult acne, extrinsic aging (from sun exposure and the environment), and problems related to hormonal fluctuations. **Dehydration** (dee-HY-dray-shun; a lack of water) and pigmentation disorders are also significant concerns to clients. Other skin conditions include comedones, hyperkeratinization, and erythema (redness). We can improve some of these conditions through regularly scheduled skin treatments, by using specialized products, and by avoiding the factors that affect the conditions. On the client's chart, you will want to note other conditions that may not be listed in **Table 5–3** and that you learn about here and in Chapter 4, Disorders and Diseases of the Skin.

▼ **TABLE 5–3** Skin Conditions and Descriptions

Skin Condition	Description
Acne	Sebaceous breakouts from hormonal changes or other factors.
Actinic keratosis	A rough area resulting from chronic sun exposure, sometimes with a layered scale or scab that sometimes falls off. Can be precancerous.
Aging	Characterized by skin laxity due to collagen and bone loss, thinner skin, dryness, photo damage, and fine lines or wrinkles (**rhytids**) (RIT-ihdz).
Asphyxiated	Smokers have asphyxiated skin from lack of oxygen. Characterized by clogged pores and wrinkles; dull and lifeless-looking. Can be yellowish or gray in color.
Comedones	*Open comedones* are blackheads and clogged pores caused by a buildup of debris, oil, and dead skin cells in the follicles. *Closed comedones, also called whiteheads,* are not open to the air or oxygen; they are trapped by dead skin cells and need to be exfoliated and extracted.
Couperose skin	Redness in the skin with no visible vascularity because the matting of blood vessels is so small and fine. Often seen with telangiectasia.
Cysts	Fluid, infection, or other matter under the skin that is encapsulated into a palpable firm mass of varying sizes, from a pea to a golf ball.
Dehydrated	Lack of water caused by the environment, medications, topical agents, aging, or dehydrating drinks such as caffeine and alcohol.
Enlarged pores	Larger follicles due to excess oil and debris trapped in the follicles or expansion due to elasticity loss or trauma.
Erythema	Redness caused by inflammation.

(Continues)

Growths	Skin cells and underlying tissue that overproduce and create an area that could be raised or flat, but can be distinguished with palpation. They may be the same color as surrounding tissue or may be pigmented. They can be present at birth or develop later.
Herpes simplex I	A communicable virus that appears as a vesicle on the lip similar to a blister. Find more information in the chapter on diseases and disorders of the skin.
Hirsutism (HUR-soo-tiz-um)	Excess body hair located in regions where hair is not normally present, such as facial hair for women. It is commonly caused by a hormonal imbalance. **Polycystic ovarian syndrome** (PCOS) is a possible cause of hirsutism. Signs and symptoms of PCOS include irregular or no menstrual periods, heavy periods, excess body and facial hair, acne, pelvic pain, difficulty getting pregnant, and patches of thick, darker, velvety skin.
Hyperkeratinization	An excessive buildup of dead skin cells/keratinized cells.
Hyperpigmentation	Overproduction of melanin due to at least one of three factors: A. UV exposure: from the sun, tanning beds, fluorescent lighting. This usually appears as diffuse brown spots of various shades on the skin B. Hormonally induced: also called melasma (refer to description in table). C. Post inflammatory hyperpigmentation: also called PIH; occurs from a surface injury to the skin. Acne lesions, insect bites, and ingrown hairs are common causes of PIH. They can appear deep red, almost purple, to dark brown in color. They can gradually fade.
Hypertrichosis (hy-pur-trih-KOH-sis)	Refers to any excess hair growth, whether it is caused from a hormonal imbalance or heredity.
Hypopigmentation	Lack of melanin production due to four possible factors: A. UV induced: intermingled with UV-induced hyperpigmentation. No treatment options, but lightening the hyperpigmentation will usually blend the hypopigmented areas so they are less noticeable. B. Posttraumatic: lack of melanocyte production due to an injury, burn, or other trauma, including a deep chemical peel. Melanocytes may begin producing again over time, but the length of time is undetermined. C. Vitiligo: an autoimmune disorder that stops melanocyte production, creating patches of depigmented skin. Topical prescription drugs can occasionally trigger rejuvenation of the melanocytes. D. Albinism: a hereditary disorder causing lack of pigment in the eyes, skin, and hair.
Irritation	Usually redness or inflammation; from a variety of causes.
Keratosis (plural: keratoses) pilaris	A buildup of cells; a rough texture.
Melasma (mel-AZ-muh)	A form of hyperpigmentation that is characterized by bilateral patches of brown pigmentation on the cheeks, jawline, forehead, and upper lip; due to hormonal imbalances, such as pregnancy, birth control pills, or hormone replacement therapy. Melasma gets worse with sun exposure.
Milia	Hardened, pearl-like collections of oil and dead skin cells trapped beneath the surface of the skin. Milia are not exposed to oxygen and have to be lanced to open and remove them. Milia are typically the size of the head of a pin. *Note:* Check with your state board, as lancets are not approved for use in all states.

(Continues)

(Continued)

Papules	Raised lesions; also called *blemishes*.
Poikiloderma of Civatte	A result of chronic sun exposure, specifically along the sides of the neck, which turn a reddish-brown color with a clear demarcation of untanned skin under the chin.
Poor elasticity	Skin laxity from damage, sun, and aging.
Pustules	An infected papule with fluid inside.
Scar	A mark on the skin where a wound, burn, or sore has healed and left a fibrous band of connective tissue, sometimes hyperpigmented or hypopigmented.
Sebaceous hyperplasia	Benign lesions seen in oilier areas of the face; described as looking like doughnut holes; cannot be extracted.
Seborrhea	Also known as *seborrheic dermatitis*. Excess oil production that causes redness, irritation, and flaking. Occurs most commonly in the hair as dandruff.
Sensitivities	Physical reactions, such as erythema, edema, wheals, itching, stinging, or discomfort, from internal or external influence on the skin.
Solar comedones (SOH-lur KAHM-uh-dohn)	Large open comedones; usually around the eyes, due to sun exposure.
Striae (strahy-ee) or stretch marks	Dermal scars due to rapid expansion or stretching of connective tissue leaving deep red, pink, or purple linear marks on the skin that gradually fade to light pink or silver over time. They often occur during growth phases in puberty, pregnancy, and weight gain.
Sun damage	UV damage to the epidermis and dermis; primary effects are wrinkles, collagen and elastin breakdown, pigmentation, and cancer.
Telangiectasia	Visible broken or distended capillaries less than 0.5 mm due to intrinsic or extrinsic causes.
Wrinkles/Aging (Rhytids)	Lines and damage from internal or external cause.

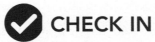 CHECK IN

17. How are skin conditions different from skin types?
18. List and define 15 common skin conditions.

Explain the Causes of Skin Conditions

Being aware of what can affect the skin will help you determine why a client may be experiencing problems. Often skin conditions are due to more than one influence. The esthetician must evaluate multiple

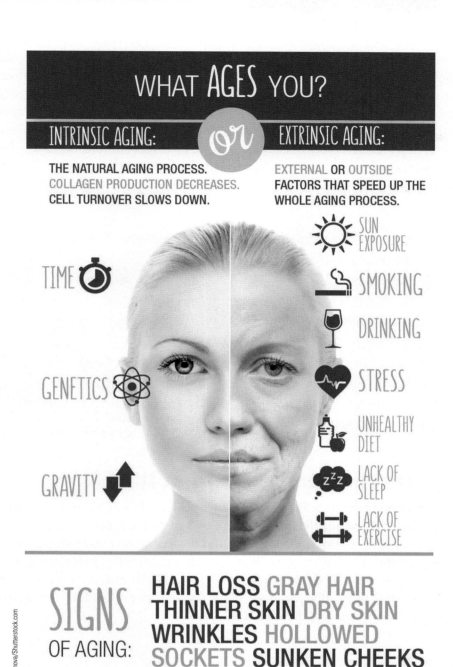

WHAT AGES YOU?

INTRINSIC AGING: or   EXTRINSIC AGING:

THE NATURAL AGING PROCESS.
COLLAGEN PRODUCTION DECREASES.
CELL TURNOVER SLOWS DOWN.

EXTERNAL OR OUTSIDE
FACTORS THAT SPEED UP THE
WHOLE AGING PROCESS.

TIME

GENETICS

GRAVITY

SUN EXPOSURE

SMOKING

DRINKING

STRESS

UNHEALTHY DIET

LACK OF SLEEP

LACK OF EXERCISE

SIGNS OF AGING: HAIR LOSS GRAY HAIR THINNER SKIN DRY SKIN WRINKLES HOLLOWED SOCKETS SUNKEN CHEEKS

Valentina Razumova/Shutterstock.com

▲ FIGURE 5–10 Intrinsic and Extrinsic Aging.

causes, both external and internal, to correct or improve a skin condition (Figure 5–10). Each client is different, and the skin of various clients may respond differently to the exact same treatment.

External Factors that Affect the Skin

Habits, diet, and stress all play a part in our health, which in turn is reflected in our skin's appearance. Skin conditions can be caused by allergies/reactions, medications, medical conditions, and other external, or **extrinsic** (EKS-trinz-ik), factors. Additionally, lack of exercise, lack of sleep, smoking, medications, and drugs will have negative effects both inside and out. Sun damage is the main external (*extrinsic*) cause of aging. These factors can also contribute to skin problems and can be detrimental to maintaining a healthy and attractive complexion. As you read through the following chart, you can understand why correct skin analysis and product and treatment recommendations are so important.

External Effects on the Skin

- UV exposure, sun damage
- Tanning beds
- Environmental exposure, pollutants, air quality
- Environment, climate, humidity
- Poor maintenance, inappropriate skin care
- Misuse of products or treatments, overexfoliation, harsh products
- Allergies and reactions to environmental factors or products
- **Photosensitivity** (FOTO-sensa-tiv-it-ee) to the sun from medications or products

Internal Factors that Affect the Skin

Our body's internal, or **intrinsic** (IN-trin-sick), health affects how we feel as well as how our body and skin look and perform. Free radicals (unstable molecules) in the body, dehydration (lack of water), vitamin deficiencies, improper nutrition, genetics, hormones, puberty, pregnancy, and menopause all affect our skin's well-being. Hormonal imbalances can lead to sensitivity, dehydration, hyperpigmentation, and microcirculation problems that affect capillaries.

Internal Effects on the Skin

- Genetics and ethnicity-influenced conditions
- Free radicals
- Dehydration
- Vitamin deficiencies
- Hormones

- Medical conditions, such as chronic illness, cancer, systemic diseases (diabetes), impaired immune function
- Puberty
- Aging
- Glycation—alters protein structures and decreases biological activity
- Pregnancy
- Menopause

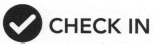

CHECK IN

19. List four intrinsic, or internal, factors that affect the skin.
20. List four extrinsic, or external, factors that affect the skin.
21. What is the main cause of premature extrinsic aging?

ACTIVITY

Protect What Matters

Download a sun factor app on your phone and tell your classmates how it helps to protect your skin from the sun.

Describe Healthy Habits for the Skin

Top 10 healthy habits for the skin:

1. Avoid sun exposure; use sunscreen daily.
2. Eat a balanced diet.
3. Do not smoke.
4. Avoid excessive alcohol.
5. Drink plenty of water.
6. Get plenty of rest.
7. Stay active and exercise regularly.
8. Use beneficial skin care products and a regular home care routine.
9. Get professional skin care treatments to maintain the results of your home care regimen and to more effectively treat the signs of aging, blemishes, or other skin conditions.
10. Implement stress relievers and maintain a calm, positive attitude.

CHECK IN

22. What are five healthy habits for the skin?

Determine Treatment Contraindications through Evaluation, Anaylsis, and Consultation

Certain treatments and skin care products may be contraindicated for a particular client, and it is your responsibility to evaluate the appropriateness of treatment and skin care products after your skin analysis and review of the client's medical history. These **contraindications** (kahn-trah-in-dih-KAY-shunz) are factors that *prohibit* a treatment from being performed or the use of a certain skin care product being used on a client's skin. Certain treatments could cause harmful or negative side effects to those who have specific medical or skin conditions.

Communicable diseases, skin disorders, medical conditions, medications, and skin irritation can all contraindicate, or prohibit, a service or use of a skin care product. The client may list a communicable disease on the client questionnaire. Recognizing diseases is vital to avoid causing harm to clients or to you.

Medications or topical exfoliating agents may make the skin too sensitive for facials or waxing.

Certain medical conditions, illnesses, and diseases, such as cancer, may contraindicate any stimulation to the face or body. Allergies and sensitivities to skin care products must be evaluated. Clients who have obvious skin conditions such as open wounds, cold sores (herpes simplex), or other abnormal-looking conditions should be referred to a medical provider for evaluation and approval for esthetic treatment. Contraindications are also discussed in other chapters.

Contraindications for Skin Treatments

- Certain skin diseases, disorders, or irritations must be considered individually based on the client's overall health.

- Use of Isotretinoin (eye-soh-TRET-i-noin). The client must have completed Isotretinoin six months prior.

- Skin-thinning or exfoliating topical medication, including Retin-A®, Renova™, Tazorac®, Differin®, or other forms of vitamin A. Avoid waxing, exfoliation, and peeling treatments for a minimum of a week.

- Pregnancy: no electrical treatments, chemical peels, or aggressive ingredients, without the client's medical provider's written permission. Some pregnant clients may experience sensitivities from waxing.

- Metal bone pins or plates in the body—avoid all electrical treatments in the area where the pin or plate is located. Medical professional consent is needed prior to treatment.

- Pacemakers or heart irregularities—avoid all electrical treatments that require a grounding pad.

- Allergies—any allergic substances listed on the health history form should be strictly avoided. Become knowledgeable about ingredients. Clients with an allergy to aspirin should not use products or have treatments using salicylic acid. They are both derived from willow bark. Clients with multiple allergies should use fragrance-free products designed for sensitive skin.

- Seizures or epilepsy—avoid all electrical and light-based treatments that pulsate. Medical professional consent is best prior to treatment if the client has a history of seizures.

- Use of oral steroids (cortisones) such as prednisone—avoid any stimulating, exfoliating treatments or waxing, as skin may be more fragile and bruise easier until the client has been off medication for a minimum of two weeks.

- Autoimmune diseases such as lupus, vitiligo—avoid any harsh or stimulating treatments or skin care products.

- Diabetes—people with diabetes who do not have good control of their insulin levels will experience slow healing. If people with diabetes are experiencing neuropathy, nerve damage to the extremities, they may not feel pain in the affected area. If you are in doubt, get approval from the client's medical provider before treatment.

- Blood thinners, including **NSAIDs** (EN-sayd-z)—use caution when performing extractions or when waxing. NSAIDs are nonsteroidal anti-inflammatory drugs; over-the-counter medication used to reduce inflammation, such as ibuprofen.

Client Consultations

A thorough client consultation is important for many reasons. The most important is to determine that a treatment is appropriate for the client or that the skin care products will benefit the client's skin. A consultation will help you to determine why a client may be unhappy with their skin or appearance. Health, lifestyle, occupation, and more affect the skin. Sometimes estheticians are like detectives, trying to determine why the client is having a certain skin problem. The more you know about your client, the more you can make appropriate recommendations for skin care and treatments.

REMINDERS ON HOW TO PREPARE FOR THE CLIENT CONSULTATION

As learned in *Milady Standard Foundations*, it is important to be prepared. To facilitate the consultation process, you should ask yourself the following questions:

1. Is the client comfortable? You are about to begin an important conversation with them that will clue you in to their needs and preferences.

2. Is your work area freshly cleaned and uncluttered?

3. Are all other appropriate tools to perform the desired service ready for use?

4. Do you have a pen or laptop/tablet along with vendor-supplied or salon-manufactured pamphlets, photos, articles, or clinical research papers? These items will help you to present the services or explain the benefits of certain ingredients that will be used to perform a treatment.

5. Do you have step-by-step photos of the actual treatment process? Photos can be helpful in letting clients know what to expect. If you have a satisfied client whose progress is significant, it is extremely important to gain their permission to use such photos for promotional purposes.

6. Will you be able to discuss whom the best candidates are for specific treatments to help decide if the treatment is suitable for a client?

FORMS

You should have at least three forms for a new client:

1. **Intake form**—also called a *client questionnaire, health history form*, or *consultation card*. Clients should complete a confidential intake form that should be updated at each visit. The form discloses the client's healthy history, all products and medications, medical conditions, any known allergies or sensitivities, along with their at-home skin care program, and skin care treatments the client has recently received that could adversely affect treatment. Information should also include important details about the client, including their name, age (optional), occupation, diet, and lifestyle habits. Refer to **Figure 5–11** for a sample intake form.

▼ **FIGURE 5–11** Client Intake Forms

Client Intake Form and Medical History

In order to provide you with the most appropriate treatment, we need you to complete the following questionnaire. All information is confidential.

Date _____

Name _____ **Date of birth** (optional) _____
      (please print)

Email address _____

Address _____
      Street   City   State   Zip

Phone number (easiest number to reach you) _____

Occupation _____

How were you referred to us? _____

Medical History

Are you currently under the care of a physician for any reason? _____ ☐ Yes ☐ No

If yes, for what? _____

History	Yes	No	Date/List/Comments
List all medications, supplements, and vitamins			
List allergies			
Accutane			
Antibiotics			
Birth control pills			
Hormones			
Aspirin, ibuprofen use			
Retin-A®, Tretinoin			
Metrogel®, MetroCream®			

(Continued)

History	Yes	No	Date/List/Comments
Glycolic acid on a regular basis			
Antidepressants			
Sun reactions			
Medication allergies			
Food allergies			
Aspirin allergy			
Latex allergy			
Lidocaine allergy			
Hydrocortisone allergy			
Hydroquinone allergy			
Diabetes			
Smoking history			
Cold sores, herpes			
Bleeding disorders			
AutoImmune, HIV			
Pregnant or planning to be			
Pacemaker			
Implants of any kind: Dental, breast, facial			
Migraine headaches			
Glaucoma			
Cancer			
Arthritis			
Hepatitis			
Thyroid imbalance			
Seizure disorder			
Active infection			
Radiation in last three months			
Skin Conditions			
Acne			
Melasma			
Tattoos, perm makeup, and microblading			
Vitiligo			
Keloid scarring			
Skin/laser treatments at another office		If so, when?	Results
Botox		If so, when?	Results
Fillers		If so, when?	Results
Hair removal		If so, when?	Results

(Continues)

History	Yes	No	Date/List/Comments
Chemical peels		If so, when?	Results
Sun exposure/tanning bed in last week? Self tanner?		If so, when?	Results
List Medical Issues Not Listed Above			

Current Skin Care and Lifestyle

1. How do you wash your face? ☐ Soap   ☐ Cleanser
2. If soap, what brand? _____
3. If cleanser, what brand name? _____
4. Do you use a moisturizer? ☐ Yes ☐ No
5. Are you on a special diet? ☐ Yes ☐ No
   If yes, please specify. _____
6. Do you consume water daily? ☐ Yes ☐ No
   If yes, how much? _____
7. Do you drink coffee, tea, or soda daily? ☐ Yes ☐ No
   Coffee ounces ___ Tea ounces ___ Soda ounces ___
8. Do you exercise? ☐ Yes ☐ No
   If yes, how often? _____
9. Have you ever had a facial? ☐ Yes ☐ No
   If yes, when was your last facial? _____
10. Do you give yourself facials at home? ☐ Yes ☐ No
    If yes, how often? _____
11. List additional cosmetics and skin care products you are currently using:

What is the primary reason for your visit today? (Select all that apply in the list below.)

☐ I'm concerned about facial or body hair and would like information on ways to get rid of it.
☐ I'm concerned about fine lines around my eyes.
☐ I'm concerned about scowl lines when I frown.
☐ I'm concerned about pigmentation or age spots.
☐ I'm concerned about broken capillaries on my face or spider veins on my legs.
☐ I'm concerned about skin laxity and sagging.
☐ I'm concerned about the lines around my mouth.
☐ I'd like more defined lips.
☐ Other (please list skin concerns below)

(Continues)

(Continued)

I certify that the preceding medical, personal, and skin history statements are true and correct. I am aware that it is my responsibility to inform the technician of my current medical and health conditions and to update this information at subsequent visits. A current history is essential for the provider to execute appropriate treatment procedures. I have signed the consent form for this procedure. I had the opportunity to ask questions prior to the treatment. I accept arbitration as a means of resolution for practice liability.

_____

Client Signature   Date

▼ **FIGURE 5–12** Client Consent Form

Client Consent Form

I hereby consent to and authorize _____ to perform the following procedure:
                                                        (esthetician)

_____

I have voluntarily elected to undergo this treatment/procedure after the nature and purpose of this treatment have been explained to me, along with the risks and hazards involved, by _____ .
                                                                                                        (esthetician)

Although it is impossible to list every potential risk and complication, I have been informed of possible benefits, risks, and complications. I also recognize there are no guaranteed results and that independent results are dependent upon age, skin condition, and lifestyle and that there is the possibility I may require further treatments of the treated areas to obtain the expected results at an additional cost.

I understand how important it is to follow all instructions given to me for post-treatment care. In the event that I have additional questions or concerns regarding my treatment or suggested home product/post-treatment care, I will consult [insert your business name] immediately.

I have also, to the best of my knowledge, given an accurate account of my medical history, including all known allergies or prescription drugs or products I am currently ingesting or using topically.

I have read and fully understand this agreement and all information detailed above. I understand the procedure and accept the risks. All of my questions have been answered to my satisfaction and I consent to the terms of this agreement. I do not hold the esthetician, whose signature appears below, responsible for any of my conditions that were present, but not disclosed, at the time of this skin care procedure, which may be affected by the treatment performed today.

Client name (printed) _____

Client name (signature) _____ Date _____

Esthetician _____ Date _____

▼ **FIGURE 5–13** Service Record Card

Service Record

Date ______________________________

Client name ______________________________

Specific concerns being targeted ______________________________

Changes to health since last visit? Yes __________ No __________

Photos taken Yes __________ No __________

Type of treatment ______________________________

Settings ______________________________

Client's skin type (circle one number)

- ☐ 1. Fair—always burns, never tans
- ☐ 2. Light skin tones—can burn, sometimes tans
- ☐ 3. Medium to olive skin tones, tans easily
- ☐ 4. Light brown to medium brown skin tones
- ☐ 5. Brown, moderately pigmented skin
- ☐ 6. Dark brown/black skin tones

Notes

____

____

Contraindications

____

____

In-Office Treatment Recommendations	Today	Future

Home care instructions given Yes __________ No __________

(Continues)

Recommended Home Skin Care Products

Product Types	AM Products Recommended	PM Products Recommended	Products Purchased
Cleanser			
Toner			
Exfoliant			
Serum			
Mask			
Protection			
Eyes/lips			
Moisturizer, sunscreen			
Other			

Skin Assessment and Analysis

Conditions

- ☐ Acne breakouts
- ☐ Actinic keratosis
- ☐ Aging
- ☐ Asphyxiation, or lacking oxygenation
- ☐ Comedones (open or closed)
- ☐ Couperose
- ☐ Cysts
- ☐ Dark circles
- ☐ Dehydration
- ☐ Enlarged pores
- ☐ Erythema
- ☐ Fine lines
- ☐ Growths

- ☐ Hirsutism
- ☐ Hyper- or hypopigmentation
- ☐ Hyperkeratinization
- ☐ Hypertrichosis
- ☐ Keratosis
- ☐ Mature
- ☐ Melasma
- ☐ Milia
- ☐ Moles
- ☐ Oiliness
- ☐ Papules
- ☐ Poikiloderma of Civatte
- ☐ Poor elasticity
- ☐ Puffiness

- ☐ Pustules
- ☐ Redness
- ☐ Rhytids
- ☐ Rosacea
- ☐ Scarring
- ☐ Sebaceous hyperplasia
- ☐ Seborrhea
- ☐ Sensitivity
- ☐ Striae, or stretch marks
- ☐ Sun damage
- ☐ Telangiectasia
- ☐ Other

Acne: ☐ 1 ☐ 2 ☐ 3 ☐ 4

Skin Type: ☐ Dry ☐ Normal ☐ Combination ☐ Oily

Skin Texture: ☐ Thin ☐ Thick ☐ Medium

Complexion Color: ☐ Pale ☐ Pink ☐ Olive ☐ Sallow ☐ Suntan ☐ Other

Pigmentation: ☐ Even ☐ Uneven ☐ Birthmarks ☐ Heavy freckling ☐ Some freckling

Muscle Tone: ☐ Good ☐ Fair ☐ Fallen

Rhytids: ☐ Deep wrinkles ☐ Crow's feet ☐ Fine lines throughout face

Broken Capillaries: ☐ Nose area ☐ Cheek area ☐ Chin area ☐ Nose ☐ Forehead

Diet Concerns _____

UV Exposure Concerns _____

Stress Concerns _____

Esthetician signature _____ **Date** _____

"**Beauty is power; a smile is its sword**"

—John Ray

2. **Consent form** (KUN-sent FORM)—also referred to as to *consent to treat release*; a customary written agreement between the esthetician and the client for applying a treatment, whether routine or preoperative (**Figure 5–12**). The client reads and signs the document, acknowledging that they understand what is being done to them as well as the risks involved in the treatment and releasing you from liability before you perform services.

3. **Client chart or service record card**—a record of all your notes from the skin analysis, the type of treatment performed, products used in the treatment, goals you are working toward, your home care recommendations, and other consultation notes (**Figure 5–13**). This information will be needed for future visits.

HOW TO USE THE CLIENT INTAKE FORM

The client intake form should be mentioned the moment a new client calls the skin care salon or spa to make an appointment. When scheduling the appointment, let the client know that you and the salon will require some information before you can begin the service. Some salons ask clients to arrive 15 minutes before their appointment time for this purpose. You will also have to allow time in your schedule to conduct a 5- to 15-minute client consultation, the verbal communication with a client to determine desired results, depending on the type of service you will be performing and the client's needs. Some schools or facilities ask clients to sign and date the intake form, especially when more advanced procedures are involved, while other facilities use the consent form for this purpose.

HOW TO USE THE CONSENT FORM

When introducing the consent form to clients, take time to review all the steps involved in the treatment process. Be sure to carefully explain any home care directions that may be necessary. Provide the client with a copy of the consent form, and keep the original for your files. It is also wise to maintain a treatment log and have the client initial and date all subsequent treatment procedures. These extra precautionary measures go a long way in safeguarding both you and the client.

QUESTIONS TO ASK DURING THE CONSULTATION

Common questions include the following:

- What is the reason for your visit? (What brought the client in? Is it for a treatment or just relaxation?)

- What are your skin concerns? (What are they bothered about?)

- What are your skin care goals? Are you preparing for a special event? When is it?

- What is your home skin care routine? (How many products does the client use at home? What are the ingredients, and how often are they used?)

- Have you had treatments before? (Is this the client's first treatment of this type?)

- Do you have allergies to products or scents?

- Is this a normal state for your skin? (Is it normally clearer? Is it usually less irritated?)

- How does your skin feel during different times of the day? (What is the degree of oiliness or dryness?)

- Do you wear sunscreen? What is the SPF value?

- Tell me about your diet. Do you eat a healthy diet? How much processed food do you eat? How often do you eat out?

- How much water do you drink?

- What is your activity level? Are you often outdoors?

- Do you smoke?

- Any other allergies?

- How stressful is your lifestyle? Are you under a lot of stress right now?

- Have you had any esthetic procedures prior? How long ago? Are you happy with the results?

The skin care consultation and skin analysis is your moment to make the clients aware of what you note about their skin condition, and what services or products you offer that could benefit them. The consultation is also a marketing and educational opportunity to introduce services and products to the client. Once you learn about ingredients and start performing skin care treatments, you will be recommending products. Think about how you can help the client through treatments, home care suggestions, and preventative measures. Conduct the consultation, discuss what you see with the client, and give recommendations during the analysis or

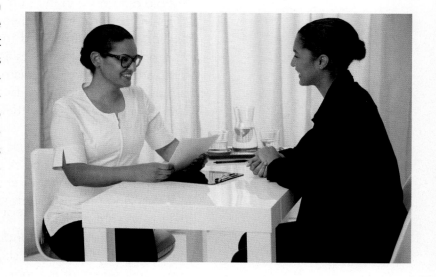

after the treatment. It is beneficial to practice skin analysis before diving into products and treatments. Each subject you study gives you a foundation to build upon for the next step.

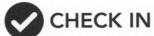

CHECK IN

23. List six contraindications for facial treatments.
24. What three forms are needed for interaction with a client?
25. List eight questions you would ask a client during a consultation.

Perform a Skin Analysis

Knowing how to analyze skin is the first step in providing successful skin care treatments and recommending effective skin care products. Identifying conditions and contraindications, as well as providing thorough consultations and charting client notes, are all elements of good esthetic practices.

Educating clients on healthy habits and the causes of skin conditions is part of the service. Products, ingredients, different types of facials, and a home care regimen for preventative maintenance are all beneficial in caring for the skin. A series of treatments may be necessary to effectively help the client's conditions. Twenty years of sun damage cannot be helped overnight. Realistically, it could take weeks or months to see a visible difference in the skin.

Even if there is no obvious visible change, skin care treatments have positive benefits and make a difference. Information on choosing products for treatments and home care is presented in Chapter 6, Skin Care Products: Chemistry, Ingredients, and Selection. Skin analysis may seem challenging, but practice and experience will build confidence in using this essential skill. Soon you will automatically notice skin conditions.

Become adept at a quick skin analysis in the waiting room because sometimes clients need quick product recommendations or are not sure what type of treatment they should schedule. This skill can be very beneficial in selling products or treatments. You can perform a more in-depth analysis when the client comes in for treatment.

Knowing skin types, conditions, and the factors affecting the skin's health, as well as interview skills that encourage your client to open up about their skin care regimen, enables you to perform an accurate skin analysis. The best tool for analyzing the skin is a magnifying lamp/light. A **Wood's lamp** (WOODZ LAMP) is a filtered black light that is used to illuminate skin disorders, fungi, bacterial disorders, and deeper levels of pigmentation (discussed in Chapter 10 Facial Devices and Technology) or an electronic photo imaging system. Other hand-held tools such as a moisture analyzation meter and devices that magnify hundreds of times are available to analyze the skin.

Client information is personal and confidential, so be objective when you write on a client's chart. Clients will appreciate you remembering their children's names or their recent trip to Hawaii, so try to recall some personal information the next time they come in and keep it in a separate file for your own personal reference. Your records could be legal documents in a dispute with a client. Write legibly. Make sure you date all entries and sign your name.

Review the steps to performing a skin analysis in **Procedure 5–1** and demonstrate your abilities to your instructor as set forth in the guidelines.

──PERFORM──
Procedure 5-1
Skin Analysis

ACTIVITY

Customize The Skin Analysis

Perform a skin analysis and practice consultations with fellow students. Complete mock health history forms with a variety of information that would be pertinent in a skin care consultation. Document your findings and record your recommendations.

 CHECK IN

26. Describe the steps in a skin analysis procedure.
27. What are the areas that the esthetician needs to review during the skin analysis?

Procedure 5-1:
Performing a Skin Analysis

Implements and Materials

Gather the following supplies and products:

SUPPLIES
- ☐ EPA-registered disinfectant
- ☐ Hand sanitizer or antibacterial soap
- ☐ Covered trash container
- ☐ Bowl
- ☐ Spatula
- ☐ Hand towels
- ☐ Headband
- ☐ Clean linens
- ☐ Bolster

SINGLE-USE ITEMS
- ☐ Gloves
- ☐ Esthetics wipes (4" × 4" for cleansing; or disposable sponges)
- ☐ Cotton rounds
- ☐ Cotton swabs
- ☐ Plastic bag
- ☐ Paper towels
- ☐ Tissues

PRODUCTS
- ☐ Eye makeup remover or cleanser
- ☐ Facial cleanser
- ☐ Toner
- ☐ Moisturizer
- ☐ Topical sunscreen

Preparation

The four components of skin analysis are **look**, **feel**, **ask**, and **listen**. *Record* your findings.

Procedure

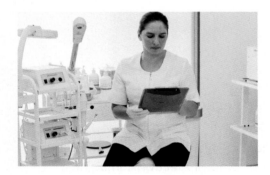

1 Review the client's health history questionnaire. Look for medical conditions, medications, allergies, or other indications that the client is not an appropriate candidate for treatment. While you are reviewing the documentation, ask your client questions for clarification, if necessary.

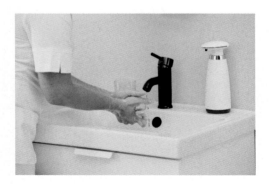

2 Wash your hands as instructed in *Milady Standard Foundations*, Procedure 5–1: Proper Handwashing.

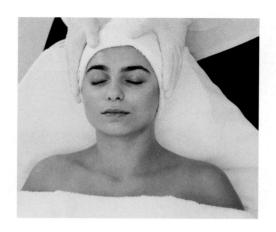

3 ***Look*** briefly at your client's skin (including the neck and chest) with your naked eye or a magnifying light. In order to achieve a more accurate analysis you will need to remove your client's makeup in the following step.

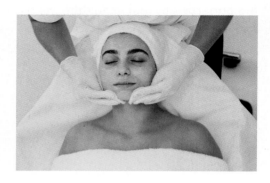

4 Cleanse the skin (a client's normal state of dryness or oiliness may not be as visible immediately after cleansing).

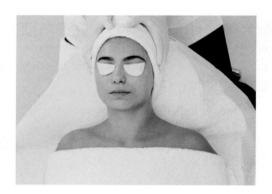

5 Cover the eyes with eye pads. Make sure the eye pads are not too large or they may block the eye area you need to analyze or treat.

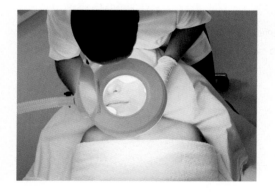

6 Use a magnifying light to examine the skin more thoroughly. A Wood's lamp or electronic imaging system may also be used.

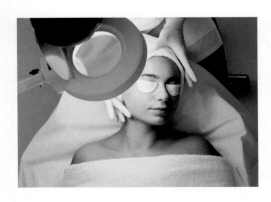

7 *Look* closely to determine the client's skin type, the conditions present, and the overall appearance.

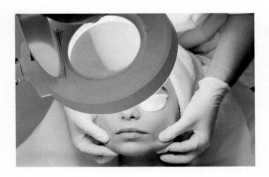

8 *Touch* the skin with the fingertips to feel its texture, its oil and water content, and its elasticity. Pay attention to the T-zone.

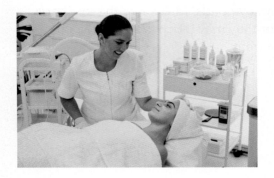

9 *Ask* and *listen*. Ask questions about the skin's appearance, the client's health, and their lifestyle to gain a better understanding. Verbally describe to your client what you are finding in your analysis.

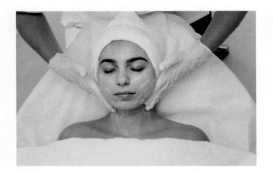

10 Apply a toner and moisturizer or sunscreen to balance and protect the skin.

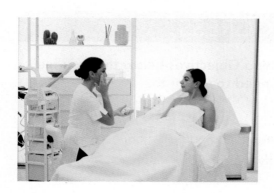

11 Recommend a skin care plan that includes professional treatments and skin care products for a home care regimen. Giving the client a treatment plan in writing and including some skin care samples is a way to build your clientele. (Refer to Chapter 6, Skin Care Products: Chemistry, Ingredients, and Selection.)

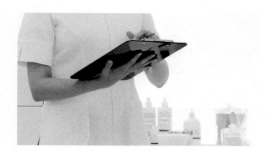

12 Record your findings and your recommendations in the client's chart—usually after the treatment is completed.

How are you doing with skin analysis? **Check the Chapter 5 Learning Objectives below that you feel you have mastered; leave unchecked those objectives you will need to return to.**

- ☐ Explain the process of skin analysis.
- ☐ Identify the four genetic skin types through visualization, palpation, and consultation.
- ☐ Differentiate the six Fitzpatrick skin types and accurately identify them.
- ☐ Distinguish the characteristics of sensitive skin.
- ☐ Recognize the intricacies involved with treating skin of color.
- ☐ Identify treatment options for the neck and décolleté.
- ☐ Illustrate examples of skin conditions.
- ☐ Explain the causes of skin conditions.
- ☐ Describe healthy habits for the skin.
- ☐ Determine treatment contraindications through evaluation, analysis, and consultation.
- ☐ Perform a skin analysis.

GLOSSARY

consent form KUN-sent FORM	pg. 186	a customary written agreement between the esthetician (salon/spa) and the client for applying a treatment, whether routine or preoperative
contraindications kahn-trah-in-dih-KAY-shunz	pg. 177	factors that prohibit a treatment due to a condition; treatments could cause harmful or negative side effects to those who have specific medical or skin conditions
décolleté dey-kol-TEY	pg. 171	also referred to as *décolletage* (dek-UH-luh-taj); pertaining to a woman's lower neck and chest
dehydration dee-HY-dray-shun	pg. 172	lack of water
extrinsic EKS-trinz-ik	pg. 176	primarily environmental factors that contribute to aging and the appearance of aging
Fitzpatrick scale FITS-pat-rick scayl	pg. 167	scale used to measure skin's reaction to the sun. There are six types: type 1 is the fairest, and type 6 is the darkest; all skin falls somewhere on this scale when evaluated on factors such as eye color, skin tone, heritage, and response to UV exposure
genetic juh-NET-ik	pg. 164	related to heredity and ancestry of origin
hirsutism HUR-soo-tiz-um	pg. 173	condition pertaining to an excessive growth or cover of hair
holistically hoh-LIS-tik-lee	pg. 166	a system of evaluating the entire individual in an interdisciplinary style, recognizing that body systems work synergistically
hypertrichosis hy-pur-trih-KOH-sis	pg. 173	condition of abnormal growth of hair, characterized by the growth of terminal hair in areas of the body that normally grow only vellus hair

intrinsic IN-trin-sick	pg. 176	skin-aging factors over which we have little control because they are a part of our genetics and familial heredity
isotretinoin eye-soh-TRET-i-noin	pg. 178	brand name: Accutane; a controlled prescription medication derived from vitamin A that is used to treat severe acne that has not responded to other treatments
melasma mel-AZ-muh	pg. 173	a form of hyperpigmentation that is characterized by bilateral patches of brown pigmentation on the cheeks, jawline, forehead, and upper lip due to hormonal imbalances such as pregnancy, birth control pills, or hormone replacement therapy
NSAIDs EN-sayd-z	pg. 179	nonsteroidal anti-inflammatory drugs; over-the-counter medication used to reduce inflammation, such as ibuprofen
palpation pal-PAY-shun	pg. 164	manual manipulation of tissue by touching to make an assessment of its condition
photosensitivity FOTO-sensa-tiv-it-ee	pg. 176	high sensitivity of the skin to UV light, usually following exposure or ingestion of certain medications, or chemicals that result in accelerated response of the skin to UV radiation
rhytids RIT-ihdz	pg. 172	wrinkles
skin type SKIN TYPE	pg. 164	classification that describes a person's genetic skin type
solar comedones SOH-lur KAHM-uh-dohn	pg. 174	large open comedones, usually around the eyes, due to sun exposure
striae strahy-ee	pg. 174	dermal scars due to rapid expansion or stretching of connective tissue leaving deep red, pink, or purple linear marks on the skin that gradually fade to light pink or silver over time. they often occur during growth phases in puberty, pregnancy, and weight gain
"tech neck" TEK NEK	pg. 171	rhytids that develop due to the repeated movement of looking down at a cell phone or other electronic device
telangiectasia tel-an-JEE-ek-tay-juh	pg. 169	visible broken or distended capillaries less than 0.5 mm due to intrinsic or extrinsic causes
TEWL too-wuhl	pg. 167	abbreviation for transepidermal water loss; water loss caused by evaporation on the skin's surface
T-zone TEE-ZOHN	pg. 164	center area of the face; corresponds to the "T" shape formed by the forehead, nose, and chin
Wood's lamp WOODZ LAMP	pg. 188	filtered black light that is used to illuminate skin disorders, fungi, bacterial disorders, and pigmentation

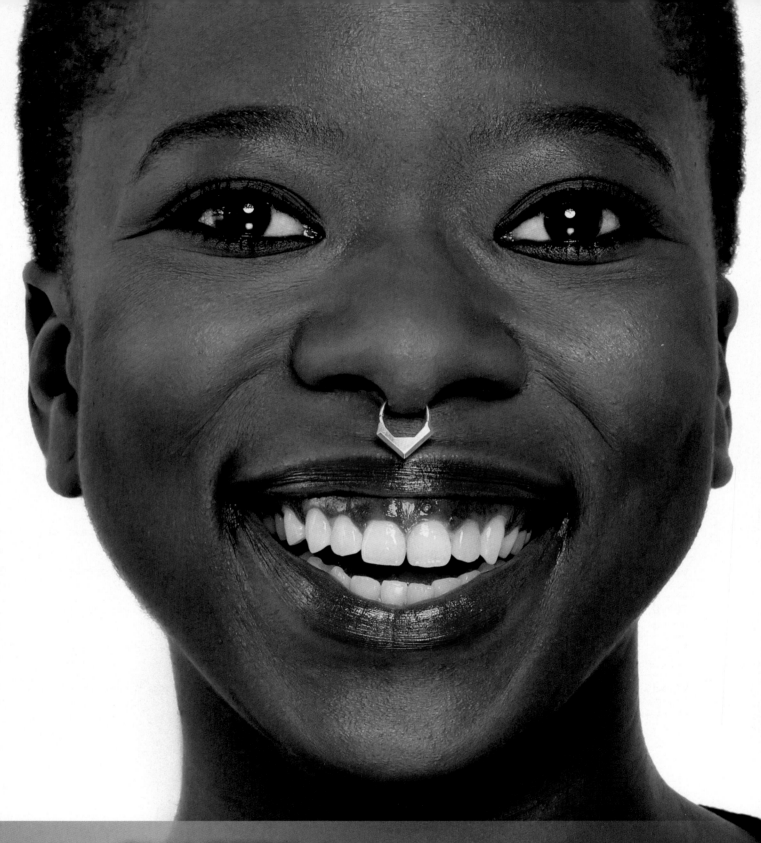

CHAPTER 6
Skin Care Products: Chemistry, Ingredients, and Selection

"Life begins at the end of your comfort zone."

–Neale Donald Walsch

Learning Objectives

After completing this chapter, you will be able to:

1. Explain how skin care products and ingredients are significant to estheticians.
2. Describe cosmetic regulations, laws, and product safety.
3. Distinguish cosmetic ingredient sources and popular terms.
4. Describe the main types of ingredients in cosmetic chemistry.
5. Identify beneficial ingredients for skin types and conditions.
6. Select appropriate products for facial treatments and home care use.
7. Recommend home care products with confidence.
8. Summarize the points to consider when choosing a professional skin care line.

Explain How Skin Care Products and Ingredients are Significant to Estheticians

Estheticians must study and have a thorough understanding of a wide range of skin care products and ingredients (**Figure 6–1**). It is very important to your career to provide clients with appropriate treatments and home care products to achieve their goal of healthy skin, as well as work within the specific laws and regulations that pertain to cosmetics and ingredients.

Estheticians should study and have a thorough understanding of skin care products because:

- It is critical to know basic chemistry of formulations, cosmetic ingredients, benefits, and potential side effects; how to select products and ingredients based on an individual's needs, skin type, and condition; and, finally, products and ingredients to avoid for certain individuals and how to handle adverse reactions.

- It is essential to educate your clients about products and ingredients that you use in a treatment or recommend for their home care use.

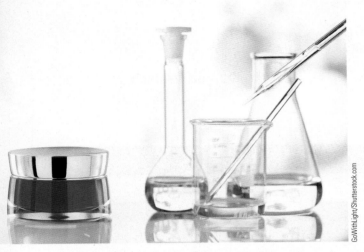

▲ **FIGURE 6–1** Estheticians must continuously study products in order to provide clients with optimal results.

- You must be able to explain what skin care products and ingredients do, why they're effective, realistic expectations, and how to properly use products at home. The more knowledgeable you are, the more confident you will be with your recommendations. Mastering this skill will bring you much success, as it creates long-term relationships with clients who depend on you for expert skin care advice.

- As new developments in cosmetic chemistry are constantly evolving, it's imperative that estheticians remain on top of the latest ingredient and product technology throughout their entire career. Postgraduate training and education is key to staying up to date and offering the best in products and services. There are many great resources available to estheticians, including industry trade shows, publications, and postgraduate workshops.

Describe Cosmetic Regulations, Laws, and Product Safety

As an esthetician, it is critical to learn laws, regulations, and safety guidelines when it comes to cosmetic products.

FDA Regulations for Cosmetics

In the United States, the Food and Drug Administration (FDA) is responsible for ensuring the safety of our nation's **cosmetics** (kahz-MET-iks), which includes makeup and skin care products. There are laws and regulations that apply to cosmetics on the market. The two most important laws pertaining to cosmetics marketed in the United States are:

- The Federal Food, Drug, and Cosmetic Act (FD&C Act)
- The Fair Packaging and Labeling Act (FPLA)

The FDA regulates cosmetics under the authority of these two laws. The law does not require cosmetic products and ingredients (other than color additives) to have FDA approval before they go on the market. In fact, no cosmetic may be labeled or advertised with statements suggesting that FDA has approved the product.

HOW DOES THE LAW DEFINE A COSMETIC?

The Federal Food, Drug, and Cosmetic Act (FD&C Act) defines cosmetics as "articles intended to be rubbed, poured, sprinkled, or sprayed on, introduced into, or otherwise applied to the human body... for cleansing, beautifying, promoting attractiveness, or altering the

DID YOU KNOW?

The FDA does not *approve* cosmetics before they go on the market. The FDA only *regulates* cosmetics in relation to safety, labeling, and the claims made for a product.

appearance."[1] Cosmetics are intended to affect the *appearance* of the skin.

HOW DOES THE LAW DEFINE A DRUG?

The FD&C Act defines drugs as "articles intended for use in the diagnosis, cure, mitigation, treatment, or prevention of disease" and "articles (other than food) intended to affect the structure or any function of the body of man or other animals."[2] Drugs in skin care products are intended to cause actual *physiological changes*, such as the structure or function of the skin.

CAN A PRODUCT BE BOTH A COSMETIC AND A DRUG?

Some nonprescription medicated products have lower doses of active ingredients and meet the definitions of both cosmetics and drugs (**Figure 6–2**). These are considered over-the-counter (OTC) drugs. This may happen when a product has two intended uses. For example, a **cleanser** (KLENZ-er) is a cosmetic because its intended use is to cleanse the skin. An acne cleanser with benzoyl peroxide is a drug because its intended use is to treat acne. This type of product is then considered both a cosmetic and a drug. Among other nonprescription cosmetic/drug combinations are **moisturizers** (MOYST-yur-yz-urz) and makeup marketed with sun-protection claims. These products must comply with FDA requirements for both cosmetics and drugs.

WHAT ARE COSMECEUTICALS?

The term **cosmeceutical** (KAHZ-muh-SUIT-ick-al) has no meaning under the law. A product can legally be a drug, a cosmetic, or a combination of both. The professional skin care industry created this term as a bridge between cosmetics and pharmaceuticals, or drugs. It can be used in many ways, but in general refers to professional skin care products and makeup that include *pharmaceutical-grade* ingredients. This pertains to higher concentrations, grade, and purity of active agents.

Product Labeling Laws and Regulations

FDA regulations for cosmetic labeling state that cosmetic companies must list the company's name, location, or distribution point as well as all the ingredients in the product. This allows consumers to check for ingredients they may be allergic to. Ingredients must be listed in descending order of predominance, starting with the ingredient having the highest concentration and ending with the ingredient having the lowest concentration. Ingredients with a concentration of less than 1 percent may be listed in any order. A fragrance must be listed as *fragrance*, but the particular ingredients used for the fragrance need not be listed.

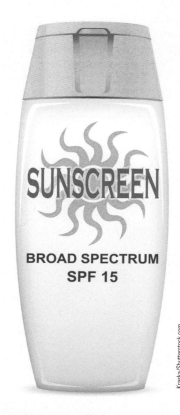

▲ **FIGURE 6–2** Nonprescription medicated products can be considered both a cosmetic and a drug.

Kraska/Shutterstock.com

---

[1] U.S. Food and Drug Administration. (April 30, 2012). Is It a Cosmetic, a Drug, or Both? (Or Is It Soap?) Retrieved from https://www.fda.gov/Cosmetics/GuidanceRegulation/LawsRegulations/ucm074201.htm#Definecosmetic

[2] Ibid.

INCI NAMES

The FDA also requires that all cosmetics labels include a list of ingredients using standardized *INCI names* for each ingredient. INCI is an acronym for *International Nomenclature Cosmetic Ingredient*. INCI names are allocated by the American Cosmetic Association, Personal Care Products Council and are used internationally. The adoption of INCI names ensures that cosmetic ingredients are consistently listed, using the same ingredient name from product to product. This allows consumers to easily compare multiple products that have the same ingredient names all around the world.

Product Safety

Companies and individuals who market cosmetics have a legal responsibility to ensure the safety and proper labeling of their products. Under the law, cosmetics must not be misbranded. For example, they must be safe for consumers when used according to directions on the label, or in the customary or expected way. Also, if a cosmetic product makes a drug claim, it is not properly labeled. The FDA can take legal action against a cosmetic on the market if they have reliable information showing that it is misbranded.

ADVERSE REACTIONS

Many ingredients used in skin care products and treatments may cause adverse skin reactions. Fragrances and some preservatives and chemical sunscreen ingredients are among the most common allergens.

Symptoms

It is often very difficult to distinguish whether a reaction is allergic or irritant. Physicians indicate that, in general, symptoms of an irritant reaction include burning, while itching is usually a sign of an allergic reaction. Additional symptoms may include inflammation of the skin, blisters, hives, or rashes. The eyes may swell, puff, or produce tears. In addition, adverse reactions may be detected immediately after product application, or may not show up until days or weeks later.

Being aware of a client's allergies and the ingredients being used in treatments is very important to avoid adverse reactions. During consultation, it's very important that a client discloses any potential allergies. This should be indicated on their skin health intake form, and then verified again by the esthetician before proceeding with a treatment.

Patch Test

If there are any concerns, the best way to guard against reactions is to pretest a small quantity of the product with a patch test. Apply the product on the inside of the arm near the elbow or behind the ear (**Figure 6–3**). If there is any reaction within 24 hours, the product should not be used.

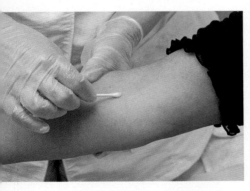

▲ **FIGURE 6–3** A patch test is the best way to determine if a client is allergic to a product.

How to Handle an Adverse Reaction

If during a facial treatment the skin becomes excessively red or the client complains of burning, immediately remove the product, rinse the skin with cold water, and apply cool compresses until the skin calms. Having products to calm skin reactions is also a recommended precaution.

If the client contacts you regarding an adverse reaction from a home care product that you've recommended, advise them to discontinue use of the product immediately. They may choose to use an over-the-counter hydrocortisone cream to help the symptoms subside. If the reaction is serious, they should seek medical care and bring the product with them so the physician can determine what caused the problem and treat accordingly. The manufacturer of the product should be notified immediately.

 CHECK IN

1. What agency in the United States is responsible for ensuring the safety of our nation's cosmetics, including makeup and skin care products?
2. By law, what is the difference between a cosmetic and a drug?
3. Why are INCI names used on product labels for ingredients?
4. What are the most common allergens in skin care products?
5. What should an esthetician do if during a facial treatment the client has an adverse reaction?

> **CAUTION!**
>
> If a client has an allergic reaction to a product that requires medical treatment, the manufacturer of the product is responsible—unless the product was purchased in bulk, repackaged by the salon in smaller containers, and resold, in which case the salon is at fault. If the product is made in the salon, the salon is responsible. Malpractice insurance does not generally cover products formulated or repackaged in the salon.

Distinguish Cosmetic Ingredient Sources and Popular Terms

Cosmetic ingredients can be derived from natural sources, including plants, vitamins, or animals. They can also be synthesized in a lab using chemical compounds.

Natural Versus Synthetic Ingredients

Products directly from nature can have powerful skin benefits; however, some of the most effective cosmetic ingredients are not derived from natural sources. Synthetically produced ingredients can be just as effective and may have certain advantages over ingredients derived from nature, such as no use of pesticides or not leaving an ecological footprint.

Manufacturers do extensive research and development to bring the latest technologies into cosmetic formulations. For example, hyaluronic acid, an ingredient used to bind moisture, was initially derived from roosters' combs. Synthetic production of this ingredient was developed, and today it is derived from synthetic sources for use in cosmetics. The synthetic version is more stable and has more effective water-binding properties.

Sometimes it can be difficult to know when to choose natural-sourced ingredients or synthetic ones because both make tremendous contributions to skin care formulations. Many manufacturers combine natural-sourced and synthetic ingredients to obtain the best of both worlds. Clients will prefer one philosophy over the other and will be attracted to either natural or more clinical products. Knowing the benefits of both is important for estheticians and for those selling products.

Popular Terms

Many of the terms used in relation to skin care products and ingredients will be found on promotional brochures, in advertisements, and in television commercials. These terms are not regulated by law but are used as descriptive words for consumer marketing purposes.

NATURAL, ALL NATURAL

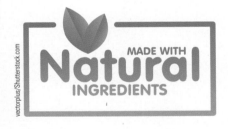

vectorplus/Shutterstock.com

The terms **natural** (NATCH-uh-rul) and **all natural** (AL NATCH-uh-rul) are often used in marketing for skin care products and ingredients derived from natural sources. Because there is no specific legal definition, they are often used loosely. Many consumers seek natural ingredients because they are concerned about the effects of chemical ingredients. Technically, *all life-forms are made of chemicals*. In fact, a single plant extract can be made up of literally hundreds of chemicals.

The true concern pertains to toxic ingredients in general, which can come from both natural and synthetic sources. There are now many resources available online to easily find toxicity ratings on ingredients in skin care products if there is a concern.

ORGANIC

Organic (or-GAN-ik) describes natural-sourced ingredients that are grown without the use of pesticides or chemicals. These ingredients are becoming more popular as consumer demand increases. The FDA does not define or regulate the term *organic* as it applies to cosmetics, body care, or personal care products. The only regulation for the term *organic* is by the U.S. Department of Agriculture (USDA) as it applies to agricultural products. If a cosmetic, body care product, or personal care product contains agricultural ingredients and can meet certain standards, it may be eligible only to be *certified organic* under the National Organic Program regulations.

CRUELTY-FREE

Cruelty-free (KROO-uhl-tee FREE) is a term used to describe products that are not tested on animals at any stage of the production process; nor are any of their ingredients tested on animals.

VEGAN

A product that is labeled **vegan** (VEE-guhn) should not contain any animal ingredients or animal by-products. This includes, but is not limited to, honey, beeswax, **lanolin** (LAN-ul-un), and collagen. However, because the term is not regulated it's often used to simply note that a product does not contain animal ingredients. This may be confusing to consumers because products may still contain animal by-products.

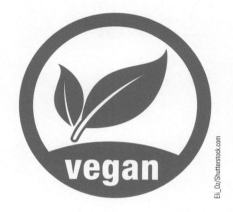

Eli_0z/Shutterstock.com

GLUTEN-FREE

Gluten is a general name for the proteins found in wheat, rye, and triticale—a cross between wheat and rye. Celiac disease is an autoimmune disorder in which eating gluten causes the lining of the body's small intestine to become inflamed. Recently, celiac disease, gluten sensitivity, and gluten intolerance cases have been on the rise and continue to grow as healthcare professionals learn more about these conditions. As a result of the mounting concern about gluten, cosmetic chemists have been asked to formulate gluten-free products.

Although there are many theories, currently there is no scientific evidence that the use of gluten-containing products is harmful to someone with celiac disease unless a product is ingested or used on the lips or in the mouth (such as lipstick, toothpaste, or mouthwash). It is possible for someone to have an allergy to wheat or another grain that could cause a skin reaction. In any case, it's always up to the client and skin care professional to make the best possible choice for their personal health.

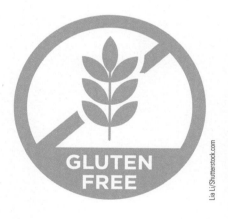

Lia Li/Shutterstock.com

On skin care ingredient labels, some primary sources of gluten are listed as hydrolyzed wheat protein, triticum vulgare (wheat germ) oil or extract, and wheat amino acids. To establish a gluten-free claim, the FDA and organizations concerned with international food standards have set preliminary thresholds of less than 20 parts per million (ppm) of gluten.

HYPOALLERGENIC, DERMATOLOGIST TESTED, NONIRRITATING

Hypoallergenic (hy-poh-al-ur-JEN-ik), *dermatologist tested*, and *nonirritating* are terms that describe ingredients or products that may be less likely to cause allergic reactions. This is not a guarantee, however, that skin will not react.

NONCOMEDOGENIC

Noncomedogenic refers to ingredients that will not clog pores.

COMEDOGENIC

Comedogenic refers to ingredients that tend to clog pores, especially by the formation of blackheads.

FRAGRANCE-FREE

A **fragrance-free** (FREY-gruhns FREE) label on a product does not mean it has no smell. Fragrance-free indicates that no additional ingredients have been added to the product to specifically provide a fragrance; however, it may already contain ingredients that have a scent. For example, a product may contain lavender for its therapeutic benefits. **Lavender** (LAV-uhn-der) has a very distinct aroma, but if it (or any other ingredient) wasn't added to the product specifically to give it a scent, the product is considered fragrance free.

UNSCENTED

Unscented (un-SENT-id) products are formulated to have no smell. Because most ingredients in a formulation do have an odor, more ingredients have to be added to mask and neutralize the smell. For example, if a product is formulated with lavender, a chemical can be added to mask or neutralize the lavender's smell so the product can then be labeled as unscented.

 CHECK IN

6. Name the sources that cosmetic ingredients can be derived from.
7. What is the difference between noncomedogenic and comedogenic ingredients?
8. What does a fragrance-free label on a product mean?
9. What has to be done to a product formulation in order for it to be labeled unscented?

Describe the Main Types of Ingredients in Cosmetic Chemistry

Every ingredient used in cosmetic chemistry has a purpose in the finished product. These ingredients are divided into two main categories:

- **Functional ingredients** (FUNK-shun-al in-GREED-ee-antz) do not affect the appearance of the skin but are necessary to the product formulation. They can act as vehicles that allow products to spread, give products body and texture, and give products a specific form such as a lotion, cream, or gel. See **Table 6–1** for a summary of some common functional ingredients.
- **Performance ingredients** (per-FOR-manz in-GREED-ee-antz) cause the actual changes in the appearance of the skin. Examples include ingredients that moisturize, exfoliate, or smooth the skin's surface. Performance ingredients are sometimes referred to as active agents—or erroneously called active ingredients. *Active ingredient* is an official

Ingredient	Types	Examples of Ingredients
Water	Vehicle, solvent	Water
Emollients	Oils, fatty acids, fatty alcohols, fatty esters, silicones	Jojoba oil, olive oil, sesame oil, mineral oil
Surfactants	Detergents, emulsifiers	Ammonium laureth sulfate, cocomidopropyl betaine, disodium lauryl sulfosuccinate, sodium laureth sulfate, sodium lauryl sulfate
Delivery systems	Vehicles, liposomes, polymers	Emollients, water, phospholipids, microsponges
Preservatives	Antimicrobials, antioxidants, chelating agents	**Urea** (yoo-REE-uh), parabens, Quaternium-15, phenoxyethanol, citric acid, disodium EDTA
Fragrances (FREY-gruh-nses)	Natural, synthetic	Synthetic perfumes, plant essential oils
Color agents	Certified, exempt, lakes	D&C organic, **zinc oxide** (ZINGK AHK-syd), mica, mineral dyes, metal salts, inorganic (iron oxide)
Thickeners	Lipids, emulsifiers, polymers, minerals, synthetic	Carbomers, gelatin, silica, stearyl alcohol, xanthan gum
pH adjusters	Buffers	Citric acid, sodium bicarbonate
Solvents	Alcohol, water	Isopropyl alcohol, butylene glycol

term used in the drug industry to indicate ingredients that chemically cause physiological changes. Refer to **Table 6-3** on page 228 for a summary of some common performance ingredients and their benefits.

Some ingredients serve multiple roles in products and can act as both functional and performance ingredients.

Main Types of Ingredients in Product Formulations

The main types of ingredients used in product formulations include a combination of both functional and performance ingredients. The following types are the most common: water, emollients, surfactants, delivery systems, preservatives, fragrances, color agents, gellants/ thickeners, pH adjusters, and solvents.

WATER

Category:
Functional and/or Performance Ingredients

Purpose:
As a functional ingredient, water helps keep other ingredients in a solution and acts as a vehicle to help spread products across the skin.

As a performance ingredient, water replenishes moisture on the surface of the skin.

EMOLLIENTS

Category:

Functional and/or Performance Ingredients

Purpose:

As functional ingredients, **emollients** (ee-MAHL-yunts) help place, spread, and keep other substances on the skin. As performance ingredients, emollients lubricate the skin's surface and guard the barrier function.

Emollients formulated in products are one of the most common performance ingredients. They are made of **lipids** (LIP-idz), which are substances such as a fat, oil, or wax. Some come from natural sources, and others are synthesized in a laboratory or derived from other oils or fatty materials. They lie on top of the skin and prevent dehydration by trapping water and decreasing transepidermal water loss (**Figure 6–4**). Emollients may be very rich or light in consistency. Dry skin that does not produce enough sebum may need heavier emollient ingredients, while oily or problematic skin can benefit from emollients that are very light in consistency.

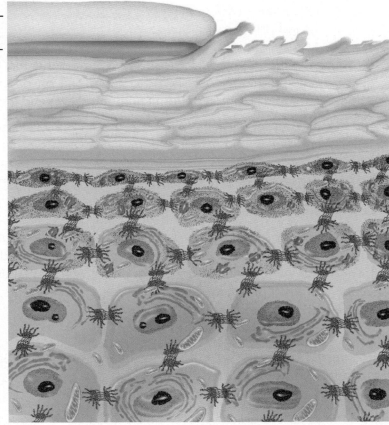

Emollient –

Trapped water –

▲ **FIGURE 6–4** Emollients trap moisture in the skin by the process of occlusion.

Types of Emollients

Oils—Oils formulated into cosmetics vary in density, fat content, and heaviness—from very light to extremely rich and heavy. For this reason, oils can be beneficial to all skin types when properly selected. Oils come from different sources. The two most common are:

- **Mineral sources**—Oils from the earth formulated in cosmetics come from highly refined and purified petroleum sources. These emollients are time tested, offer excellent protection against dehydration, and help prevent skin contact with irritants. They are completely nonreactive and biologically inert, which means that they do not react with other chemicals involved in the skin's function. They can be used with no added preservatives because they do not harbor bacteria or other organisms.

  Examples:
  - **Liquid paraffin** (LIK-wud PAYR-uh-fin)—emollient ingredient derived from petroleum sources
  - Mineral oil
  - Petrolatum

- **Botanical oils**—Dozens of plant oils are used in skin care products. Plant oils vary in fatty acid content and heaviness. **Coconut oil** (KOH-kuh-nuht OYL) and **palm oil** (PAHM OYL) are two of the fattiest and heaviest oils. Some light and less comedogenic plant oils are argan oil and **hemp seed oil** (HEMP SEED OYL), which are highly beneficial to oily and problematic skin.

DID YOU KNOW?

Botanical oils vary in fatty acid content and heaviness. Many estheticians refer to comedogenic ratings to guide them in selecting botanical oils for certain skin types. There are a few rating scales available on the Internet, which may differ slightly because they are often updated. Use **Table 6–2** to compare comedogenic ratings of common oils. This list has been compiled from various sources, including the American Academy of Dermatology.

▼ **TABLE 6–2** Comedogenic Ratings

Comedogenic Ratings							
SCALE	Almond oil	2	Coconut oil	4	Linseed oil	4	Rosehip oil	1
0 – Will not clog pores	Argan oil	0	Evening primrose oil	2	Mineral oil	0	Safflower oil	0
1 – Low	Avocado oil	2	Flax seed oil	4	Neem oil	1	Sea buckthorn oil	1
2 – Moderately low	Baobab oil	2	Grape seed oil	2	Olive oil	2	Shea butter	0
3 – Moderate	Borage oil	2	Hazelnut oil	2	Palm oil	4	Sunflower oil	2
4 – Fairly high	Calendula oil	1	Hemp seed oil	0	Pomegranate oil	1	Tamanu oil	2
5 – High	Cocoa butter	4	Jojoba oil	2	Pumpkin seed oil	2	Wheat germ oil	5

Silicones—a group of oils that are chemically combined with silicon and oxygen and leave a noncomedogenic protective film on the surface of the skin. They also act as vehicles (for spreading) in some products. They are excellent protectants, helping to keep moisture trapped in the skin yet allowing oxygen into and out of the follicles. Silicones also add a silky, nongreasy feel to products and are frequently used in sunscreens, foundations, and moisturizers.

Examples:

- Cyclopentasiloxane
- Dimethicone
- Phenyl trimethicone

Fatty acids (FADDY ASUDS)—**lubricant** (LOO-bri-kuh nt) ingredients derived from plant oils or animal fats. Although these ingredients are acids, they are not irritating and are actually more like oils.

Examples:

- Caprylic acid
- Oleic acid
- Stearic acid

Fatty alcohols (FAT-ee AL-kuh-hawlz)—fatty acids that have been exposed to hydrogen. They are not drying; they have a wax-like consistency and are used as emollients or spreading agents.

Examples:

- Cetyl alcohol
- Lauryl alcohol
- Stearyl alcohol

Fatty esters (FAT-ee ES-terz)—produced from combining fatty acids and fatty alcohols. Esters are easily recognized on labels because they almost always end in -*ate*. They often feel better than natural oils and lubricate more evenly.

Examples:

- Glyceryl stearate
- Isopropyl myristate
- Octyl palmitate

SURFACTANTS

Category:
Functional Ingredients

Purpose:
Surfactants reduce tension between the skin and the product, and also increase the ability of cosmetic products to spread. They can act as cleansing agents, foaming agents, and emulsifiers to create stable mixtures of oil and water, and more.

Surfactants work by becoming infused in both water and oil mixtures. They do this by having molecules with a water-loving head and an oil-loving tail. Surfactants play many roles in cosmetic formulations and are some of the most versatile ingredients in skin care.

Types of Surfactants

Detergents (dee-TUR-jents)—the main types of surfactants and are used primarily in cleansing products. They are the agents that cause cleansers to foam and remove oil, dirt, makeup, and debris from the surface of the skin (**Figure 6–5**). More gentle detergents can be derived from natural sources such as coconut.

Oil and dirt –

Surfactant –

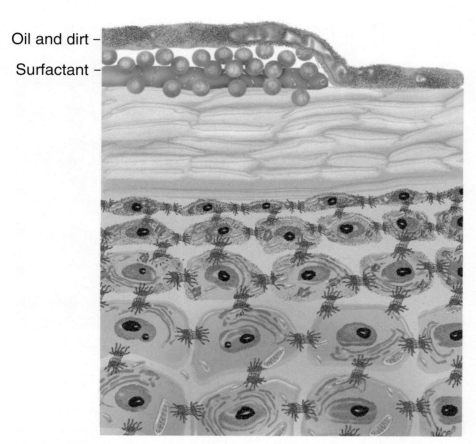

▲ **FIGURE 6–5** Detergents reduce the surface tension of dirt and oils and lift them from the skin.

Examples:

- Ammonium laureth sulfate
- Cocomidopropyl betaine
- Disodium lauryl sulfosuccinate
- Sodium laureth sulfate
- Sodium lauryl sulfate

Emulsifiers (ee-MUL-suh-fy-urz)—surfactants that cause oil and water to mix. Almost all skin care products are a mixture of oil and water, or emulsions. Without emulsifiers, oil and water in products would separate into layers. Emulsifiers surround oil particles, allowing them to remain evenly distributed throughout the water (**Figure 6–6**).

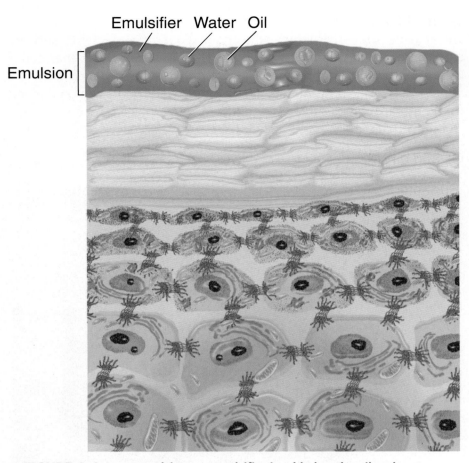

Emulsifier   Water   Oil

Emulsion

▲ FIGURE 6–6 In an emulsion, an emulsifier is added to the oil and water process.

There are two types of emulsifiers: Oil-in-water (o/w) emulsifiers keep oil drops mixed in water, while water-in-oil (w/o) emulsifiers keep water drops mixed in oil. W/O emulsifiers are used in rich moisturizers, such as night creams. O/W emulsifiers are used more in hydrating products such as light lotions and serums.

Examples:

- Polysorbate
- Potassium cetyl sulfate
- Cetearyl alcohol

DELIVERY SYSTEMS

Category:
Functional Ingredients

Purpose:
The skin's job is to protect our body from outside irritants, so it's designed to keep everything out—including skin care ingredients. How ingredients are delivered into the skin can be just as important as the ingredients themselves. **Delivery systems** (Del-IV-er-ee SIS-tems)

are used to distribute a product's key performance ingredients into the skin once it's applied.

Types of Delivery Systems

Vehicles (VEE-hik-uhls)—carrying bases and spreading agents necessary for the formulation of a cosmetic. Vehicles carry or deliver other ingredients into the skin and make them more effective.

Examples:

- Emollients
- Silicones
- Water

Liposomes (LY-puh-zohms)—microscopic hollow, fluid-like spheres (like bubbles) filled with performance ingredients to encapsulate and protect them. The bilayer structure of liposomes mimics cell membranes, allowing for easy penetration beyond the stratum corneum. Liposomes bring key ingredients to a targeted depth of the skin and slowly release them. One liposome may contain many lipid layers within, filled with multiple performance ingredients (**Figure 6–7**). Liposomes also protect the quality and integrity of performance ingredients in a product. The liposome itself is made of several ingredients, and *phospholipid* will be on product labels.

Polymers (PAHL-imerz)—chemical compounds formed by a number of small molecules. One use of polymers is in delivery systems. They are used as advanced vehicles that release ingredients onto the skin's surface at a microscopically controlled rate.

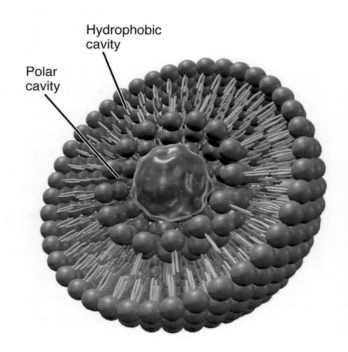

▲ **FIGURE 6–7** Liposomes can encapsulate and transport water-soluble ingredients in their polar cavity and oil-soluble ingredients in their hydrophobic cavity.

Examples:

- Hydrogels
- Microsponges

PRESERVATIVES

Category:
Functional Ingredients

Purpose:
Preservatives (Pre-SERV-uh-tifs) prevent bacteria, fungi, molds, and other microorganisms from living in a product. Preservatives also extend the shelf life of a product and offer protection from chemical changes that can adversely affect the product. Most products contain a blend of preservatives to cover the range of bacteria, fungi, and so on that might be encountered.

Types of Preservatives

Traditional—include formaldehyde-releasers and **parabens** (PAYR-uh-beenz). A formaldehyde-releaser is a chemical compound that slowly releases formaldehyde, an antimicrobial chemical, as it decomposes in a product formulation. Some of these chemical preservatives remain controversial due to the potential of irritancy and other health concerns. Cosmetic regulatory organizations around the world suggest that parabens, especially in the small amounts used in cosmetics, do not pose a significant health risk; others feel there may be reason for concern.

Examples:

- Butylparaben
- **Methylparaben** (Meth-ul-PARA-bin)—most frequently used preservatives because of its very low sensitizing potential; combats bacteria and molds; noncomedogenic
- Propylparaben
- Imadozolidinyl urea
- Diazolidinyl urea
- **Quaternium-15** (kwah-TAYR-nee-um fif-TEEN) - all-purpose preservative active against bacteria, mold, and yeast. probably the greatest formaldehyde-releaser among cosmetic preservatives; may cause dermatitis and allergies

Organic acids and natural alternatives—available for use as preservatives; typically combined together in a product to provide a wide range of protection from the growth of bacteria and fungi.

Examples:

- Phenoxyethanol
- Sodium benzoate
- Potassium sorbate
- Benzyl alcohol
- Benzoic acid
- Sorbic acid

Antioxidants—When used as a preservative, an antioxidant extends the shelf life of a product and reduces the rate of oxidation in formulas. *Oxidation* is a chemical process that occurs when oils or other natural ingredients are exposed to oxygen and causes degradation.

Examples:

- BHA (synthetic) butylated hydroxyanisole
- BHT (synthetic) butylated hydroxytoluene
- Citric acid

Chelating agents (KEY-layt-ing AY-jents)—ingredients added to cosmetics that boost the efficacy of preservatives. Although they are not preservatives in their own right, they play a crucial role in the stability and quality of skin care products. Chelating agents work by breaking down the cell walls of bacteria and other microorganisms. This allows preservatives to be more effective for a longer period of time.

Examples:
- Disodium EDTA
- Tetrasodium EDTA
- Trisodium EDTA

FRAGRANCES

Category:
Functional Ingredients

Purpose:
Ingredients may be added to mask a formulation's unpleasant natural smell, neutralize the smell, or improve the consumer's experience and use of the product.

Types of Fragrances
Synthetic fragrances—created by combining chemical ingredients in a laboratory, and can consist of as many as 200 ingredients. There is no way to know what the chemicals are, since the label will simply say *fragrance*.

Natural fragrances—Botanicals comprise the basic elements of natural scents in skin care product formulations. There are countless extracts and individual scents to choose from.

- **Essential oils** (ih-SEN-shul OYLZ) are highly concentrated plant oils used for their natural aromas and are referred to as the fragrant "soul" of the plant (**Figure 6–8**). Manufacturers often formulate products with specific essential oils to provide the benefits of aromatherapy in addition to giving the product a pleasant smell.
  - **Aromatherapy** (uh-ROH-muh-THAIR-uh-pee) is derived from the ancient practice of using natural plant essences to promote health and well-being. It consists of the use of pure essential oils obtained from a wide assortment of plants and **herbs** (URBS) that have been steam distilled or cold pressed from flowers, fruit, bark, and roots.

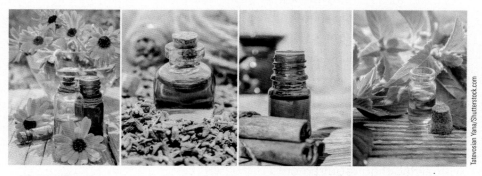

▲ **FIGURE 6–8** Essential oils are highly concentrated plant oils used for their natural aromas.

FOCUS ON

Aromatherapy

In the practice of aromatherapy, when essential oils are inhaled through the nose, aromatic molecules are carried through the lining of the nasal cavity via tiny **olfactory nerves** (ohl-FAK-tuh-ree NURVZ) located in the roof of the inner nose. These "smell" receptors communicate with parts of the brain that serve as storehouses for emotions and memories. They may be applied to pulse-points or mixed with a carrier oil or cream used in massage or a facial mask. Whether inhaled or applied topically, researchers believe that essential oils can help influence changes in physical, emotional, and mental health. For estheticians interested in the practice of aromatherapy, it's very important to first check with your state board regulations to determine if it falls within your scope of licensure. Additional training and education is required as well because essential oils are extremely volatile and can cause adverse effects (i.e. allergies), including burns, when used incorrectly.

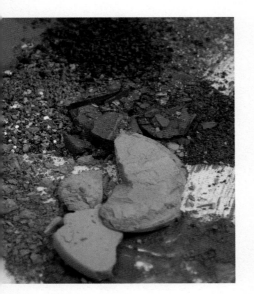

COLOR AGENTS

Category:

Functional and/or Performance Ingredients

Purpose:

As functional ingredients, color agents in skin care formulations enhance a product's visual appeal. As performance ingredients, they're found in makeup such as eyeshadow, foundation, and lipstick to change the appearance of the skin. **Color agents** (KUL-ur AY-jents) are substances such as vegetable, pigment, or mineral dyes that give products color.

Types of Color Agents

Colors subject to certification—These color additives are subject to FDA batch certification and include synthetic organic dyes, lakes, or pigments. They are synthesized mainly from raw materials obtained from petroleum. These **certified colors** (SUR-tih-fyd KUL-urz) are listed on ingredient labels as *D&C*, which stands for drug and cosmetic, or *FD&C*, which stands for food, drug, and cosmetic.

- **Lakes** (LEYKS) are insoluble pigments made by combining a dye with an inorganic material and are commonly used in colorful cosmetics. Because lakes are not soluble in water, they are often used when it is important to keep a color from "bleeding", as in lipstick.

Colors exempt from certification—These color additives are obtained primarily from mineral, plant, or animal sources. Although **noncertified colors** (NAHN-sir-tif-eyed COLORZ) are not subject to FDA batch certification requirements, they are still considered artificial colors. When used in cosmetics or other FDA-regulated products, they must comply with all labeling requirements.

THICKENERS

Category:

Functional Ingredients

Purpose:

Thickeners are added to products to give them a specific consistency, or to help suspend ingredients that are hard to mix into a product. They're derived from various sources such as lipids, emulsifiers, polymers, minerals, and synthetic ingredients.

Examples:

- **Carbomers** (KAHR-boh-murz)—ingredients used to thicken creams; frequently used in gel products
- Carnauba wax
- Gelatin
- Silica
- Stearyl alcohol
- Xanthan gum

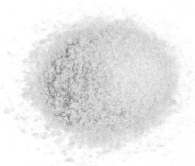

PH ADJUSTERS

Category:

Functional Ingredients

Purpose:

Also called buffering agents, **pH adjusters** (P-H ah-JUST-uhrz) stabilize products and prevent changes in pH. Acids or alkalis (bases) are used to adjust the pH of products.

Examples:

- Acetic acid
- Citric acid
- Sodium hydroxide
- **Sodium bicarbonate** (SOH-dee-um bye-KAR-buh-nayt)—baking soda; an alkaline inorganic salt used as a buffering agent, neutralizer, and pH adjuster

SOLVENTS

Category:

Functional Ingredients

Purpose:

Solvents are added to a product formulation to help dissolve other ingredients.

Examples:

- **Alcohol** (AL-kuh-hawl)—Antiseptic and solvent used in perfumes, lotions, and astringents. Specially denatured (SD) alcohol is a mixture of ethanol with a denaturing agent.
- Polyethylene glycol
- Water

BOTANICALS

Category:
Performance Ingredients

Purpose:
Botanicals (bow-TAN-ee-calz) have become a major source of ingredients in skin care products and treatments. Botanicals can provide many benefits to support the health, texture, and integrity of the skin, including healing, soothing, and brightening. Many botanical ingredients also provide antimicrobial and antioxidant benefits.

A botanical ingredient originates from a plant, including herbs, roots, flowers, fruits, leaves, and seeds (**Figure 6–9**). The actual composition of a botanical ingredient can depend on many things. For example, a botanical ingredient can be extracted from the plant by using a solvent. Different parts of the plant might be processed for use such as the flowers, seeds, roots, or leaves. Some ingredients are obtained directly without extraction. The plant part might be dried and ground into a powder. In other cases, the plant might be squeezed or pressed to obtain the juice or oil.

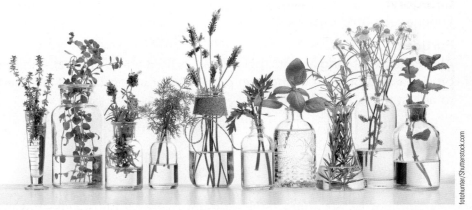

▲ **FIGURE 6–9** Botanicals have become a major source of ingredients in skin care products.

Examples:
The list of botanical ingredients used in skin care products is endless. Throughout this chapter you will find many common botanicals used in product formulations along with their distinct benefits.

INGREDIENTS FOR EXFOLIATION

Category:
Performance Ingredients

Purpose:
Exfoliating ingredients provide exfoliation (eks-foh-lee AY-shun), the removal of dead skin cells on the skin's outermost surface. Exfoliation can also help skin appear brighter and can clear the path for other skin care products to work more effectively.

Types of Ingredients for Exfoliation

Mechanical—Also referred to as physical, these are ingredients used to polish away dead cells from the skin's surface. Gentle massage actions of the specific ingredient onto the skin loosen dead surface skin cells so that they can be sloughed away.

Examples:

- Beeswax
- Ground nuts and seeds
- Jojoba beads
- Magnesium crystals
- Oatmeal
- Rice bran

Chemical—Chemical agents are used to dissolve dead skin cells on the surface and the intercellular matrix, or "glue", that holds them together (desmosomes). In addition to smoothing the skin, they can also help brighten the overall skin tone and improve conditions such as acne.

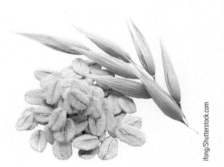

ifong/Shutterstock.com

Types of Chemical Ingredients for Exfoliation

- **Enzymes** (EN-zymz) provide gentle exfoliation and dissolve keratin proteins within dead skin cells on the surface to make skin softer and smoother, and to help maintain the hydration level of the epidermis.

  Examples:

  - Bromelain (pineapple)
  - Papain (papaya)
  - Pumpkin
  - Pancreatin (beef by-products)

- **Alpha hydroxy acids** (AL-fah Hy-DROK-see AS-udz) *(AHAs)* are naturally occurring acids derived from fruit, nuts, milk, or sugars. Today, some AHAs may also be synthetically produced. AHAs are **water soluble** (WAW-tur SAHL-yoo-buhl) and dissolve the "glue" that holds dead skin cells together, allowing them to slough off. They brighten skin, smooth the surface, and aid in cell turnover and collagen production.

  Examples:

  - Citric acid (oranges, lemons)
  - Glycolic acid (sugar cane)
  - Lactic acid (milk proteins)
  - Malic acid (apples)
  - Mandelic acid (bitter almonds)
  - Tartaric acid (grapes)

It's very important to understand how alpha hydroxy acids work in the skin. How deep they penetrate and the amount of exfoliation they provide depends on their molecular structure as well as the concentration of the acid in the product. The most common AHAs found in skin care products include the following:

○ *Glycolic acid* has the smallest molecular structure and therefore has the ability to penetrate the deepest of all AHAs. For this reason, it's considered the most active AHA and highly effective to exfoliate, brighten, and smooth the skin's texture. Products with high concentrations of glycolic acid should be used with caution, especially on very thin or sensitive skin.

○ *Lactic acid* is one of the most popular AHAs. With its larger molecular structure, it is gentler and potentially less irritating than glycolic acid. In addition to exfoliating, lactic acid has its own unique properties that enable it to increase natural moisturizers and epidermal barrier lipids within the skin. It also has lightening benefits for those with discoloration.

○ *Mandelic acid*, having the largest molecular structure, is very gentle yet has been found to be effective to improve overall skin tone and texture and helpful in treating oily and problematic skin due to its natural antibacterial and sebum-regulating properties.

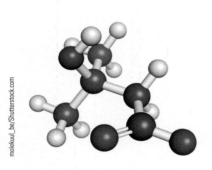

molekuul_be/Shutterstock.com

- **Beta hydroxy acids** (BA-ta Hy-DROK-see AS-udz) *(BHAs)*—**Salicylic acid** (sal-uh-SIL-ik AS-ud) is the most common BHA found in skin care products. Like AHAs, salicylic acid works by dissolving the bond between cells in the epidermis so dead cells can slough off. The main difference is that salicylic acid is oil soluble (OYL sol-yoo-bull) so it can get down into the pores to cut through the oil that's clogging them. It also has antibacterial and anti-inflammatory properties, so it's perfect for treating oily and problematic skin. Certain botanicals are high in natural salicylic acid and are often used for oily and problematic skin.

  Examples:
  ○ Meadowsweet
  ○ Willow bark

- **Retinol** (RET-in-awl; a vitamin A derivative) has gained popularity in skin care products and professional treatments because when applied, it does not induce immediate redness or irritation like high concentrations of hydroxy acids potentially can. Visible sloughing may not be seen for several days after application. The amount of retinol in a product will vary, with higher concentrations available through licensed skin care and medical professionals. More details on retinol are provided in this section under Vitamins on page 221.

LIGHTENERS AND BRIGHTENERS

Category:

Performance Ingredients

Purpose:

Brightening ingredients provide and maintain a natural radiance and glow to the skin. Botanicals are a very popular source of brightening agents.

Lightening ingredients are used to improve discoloration in the skin (hyperpigmentation) which can be caused by many things including sun damage, hormone imbalance, injury, and acne breakouts. They help return skin back to its normal, healthy color. They are also known as melanin suppressants, or tyrosinase inhibitors. Tyrosinase is the enzyme that converts tyrosine, an amino acid, into melanin. Areas of discoloration are caused by the overproduction of melanin. Tyrosinase inhibitors slow down this process, helping skin return back to its normal color.

Examples:

- Azelaic acid
- Bearberry
- Hexylresorcinol
- Kojic acid
- Licorice
- Vitamin C

In addition, *hydroquinone* is proven to be one of the most effective skin lightening ingredients available but also one of the most controversial due to health concerns, particularly if used long term. In the Unites States it is classified as a drug. Up to 2 percent concentrations are available over the counter, and higher concentrations are available by prescription only.

FOCUS ON

Controversial Ingredients

Controversial ingredients used in products include the surfactant sodium lauryl sulfate; preservatives, including parabens and formaldehyde-releasers; the lightening agent hydroquinone; color agents; nanoparticles; and plasticizers called **phthalates** (THAL-ates).

Scientific research and testing continue to determine potential side effects from using certain chemicals. Some concerns are valid, while others are not yet proven. There are many rumors, and incorrect information is prevalent on the Internet. Estheticians and consumers need to research and verify facts from reliable sources to determine what true concerns there may be.

NUTRITION, HEALING, AND REJUVENATION

Category:

Performance Ingredients

Purpose:

When applied topically, ingredients that provide vital nutrients and hydration to the skin also play a crucial role in healing and repair. A number of high-tech ingredients also serve to reduce inflammation, stimulate metabolic processes, and help restore skin to a healthy state while preventing further damage. These performance ingredients are key to maintaining healthy skin, preventing premature aging, and improving the signs of existing skin damage.

Types of Ingredients

Many ingredients are used, and thousands of possible formula combinations exist. Combining them with specific emollients will determine the difference between a very rich cream, light lotion or serum, or targeted skin type and condition.

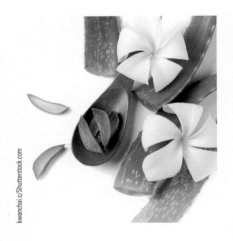

Humectants (hyoo-MEK-tents), **hydrators** (HY-drayt-urs), and **hydrophilic agents** (hy-drah-FIL-ik AY-jents)—ingredients that attract water to the skin's surface. They can lock water on the skin, reducing dehydration.

Examples:

- Algae extract
- Aloe vera
- Glycerin
- Hyaluronic acid
- Honey
- Sodium PCA

Antioxidants—among the most effective ingredients *for all skin types and conditions*; include vitamins, amino acids, botanicals, and other natural substances. Antioxidants help to protect the skin from free radicals and the damaging effects of pollution, stress, UV rays, and the strong blue light waves emitted by LED screens on smartphones and computers. When applied topically, antioxidants neutralize free radicals before they can attach themselves to cell membranes and destroy the cells. Daily application of antioxidants can help prevent premature skin aging, improve the visible signs of aging, and help prevent the inflammation process that leads to cell and skin damage. Many antioxidant ingredients are available, and when used in combination, these formulas are called broad-spectrum antioxidants and give a greater range of protection.

Examples:

- Alpha lipoic acid
- Coenzyme Q10

- Green tea
- Resveratrol
- Pomegranate
- Vitamins A, C, & E

Vitamins—essential to your health and body functions; deficiencies can cause adverse effects on the skin. Vitamins in product formulas provide essential nutrition for preventing and improving the signs of aging and other skin disorders.

Examples:

- *Vitamin A* is a potent antioxidant ingredient, protecting skin against UV damage and slowing down the signs of aging. Vitamin A is composed of two parts. The first part is provitamin A carotenoids, like beta-carotene, which help to maintain healthy skin. The second part is its active forms called retinoids. There are many different types of retinoids including retinyl esters, retinol, retinaldehyde, and retinoic acid. Choosing the best form of retinoid for each client (and its concentration in a product) is imperative. The most common retinoids found in skin care products to improve conditions such as acne, hyperpigmentation, and the signs of aging, are retinoic acid and retinol.
  - ○ *Retinoic* acid is the most potent retinoid approved as an active drug ingredient in the US. It is prescribed by physicians to treat wrinkles, sun damage, and acne. It is of the **keratolytic** (kair-uh-tuh-LIT-ik) group, meaning it causes sloughing, or exfoliating, of skin cells. Retinoic acid is available by prescription in different strengths as a cream or gel. Brand names include Retin-A® and Renova® (tretinoin), Tazorac® (tazarotene), and Differin® (adapalene). Although retinoic acid is very effective, it may cause side effects such as redness, inflammation, irritation, photosensitivity, and excessive peeling.
  - ○ *Retinol* (RET-in-awl) is found in many over-the-counter skin care products, including creams, lotions, and serums. Concentrations vary, and once applied retinol converts into retinoic acid in the skin. Retinol aids damaged cells to mature normally, encourages skin exfoliation, stimulates cell proliferation, and brightens skin. Retinol is referred to by many experts as the gold standard in antiaging to smooth out lines, wrinkles, and texture concerns. Retinol is also used to improve acne, rosacea, and hyperpigmentation. Adverse reactions are less common than those associated with prescription retinoic acid; however, high concentrations of retinol in professional skin care products should be used with caution as they can also cause side effects including photosensitivity.

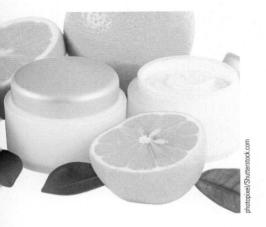

photopixel/Shutterstock.com

- *Vitamin C* has been referred to by some experts as an anti-aging superstar. In addition to being a potent antioxidant, vitamin C performs a variety of other functions within the skin, including stimulating collagen, smoothing texture, brightening and evening out the skin tone, reducing inflammation, and enhancing protection against UV exposure. There are different forms of vitamin C used in skin care products. It's very important to understand how each differs in order to select the appropriate form for individual skin types.
  - *Ascorbic acid* (L-ascorbic acid) is the acidic, water-soluble form of vitamin C. It is considered the most active form of vitamin C and also encourages exfoliation. Due to its low pH, it is a very effective anti-aging ingredient; however, daily use of high concentrations may be irritating or cause inflammation in sensitive skin types.
  - *Ester of vitamin C* (also called ester C) is a pH-neutral, oil-soluble derivative of vitamin C joined by a chemical ester bond with a fatty acid from palm oil (palmitic acid). It's absorbed into the skin much more easily than water-soluble ingredients are. It's highly stable and maintains its effectiveness when mixed with other ingredients. Vitamin C ester stimulates fibroblasts and cell metabolism. It is considered nonirritating and includes the ingredient ascorbyl palmitate.
  - *Vitamin C phosphate* derivatives are pH neutral and water soluble, and they are considered very stable and nonirritating. These include magnesium ascorbyl phosphate and sodium ascorbyl phosphate.
  - *Tetrahexyldecyl ascorbate* is an oil-soluble form of vitamin C found to increase collagen synthesis while brightening and evening out the skin tone. It is pH neutral and easily absorbed into the skin. This is considered one of the most stable forms of vitamin C.
- *Vitamin E* is also a potent antioxidant. Its main function in skin care is to protect against UV damage, strengthen the skin's natural barrier, heal and repair tissue, and prevent moisture loss. Tocopherol and tocopheryl acetate are common derivatives found in skin care products.
- *B vitamins* commonly found in skin care formulations include the following:
  - *Vitamin B5* is also known as pantothenic acid. The alcohol form of vitamin B5 is called panthenol. When panthenol is applied to and absorbed by the skin, it converts into pantothenic acid, which has natural abilities to deeply hydrate, soothe, heal, and regenerate the skin.

○ *Vitamin B3* helps to increase the production of ceramides and fatty acids, two key components of the skin's protective barrier. This in turn helps skin retain its natural moisture and reduces redness and irritation. *Niacinamide* is a derivative of vitamin B3 that also has anti-aging benefits, including reducing fine lines and wrinkles, minimizing pores, and helping to brighten a dull complexion.

- *Vitamin K* is essential in aiding the body's process of blood clotting, which helps the body heal wounds and bruises. When applied topically in a product, vitamin K can help reduce swelling and bruising of the skin and is often recommended by physicians for use after surgical procedures. It can also improve the appearance of conditions such as stretch marks, spider veins, and scars. Vitamin K is also popular in product formulations for the eye area. Fragile capillaries under the eyes that allow blood to leak into the skin are considered one cause of under-eye circles, and vitamin K may improve this condition by controlling blood clotting.

Minerals—needed by the skin for optimal health and function. Minerals also provide therapeutic benefits when applied topically through skin care products.

Examples:

- *Copper* is a powerful antioxidant and helps protect skin. Copper stimulates collagen and elastin synthesis helping to maintain skin elasticity, tone, and texture.

- *Magnesium* helps maintain moisture levels.

- *Zinc* boosts immune function, heals, reduces inflammation, is antimicrobial, and protects against environmental stressors such as UV exposure and pollution.

- *Selenium* is a powerful antioxidant and may also help to balance oily skin.

- *Silica* is important for firming and tightening as well as keeping skin looking smooth.

- *Sulfur* is known to have natural antibacterial and anti-inflammatory properties, and is often used to treat acne and rosacea.

- *Silver* provides anti-inflammatory, antimicrobial, and wound-healing properties and also helps to strengthen the skin's immune system. Colloidal silver is tiny silver particles suspended in water.

- *Gold* contains healing and anti-inflammatory qualities. Gold helps to revitalize and firm skin.

Peptides (PEP-tydz)—short chains of amino acids; the building blocks of proteins. The most commonly known proteins in the skin are collagen, elastin, and keratin, which are responsible for skin firmness and texture. There are hundreds of different peptides, all of which are made from different combinations of amino acids.

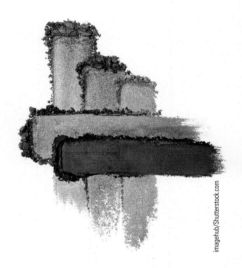
imagehub/Shutterstock.com

In skin care products, many peptide ingredients are used to help reinforce those proteins naturally occurring in the skin, therefore revitalizing the skin's building blocks so it becomes more resilient. Distinct peptides, and peptide blends, can improve many conditions. They can smooth lines and wrinkles, brighten skin tone, repair the barrier function, increase firmness and hydration, reduce swelling under the eyes, and provide antimicrobial effects to treat acne lesions.

A specific group of peptides, called *neuropeptides*, act by affecting neurotransmitters in the skin. When this happens, nerve cells in the skin cease communicating and relax, slowing down muscle contractions. This in turn softens lines and wrinkles and can help prevent them from forming.

Examples:

- Palmitoyl pentapeptide
- Palmitoyl oligopeptide
- Palmitoyl-tripeptide
- Acetyl hexapeptide
- Acetyl glutamyl heptapeptide

Ceramides (a family of lipid molecules)—in skin care products, restore moisture, reinforce the skin's natural barrier, and help protect it against harm from foreign elements. Ceramides replenish the natural lipids in skin that are lost from exposure to harsh environmental factors, from use of drying products, and during the natural aging process.

Examples:

- Sphinogsine
- Sphinganine
- Phytosphingosine
- Ceramide EOP, Ceramide AP

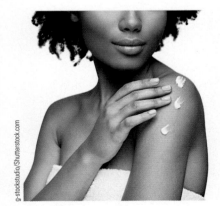

Healing botanicals (HEE-ling bow-tan-ee-calz)—Botanicals such as calendula, chamomile, rose, and aloe vera have all been used in skin care for many years for their natural healing properties. In addition, certain botanical oils and stem cell extracts have become increasingly popular in product formulations because they provide additional benefits for ultimate healing and repair.

Botanical oils rich in *essential fatty acids* (EFAs) not only provide their own distinct therapeutic benefits, because they contain EFAs, they also promote healthy cell membranes and barrier function. Without enough EFAs skin can suffer from dryness, irritation, inflammation, and premature aging. EFAs help cells stay fluid and flexible, allowing water and vital nutrients to enter the cells and wastes to exit. EFAs also create an antimicrobial barrier against the elements. There are two kinds of EFAs, *linoleic acid* (omega-6 fatty acids) and *alpha-linoleic acid* (omega-3 fatty acids). Because skin cannot manufacture these, they must be obtained from outside sources—through either diet or topical applications. All skin types and conditions, especially skin that is sensitive or inflamed, and even skin with acne, can benefit from some of these oils because they mimic the skin's own sebum, will not clog pores, and prevent overproduction of oil.

Examples:

- Abyssinian seed oil
- Argan oil
- Baobab seed oil
- Borage seed oil
- Evening primrose oil
- Meadowfoam seed oil
- Pomegranate seed oil
- Safflower seed oil
- Sea buckthorn oil
- Camellia oil

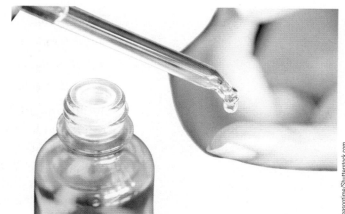

Plant stem cells are naturally occurring botanicals extracted from the meristems of plants (their rejuvenation centers). Their substantial antioxidant activity has been proven to protect skin stem cells from UV-induced oxidative stress, inhibit inflammation, neutralize free radicals, and help reverse the effects of photoaging. **Plant stem cells** (PLANT STEM SELLZ) can uniquely assist in increasing production of human skin cells and collagen by delivering potent nutrients to the skin. Botanical stem cell ingredients can be derived from several sources, and with advances in this technology the list of sources continues to grow.

Examples:

- Alpine rose stem cell
- Echinacea stem cell
- Edelweiss stem cell
- Orange stem cell
- Grape stem cell
- Lilac stem cell
- Madonna lily stem cell
- Sea fennel stem cell
- Swiss apple stem cell

Probiotics—Topically applied probiotics are considered one of the latest beauty breakthroughs, especially for skin prone to acne, rosacea, and eczema. The skin's environment, known as the microbiome, consists of millions of bacteria and immune cells that all work together to maintain the protective barrier, which is critical as skin is the first line of defense against the outside world. Just as internal probiotics help to balance the beneficial and harmful bacteria in your gut, topical probiotics act to balance and retain healthy bacteria on your skin while combatting harmful bacteria. This results in strengthening the skin's barrier function while promoting a healthy, active immune system. In addition, topical probiotics help to decrease sensitivity and contain anti-inflammatory and antibacterial properties.

Examples:
- Lactobacillus plantarum
- Lactobacillus ferment
- Bifidobacterium longum

Polyglucans (POLY-glue-canz) and beta-glucans (BA-ta GLOO canz)—Used to enhance the skin's defense mechanism and stimulate cell metabolism. They are normally derived from yeast cells and have a natural affinity for the skin. Polyglucans are hydrophilic, absorbing more than 10 times their weight in water. Polyglucans also help preserve hydration, collagen, and elastin by forming a protective film on the skin. Beta-glucans help reduce the appearance of fine lines and wrinkles by stimulating the formation of collagen.

Glycoproteins (GLY-co-PRO-teenz; also called *glycopolypeptides*)—yeast cell derivatives that have been found to enhance moisture content, immune response, and cellular metabolism, which boosts cellular oxygen uptake. This revitalizing capacity strengthens the skin's natural ability to protect itself against damaging environmental influences. Glycoproteins are skin conditioning agents derived from carbohydrates and proteins. These are especially beneficial to skin that appears unhealthy, is dull from smoking, has diffused redness, or has environmental damage.

Growth factors (also called *cytokines*)—protein ingredients that regulate cellular growth and proliferation to promote skin tissue repair and regeneration. They play an important part in healing and maintaining a healthy skin structure, including firmness and elasticity. Advances in technology have created multiple sources of growth factors, and each may have its own benefits. They can be derived from human cells grown in a laboratory (epidermal growth factor [EGF] and transforming growth factor-beta [TGF-β]), as well as from nonhuman sources such as plants. This is an area of ingredient technology that has faced both controversy and excitement but continues to grow as new research emerges.

SUNSCREEN INGREDIENTS
Category:
Performance Ingredients

Purpose:
Sunscreen ingredients help prevent ultraviolet radiation (UV) from harming the skin. Both UVA and UVB rays, damage skin and increase

the risk of skin cancer. In addition to causing cancer, excessive unprotected sun exposure also leads to premature aging, including wrinkles, sagging, leathery texture, and hyperpigmentation.

Types of Ingredients

Chemical—Chemical sunscreen ingredients are organic (carbon-based) compounds that work by absorbing UV rays into the skin, changing them to heat, then releasing them from the skin. Caution should be used, as chemical sunscreen ingredients may cause irritation as well as an increase in existing brown spots, discoloration, and cell damage due to a higher internal skin temperature. They also vary in protection from specific UV rays as well; some protect only from UVB rays and do not provide protection from UVA rays.

Examples:

- Avobenzone (butyl methoxydibenzoylmethane)
- Oxybenzone (benzophenone)
- Octinoxate (octyl methoxycinnimate)
- Octisalate (octyl salicylate)
- Homosalate

Physical—Physical sunscreen ingredients, also called mineral sunscreens, are inorganic (without carbon) mineral compounds that physically reflect or scatter ultraviolet radiation. They naturally provide broad-spectrum protection against both UVA and UVB rays. These are typically the preferred sunscreen ingredients for sensitive or reactive skin, as well as inflamed conditions such as acne and rosacea.

Examples:

- Zinc oxide
- **Titanium dioxide** (ty-TAYN-eeum dy-AHK-syd)—inorganic physical sunscreen that reflects UV radiation

 CHECK IN

10. What are the two main categories of ingredients in cosmetic chemistry?
11. Why are preservatives necessary in cosmetics?
12. Where do botanical ingredients originate?
13. What is the main difference between a mechanical exfoliating ingredient and a chemical exfoliating ingredient?
14. What are the two types of sunscreen ingredients, and how does each work?

Identify Beneficial Ingredients for Skin Types and Conditions

Products are precisely formulated with ingredients to treat dry, normal, combination, and oily skin types. Many products may also include ingredients to improve skin conditions such as acne, hyperpigmentation, rosacea, and the signs of aging.

Determining which ingredients are best for an individual's needs is an important step in product selection. It's also very important to remember that best results are achieved by combining multiple performance ingredients within products. Choosing just one ingredient will never provide the results that you'll achieve when using a powerful blend of performance ingredients.

Many ingredients in skin care formulations have multiple benefits and can treat several skin types and conditions at the same time. See **Table 6–3** for common performance ingredients found in cosmetics along with benefits and the most recommended skin types and conditions.

▼ **TABLE 6–3** Common Performance Ingredients in Skin Care Products

Ingredient	Benefits	Dry	Dehydrated	Combination	Oily	Acne/Problematic	Sensitive/Reactive	Hyperpigmentation	Mature/Aging
Acai berry (ah-SAH-ee BER-ee)	Potent antioxidant; anti-inflammatory; brightens skin tone; anti-aging						•	•	•
Algae (AL-jee) extract	Commonly referred to as **seaweed** (SEE-weed); humectant; hydrates; detoxifies; replenishes essential vitamins and minerals; rich in antioxidants		•	•	•				•
Allantoin (al-AHN-toyn)	Moisturizes; soothes, softens, protects, aids in wound healing; promotes cell proliferation and longevity	•						•	•
Aloe vera (AL-oh VAIR-uh)	Humectant; hydrates, softens, heals; antimicrobial; anti-inflammatory; soothes; calms	•	•	•	•	•	•		•
Alpha lipoic acid (AL-fah Lip-OH-ic ASs-ud)	Universal antioxidant; anti-inflammatory; anti-aging; enhances natural exfoliation; minimizes pores; soothes; reduces puffiness	•	•	•	•	•	•	•	•
Alpine rose plant stem cell	Repairs cells; improves barrier function; boosts epidermal regeneration	•					•		•
Arbutin	Natural skin lightener; melanin suppressant							•	

(Continued)

(Continued)

Ingredient	Benefits	Dry	Dehydrated	Combination	Oily	Acne/Problematic	Sensitive/Reactive	Hyperpigmentation	Mature/Aging
Argan oil (AR-gon OYL)	Light emollient plant oil; contains beneficial lipids and fatty acids for skin, including oleic acid, palmitic acid, linoleic acid; antioxidant; replaces natural skin hydration	•	•						•
Argireline®	Trade name for neuropeptide blend; slows muscle contractions; smooths texture								•
Arnica montana	Antiseptic; astringent; anti-inflammatory; soothes; calms			•	•	•	•		
Avocado oil	Emollient; soothes; high in vitamins A, D, E; antioxidant	•							•
Azelaic acid	Anti-inflammatory; skin lightener; antibacterial					•	•	•	
Azulene (azz-U-leen)	Anti-inflammatory; soothes						•		
Bamboo	Prevents moisture loss; antioxidant; soothes; astringent		•	•	•	•	•		
Bearberry	Natural skin lightener; melanin suppressant; soothes						•	•	
Benzoyl peroxide (BEN-zoyl puh-RAHK-syd)	Effective antibacterial agent targeting *Propionibacterium acnes*					•			
Calendula (ca-LEND-yoo-lah)	Emollient; soothes; heals; anti-inflammatory; antiseptic; anti-itching	•					•		
Caviar	Repairs cells; hydrates; nourishes; restores; high in amino acids, vitamins, and minerals	•							•
Centella asiatica	Also known as Indian pennywort and gotu kola; nourishes; heals; anti-inflammatory; anti-irritant; stimulates new cell growth; builds collagen; improves circulation	•					•		•
Ceramides	Help repair barrier function; moisturize; improve hydration; soften	•					•		•
Chamomile (KAM-uh-meel)	Soothes; anti-inflammatory; anti-itching; antiseptic; purifies			•	•	•	•		
Charcoal	Detoxifies; absorbs oil and debris			•	•	•			

(Continued)

(Continued)

Ingredient	Benefits	Dry	Dehydrated	Combination	Oily	Acne/Problematic	Sensitive/Reactive	Hyperpigmentation	Mature/Aging
Coenzyme Q10 (KOE-en-zhym KUE TEN)	Powerful antioxidant; protects and revitalizes skin cells								•
Colloidal gold	Heals; firms; gives skin a healthy glow						•		•
Colloidal silver	Anti-inflammatory; heals; antibacterial					•	•		
Cucumber	Humectant; antioxidant; anti-inflammatory; soothes; reduces swelling		•				•		
Echinacea (ek-uh-NEY-see-uh)	Heals; astringent; antibacterial			•	•	•			
Edelweiss plant stem cell	Repairs cells; potent antioxidant; heals damaged tissue caused by inflammation or trauma; stimulates collagen regeneration						•	•	•
Enzymes	Gentle surface exfoliation; softens; increases hydration	•	•	•			•		•
Eucalyptus	Anti-inflammatory; antibacterial					•	•		
Evening primrose oil	Emollient; moisturizes; enhances barrier function; soothes; heals; anti-inflammatory	•					•		
Geranium	Anti-inflammatory; anti-irritant; astringent; antibacterial; heals			•	•	•	•		
Ginger	Antibacterial; anti-inflammatory; calms; soothes					•	•		
Ginseng	Nourishes; boosts collagen; brightens; promotes healthy cell regeneration; heals; anti-inflammatory; balances oil production			•	•	•	•	•	•
Glycerin (GLIS-ur-in)	Humectant; hydrates	•	•						
Glycolic acid	Water-soluble alpha hydroxy acid; exfoliates; improves hydration; diminishes the signs of aging	•		•	•			•	•
Gooseberry	Antioxidant; natural skin lightener; melanin suppressant							•	
Grape plant stem cell	Repairs cells; protects against UV stress; fights photoaging; delays natural aging process						•	•	•

(Continued)

(Continued)

Ingredient	Benefits	Dry	Dehydrated	Combination	Oily	Acne/Problematic	Sensitive/Reactive	Hyperpigmentation	Mature/Aging
Grape seed oil	Light emollient; nourishes; moisturizes; rich in vitamins and essential fatty acids (EFAs); antioxidant; balances oil	•		•					•
Green tea (GREEN TEE)	Potent antioxidant with many anti-aging benefits; brightens; enhances photoprotection; anti-inflammatory; soothes; antibacterial; reduces swelling	•	•	•	•	•	•	•	•
Hexylresorcinol	Skin lightener; antiseptic; firms					•		•	•
Hibiscus	Antioxidant; humectant; antimicrobial		•				•		
Honey	Humectant; antioxidant; soothes; softens; antibacterial; clarifies			•	•	•	•		
Hyaluronic acid	Humectant; prevents transepidermal water loss		•						
Hydroquinone	Chemical bleaching agent; tyrosinase inhibitor							•	
Irish moss	Also known as red algae; emollient; humectant; softens; soothes; anti-inflammatory	•	•				•		
Juniper	Antiseptic; astringent				•	•			
Kaolin	Oil-absorbing clay; calms; soothes				•	•	•	•	
Kojic acid (KOE-jik AS-ud)	Natural skin lightener; melanin suppressant							•	
Lactic acid	Water-soluble alpha hydroxy acid; exfoliates; brightens skin tone; increases hydration	•	•		•			•	•
Lactobacillus ferment	Probiotic; balances and retains healthy bacteria on skin while combatting harmful bacteria; strengthens barrier function; promotes a healthy immune system; decrease sensitivity; anti-inflammatory; increases hydration	•	•		•	•	•	•	•
L-ascorbic acid	Acidic form of vitamin C; natural skin lightener; stimulates collagen synthesis; exfoliates					•	•	•	•
Lemon extract	Astringent; brightens					•	•		
Licorice (LIK-uh-rish)	Antioxidant; anti-inflammatory; natural skin lightener and melanin suppressant						•	•	

(Continued)

Ingredient	Benefits	Dry	Dehydrated	Combination	Oily	Acne/Problematic	Sensitive/Reactive	Hyperpigmentation	Mature/Aging
Lilac plant stem cell	Repairs cells; antioxidant; brightens; anti-inflammatory; reduces acne lesions				•	•	•	•	
Madonna lily plant stem cell	Repairs cells; skin brightener; inhibits melanosome transfer; evens out skin tone; encourages epidermal regeneration; stimulates collagen and elastin production							•	•
Mandelic acid	Gentle, water-soluble alpha hydroxy acid; exfoliates; brightens; smooths texture; antibacterial; regulates sebum production	•	•	•	•	•		•	•
Mastiha	Antioxidant; anti-inflammatory; strengthens immune system; antimicrobial; minimizes pores; natural skin brightener	•	•	•	•	•		•	•
Matrixyl®	Trade name for anti-aging peptide; nonirritating; stimulates collagen synthesis and elastin production; strengthens; repairs; smooths texture; firms								•
Meadowsweet	High in natural salicylic acid; astringent; antioxidant; anti-inflammatory			•	•	•			
Mineral oil (MIN-ur-ul OYL)	Emollient; helps improve barrier function; soothes; considered one of the safest, most non-sensitizing moisturizing ingredients	•							
Mulberry	Natural skin lightener; melanin suppressant							•	
Niacinamide	Also known as vitamin B3 and nicotinic acid; boosts barrier function; anti-inflammatory; protects skin from UV rays; improves texture; brightens; minimizes pores	•	•	•	•	•		•	•
Oligopeptide-8	Peptide; antimicrobial targeting *P. acnes*					•			
Olive oil	Emollient; antioxidant; moisturizes	•							•
Orange plant stem cell	Repairs cells; increases dermal fibroblast activity; strengthens; restores	•							•
Panthenol	Vitamin B5; humectant; moisturizes; anti-inflammatory; softens; stimulates cell proliferation; aids in tissue repair	•	•				•		•
Passion flower	Antioxidant; relaxes muscle contractions; smooths wrinkles								•

(Continued)

Ingredient	Benefits	Dry	Dehydrated	Combination	Oily	Acne/Problematic	Sensitive/Reactive	Hyperpigmentation	Mature/Aging
Petrolatum (peh-troh-LAY-tum)	Emollient and skin protectant; replenishes moisture; soothes	•							
Pomegranate	Potent antioxidant; anti-inflammatory; anti-aging; soothes						•		•
Pumpkin	Antioxidant; rich in vitamins and minerals; soothes; softens; balances oil production; minimizes pores; exfoliates; brightens			•	•	•			
Red raspberry	Potent antioxidant; anti-inflammatory; soothes; enhances natural UV protection						•		•
Resveratrol	Potent antioxidant, anti-inflammatory; stimulates collagen production; smooths texture						•		•
Retinol	Vitamin A derivative; antioxidant; rejuvenates; exfoliates; brightens; smooths; firms; improves all skin conditions; encourages cells to mature normally	•	•	•	•	•	•	•	•
Rumex	Melanin suppressant; anti-inflammatory; brightens							•	
Salicylic acid	Oil-soluble beta hydroxy acid; exfoliates; helps unclog pores; antibacterial; astringent			•	•	•			
Sea buckthorn oil	Light emollient; anti-inflammatory; antimicrobial; balances sebum production; heals	•			•	•	•		
Sea fennel plant stem cell	Repairs cells; organic skin brightener; helps repair melanocyte damage							•	•
Sea oak extract	Enhances natural UV protection; brightens; antibacterial					•	•	•	
Sea whip	Anti-inflammatory; soothes						•		
Shea butter	Noncomedogenic emollient; hydrates; softens and smooths; rich in antioxidants	•	•	•	•	•	•	•	•
Silver ear mushroom	Also known as Tremella; humectant; hydrates; anti-inflammatory; softens	•	•			•	•		
Snow crocus bulb	Anti-aging; boosts collagen and elastin production; stimulates growth factors; smooths; firms								•
Squalane (SKWA-lane)	Emollient; moisturizes and lubricates; softens; smooths; anti-irritant	•					•		•

(Continued)

(Continued)

Ingredient	Benefits	Dry	Dehydrated	Combination	Oily	Acne/Problematic	Sensitive/Reactive	Hyperpigmentation	Mature/Aging
Sulfur (SUL-fur)	Antiseptic; reduces oil gland activity; dissolves surface layer of dead cells					•			
Summer snowflake	Slows skin cell aging process; increases natural skin defense from oxidative damage; smooths; brightens							•	•
Swiss apple plant stem cell	Repairs cells; restores; potent antioxidant; slows skin cell aging process; heals; anti-inflammatory	•					•		•
SYN®-AKE	Trade name for neuropeptide blend; slows muscle contractions; smooths texture								•
Tea tree oil (TEE TREE OYL)	Antimicrobial; antibacterial; antifungal; promotes healing			•	•	•			
Tetrahexyldecyl ascorbate	Also known by the trade name BV-OSC; oil-soluble form of vitamin C; antioxidant; anti-inflammatory; brightens; melanin suppressant; stimulates collagen synthesis						•	•	•
Thyme	Antioxidant; anti-inflammatory; antibacterial					•	•		
Vitamin A	Antioxidant; protects against UV damage; slows signs of aging; encourages healthy skin cell production; boosts immune system	•	•	•	•	•	•	•	•
Vitamin C	Antioxidant; anti-inflammatory; brightens; stimulates collagen synthesis	•	•	•	•	•	•	•	•
Vitamin E	Oil-soluble antioxidant and free radical scavenger; anti-inflammatory; moisturizes; hydrates; helps restore barrier function	•						•	•
White tea	Humectant; antifungal; antimicrobial; antioxidant; astringent		•	•	•	•		•	
Willow bark	Contains natural salicylic acid compounds; antimicrobial; astringent			•	•	•			
Witch hazel (WICH HAY-zul)	Anti-inflammatory; astringent; antimicrobial; heals wounds; softens; humectant		•	•	•	•		•	

All Skin Types and Conditions

Everybody, regardless of skin type or condition, needs ingredients applied daily to maintain optimal skin health. Skin must have adequate hydration, essential nutrition, and protection from environmental assaults every day of the year. Providing this healthy balance will also prevent premature skin aging and cell damage.

Ingredients for exfoliation can also be highly beneficial and are selected by individual skin types. These are typically found in skin care products that are used on a weekly basis, although some products may be formulated to be used more frequently.

TYPES OF UNIVERSAL INGREDIENTS

- Antioxidants
- Vitamins
- Minerals
- Physical sunscreen ingredients

COMBINATION SKIN

The goal in treating combination skin is to maintain a healthy balance of water and oil. Dry or dehydrated areas need moisturizing and increased internal hydration, while oily areas require special care to reduce the overactivity of the oil glands and keep pores from becoming clogged, leading to acne.

Types of Ingredients

- Emollients
- Humectants
- Oil balancing/regulating

DRY

The goal in treating dry skin is to provide moisturizing, replenishing, and skin-restoring ingredients.

Types of Ingredients

- Ceramides
- Emollients
- Humectants

DEHYDRATED

The goal in treating dehydrated skin is to restore internal skin hydration and retain inner moisture by preventing transepidermal water loss (TEWL).

Types of Ingredients

- Humectants
- Light to rich emollients based on skin type

OILY

The goal in treating oily skin is to provide ingredients that reduce the overactivity of the oil glands, promote a healthy oil–water balance, and keep pores from becoming clogged, leading to acne.

Types of Ingredients

- Hydroxy acids
- Humectants, light emollients
- Oil balancing/regulating
- Clarifying, detoxifying

ACNE/PROBLEMATIC

The goal in treating acne and problematic skin is to reduce the overactivity of the oil glands, promote a healthy oil–water balance, keep pores from becoming clogged, inhibit acne-causing bacteria, and reduce inflammation associated with inflamed lesions. Clients may also want to consider seeking assistance from a professional regarding internal factors such as diet, stress, and hormone fluctuations because they contribute to acne conditions.

Types of Ingredients

- Antibacterial/antimicrobial
- Anti-inflammatory, soothing
- Humectants, light emollients
- Oil balancing, clarifying, detoxifying
- Retinoids
- Topical probiotics

SENSITIVE/REACTIVE

The goal in treating sensitive and reactive skin is choosing products with ingredients to soothe, calm, reduce inflammation, heal, and help restore the skin's barrier function. Many clients with rosacea may also benefit from these types of ingredients.

Types of Ingredients

- Anti-inflammatory, soothing
- Anti-irritant
- Ceramides
- Humectants, emollients based on skin type
- Topical probiotics
- Healing, high in EFAs (essential fatty acids)

HYPERPIGMENTATION

The goal in treating hyperpigmentation is to use products with a blend of ingredients that will reduce heat and inflammation within the skin accompanied by lighteners and brighteners to reduce pigmented areas and minimize melanin production. In addition to these ingredients, daily use of a broad-spectrum sunscreen, preferably physical SPF 30 or greater, is highly recommended to prevent further darkening of pigmented areas.

Types of Ingredients

- Anti-inflammatory, soothing
- Retinoids
- Lighteners and brighteners

MATURE/AGING SKIN

Mature and aging skin can suffer from many conditions, including dryness, dehydration, inflammation, and hyperpigmentation. In addition, lines, wrinkles, sagging skin, and sun damage may be visible. Key ingredients have been proven beneficial (especially when combined) in helping increase collagen synthesis and improving the appearance of aging skin. Some also have potent properties to restore, rejuvenate, and protect cell membranes from oxidative damage and prevent collagen from being destroyed.

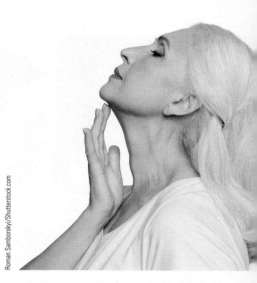

Roman Samborskyi/Shutterstock.com

Types of Ingredients

- Ceramides
- Humectants, emollients based on skin type
- Growth factors
- Vitamin C
- Peptides
- Retinoids

 CHECK IN

15. What four types of universal ingredients are beneficial for all skin types and conditions?
16. What is the goal when treating combination skin, and what care is required?
17. What main types of ingredients are beneficial for treating dehydrated skin?
18. What skin conditions and visible signs of aging can be seen in mature/aging skin?

Select Appropriate Products for Facial Treatments and Home Care Use

Products used in treatments and for home care can make a significant difference in the skin's health and appearance. Understanding and selecting the right products play a huge role in a skin care program and ultimately determine overall results (**Figure 6–10**). This is the reason products are the lifeblood of an esthetician's career.

Products come in many forms and there are literally hundreds of ingredients available to create formulations. Through continued research and advances in technology, cosmetic chemists constantly develop new products for use in professional skin care.

Most skin care products can be grouped into the following main categories:

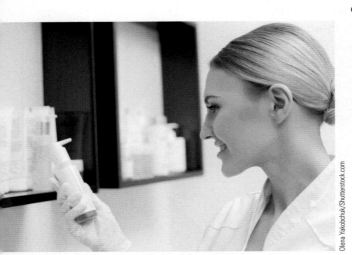

- Cleansers
- Toners
- Exfoliants
- Masks
- Massage products
- Serums and ampoules
- Moisturizers
- Specialty products for eyes and lips
- Sun protection

▲ **FIGURE 6–10** For optimal skin health and results, estheticians must choose the right products for every client's treatment and home care regimen.

Cleansers

From gentle, soothing cleansers to deep-cleansing formulas, cleansers can be found in many forms and contain an assortment of ingredients to target specific skin types and conditions.

Benefits:

- Dissolve makeup, oil, and dirt to keep pores clean and prepare the skin for other products.
- Additional ingredients can benefit certain skin conditions such as dryness, sensitivity, dehydration, and acne.

TYPES OF CLEANSERS

Cleansing waters (also known as *micellar* (my-SELL-ar) *water*)—liquids to cleanse, tone, and condition the skin in one step; formulated for all skin types. These cleansers are made of microscopic oil molecules (called micelles) that are suspended in purified water. They are wiped across the skin with a cotton pad and not rinsed off. They easily lift dirt, oil, and makeup without disturbing the skin's natural pH balance.

Cleansing gels—water-based foaming cleansers; generally the most popular type of cleanser. Cleansing gels may be formulated for all skin types.

Cleansing lotions—light emulsions typically best for normal to dry skin types. These cleansers do not strip the skin's natural oil or pH balance.

Cleansing creams—rich water-in-oil emulsions used primarily to dissolve makeup and dirt. They are suitable for very dry and mature skin. Actors and other performers use these products to remove heavy stage makeup.

Cleansing oils—have become quite popular for use on all skin types. These formulas contain beneficial, or "good", oils to break down makeup, dirt, excess sebum, and pollutants on the skin's surface. They can be used alone, or as the first step in a "double-cleansing" method. For this method, a cleansing oil is used first to easily dissolve makeup, sunscreen, dirt, and oil that water-based cleansers are unable to fully dissolve. After rinsing off the cleansing oil, a second cleanser, specific to the skin type, is then used to complete the cleansing process.

Toners

Toners (TOH-nurz) are water-based liquids applied to the skin after cleansing with a cotton pad or spritzed directly onto the skin, avoiding the eyes. Alcohol-free toners, also referred to as **fresheners** (FRESH-un-urz) or freshening lotions, contain botanicals and hydrators to soothe the skin. Toners formulated for oily or acne-prone skin, also referred to as **astringents** (uh-STRIN-jents), may also contain hydroxy acids and various amounts of alcohol.

Benefits:

- Remove residue left behind by cleansers or other products
- Soften the skin and allow for better absorption of other products to be applied
- Restore the skin's natural pH after cleansing and hydrate the skin
- Have a temporary tightening effect on both the skin and follicle openings

Exfoliants

Products used to exfoliate the skin may include a single exfoliating ingredient, or blends of multiple exfoliants plus botanicals and hydrators.

CAUTION!
As a student, you should always receive hands-on training from your instructor before attempting exfoliation procedures. Exfoliation can cause irritation and damage to the skin and capillaries if overused, or used incorrectly.

CAUTION!

To avoid damaging skin, do not use scrubs or any harsh exfoliation techniques on clients with these skin conditions:

- Sensitive skin
- Skin with many visible capillaries
- Thin skin that reddens easily
- Older skin that is thin and bruises easily
- Acne-prone skin with inflamed papules and pustules
- Clients using daily skin care products containing retinol or hydroxy acids
- Skin medically treated with prescription drugs such as tretinoin (Retin-A®), isotretinoin (Amnesteem®), adapalene (Differin®), tazarotene (Tazorac®), other acne drugs, azelaic acid, alpha hydroxy acids (AHAs), or salicylic acid (found in many common skin products).

For home care, **exfoliants** (Ex-FOLEY-antz) are often used after cleansing. Frequency of use depends on the skin type or condition, and the manufacturer's instructions. In facial treatments, exfoliants are generally used after cleansing and toning.

It's very important to select the right exfoliant according to the client's skin type and condition. Use caution when exfoliating the skin. It is also important to note that the esthetician's domain is addressing the superficial epidermis, not providing treatments that involve the live layers of the skin below the epidermis.

Benefits:

- Softer, smoother, and brighter complexion
- Improve skin's ability to retain moisture and lipids
- Cell turnover rate is increased; blood flow and circulation are stimulated
- Follicle openings are cleaner; deep pore cleansing and extractions are easier
- Product penetration is improved and delivery of ingredients into the epidermis is more effective
- Makeup application is smoother and more even

TYPES OF EXFOLIANTS

Mechanical Exfoliants (Muh-KAN-ih-kul Ex-FOLEY-antz)—often referred to as physical exfoliants; polish dead cells off of the surface of the skin (**Figure 6–11**). Examples of mechanical exfoliants include cleansers, scrubs, and masks made with ingredients such as rice bran, almond meal, jojoba beads, or magnesium crystals.

Chemical Exfoliants (KEM-uh-kul Ex-FOLEY-antz)—contain ingredients such as hydroxy acids, chemical compounds, and retinol. For home care use, chemical exfoliants can be found as cleansers, serums, creams, and masks and are used according to the manufacturer's instructions.

Professional chemical exfoliating solutions, often called chemical resurfacing solutions, may be in liquid or gel form (**Figure 6–12**) and contain much higher concentrations of exfoliating agents. Chemical exfoliation products and procedures are discussed in Chapter 13, Advanced Topics and Treatments.

Enzyme—include ingredients such as pineapple, **papaya** (puh-PAH-yuh), and pumpkin enzymes. These exfoliants are gentle and can be beneficial for use in both professional treatments and home care, particularly for sensitive and reactive skin. The most popular types of enzyme exfoliants used in facial treatments are a powdered form that is

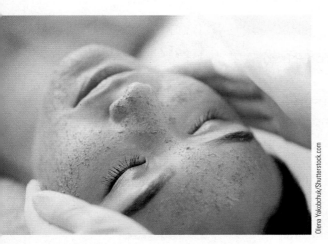

▲ **FIGURE 6–11** Mechanical exfoliants physically polish away dead skin cells.

Olena Yakobchuk/Shutterstock.com

mixed by the esthetician with warm water and one already premixed in a base similar to a mask or gel.

- **Gommage** (goh-MAJ) is a type of enzyme exfoliant product also known as *roll-off mask*. Gommage is a cream or paste containing enzymes. It is applied to the skin, then left to dry slightly, allowing the enzymes to digest the dead skin cells on the surface. It is then rubbed, or "rolled", off the skin, taking dead skin cells with it. This treatment is actually a combination of an enzyme and mechanical exfoliant.

Masks

A good **mask** (MASQUE), also known as *pack* or *masque*, can do wonders for the skin. Mask ingredients can range from soothing and hydrating botanicals, to oil-absorbing, acne-fighting hydroxy acids and more. Masks can be formulated in clay, seaweed, or hydrating bases and come in powder form and premixed. Masks allow an esthetician to treat several skin conditions at the same time, and are also beneficial for weekly home care use.

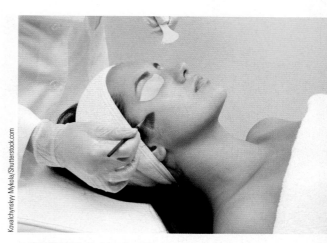

▲ **FIGURE 6–12 Application of an AHA solution for chemical exfoliation.**

Benefits:
- Tighten and tone, brighten the complexion, and rejuvenate
- Hydrate, nourish, calm, and soothe
- Clarify, detoxify, draw impurities out of the pores, and clear up blemishes

TYPES OF MASKS

Nonsetting—designed to remain moist on the skin to provide nourishment. They do not dry, harden, or "set up". They are highly beneficial for sensitive, inflamed, aging, dry, and dehydrated skin. They can come in a gel form containing soothing ingredients such as cucumber and aloe, or in a cream consistency containing moisturizing plant oils and other emollients.

- *Sheet masks* are considered nonsetting masks. They are available as a single packaged moist or freeze-dried sheet. Prepackaged moist sheet masks are simply applied directly to the skin until removal (**Figure 6–13**). Freeze-dried sheet masks are similar to a piece of paper and infused with performance ingredients. After the freeze-dried sheet is pressed onto the skin, it's moistened and remains wet until removal. Collagen sheet masks are very popular, as they are plumping, calming, and hydrating, and they diminish the appearance of wrinkles.

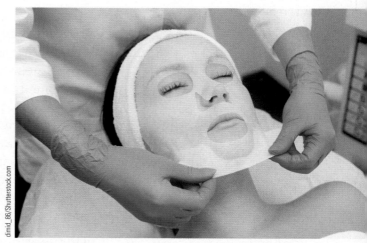

▲ **FIGURE 6–13 Nonsetting moist sheet masks are popular for professional and home care use.**

Setting—in a base that dries and hardens after application. There are several different types of setting masks.

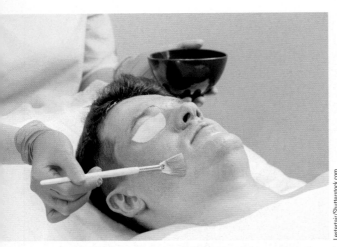

▲ **FIGURE 6–14** Clay setting masks draw excess oil and impurities to the surface of the skin as it dries and hardens.

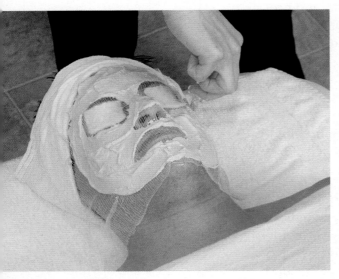

▲ **FIGURE 6–15** Alginate setting masks are easily removed.

- **Clay masks** (KLAY MASKZ) draw excess oil and impurities to the surface of the skin as the mask dries and tightens (**Figure 6–14**). Clay also stimulates circulation and temporarily contracts the pores of the skin. These masks typically contain kaolin, bentonite, or silica for their tightening and sebum-absorbing effects. Clay masks are typically used on combination, oily, and problematic skin. Setting masks with charcoal help detoxify skin while those with sulfur have healing and antiseptic properties to help with acne.

- **Alginate** (AL-jun-ate) masks are often seaweed based and applied after a serum or treatment cream in a facial treatment. They come in powder form and are mixed with water or serums. After mixing, they are quickly applied to the face and then dry to form a rubberized texture (**Figure 6–15**). Alginate masks form a seal that encourages the skin's absorption of the serum or cream underneath.

- **Modelage masks** (MAHD-ul-ahj MASKZ), also known as *thermal masks*, are applied after a nourishing serum in a facial treatment. These masks contain special crystals of gypsum, a plaster-like ingredient. Modelage masks are mixed with water immediately before application, then applied over gauze about ¼-inch (0.6 cm) thick. As the modelage mask sets up and hardens, a chemical reaction occurs to gradually increase the mask's temperature to approximately 105 degrees Fahrenheit (40.5 degrees Celsius). This helps serums applied underneath penetrate while also increasing blood circulation. After approximately 20 minutes the mask cools and is removed. These professional masks can become heavy on the face and should not be applied to the lower neck or to clients who suffer from claustrophobia.

- **Paraffin wax masks** (PAYR-uh-fin WAKS MASKS) are facial masks that contain paraffin wax and are specially prepared in the salon. The wax is melted at a little more than body temperature (98.6 degrees Fahrenheit [37 degrees Celsius]) before application. When applied, the paraffin quickly cools to a lukewarm temperature and sets. Paraffin masks are applied on top of a nourishing cream, as the warm paraffin allows for deeper penetration of the ingredients into the skin. The heat from the paraffin wax also increases blood circulation and is beneficial for dry, mature skin, or skin that is dull and lifeless. It has a plumping and softening effect on the skin. The paraffin mask procedure is presented in Chapter 8, Facial Treatments.

Custom-designed—"homemade" masks mixed with fresh ingredients such as fruits, vegetables, milk, yogurt, honey, and oatmeal. These masks are beneficial unless the person is allergic to a particular ingredient. Custom-designed masks can be fun to experiment with, but they are usually made and used at home rather than in a professional setting. Sanitation, regulations, and convenience hinder the use of home-made masks in the salon. Additionally, products not packaged by a manufacturer may not be covered under an employer's insurance.

Massage Products

Massage products are designed to provide slip and glide during facial massage in a professional treatment. Some also contain performance ingredients to nourish and treat the skin during the massage procedure.

Benefits:

- Improve microcirculation of blood flow to the skin, which brings a healthy, youthful glow
- Help to encourage the optimum flow of lymph, which assists in the elimination of toxins
- Reduce puffiness and improve the overall quality of the complexion
- Nourish and hydrate skin

TYPES OF MASSAGE PRODUCTS

Massage oils—Oils used for facial massage vary in thickness. These products typically contain a blend of botanical oils with additional ingredients to target specific skin types and conditions. Examples include sweet almond oil for normal to dry skin and **jojoba** (hoh-HOH-buh) oil for combination to oily skin. Experienced estheticians that have taken additional courses and training in aromatherapy may also create custom essential oil blends if allowed by their state board regulations.

Massage creams—rich in consistency, feel very luxurious, and contain moisturizing emollients. They provide great slip for a longer period of time, as they do not absorb quickly into the skin. Massage creams are typically preferred for dry and mature skin.

Massage lotions—light in consistency and contain a combination of emollients and humectants. These are the most universal type of product for facial massage due to a wide selection of ingredient blends for all skin types.

Massage gels—water-soluble blends containing humectants and a variety of botanicals. These are preferred for oily skin, especially if it is also dehydrated.

Serums and Ampoules

Serums (SE-rum) and **ampoules** (AM-pyoolz) contain highly concentrated performance ingredients designed to target specific skin conditions and effectively penetrate the skin. They can be applied under

CAUTION!
Remember that some people are allergic to seaweed and even shellfish, which is usually a contraindication for seaweed products. Serious reactions to marine-based products do occur, so exercise caution when using these ingredients.

a moisturizer, mask, or massage cream; or they may be used with machines in a facial treatment. These products are also an important step in home care routines.

Serums and ampoules are essentially the same type of product. The difference between a serum and an ampoule is simply the packaging. Serums are typically packaged in a pump container or dropper bottle. Ampoules are small, sealed vials containing a single premeasured application.

Benefits:

- Increase hydration and nourishment
- Aid in skin strengthening, healing, and repair
- Anti-aging; exfoliate, brighten, and even out the skin tone
- Balance oil production and acne prevention

Moisturizers and Hydrators

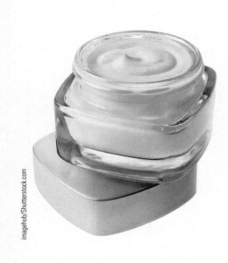

imagehub/Shutterstock.com

Moisturizers and hydrators both address the importance of maintaining healthy skin. They ensure that skin is getting the essential moisture it needs to remain healthy. They are applied at the end of the facial and are intended for twice daily use at home.

Although the two words are often used interchangeably, there is a big difference in how they work to achieve this result as well as the ingredients in their formulations. It is very important to select the best moisturizer or hydrator based on skin type and condition for use in a facial treatment as well as for home care. How naturally dry or oily the skin is and how humid or dry the environment is will help determine which type of product is best.

Benefits:

- Nourish skin by increasing and maintaining essential water content
- Protect skin from the elements
- Prevent premature aging; fight dryness and dehydration
- Balance the oil–water content of skin, preventing overproduction of oil
- Improve various skin conditions such as redness and the signs of aging

TYPES OF MOISTURIZERS AND HYDRATORS

Moisturizers—include creams and lotions formulated to create a protective barrier on the surface of the skin to seal in moisture and soften the skin. Moisturizers help trap the skin's natural oils and lipids on the surface of the skin. Oil-based moisturizers with heavier emollients are best for dry skin, while light emulsions that absorb quickly are best for combination to oily skin.

Hydrators—typically oil-free products formulated with humectants to attract water to the skin; particularly beneficial for dehydrated, oily, and problematic skin.

Treatment creams (also referred to as *nourishing creams or night creams*)—designed to moisturize, condition, and restore the skin—especially during sleep, when normal tissue repair is taking place. Treatment creams are often heavier in texture than daytime moisturizers and contain diverse performance ingredients to target specific skin conditions.

Specialty Products for Eyes and Lips

Products specifically for the areas around the eyes and lips can address many issues on these areas and are for use at home, as well as for use in a facial treatment.

PRODUCTS FOR EYES

The skin around the eyes is the thinnest, most delicate skin on the entire body and requires special attention. It's fragile, more prone to dryness, and quicker to show signs of aging and fatigue. Constant movement and squinting speeds up the creation of "crow's feet", and fluids can collect under the eyes and cause puffiness and dark circles. Unfortunately thinning eyelashes and eyebrows are also part of the aging process, losing the length and fullness they once had.

Benefits:

- Protect delicate tissue, provide a more youthful appearance, and prevent early signs of aging
- Help to reduce lines, wrinkles, puffiness, dark circles, dehydration, and dryness
- Enhance eyelash and eyebrow growth, length, and volume

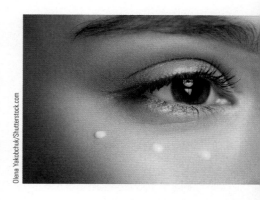

Olena Yakobchuk/Shutterstock.com

Eye balms, creams, and gels—formulated to treat specific concerns and maintain healthy skin around the eye area. A variety of performance ingredients may be found in eye products, including peptides, antioxidants, and ceramides. Eye balms are very rich in texture and include ingredients such as macadamia oil or coconut oil. Eye creams are lighter in consistency and may include shea butter, silicones, or plant oils. Eye gels are very light and contain humectants such as hyaluronic acid, aloe, or glycerin.

Eye makeup removers—help to gently clean away eye makeup, especially waterproof mascara. Eye makeup removers are available in both oil-based and oil-free formulas. They may also contain soothing botanicals such as cucumber and allantoin.

Eyelash and eyebrow enhancers—used at home daily to nourish, condition, and enhance growth and volume. Most users begin to see results within four to eight weeks, with the most dramatic results appearing between weeks 12 and 16. Use of these products must be continued to maintain results. If use is stopped then lashes and brows will eventually return to their original state. Products available include the prescription drug Latisse® (bimatoprost ophthalmic solution) as

With all product usage, choose the right formulas for your client's skin. Be sure to apply the appropriate amount of product; using too much can have adverse effects on the skin and also wastes product and money.

well as over-the-counter brands formulated with various vitamins, botanicals, and peptides.

PRODUCTS FOR LIPS
Aging and environmental assaults cause lines to form around the vermillion border. Lips can easily lose moisture and volume, and become dry, chapped, or cracked.

Benefits:
- Protect delicate tissue, provide a more youthful appearance, and prevent early signs of aging
- Provide nutrients and hydration to protect from moisture loss and improve dry, chapped lips.
- Restore natural lip volume and color, and soften lines around the vermillion border

Lip balms, creams, and oils—formulated to hydrate and soften lips. When applied to the vermillion border they help to smooth out lines and soften wrinkles. Some lip treatment products contain collagen derivatives or other agents to plump up the lips and restore natural volume. Exfoliating and healing ingredients are also used in lip conditioners.

Sun Protection Products (Sunscreens)

By damaging the skin's cellular DNA, excessive UV exposure causes signs of premature aging in the skin and produces genetic mutations that can lead to skin cancer. Both the U.S. Department of Health and Human Services and the World Health Organization have identified UV as a proven human carcinogen. The role of a sun protection product is to absorb, scatter, or reflect damaging UV rays before they have a chance to interact with the skin. Sun protection products may be used as the last step of a facial treatment, and are essential for daily home care use, all year long.

Benefits:
- Protect skin from UV radiation exposure, skin cancer, premature aging, and skin damage

SUN PROTECTION FACTOR (SPF) RATING
A **sun protection factor** (SUN-proh-TEK-shun FAK-tur) (SPF) rating is a measure of time, determining *how long* a sunscreen product will protect you from UVB rays, the chief cause of sunburn. The individual SPF rating number on a product is used to calculate this length of time. For example, if somebody normally burns after 20 minutes in the sun with no protection, an SPF 30 sunscreen multiplies that 20 minutes by 30 (the SPF rating), which is equal to 600 minutes of protection, assuming it's applied correctly. It's still necessary, however, to reapply sunscreen

much more frequently, especially if there is direct exposure to UV rays for long periods of time.

As far as the actual *amount of UVB rays being blocked*, it's estimated that SPF 15 sunscreen blocks approximately 93 percent of UVB radiation, while an SPF 30 blocks nearly 97 percent. An SPF 50 blocks an estimated 98 percent of UVB rays. Products with even higher SPF ratings provide very minimal additional coverage, and most often contain high amounts of added chemical sunscreen ingredients.

It's also important to remember that the SPF rating does not apply to UVA rays, which penetrate the skin more deeply than UVB rays do. UVA rays have long been known to play a major part in skin aging and wrinkling (photoaging). UVA exposure also contributes to, and may even initiate the development of, skin cancers.

Always use and recommend broad-spectrum sun protection products to protect against both UVA and UVB rays. Educate your clients on the importance of year-round daily use, as well as proper application. The biggest misconception regarding sun protection is that it's needed only for sunny summer days. We are constantly being exposed to UV rays, and they are just as strong when passing through clouds any time of year.

TYPES OF SUN PROTECTION PRODUCTS

Basic sunscreens—Basic sunscreen creams, lotions, oils, and sprays provide only the specified UV protection and are applied as the final step in any skin care regimen.

Combination day cream or lotion/sun protection—very popular, easy to use multipurpose products. They provide the benefits of a day cream or lotion with built-in sun protection in one easy step. They may also include other performance ingredients such as antioxidants and botanicals. Products may be oil free or rich in consistency, as they are formulated for all skin types.

Tinted sunscreen/moisturizers and lotions—take a combination sun protection product one step further by also providing sheer to light makeup foundation coverage to even out the skin tone. Healthy minerals are often used to give the product a natural tint or shade.

BB creams—multitasking products for daytime use that include a day cream, sunscreen, makeup foundation coverage, age prevention, and corrective ingredients all in one easy step and can be found for all skin types.

BB creams, often short for "beauty balm" or "blemish balm," originated in Korea. A spinoff, CC cream (color and correct) is similar to a BB cream but provides heavier coverage, similar to a concealer. CC creams have added performance ingredients to help improve skin imperfections like dark spots or redness.

CHECK IN

19. What are the main categories of skin care products?
20. What are five benefits of exfoliation?
21. What is the difference between a nonsetting and a setting mask?
22. Why does the area around the eyes require special attention, and what are some causes of problems with the skin around the eyes?
23. What is a sun protection factor (SPF) rating?

Recommend Home Care Products With Confidence

Did you know that how your clients treat their skin at home every day is more important than having a professional facial treatment? Some experts estimate that 80 percent of results in a skin care program are determined by daily, year-round home care. Professional facial treatments will certainly enhance and boost those results; however proper daily care is most important for healthy, beautiful skin.

Retailing products is a very important part of an esthetician's job. It's necessary for you and the business to be financially successful, and having products available for clients to purchase will help them achieve their goals of healthy, bright, and beautiful skin.

If the word *sales* makes you uncomfortable, then don't "sell"—recommend! If your client has a specific goal or skin concern, it would be a huge disservice to let them leave without providing your professional recommendations for home care. Consider yourself their skin care consultant, skin therapist, or personal skin care trainer. Clients expect your expert advice! (See **Figure 6–16**.) The more you know about your products and ingredients, the more confident and successful you will become at retailing because it will happen naturally.

Three Steps to Successful Retailing

1. PROVIDE PRODUCT EDUCATION

Education is key to your success, and this is especially true when recommending home care products. Keep it simple and to the point. Providing too much information will overwhelm most clients. Highlight key product features, ingredients, and how it will benefit their skin. You should also be able to explain why professional products available only from licensed estheticians are more beneficial to the health of their skin compared to over-the-counter products that can be purchased in any drug store, department store, online, or from anyone not licensed and educated in professional skin care:

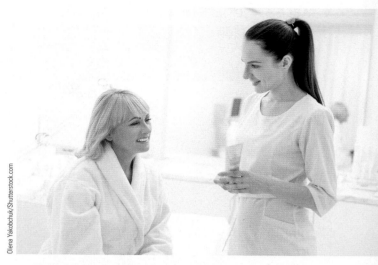

▲ **FIGURE 6–16** Clients expect an esthetician's expert advice to achieve their goals. Don't sell—recommend!

- **Ability to customize for specific skin types and conditions**—Over-the-counter brands are made for the masses. Professional products are designed for distinct skin types and conditions, and estheticians have the ability to create a totally customized program for anyone that walks through the door.

- **Higher quality and quantity of performance ingredients**—Professional products with a higher quality and quantity of performance ingredients and active agents mean more effective and better results.

- **Concentrated and cost-effective**—Although professional products may cost more up front than over-the-counter brands, they can be much more affordable over time because they are concentrated, not "watered down". When less needs to be used, the product lasts longer. Some professional skin care products actually cost far less than many high-end department store brands.

2. PRESENT PRECISE INSTRUCTIONS

Give clients simple, precise instructions as to how and when to apply, and also how much to use of each product. It's also a great idea to give clients a home care instructions sheet with your name and contact information listed (**Table 6–4**) to take with them. Remember to instruct them to contact you if they have any questions or concerns with their home care products, and that you're happy to assist them.

3. PRACTICE PROFESSIONAL FOLLOW-UP

A good practice is to follow up with clients after they've purchased products that you've recommended, especially if they're new and switching

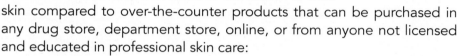

HERE'S A TIP

To save time and be ready for the post-consultation, pull out recommended home care products while the client is getting dressed after a facial. Show them what you recommend before they check out at the front desk.

▼ TABLE 6–4 Client Home Care Instruction Sheet

CLIENT HOME CARE INSTRUCTIONS SHEET Write recommendations for clients from the product lines you carry. Most product companies provide home care sheets to give to clients.			
Day	**Night**	**Weekly**	**Product Notes**
Cleanser:	Cleanser:	Mask:	
Toner:	Toner:	Exfoliant:	
Serum:	Serum:		
Eye Cream:	Eye Cream:		
Moisturizer:	Moisturizer:		
Sunscreen:			
Other:			

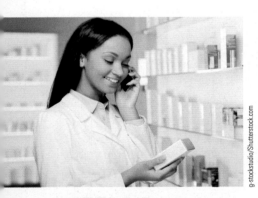

▲ FIGURE 6–17 Contacting clients within 1 week after product purchases and treatments builds trust.

from over-the-counter brands. This truly distinguishes you as a skin care professional. Contact them within a week and let them know that you're checking in to see how they like the products, if they have any questions, and how they're doing (**Figure 6–17**).

Many times, if problems or questions do arise, clients choose not to contact you and simply disappear. Remind them that this is a starting point and you may have to fine-tune their regimen as changes occur and you get to know their skin, and their personal preferences, much better. This will also help build a wonderful long-term relationship, as they know you will be with them every step of the way.

 CHECK IN

24. Why is retailing an important part of an esthetician's job?
25. What are the three steps to successful retailing?
26. What are three benefits of professional skin care products compared to over-the-counter brands?

Summarize the Points to Consider When Choosing a Professional Skin Care Line

Most estheticians will be faced with choosing a professional skin care line at some point in their career. This is one of the biggest business decisions an esthetician can make (**Figure 6–18**). Whether a technician is self-employed or involved in choosing product lines for a salon owner, the product line and its retail sales affect the success of the business. It's also important to remember that when you choose a product line, you are also choosing a company that you will be in a long-term business partnership with. A manufacturer may offer the most amazing products, but if they do not provide any support in education and marketing to help your business grow and be successful, it may not be the right partnership for you.

When choosing a product line, take into consideration the following points:

- Is the range of products versatile—that is, are products available for all skin types and conditions?
- Are the ingredients high quality and beneficial?
- Are the wholesale costs and retail prices affordable for you and your clients?
- Does the manufacturer require minimum order amounts or product quantities?
- What support in product training and education does the manufacturer provide? Educational opportunities and training classes help you become more knowledgeable, confident, and successful.
- What support in business and marketing does the manufacturer provide? The costs of samples and brochures, return policies, and marketing items affect your business.
- Is the product name recognizable and reputable? Many clients choose a product based on its name and how it is marketed.
- Is the packaging appealing and easy to use? Shelf appeal can be a very important factor in successful retailing.
- Does the manufacturer sell exclusively to licensed skin care professionals, or do they also sell directly to consumers through their own website or authorized online retailers? This is very important to know because the convenience of online shopping will continue to grow! If you're spending time educating your clients on product recommendations, it may really hurt your business if they can

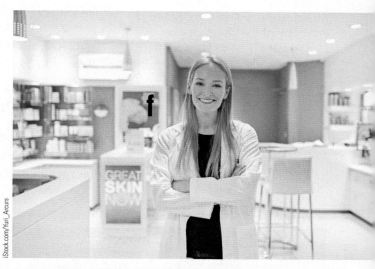

▲ **FIGURE 6–18** One of the biggest decisions in an esthetician's career is choosing a professional skin care line.

easily purchase those products directly from the manufacturer or an authorized online retailer. Professional brands are now recognizing this and some have implemented programs to assist licensed professionals in this process. Also keep in mind when researching that there are many *unauthorized* sales of professional brands on the Internet. Although manufacturers enforce very strict guidelines prohibiting the sale of their products online, unscrupulous individuals will continue to find unethical ways to earn some easy money. Warn your clients that unauthorized products for sale may actually harm their skin as most are old, expired, or counterfeit.

Product Prices and Costs

Pricing and costs of products are important considerations for both you and your clients. Generally, the markup for retail products is 100 percent, or double the salon's wholesale cost. Also keep in mind that

▼ **TABLE 6–5** Chart for Comparing and Rating Product Lines

COMPARING AND RATING PRODUCT LINES Use your own rating system—for example, rate products from 1 to 5 or from excellent to fair.								
Product line:				**Minimum order requirements:**				
Training and education provided: YES ○ NO ○				**Available marketing items:**				
	Cleansers	**Toners**	**Serums**	**Moisturizers**	**Exfoliants**	**Masks**	**Sunscreens**	**Other**
Skin Types								
Key Ingredients								
Cost Range								
Quality								
Texture								
Scent								
Packaging								
Sold online? If yes, are these authorized retailers? List websites:								
Overall rating/notes:								

in addition to the wholesale cost of products, salon owners have other business expenses related to products, including shipping, stocking and inventory, and employee wages.

A good way to determine actual product cost is to break down the purchase price into daily or weekly costs. This gives clients a better idea of how affordable the product really is, and how much they are actually spending (which is usually not more than a cup of coffee per day).

For example, if you have a product priced at $50 for 2 ounces (56 g) and it is estimated to last six months:

- The cost per month is $8.33 (the price of $50 divided by six months).
- The cost per week is $2.08 ($8.33 for one month divided by four weeks in a month).
- This is only $0.30 per day ($2.08 per week divided by seven days per week).

A very good price for maintaining beautiful skin!

Web Resources

For more information on regulations, skin care ingredients, and product formulations please visit these websites:
www.fda.gov
www.ams.usda.gov
www.personalcarecouncil.org
www.aad.org
www.cir-safety.org
www.cosmeticsdatabase.org
www.cosmeticsdesign.com
www.medscape.com
www.nsf.org
www.skincancer.org
www.rosacea.org

CHECK IN

27. List your top three most important considerations when choosing a product line.
28. What is a good way to determine actual product cost?

COMPETENCY PROGRESS

How are you doing with Skin Care Products: Chemistry, Ingredients, and Selection? **Check the Chapter 6 Learning Objectives below that you feel you have mastered; leave unchecked those objectives you will need to return to:**

☐ Explain how skin care products and ingredients are significant to estheticians.

☐ Describe cosmetic regulations, laws, and product safety.

☐ Distinguish cosmetic ingredient sources and popular terms.

☐ Describe the main types of ingredients in cosmetic chemistry.

☐ Identify beneficial ingredients for various skin types and conditions.

☐ Select appropriate products for facial treatments and home care use.

☐ Recommend home care products with confidence.

☐ Summarize the points to consider when choosing a professional skin care line.

acai berry ah-SAH-ee BER-ee	pg. 228	berry rich in antioxidants, vitamins A, B, C, and E; protects, replenishes; helps heal damaged skin
alcohol AL-kuh-hawl	pg. 125	antiseptic and solvent used in perfumes, lotions, and astringents; specially denatured (SD) alcohol is a mixture of ethanol with a denaturing agent
algae AL-jee	pg. 228	seaweed derivatives used as thickening agents, water-binding agents, and antioxidants; also nourishes the skin with vitamins and minerals
alginate AL-jun-ate	pg. 242	often seaweed based mask applied after a serum or treatment cream. They come in powder form and are mixed with water or serums, and dry to form a rubberized texture.
allantoin al-AHN-toyn	pg. 228	derived from the root of the comfrey plant, helps to soften and protect while actively soothing skin
aloe vera AL-oh VAIR-uh	pg. 228	popular botanical used in cosmetic formulations; emollient and humectant with hydrating, softening, healing, antimicrobial, and anti-inflammatory properties
alpha hydroxy acids AL-fah Hy-DROK-see AS-udz	pg. 217	abbreviated AHAS; derived naturally from various plant sources and from milk; used for improving signs of aging, dry skin, and an uneven skin tone
alpha lipoic acid AL-fah Lip-OH-ic ASs-ud	pg. 228	a natural molecule found in every cell in the body; it is a powerful antioxidant and is soluble in water and oil
ampoules AM-pyoolz	pg. 243	small, sealed vial containing a single application of highly concentrated serum of extracts in a water or oil base
anhydrous an-HY-drus	pg. 206	describes products that do not contain any water
argan oil AR-gon OYL	pg. 229	derived from the kernels of the argan tree; very light botanical oil used as an emollient
aromatherapy uh-ROH-muh-THAIR-uh-pee	pg. 213	therapeutic use of plant aromas and essential oils for beauty and health treatment purposes; involves the use of highly concentrated, nonoily, and volatile essential oils to induce such reactions as relaxation and invigoration, or to simply create a pleasant fragrance during a service
astringents uh-STRIN-jents	pg. 239	also called toners, these liquids help remove excess oil on the skin
azulene azz-U-leen	pg. 229	derived from the chamomile plant and characterized by its deep blue color; has anti-inflammatory and soothing properties
benzoyl peroxide BEN-zoyl puh-RAHK-syd	pg. 229	ingredient with antibacterial properties commonly used to treat inflamed acne lesions
beta-glucans BA-ta GLOO-canz	pg. 226	ingredients used in anti-aging cosmetics to help reduce the appearance of fine lines and wrinkles by stimulating the formation of collagen
beta hydroxy acids BA-ta Hy-DROK-see AS-udz	pg. 218	abbreviated BHAS; exfoliating organic acid; salicylic acid; milder than alpha hydroxy acids (AHAS); BHAS dissolve oil and are beneficial for oily skin
botanicals bow-TAN-ee-calz	pg. 216	ingredients derived from plants
calendula ca-LEND-yoo-lah	pg. 229	anti-inflammatory plant extract
carbomers KAHR-boh-murz	pg. 215	ingredients used to thicken creams; frequently used in gel products
certified colors SUR-tih-fyd KUL-urz	pg. 214	inorganic color agents also known as *metal salts*; listed on ingredient labels as D&C (drug and cosmetic)

chamomile KAM-uh-meel	pg. 229	plant extract with calming and soothing properties
chelating agents KEY-layt-ing AY-jents	pg. 212	a chemical added to cosmetics to improve the efficiency of the preservative
chemical exfoliants KEM-uh-kul Ex-FOLEY-antz-antz	pg. 240	products with chemical agents used to dissolve dead skin cells and the intercellular matrix, or "glue", that holds them together (desmosomes)
clay masks KLAY MASKZ	pg. 242	oil-absorbing purifying masks made with a clay base (such as kaolin or bentonite) that draw impurities to the surface of the skin as they dry and tighten
cleanser KLENZ-er	pg. 199	soap or detergent that cleans the skin
coconut oil KOH-kuh-nuht OYL	pg. 207	derived from coconut, one of the fattiest and heaviest oils used as an emollient
coenzyme Q10 KOE-en-zhym KUE TEN	pg. 230	powerful antioxidant that protects and revitalizes skin cells
color agents KUL-ur AY-jents	pg. 214	substances such as vegetable, pigment, or mineral dyes that give products color
cosmeceutical KAHZ-muh-SUIT-ick-al	pg. 199	term used to describe high-quality products or ingredients intended to improve the skin's health and appearance
cosmetics kahz-MET-iks	pg. 198	as defined by the U.S. Food And Drug Administration (FDA): articles that are intended to be rubbed, poured, sprinkled, or otherwise applied to the human body or any part thereof for cleansing, beautifying, promoting attractiveness, or altering the appearance
cruelty-free KROO-uhl-tee FREE	pg. 203	term used to describe products that are not tested on animals at any stage of the production process; nor are any of its ingredients tested on animals
delivery systems del-IV-er-ee SIS-tems	pg. 210	systems that deliver ingredients to specific tissues of the epidermis
detergents dee-TUR-jents	pg. 209	type of surfactant used as cleansers in skin-cleansing products
echinacea ek-uh-NEY-see-uh	pg. 230	derivative of the purple coneflower; prevents infection and has healing properties; used internally to support the immune system
emollients ee-MAHL-yunts	pg. 206	oil or fatty ingredients that lubricate, moisturize, and prevent water loss
emulsifiers ee-MUL-suh-fy-urz	pg. 209	surfactants that cause oil and water to mix and form an emulsion; an ingredient that brings two normally incompatible materials together and binds them into a uniform and fairly stable blend
enzymes (for exfoliation) EN-zymz	pg. 217	provide gentle exfoliation and dissolve keratin proteins within dead skin cells on the surface
essential oils ih-SEN-shul OYLZ	pg. 213	oils derived from herbs; have many different properties and effects on the skin and psyche
exfoliants ex-FOLEY-antz	pg. 240	mechanical and chemical products or processes used to exfoliate the skin
exfoliation eks-foh-lee AY-shun	pg. 216	peeling or sloughing of the outer layer of skin
fatty acids FADDY ASUDS	pg. 208	emollients; lubricant ingredients derived from plant oils or animal fats

fatty alcohols FAT-ee AL-kuh-hawlz	pg. 208	emollients; fatty acids that have been exposed to hydrogen
fatty esters FAT-ee ES-terz	pg. 208	emollients produced from fatty acids and alcohols
fragrance-free FREY-gruhns FREE	pg. 204	this term indicates that no additional ingredients have been added to a product to specifically provide a fragrance; however, it may already contain ingredients that have a scent
fragrances FREY-gruh-nses	pg. 205	give products their scent
fresheners FRESH-un-urz	pg. 239	toners, skin-freshening lotions, and liquids applied after cleansing to soothe and hydrate
functional ingredients FUNK-shun-al in-GREED-ee-antz	pg. 204	ingredients in cosmetic products that allow the products to spread, give them body and texture, and give them a specific form such as a lotion, cream, or gel; preservatives are also functional ingredients
glycerin GLIS-ur-in	pg. 230	formed by a decomposition of oils or fats; excellent skin softener and humectant; very strong water binder; sweet, colorless, oily substance used as a solvent and as a moisturizer in skin and body creams
glycoproteins gly-co-PRO-teenz	pg. 226	skin-conditioning agents derived from carbohydrates and proteins that enhance cellular metabolism and wound healing
gommage goh-MAJ	pg. 241	also known as *roll-off mask*; enzyme exfoliating masks that are rubbed off the skin
green tea GREEN TEE	pg. 231	powerful antioxidant and soothing agent; antibacterial, anti-inflammatory, skin brightening, and a stimulant
healing botanicals hee-ling bow-TAN-ee-calz	pg. 224	substances from plants such as chamomile, aloe, plant stem cells, and botanical oils that help to heal the skin
hemp seed oil HEMP SEED OYL	pg. 207	derived from hemp seeds, very light botanical oil used as an emollient
herbs URBS	pg. 213	hundreds of different herbs that contain phytohormones are used in skin care products and cosmetics; they heal, stimulate, soothe, and moisturize
humectants hyoo-MEK-tents	pg. 220	ingredients that attract water; humectants draw moisture to the skin and soften its surface, diminishing lines caused by dehydration
hydrators HY-drayt-urs	pg. 220	ingredients that attract water to the skin's surface
hydrophilic agents hy-drah-FIL-ik AY-jents	pg. 220	ingredients that attract water to the skin's surface
hypoallergenic hy-poh-al-ur-JEN-ik	pg. 203	refers to ingredients or products that may be less likely to cause allergic reactions
jojoba hoh-HOH-buh	pg. 243	oil widely used in cosmetics; extracted from the bean-like seeds of a desert shrub; used as a lubricant and noncomedogenic emollient and moisturizer
keratolytic kair-uh-tuh-LIT-ik	pg. 221	agent that causes exfoliation, or sloughing, of skin cells
kojic acid KOE-jik AS-ud	pg. 231	skin-brightening agent
lakes LEYKS	pg. 214	insoluble pigments made by combining a dye with an inorganic material
lanolin LAN-ul-un	pg. 203	emollient with moisturizing properties; also, an emulsifier with high water-absorption capabilities
lavender LAV-uhn-der	pg. 204	antiallergenic, anti-inflammatory, antiseptic, antibacterial, balancing, energizing, soothing, and healing

licorice LIK-uh-rish	pg. 231	anti-irritant used for sensitive skin; helps lighten pigmentation
lipids LIP-idz	pg. 206	fats or fat-like substances; lipids help repair and protect the barrier function of the skin
liposomes LY-puh-zohms	pg. 211	closed-lipid bilayer spheres that encapsulate ingredients, target their delivery to specific tissues of the skin, and control their release
liquid paraffin LIK-wud PAYR-uh-fin	pg. 207	emollient ingredient derived from petroleum sources
lubricant LOO-bri-kuh nt	pg. 208	coats the skin and reduces friction; mineral oil is a lubricant
mask MASQUE	pg. 241	also known as *pack or masque*; concentrated treatment product often composed of herbs, vitamins, mineral clays, moisturizing agents, skin softeners, aromatherapy oils, beneficial extracts, and other beneficial ingredients to cleanse, exfoliate, tighten, tone, hydrate, and nourish and treat the skin
mechanical exfoliants muh-KAN-ih-kul Ex-FOLEY-antz	pg. 240	products used as a physical method of polishing dead cells off the skin
methylparaben meth-ul-PARA-bin	pg. 212	one of the most frequently used preservatives because of its very low sensitizing potential; combats bacteria and molds; noncomedogenic
mineral oil MIN-ur-ul OYL	pg. 232	lubricant derived from petroleum
modelage masks MAHD-ul-ahj MASKZ	pg. 242	also known as *thermal masks or thermal heat masks*; facial masks containing special crystals of gypsum, a plaster-like ingredient
moisturizers MOYST-yur-yz-urz	pg. 199	products formulated to add moisture to the skin
natural, all natural NATCH-uh-rul, AL NATCH-uh-rul	pg. 202	terms often used in marketing for skin care products and ingredients derived from natural sources.
noncertified colors NAHN-sir-tif-eyed COLORZ	pg. 214	colors that are organic, meaning they come from animal or plant extracts; they can also be natural mineral pigments
oil soluble OYL sol-yoo-bull	pg. 218	compatible with oil
olfactory nerve ohl-FAK-tuh-ree NURV	pg. 214	"smell" receptors in the nose that communicate with parts of the brain that serve as storehouses for emotions and memories
organic or-GAN-ik	pg. 202	term used to describe natural-sourced ingredients that are grown without the use of pesticides or chemicals
palm oil PAHM OYL	pg. 207	derived from the oil palm tree; one of the fattiest and heaviest oils used as an emollient
papaya puh-PAH-yuh	pg. 240	natural enzyme used for exfoliation and in enzyme peels
parabens PAYR-uh-beenz	pg. 212	one of the most commonly used groups of preservatives in the cosmetic, pharmaceutical, and food industries; provide bacteriostatic and fungistatic activity against diverse organisms
paraffin wax masks PAYR-uh-fin WAKS MASKS	pg. 242	mask used to warm the skin and promote penetration of ingredients through the heat trapped under the surface of the paraffin
peptides PEP-tydz	pg. 223	chains of amino acids that stimulate fibroblasts, cell metabolism, collagen; improve skin's firmness. Larger chains are called polypeptides
performance ingredients per-FOR-manz in-GREED-ee-antz	pg. 204	ingredients in cosmetic products that cause the actual changes in the appearance of the skin

petrolatum peh-troh-LAY-tum	pg. 233	emollient ingredient derived from petroleum sources
pH adjusters P-H ah-JUST-uhrz	pg. 215	acids or alkalis (bases) used to adjust the pH of products
phthalates THAL-ates	pg. 219	plasticizers used in skin care formulas to moisturize and soften skin, and to dissolve or blend ingredients
plant stem cells PLANT STEM SELLZ	pg. 225	derived from plants to protect or stimulate our own skin stem cells; health and anti-aging benefits
polyglucans poly-GLUE-canz	pg. 226	ingredients derived from yeast cells that help strengthen the immune system and stimulate metabolism; hydrophilic and help preserve and protect collagen and elastin
polymers PAHL-imerz	pg. 211	chemical compounds formed by combining a number of small molecules (monomers) into long chain-like structures; advanced vehicles that release substances onto the skin's surface at a microscopically controlled rate
preservatives pre-SERV-uh-tifs	pg. 211	chemical agents that inhibit the growth of microorganisms in cosmetic formulations; they kill bacteria and prevent products from spoiling
quaternium 15 kwah-TAYR-nee-um fif-TEEN	pg. 212	all-purpose preservative active against bacteria, mold, and yeast. Probably the greatest formaldehyde-releaser among cosmetic preservatives; may cause dermatitis and allergies
retinol RET-in-awl	pg. 218	natural form of vitamin A; stimulates cell repair and helps to normalize skin cells by generating new cells
salicylic acid sal-uh-SIL-ik AS-ud	pg. 218	beta hydroxy acid with exfoliating and antiseptic properties; natural sources include sweet birch, willow bark, and wintergreen
seaweed SEE-weed	pg. 228	seaweed derivatives such as algae have many nourishing properties; known for its humectant and moisturizing properties, vitamin content, metabolism stimulation and detoxification, and aiding skin firmness
serums SE-rum	pg. 243	concentrated liquid ingredients for the skin designed to penetrate and treat various skin conditions
sodium bicarbonate SOH-dee-um bye-KAR-buh-nayt	pg. 215	baking soda; an alkaline inorganic salt used as a buffering agent, neutralizer, and pH adjuster
squalane SKWA-lane	pg. 233	derived from olives; desensitizes and nourishes; an emollient
sulfur SUL-fur	pg. 234	reduces the activity of oil glands and dissolves the skin's surface layer of dry, dead cells; commonly used in acne products
sun protection factor SUN-proh-TEK-shun FAK-tur	pg. 246	abbreviated SPF; indicates the ability of a product to delay sun-induced erythema, the visible sign of sun damage; the SPF rating is based only on UVB protection, not UVA exposure
tea tree oil TEE TREE OYL	pg. 234	soothing and antiseptic; antifungal properties
titanium dioxide ty-TAYN-eeum dy-AHK-syd	pg. 227	inorganic physical sunscreen that reflects UV radiation
toners TOH-nurz	pg. 239	also known as *fresheners or astringents*; liquids designed to tone and tighten the skin's surface
unscented un-SENT-id	pg. 204	products formulated to have no smell; because most ingredients in a formulation do have an odor, more ingredients have to be added to neutralize the smell
urea yoo-REE-uh	pg. 205	properties include enhancing the penetrative abilities of other substances; anti-inflammatory, antiseptic, and deodorizing action that protects the skin's surface and helps maintain healthy skin

vegan VEE-guhn	pg. 203	a product that is labeled vegan should not contain any animal ingredients or animal by-products
vehicles VEE-hik-uhls	pg. 211	spreading agents and ingredients that carry or deliver other ingredients into the skin and make them more effective
water soluble WAW-tur SAHL-yoo-buhl	pg. 217	mixable with water
witch hazel WICH HAY-zul	pg. 234	extracted from the bark of the hamanelis shrub; can be a soothing agent or, in higher concentrations, an astringent
zinc oxide ZINGK AHK-syd	pg. 205	mineral physical sunscreen ingredient that reflects UVA and UVB rays; also used to protect, soothe, and heal the skin; is somewhat astringent, antiseptic, and antimicrobial

PART 2
Skin Care Treatments

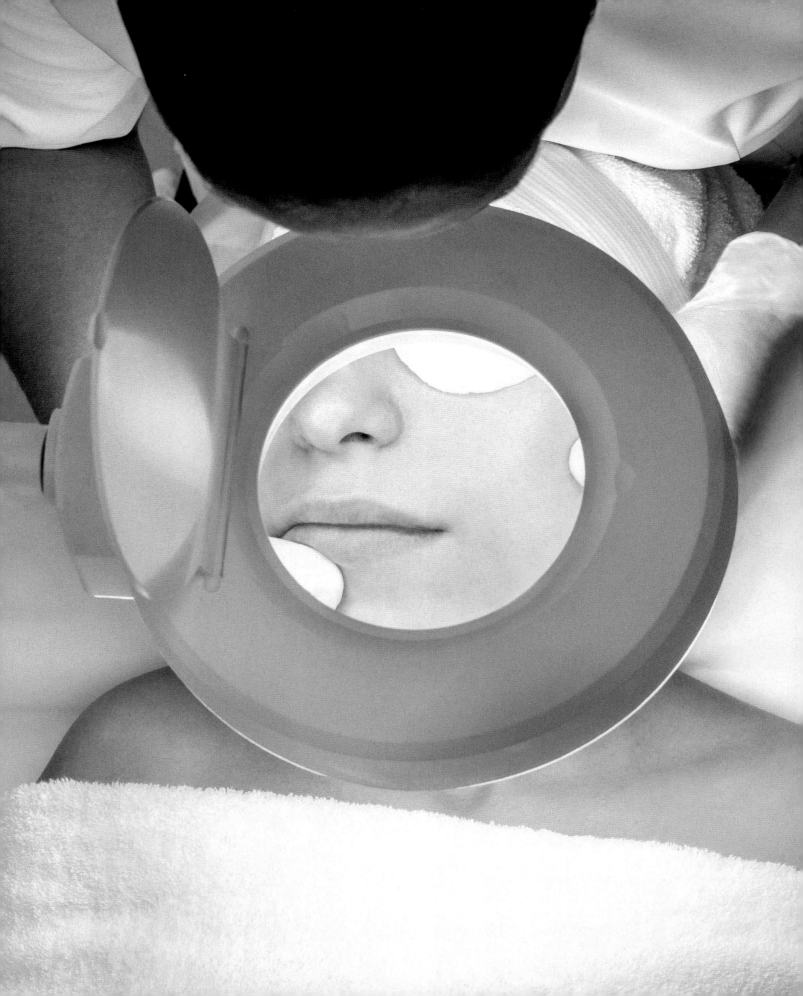

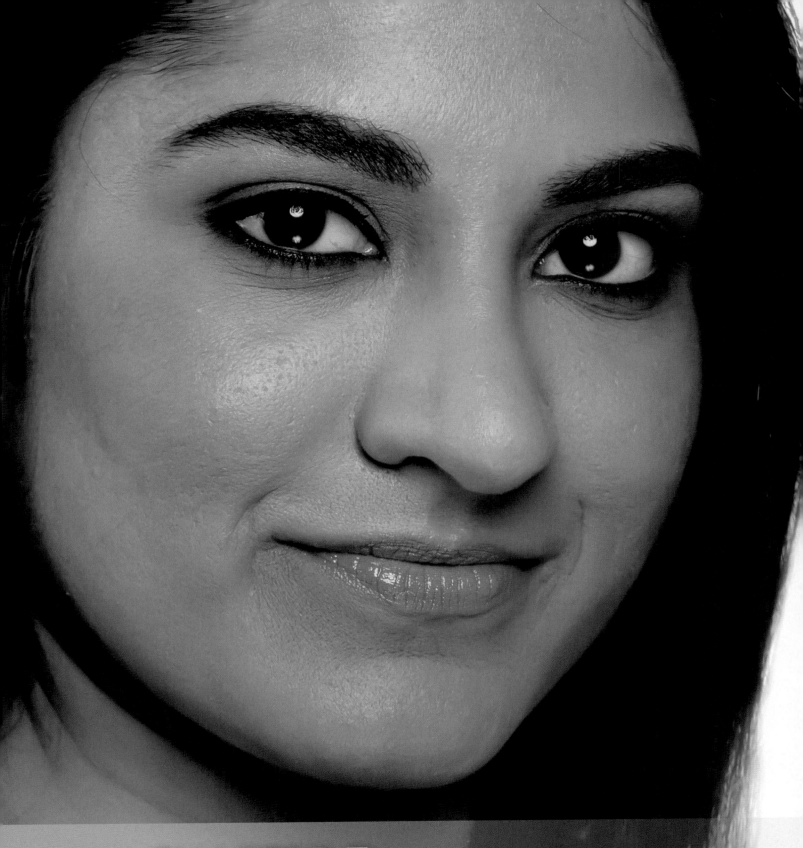

 CHAPTER 7
The Treatment Room

"The beautiful thing about learning is nobody can take it away from you."

–B. B. King

Learning Objectives

After completing this chapter, you will be able to:

1. Explain why treatment room preparation is an integral part of providing treatments.
2. Review the elements of an esthetician's professional appearance.
3. Outline essential room and station structural features.
4. Describe the ideal ambience, furniture, and equipment for facials.
5. Properly manage treatment room supplies and products.
6. Be able to set up a facial treatment area, such as a facial bar or station.
7. Prepare the treatment room for services.
8. Properly clean and disinfect the treatment room.
9. Perform pre- and post-service procedures to meet safety and health requirements.

Explain Why Treatment Room Preparation is an Integral Part of Providing Treatments

This chapter is designed to help estheticians learn to properly prepare the treatment room or facial bar station for services as an integral part of giving treatments (**Figure 7–1**). Treatment room setup includes choosing and properly installing and arranging furniture, equipment, supplies, and products. Included in this chapter are easy-to-use checklists and advice for setting up, cleaning and disinfecting, and keeping the room well stocked. Whether you intend on becoming a salon or spa owner, being a member of an esthetic staff, or performing treatments at a spa or salon on a freelance basis, maintaining the highest standards in professionalism, personal hygiene, and image, as well as following proper protocol, is vital to your success. After the facial service, it is critical to follow proper cleaning and disinfection protocols to prepare the treatment room or station for the next client.

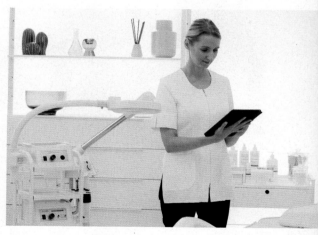

▲ **FIGURE 7–1** Review the checklists while setting up your treatment room.

Estheticians should study and have a thorough understanding of the treatment room because:

- It is essential to provide a consistent, comfortable, relaxing, and clean environment for the client.
- Planning and preparing a well-stocked and organized room is necessary to function efficiently and provide good service.
- Complying with your state board regulations regarding the cleanliness of the treatment rooms assures your safety as well as your client's.
- You will feel confident if you are organized and prepared by maintaining a professional appearance and demeanor and an organized environment.

Review the Elements of an Esthetician's Professional Appearance

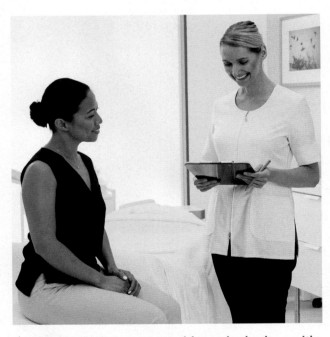

▲ FIGURE 7–2 Convey a positive attitude along with a credible image that conveys your knowledge and professionalism.

Making a good first impression is important in any business setting. Your success depends on many factors, including your image and attitude. An esthetician's appearance and professionalism reflect on the business. Practicing *good hygiene*, dressing professionally, and having a *neat appearance* all convey a polished image (**Figure 7–2**). Additionally, employers, coworkers, and clients appreciate working with someone who has a *positive attitude*. This positive attribute will contribute favorably to the team.

Being *dependable* and *providing excellent customer service* is imperative. Professionalism includes being *prepared*, that is, taking the initiative to plan enough time to set up the room before the day begins. Plan on arriving at least 30 minutes prior to the start of your shift to make sure your room is well stocked and that all your electrical equipment is in working order. You will project a calm, confident image if you and your treatment room or station are clean, organized, and fully prepared for you to provide treatments.

Refer to *Milady Standard Foundations* Chapter 2, Professional Image, for more information on professionalism.

Professional Image Checklist

Your job is to provide skin care services and to recommend professional home care to your client in order to support the services you provide. To accomplish this, you must portray a credible image that conveys your knowledge and professionalism, as well as reflects the professionalism and cleanliness of the work establishment. Consider these points when assessing your appearance:

- **Well-groomed hair.** Hair should be clean and neatly styled and pulled back if worn long. A good cut and color are key to a professional appearance in esthetics. Be diligent about keeping hair in healthy condition. Healthy, beautiful hair is linked to healthy, beautiful skin. Keep hair up and away from clients at all times during treatment. Never let your hair brush against your client's skin.

- **Minimal accessories.** Jewelry should be kept to a minimum—no jangling bracelets, dangling earrings, long necklaces, or large rings.

- **Skin.** A professional esthetician's skin is a reflection of their own expertise and the proficiency of their skin care establishment. We must be a reflection of the skin care industry by using professional skin care and taking care of our skin.

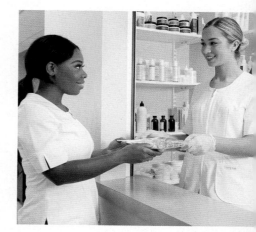

- **Well-groomed nails.** Short nails are a must so that the client is never scratched. Well-manicured, short nails with no polish or light polish are acceptable in most working environments.

- **Makeup.** Wear makeup to reflect the image of the spa or salon you are working for. Light makeup is acceptable with well-groomed brows.

- **Proper uniform.** Your lab coat, scrubs, uniform, or apron should be spotless, freshly laundered, crisp, and ironed. Comfortable, closed-toed shoes, in accordance with your state board guidelines, are also part of the uniform.

- **Positive energy and a healthy lifestyle.** A genuine smile, good posture, eye contact, and an engaging handshake will convey that you have a positive attitude, vitality, and energy. Energy may be hard to come by with a busy schedule. One way to maintain it is with healthy eating and drinking plenty of water. Working on multiple clients relies on having plenty of energy throughout your shift. The last client should have the same experience as the first client of the day. Rest, relaxation, hobbies and healthy eating will assist the esthetician to have longevity in the spa industry.

 CHECK IN

1. What are the essential qualities necessary to convey professionalism?
2. What six elements constitute a professional image?

Outline Essential Room and Station Structural Features

Aside from aesthetically pleasing interior design, a properly constructed and equipped treatment room or area is an essential part of a successful business (**Figure 7–3**). The most important structural features in a treatment room or area are outlined in the following section.

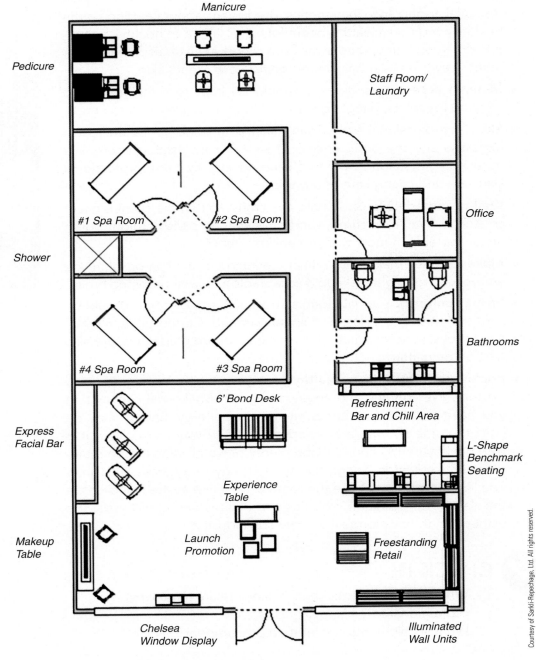

▲ **FIGURE 7–3** Sample layout of spa or salon.

Structural Features

SIZE

The treatment room or area should be large enough to ensure proper movement of the esthetician in the space. Neither the professional nor the client should ever feel cramped.

PROPER VENTILATION

A properly ventilated work space ensures a healthy esthetician and healthy clients. The Occupational Safety and Health Association (OSHA), provides important guidelines for ventilation in regards to nail service rooms and areas, as well as the use of formaldehydes in hair care, but proper ventilation is also key for the health of the skin care practitioner as well as the client. Fumes from skin care treatments, as well as cleaning and disinfecting materials, must be properly eliminated. Air vents must be present in the room, providing air input and output. This means two separate vents. These vents must be properly functioning and calibrated for two or more people within the room.

ELECTRICAL OUTLETS

With the use of more and more machines as well as electronic devices within the treatment room or area, the proper number of electrical outlets, with subsequent appropriate electrical service capability, is essential to the proper functioning of the treatment room or area. Treatment rooms should have a minimum of four separate electrical outlets. Avoid the use of extension cords or multiple plug appliances within the room, as these can overheat and become a fire hazard. Always be sure that no wires are in your way or in the way of the client.

RUNNING WATER

Having a sink within the treatment rooms and a separate shower area is ideal for a full-service skin care salon. It is essential for the thorough removal of facial and body products, proper hand washing, and proper cleansing and disinfection of the work areas.

Many spas and salons today do not have a sink in the room. The access to water may be in the hall or breakroom area. In these cases, a hot towel cabinet and bringing in two bowls of water will alleviate any need to leave the treatment room on multiple occasions during a facial treatment.

WASHABLE FLOORING AND WORKSTATION SURFACES

Carpeting or rugs can harbor germs and dirt; therefore, treatment room flooring and workstation surfaces (including treatment tables and chairs) need to be easily washable and able to tolerate daily washing with antimicrobial cleansers without degrading. Flooring and workstation areas should be tile or stone, re-engineered wood, bamboo or vinyl, while facial chairs and stools should be made of nonabsorbent washable synthetic materials.

DID YOU KNOW?

Successful skin treatments are not confined to a treatment room. You can expect treatment room sizes will vary, especially with the influx of the rental studio prototypes, pop-up shops, and mobile spas.

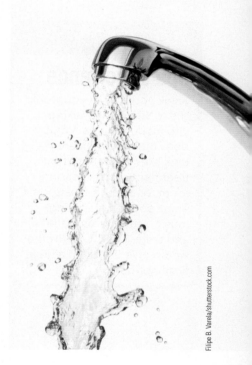

Filipe B. Varela/shutterstock.com

PROPER LIGHTING

Dim lights may help relax the client and set the mood for the treatment, but the lighting should be able to be increased or decreased during skin analysis and product removal. Light fixtures should also be able to be adjusted to point up toward the ceiling or down. Uplighting provides the most efficient light for a treatment room, and also helps create a better esthetic atmosphere.

 CHECK IN

3. What are the key structural features to look for in a skin care treatment room or area?
4. What kind of vents must be present in a treatment room?
5. What is the minimum number of electrical outlets in a treatment room?
6. Of what type of materials should flooring and workstations be made?

ACTIVITY

Spa Experience

Think about what you would like to see when walking into a salon or spa. What does the reception area look like? What about the treatment room, dressing room, or even the restroom? Think about the lighting, music, scent, temperature, and taste. List five items that would give the client a great first impression.

Describe the Ideal Ambience, Furniture, and Equipment for Facials

The first seven seconds of a potential client's initial encounter with your spa is critical to conveying your professional image.

Ambience

The ambience including the sight, sound, smell, and feel of your spa, plays a factor in selling your facility and services to potential customers (**Figure 7–4a and b**).

The proper spa environment should engage all five of the senses. As learned, *proper lighting* is key to illuminating a well-designed spa environment. The *music selection* that has spa sounds will add a definitive flavor to your spa's identity. *Temperature* is very important as well to keep clients feeling warm enough in the treatment room, or properly cooled if it is hot outside. *Scent* is crucial in a spa environment. Stale or foul odors can imply lack of proper cleaning and disinfection, while overly chemical smells can be off-putting. Scents should be soothing and natural. Finally, a spa or salon should not overlook the sense of *taste*. Offer naturally flavoured waters and small healthy snacks for refreshment in the reception area to promote the energy and well-being of your clients. All these engagements will heighten the client's positive perception of the spa.

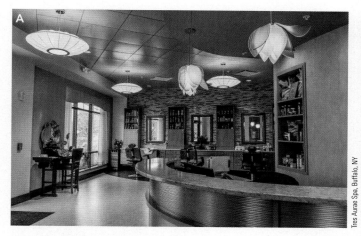
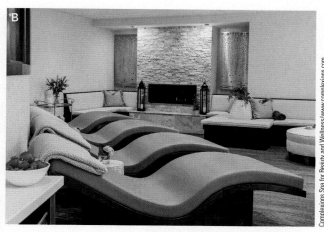

▲ **FIGURE 7–4** The design and ambience of your spa environment plays an important role in enticing and maintaining clientele.

Room esthetics is vital to creating a relaxing, professional atmosphere. Treatment room furnishings can range from the basics to high-end designer equipment. Relaxing colors, music, and décor are preferable in a spa. When setting up a room for treatments, think about the services you will perform and how you will work at the station. Another consideration is how comfortable the client will be on the treatment table (be sure to consider the needs of all genders as well). Ensuring client safety and following health regulations are the two most important considerations before, during, and after treatments.

(Facial equipment and machines are discussed in Chapter 10, Facial Devices and Technology.)

A Checklist of Furniture and Equipment

Equipment for the facial treatment consists of the following items (**Figure 7–5**):

A. *Treatment table* (also called a facial chair, table, or bed) —A treatment table may come equipped to have adjustable height, removable headrests, adjustable head- and footrests, electrical controls, and built-in electrical outlets.

B. *Esthetician's chair*, or operator's stool —The esthetician's stool needs to be *ergonomically correct*: healthy for the body and spine. Make sure it is both adjustable and comfortable for you while you perform services and that it can roll around easily. You need to adjust the chair so that it is waist height to the treatment table. This will ensure that you will not be working at an awkward angle to the client while you are sitting (see the section titled "Ergonomics in the Treatment Room"). An incorrect angle can cause injury to the client, while constant repetitive movements at the wrong height can cause neck and back problems for the esthetician.

CAUTION!
A workstation that is uncomfortable for the body could cause neck, back, and hand problems over time.

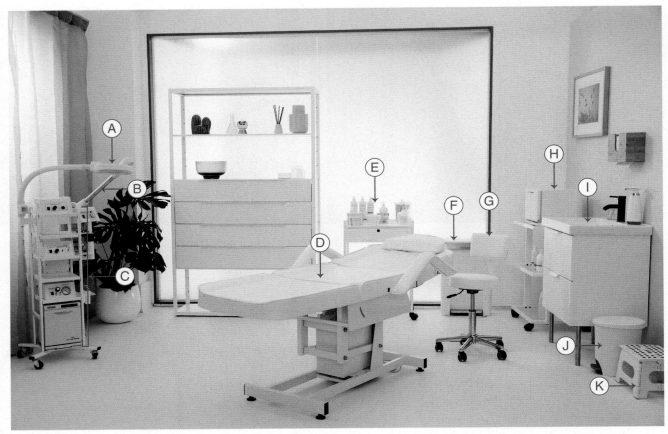

(A) Magnifying Lamp   (E) Trolley   (I) Sink

(B) Steamer   (F) Covered Laundry Hamper   (J) Covered Waste Container

(C) Multifunctional Machine   (G) Esthetician's Chair   (K) Step Stool

(D) Treatment Table   (H) Towel Warmer

▲ **FIGURE 7–5** Facial treatment rooms have some essential pieces of furniture and equipment.

C. *Step stool*—If you do not have an electric treatment table, a step stool helps clients get on and off the table safely. Make sure the stool is stable. Assist clients if they need help.

D. **Trolley** (TROL-ee) or utility cart—A cart holds tools, supplies, and products. This can be a stationary table or roll cart.

E. *Magnifying lamp* or *light* —To properly analyze a client's skin, you need magnification and good light. A magnifying lamp provides both of these attributes and is necessary for use during many parts of procedures, especially extractions. A magnifying lamp gives you a clear view of the skin, and also protects you from exposure to debris from procedures such as extractions. Because of optical sensitivity, always place cotton pads over the client's eyes when using the lamp. To properly analyze a client's skin, a 3 or 5 diopter lens magnification and good light is sufficient. A magnifying lamp with a circular bulb, rotating head, and mobile base is ideal so that you can angle the lamp properly to examine the client's skin to determine type and condition, as well as treat skin.

F. *Steamer*—Steam is part of a standard facial procedure. Follow the manufacturer's advice on what water to use in the steamer and make sure it is UL approved. Clean the steamer daily. Facial steaming aids in the deep cleansing effect of the facial and should be performed before extractions. Skip on sensitive or rosacea-prone skin.

G. *Galvanic, high-frequency, brush, vacuum, and spray machines*— These can be either individual machines or multifunctional machines all on one stand. All jewelry should be removed from the client and esthetician before treatments.

H. *Towel warmer*, or "hot cabi"—Hot towel cabinets keep warm, moist towels ready for use throughout the day in the skin care treatment room. Moist towels can be used to remove products from the skin during a facial and body treatments.

I. Closed, covered *waste container for trash*—A fire retardant receptacle (metal) with a self-closing lid and foot pedal is required for preventing contamination, especially if disposing of chemical waste material.

J. Closed, covered *laundry hamper* with foot pedal is ideal for preventing contamination.

K. A sink or basin for water is essential in a treatment room. You should always have access to clean water during treatments.

ADDITIONAL ITEMS

These are some additional items that may be in your treatment room:

L. *Wax heater*—The wax heater is an electric warming device used for soft-wax, paraffin, and hard-wax applications (Figure 7–6). It is usually kept activated during the day for walk-ins or unexpected requests. Waxing is discussed in Chapter 11, Hair Removal.

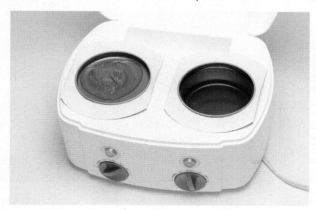

▲ **FIGURE 7–6** Wax heater

> ## CAUTION!
> An ultraviolet (UV) sanitizer unit does not disinfect tools and is used only for storage after tools have been disinfected.

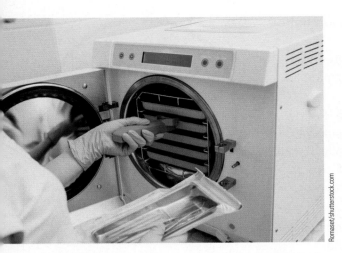

▲ **FIGURE 7–7** Autoclaves completely kill all microorganisms.

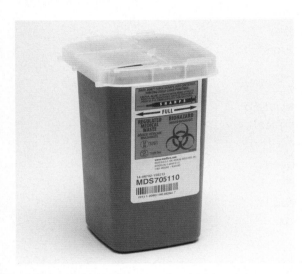

▲ **FIGURE 7–8** Sharps disposal container

M. *Autoclave*—An autoclave is a sterilizer for implements, meaning it completely kills all microorganisms, including bacteria, fungi, viruses, and bacterial spores (**Figure 7–7**). An autoclave sterilizes by providing pressurized steam. Reusable implements need to be sterilized between treatments. Use disposable supplies to avoid the chance of cross-contamination. While this piece of equipment may be costly, there are now relatively inexpensive models available. While autoclaves may not be required in every state (check your state board), you should self-mandate use of these sterilizers. They are worth the investment: They assure your clients of the quality of your services and salon or spa.

N. *Sharps disposal container*—A sharps disposal container is a puncture-proof biohazard container for disposal of lancets, syringes, needles and other sharp objects that can be used during procedures (**Figure 7–8**). Follow OSHA and state regulations for proper disposal. Not all facilities perform services that require a sharps disposal container.

O. A small *hand-held mirror* for the client to see before and after treatment results is beneficial to their service (**Figure 7–9**).

P. *Binder for Safety Data Sheets* (SDS)—These forms should be kept in a binder or on the computer within the treatment room for easy access when needed *(Figure 7–10)*. (See "Focus On: What Are SDSs?")

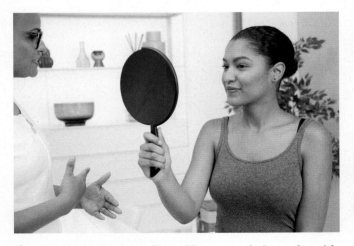

▲ **FIGURE 7–9** Many clients like to see their results with a hand-held mirror.

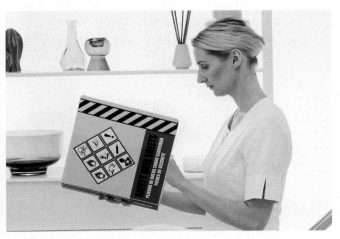

▲ **FIGURE 7–10** Always have Safety Data Sheets available to review details on every skin care product.

Ergonomics in the Treatment Room

Ergonomics is the study of adapting work conditions to suit the worker. The equipment and the positions we use should be healthy for the spine and other parts of the body. Adjust the treatment table height, if possible. When setting up, remember:

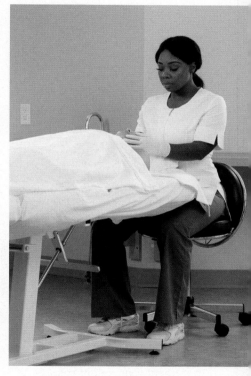

▲ FIGURE 7–11 Practice proper ergonomics by adjusting the treatment table to suit your height.

- Align the stool with the treatment table for the correct height and position to perform services.
- The esthetician's feet should be flat on the floor, and hands should be below chest level.
- A good stool with back support is essential for esthetic work. It is worth paying a little more for a well-padded and quality stool.
- The room setup should be comfortable for the esthetician to avoid strain on the hands, body, and back (**Figure 7–11**).
- No part of your body should be touching the client except your hands and perhaps arms during the service.
- Arrange the supply cart or counter as close to the treatment table as possible. When reaching for a product or implement, or to adjust equipment, get up out of the chair. Do not overstretch your back to reach for something.
- Be aware of the position of your back and remind yourself to sit up straight. Pay attention to your posture.
- Stretching and loosening up the hands before and after working is helpful in maintaining the health and flexibility of the wrists and hands.
- In between clients, stretch and take 12 deep breaths.

Costs of Starting Your Own Business

After reviewing the list of furniture and equipment required, you may be curious about what costs are involved in setting up a spa or salon business. When deciding whether or not to open your own skin care salon or spa, many factors come into consideration, not least of them being *cost*. When estimating cost, it is important to break down everything you will need and the cost associated with that need. Pricing fluctuates from area to area and spas come in all shapes and sizes. Research the supplies and equipment costs to determine what you would need to spend to set up your own room. Consider Tonya's story as an example of the importance of research and cost estimating.

Tonya is considering building a new facility and the cost in her location is $225 to $375 per square foot, with a minimum space requirement of 1,500 square feet (**Figure 7–12**). That means $450,000 for the salon or spa space. After some research, the cost for the equipment in the treatment room, excluding any reception and retail areas, adds up to between $6,400.00 to $9,200.00. She took into consideration the treatment table, mobile facial bar, workstation, the facial stool, hot towel cabinet and single-use and multiuse items to start.

Tonya has now estimated the start-up cost to build her own facility to be between $456,400 to $459,200. She can now make a more informed decision between building or renting in her area. This is an exercise that any esthetician can do to determine what you would need to spend to set up your own room.

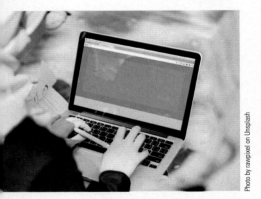

Photo by rawpixel on Unsplash

▲ **FIGURE 7–12** Research to find out what setting up a treatment room might cost.

✓ CHECK IN

7. What are the two most important factors to consider when furnishing a treatment room?
8. What are the two main functions of a magnifying lamp?
9. What is a sharps container?
10. Why do laundry hampers and trash receptacles ideally need to be pedal activated with closed lids?

Properly Manage Treatment Room Supplies and Products

Part of your success as an esthetician involves properly managing supplies. Like a great chef, having a clean, uncluttered workspace with all the items you need to perform the service easily within reach is key to performing a successful treatment or procedure (**Figure 7–13**). If you have to stop a procedure to find supplies, it decreases the client's satisfaction. Also, supplies such as facial masks, moisturizers, and other high-end products can be costly, so proper inventory control is

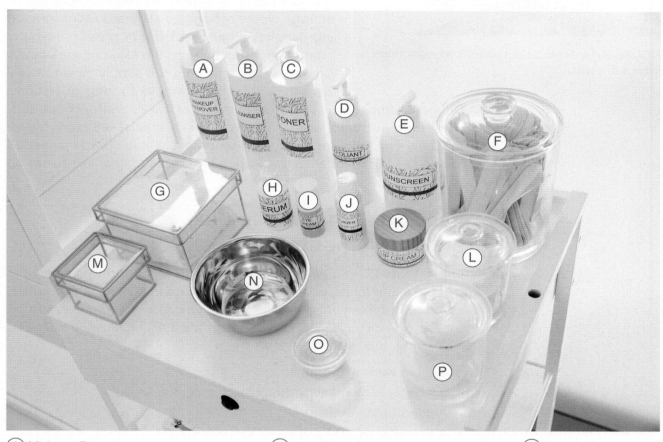

(A) Makeup Remover

(B) Cleanser

(C) Toner

(D) Exfoliant

(E) Sunscreen

(F) Disposable Spatulas

(G) 4x4 Esthetic Wipes

(H) Serum

(I) Eye Cream

(J) Moisturizer

(K) Lip Cream

(L) Sponges

(M) 2x2 Esthetic Wipes

(N) Basin for Water

(O) Dispensed Product

(P) Cotton Rounds

▲ **FIGURE 7–13** Set up the cart with facial treatment supplies in the order of procedure application.

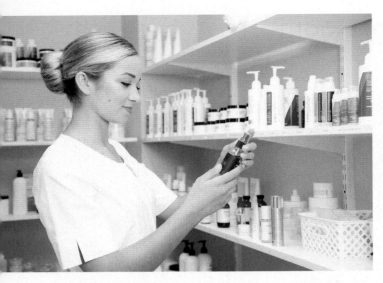

▲ **FIGURE 7–14** Products and supplies are sometimes stored in a dispensary.

important to either helping sustain your employer's business or keeping to your own budget if you are self-employed.

Supplies can be multiuse, as in sheets or a hand-held mirror, or single-use, such as a cotton swab or lancet. Single-use items must be disposed of immediately after use in a closed-lid trash can or sharps container. Proper storage is necessary to keep items clean and sterile, so they must be kept in clean, covered, labeled containers. If supplies and products are not kept in the treatment room or at workstations, then they are typically kept in a **dispensary** (dis-PEN-suh-ree) or storage closet, which is a separate room for storing supplies (**Figure 7–14**). For proper inventory control, please adhere to the salon or spa's policy on removing items from the supply closet or dispensary for stocking treatment rooms or stations.

Different setups require different numbers of towels and/or cotton supplies. Each instructor or manager will have a special setup procedure to follow. The following section presents an example of what is needed for a basic facial. Refer to the waxing and makeup chapters to set up for those services.

Facial Treatment Supplies and Implements

Implements (IM-pluh-mentz) are tools used to perform your services and are either multiuse or single-use. Multiuse implements, also known as reusable implements, must be properly cleaned and disinfected after use on one client and prior to use on another. Multiuse implements include the following:

- A table warmer (optional)
- A bolster for back support, placed under the knees
- A hand-held mirror
- A pillow or rolled hand towel for neck support
- An extraction tool such as a comedone extractor
- Blankets to cover the client
- Bowl or basin for water
- Client chart and home care prescription card/pad or computer for database
- Client gown/wrap for the client to change into
- Facial kits
- Glass or plastic containers to hold cotton pads or other supplies

- Linens such as sheets and face and hand towels (either cloth or disposable)
- Rubber mixing bowls to warm or mix product in
- Metal spatulas to disperse products from jars
- Retail product brochures
- Scissors
- Tongs to handle hot towels and retrieve clean items (**Figure 7–15**)
- Tweezers.

Single-Use Items

Single-use items are disposable and can be used only once. This supply usage depends on your facility and may include the following (**Figure 7–16**):

- Client headband to protect the hair and hold it out of the way
- 2" × 2" (5 cm × 5 cm) esthetics wipes, for cleaning and for product application
- 4" × 4" (10 cm × 10 cm) esthetics wipes or single-use sponges to remove product from the skin (sponges are porous and cannot be disinfected or reused)
- Disposable hair wraps/protective caps
- Disposable lancets (see state regulations for extraction rules)
- Disposable vinyl or nitrile gloves (latex is not recommended, as many people are allergic to latex and oil can break down the latex, compromising the protection of the gloves)
- Fan and mask brushes to apply masks or massage lotions. Note: Because brushes are porous, they cannot be disinfected. Brushes should be disposable.
- Fragrance-free tissues, which are available in medical supply stores or online, and can make a significant difference in the treatments; these do not contain fragrance or dyes, so do not cause reactions on the skin
- Gauze squares for use with certain facial treatments
- Makeup sponges for applying makeup post procedure and for applying product
- Paper towels
- Personal service towels (PST) to drape clients and to keep work area clean

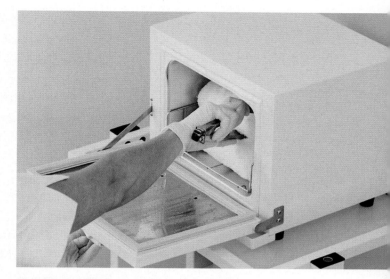

▲ **FIGURE 7–15** Use tongs to handle hot towels.

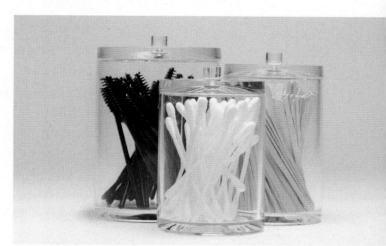

▲ **FIGURE 7–16** Always keep single-use items in covered containers.

- Plastic liners for electric mittens and booties
- Sealable plastic bag for proper disposal of single-use items
- Sterile cotton swabs for performing extractions; it is important that these are sterile when using for extraction; can have wooden handles for extra strength
- Wax supplies (see Chapter 11, Hair Removal).

Products

Products are the main ingredients in performing services. Chapter 6, Skin Care Products: Chemistry, Ingredients, and Selection, addresses the guidelines for choosing products. Have the correct products for all client services on hand (**Figure 7–17**). Some of the basic products used in facials include the following:

- Body massage creams
- Body oil
- Cleanser
- Desincrustation solution
- Essential oils
- Exfoliants (mechanical, chemical)
- Eye cream
- Eye pads
- Face massage cream or lotion
- Facial peel kits
- Galvanic gel to be used with galvanic treatment
- Hand cream
- Lip balm
- Makeup remover
- Masks (cream, mud/clay, seaweed, sheet, paraffin)
- Moisturizer (cream, lotions, gel)
- Serums and ampoules
- Sunscreens
- Toner and astringent.

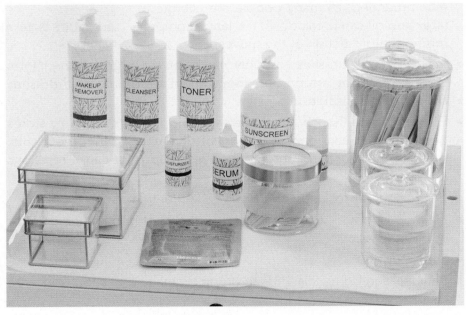

▲ **FIGURE 7–17 Always have your products organized on your cart before each service.**

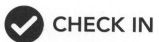
11. Why is it important to stock and organize supplies prior to treating your clients?
12. How are multiuse supplies different from single-use supplies?
13. How do you dispose of single-use supplies?

Be Able to Set Up a Facial Treatment Area, Such as Facial Bar or Station

Many salons and spas are now utilizing a **facial station** (FAY-shul STAY-shun) or facial bar concept in their facilities in addition or in place of treatment rooms. These are treatment areas within the reception or retail area of the facility, usually located within 20 feet of the front door to allow for maximum visibility. Intensive peels, full facial or body treatments that include extensive extractions, and full body massage are not performed in this space. Express or mini shortened facial treatments such as eye treatments and facial sheet masks, men's treatments such as beard facials, and even targeted body treatments such as hand and foot treatments, can be performed at these stations. The client does not need to disrobe or change for these treatments, and not all equipment and supplies are needed. Sheet masks continue to show growth in popularity, and are particularly well suited for the facial bar environment in that they do not require mixing, and can be performed in conjunction with other services (**Figure 7–18**). The facial bar or station will consist of a workstation or several workstations. Each workstation should be set up in an orderly way with all of the products and items needed. Be sure the stations are fully supplied, which ensures a smooth transition between clients and maintains the cleanest environment for you and your clients. Here's a list of the abbreviated supplies:

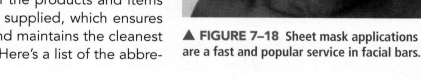

▲ FIGURE 7–18 Sheet mask applications are a fast and popular service in facial bars.

- Facial chair
- Magnifying lamp
- Consultation chart
- Unscented facial tissues
- Gloves
- Esthetics wipes
- Disposable headbands
- Hand sanitizer
- Spatulas
- Closed-lid garbage cans
- Disposable towels
- Rubber mixing bowls
- Small bowls
- Bottled water for quick water changes
- Hand-held mirror

- Makeup sponges for application of masks and makeup
- Facial cape to drape the client
- Cotton swabs
- Trolley or workstation set up with aforementioned products listed.

 CHECK IN

14. How is a facial station or bar different from a treatment room?
15. What treatments are not performed at a facial station or bar?

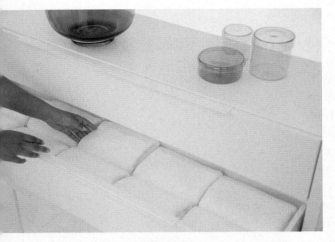

▲ FIGURE 7–19 Have clean laundry and supplies at hand based on your schedule for the day.

—PERFORM—
Procedure 7-1
Pre-Service—Preparing the Treatment Room

ACTIVITY

Perfect Timing

Time yourself to see how fast you can set up the workstation for a facial. See if you can set up from memory after practicing for a while.

Prepare the Treatment Room for Services

Before setting up the room, refer to the setup checklist that the facility uses. Look at your schedule to see what supplies are needed. Remember walk-ins or add on clients can be added at any time. If specified, put the clean laundry away (**Figure 7–19**). Have the client's chart notes ready, and review the product retail consultation forms if applicable. After practicing for a while, you will find that setting up becomes easier. The following guidelines are for a standard facial setup. It takes approximately 10 minutes to set up for a service and 10 to 15 minutes to clean up after a service. A checklist of equipment, supplies, and single-use items are also summarized in Chapter 8, Facial Treatments. Once you have gathered all that you need for treatments, you can start setting up. Perform Procedure 7–1: Pre-Service—Preparing the Treatment Room on page 285.

Setting Out Single-Use Items

Single-use items are kept in clean, covered containers, drawers, or closed cupboards to prevent contamination. After washing your hands, dispense only the amount needed for the service. Use clean forceps or tongs to retrieve additional supplies during a service.

Set out single-use supplies on a clean towel in the order they will be used. Do not put clean or soiled supplies on bare counter surfaces. Contaminated, single-use items must be disposed of properly in a covered waste receptacle.

Arranging the Products

Set out the treatment products in order of the procedure application: cleanser, massage cream or lotion, mask, toner, moisturizer, and other products as determined by the client's skin analysis.

Setting Up the Dressing Area

Set up the dressing room for the client. If possible, it is more efficient to have the client change in a room separate from the treatment room, so that the room can be reset easily between clients. See individual chapters on facial treatments and waxing to review the protocol for each treatment, but the following are general guidelines:

- Arrange a place for the client to sit while changing.

- Have a clean robe or spa wrap hanging on a hook on the door or folded on a small table for the client to change into (**Figure 7–20**).

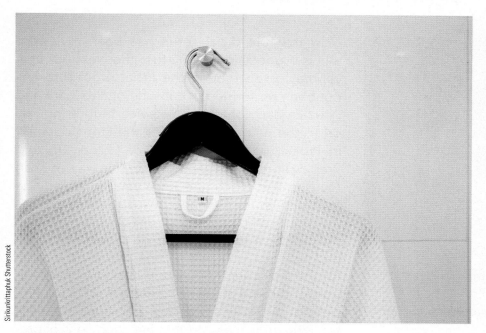

Sirikunkrittaphuk Shutterstock

▲ **FIGURE 7–20** Have a clean robe or spa wrap ready before the client arrives.

- Get water or tea ready for the client, and have a client chart and release form prepared.

- Remember to explain to the client where to put their personal belongings, including jewelry and purse, and how to put on the spa wrap. Never touch the client's jewelry or assist them with the removal of the jewelry.

- Explain to the client how to get onto the table and where to position their head.

- Explain exactly what clothes need to be removed and how to put the gown on. This can vary from treatment to treatment. For a facial bar, no clothing will need to be removed. Some clients have not had a facial or wax service and do not know exactly what they are expected to do.

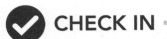
16. What are a few guidelines to follow when setting up single-use supplies?
17. What are a few instructions you will need to provide to your client before the service?

Properly Clean and Disinfect the Treatment Room

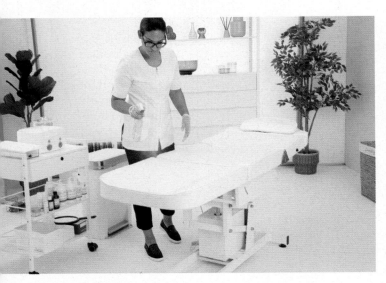

▲ FIGURE 7–21 Practice clean-up procedures to efficiently prepare for the next client.

Now that the facial setup has been reviewed, this is a good time to discuss the clean-up procedures, even though the facial procedure has not been performed yet. It is helpful to learn and practice each phase of a service before moving on to the next step. Practice the steps outlined in Procedure 7–2: Post-Service—Clean-Up and Preparation for the Next Client. This way you can focus on the procedure since you will already be familiar with the pre- and post-service steps.

After completing the post-consultation with the client, be sure to record the client chart notes and write up retail sales. Then prepare the room for the next client, or clean the room in preparation for the end of the day (Figure 7–21). Remember that the order of the clean-up varies with each facility's guidelines and that infection control procedures improve as laws and technology evolve.

---PERFORM---
Procedure 7-2
Post-Service—Clean-Up and Preparation for the Next Client

As discussed in *Milady Standard Foundations* Chapter 5, Infection Control: Principles and Practices, there are two methods of proper infection control:

- Method 1: clean and then disinfect with an appropriate disinfectant

- Method 2: clean and then sterilize

Refresher on Cleaning and Disinfecting Implements

In addition to reviewing *Milady Standard Foundations*, Chapter 5, Infection Control, here are a few other cleaning and disinfection considerations and reminders:

• Wear gloves for all procedures to prevent contamination and protect hands from strong chemicals. Wash hands after completing infection control procedures.

- Wash and disinfect all synthetic brushes, tweezers, and other non-disposables. Implements are multiuse items and include tools such as synthetic brushes, tweezers, and comedone extractors.
- Change the disinfectant to comply with the manufacturer's directions and infection control regulations. If required, record on a dated log when the disinfectant is changed (Table 7–1).

▼ TABLE 7–1 Example of a Disinfectant Log

DISINFECTANT LOG	
Change the disinfectant solution in the container according to the manufacturer's directions or if it is cloudy and seems to require changing. Record when it is changed.	
DATE CHANGED	**YOUR INITIALS**
March 5th	J.S.

- To avoid cross-contamination, roll the used side of linens and sheets inward so the dirty side is inside the laundry bundle. This also helps keep product and hair off the floor and saves cleaning time. For additional cleanliness, do not let linens or other items touch your clothing before or after use.
- Turn off the table warmer if used.
- Clean the wax machine (and turn it off and unplug it at the end of the day).
- Disinfect the steamer and magnifying lamp.
- Disinfect the bottom tray and the inside of the towel warmer after removing all used items.
- Disinfect any other equipment that was used and turn it off.
- Clean all containers and wipe off dirty product containers with a disinfectant.
- Clean all counters, sinks, surfaces, and floor mats with disinfectant.

Appropriate Handling of Single-Use Items

- Soiled items such as gloves and extraction supplies must be placed in a covered waste container.
- While in use, single-use items must be placed on surfaces that can be disinfected or disposed of, such as a paper towel.

CAUTION!
Check with the appropriate regulatory agencies about extraction laws and the disposal of extraction supplies.

- Keep the clean supplies separate from the used ones. Take out only what is needed for each service.
- Disposable extraction lancets go in a sharps disposal container. (Check OSHA and state rules for proper handling.)

End-of-the-Day Clean-Up

In most facilities, estheticians/students are responsible for the cleanliness of the treatment rooms. Estheticians must be prepared to clean up areas they use. Be sure to alert the manager about areas of the facility that may need repair or deep cleaning. Clean-up procedures are regulated by regional laws, so be aware of these regulations. Follow the *End-of-Day Checklist* outlined in Procedure 7–2: Post-Service—Clean-Up and Preparation for the Next Client on page 291.

You now have a good idea about how much work goes into preparing for services. Once you have a good setup and all of the tools needed, it is easy to stay organized and work efficiently. A clean environment is necessary for client safety and to comply with the laws of your local regulatory agencies. Clients will be confident in your ability and feel safe in your hands when they know your facility is clean. Keeping the room organized is necessary for a smooth, efficient operation. Now you are ready to welcome clients. The other chapters will cover facial, waxing, and makeup procedures.

 CHECK IN

18. Explain how to avoid cross-contamination when cleaning up linens and sheets after a service.

Perform Pre- and Post-Service Procedures

It is easier to keep track of what you are doing, remain organized, and give consistent service when you practice setting up. Practice should be applied to a treatment room or station and a supply trolley. Review of proper procedures for cleaning and resetting a room, both for between clients and at the end of the day is also imperative. Following are two practice procedures to master each of these activities: (1) pre-service (preparing the treatment room) and (2) post-service (cleaning up and preparing for the next client). Like an actor rehearsing their lines, repetitive practice will enhance your performance as an esthetician and increase your value as a skin care professional.

Procedure 7-1:
Pre-Service—Preparing the Treatment Room

Check your room supply of linens (towels and sheets) and replenish as needed. For the first appointment of the day, preheat your towel warmer, towels, wax heater, steamer, and any other equipment as needed.

Time Needed: 10–15 minutes

Materials, Implements, and Equipment

(Please note: actual products will vary depending on the client's recommended treatment plan. Additional equipment and supplies to consider is mentioned earlier in the chapter.)

EQUIPMENT
- [ ] Facial equipment (treatment table, stool, towel warmer, steamer, magnifying lamp)
- [ ] Trolley
- [ ] Client charts
- [ ] Close-lid garbage cans

SUPPLIES
- [ ] 2 Twin-size flat bed sheets (backup is needed)
- [ ] EPA-registered disinfectant
- [ ] Hand sanitizer and liquid soap
- [ ] Dish soap
- [ ] Mixing bowls
- [ ] 2 Bowls of warm water (without sink in room)
- [ ] Hand-held mirror
- [ ] Spatula
- [ ] Hand towels (2-4)
- [ ] Linens
- [ ] Bolster
- [ ] Pillows
- [ ] Facial cape to drape the client

SINGLE-USE ITEMS
- [ ] Disposable or synthetic brushes (2)

- [ ] Gloves
- [ ] Esthetics wipes (4" × 4" for cleansing; or disposable sponges)
- [ ] Cotton rounds or squares
- [ ] Cotton swabs
- [ ] Makeup sponges for application of masks and makeup
- [ ] Headband or protective cap
- [ ] Plastic bag
- [ ] Paper towels
- [ ] Spatulas
- [ ] Tissues (unscented)

PRODUCTS
- [ ] Eye makeup remover or cleanser
- [ ] Facial cleanser (one cream and one gel)
- [ ] Masks
- [ ] Moisturizer
- [ ] Serum
- [ ] Astringent/Toner
- [ ] Sunscreen

A. Review the Daily Schedule

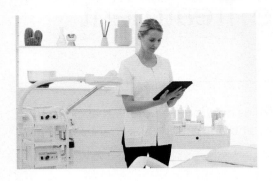

1 Review your client schedule for the day and decide which products you are likely to need for each service. Make sure you have enough of all the products you will be using that day. You may have to retrieve additional product from the dispensary. This is also a good time to refresh your mind about each repeat client you will be seeing that day and their individual concerns.

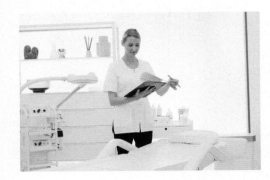

2 Retrieve the client's intake form or service record card and review it. If the appointment is for a new client, the client will need a new intake form.

B. Equipment Preparation

Time Needed: Preheating equipment can take up to 15 minutes.

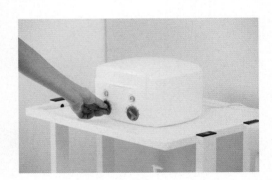

3 Turn on the wax heater as needed. Check and adjust the temperature.

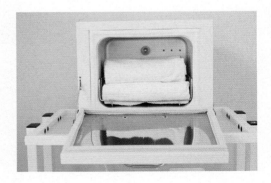

4 Preheat the towel warmer and put in wet towels. Note: Towels should not be dripping wet.

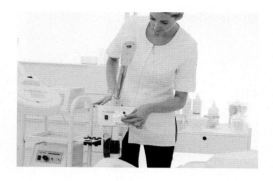

5 Preheat the steamer. First check the steamer water level (it should be just slightly below the fill line). If necessary, refill the steamer. Follow the manufacturer's directions for care. Refer to Chapter 10, Facial Devices and Technology, for steamer information.

6 Preheat any other equipment needed.

C. Prepare the Treatment Table

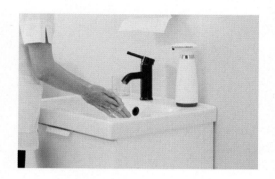

7 Wash your hands with soap and warm water before setting up and touching clean items.

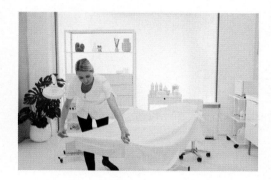

8 Place one sheet lengthwise on the treatment table.

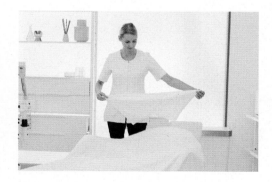

9 Place one hand towel lengthwise on top of the sheet at the head of the table. Lay out another hand towel for placement over the décolleté on the upper chest area if applicable.

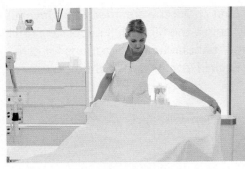

10 Place the second sheet lengthwise on top of the first.

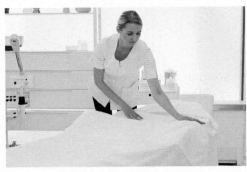

11 Fold the top one-quarter of the second sheet back horizontally. Then fold the sheet diagonally across the table.

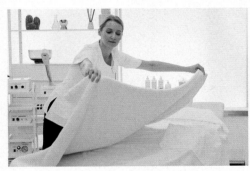

12 Place a blanket on top of the linens to keep the client warm and comfortable.

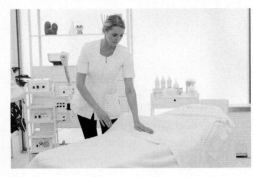

13 Have a clean headband and gown or wrap ready for the client.

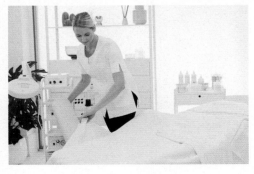

14 Have a bolster and pillow available.

D. Setting Up Supplies

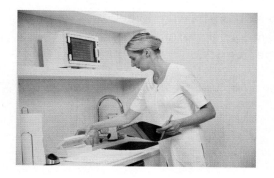

15 Check to make sure the disinfectant is ready. Wet disinfectants are filled and changed according to the manufacturer's instructions (check to see that the strength is maintained by regular refilling).

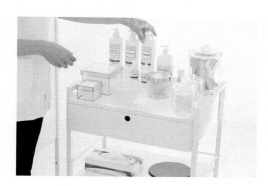

16 Place supplies on a clean towel (paper or cloth) on the clean and disinfected workstation. Put out supplies in the order used, line up neatly, and if any supplies or products are uncovered, cover with another towel until you are ready to use them.

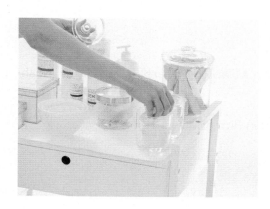

17 Set up the professional trolley with supplies and disposables. See the list of materials needed and the visual for reference.

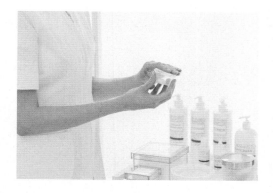

18 Dispense only the amount of product needed for the service.

E. Setting Up the Dressing Area

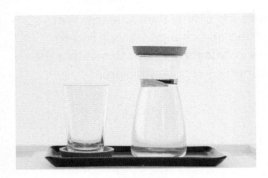

19 Arrange a clean robe or spa wrap folded on a small table for the client to change into. (*Note:* for a facial bar, clothing is not removed.)

20 Have cold water or tea water ready for the client.

F. Preparing for the Client

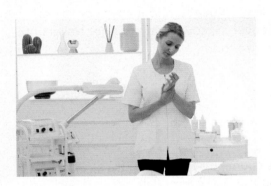

21 Organize yourself by taking care of your personal needs before the client arrives— stretch, use the restroom, get a drink of water, return personal calls— so you can focus your full attention on their needs. Remember to turn off electronic devices to eliminate any distractions. Take a moment to clear your head of all your personal concerns and issues.

22 Referencing Procedure 5–3: Proper Hand Washing located in *Milady Standard Foundations*, wash your hands before going to greet your client.

23 Your client has arrived! Proceed to follow the steps outlined in Procedure 8–1: Pre-Service: Prepare the Client for Treatment.

Procedure 7-2:
Post-Service—Clean-Up and Preparation for the Next Client

Time Needed: 10–15 minutes

A. End-of-Service Checklist

At the end of the service, the esthetician must clean the treatment room and ready it for the next client.

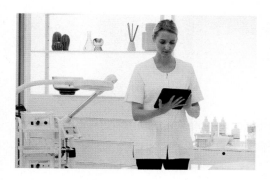

1 Create an end of service checklist that works for your space. Not everyone will complete the post-service steps in the same order.

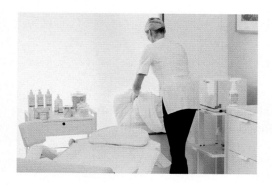

2 Place all soiled laundry linens (towels and sheets) in a covered receptacle.

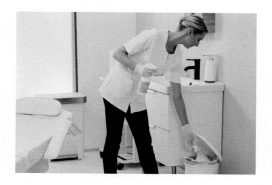

3 Discard any used disposables into a covered trash container.

4 Disposable extraction lancets go in a sharps disposal container. (Check OSHA and state rules for proper handling.)

DID YOU KNOW?

Do not put wet brushes in a closed drawer or container because moisture may cause mildew and not dry properly. Lay brushes out to dry, covered with a clean towel before storing in a closed container.

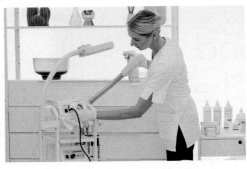

5 Wipe down all equipment with an EPA-approved disinfectant.

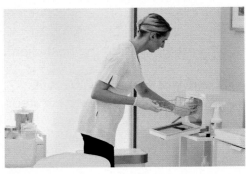

6 Clean trolley and workstation surfaces. Clean and disinfect the bottom tray and the inside of the towel warmer after removing all used items.

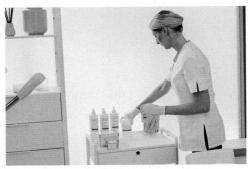

7 Reset products and disposable items and replenish clean robes and spa wraps.

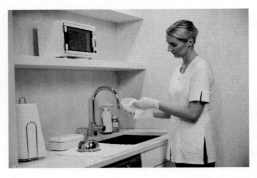

8 Use an antibacterial dish soap and warm water to wash the used bowl(s). Rinse and dry thoroughly.

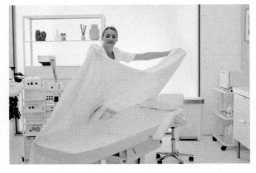

9 Change linen on the treatment table.

B. End-of-Day Checklist

At the end of the day, be sure to follow these procedures:

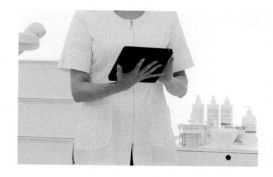

1 Complete the end of service checklist and check the schedule for the next shift or workday.

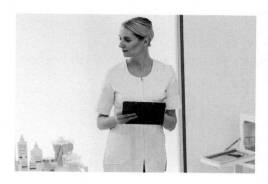

2 Use an end-of-day checklist to make sure you do not forget anything.

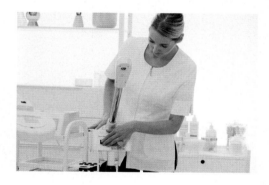

3 Turn off and unplug all equipment.

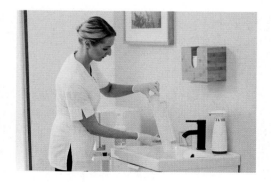

4 Leave the towel-warmer door open to dry and empty the tray underneath before cleaning and disinfecting it.

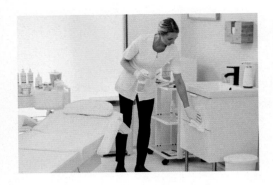

5 Clean anything that has not been cleaned after the last service, including the equipment, table, sink, counters, and doorknobs.

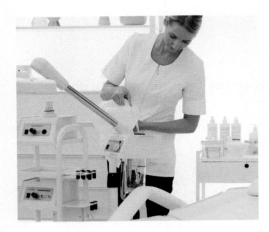

6 Refill all containers, supplies, and the steamer.

7 Check floors; sweep or mop as required. Check for wax spills.

8 Empty waste containers. Replace with clean trash liners.

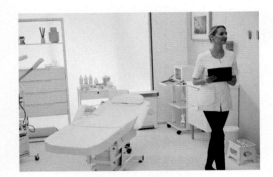

9 Remove personal items from the area.

How are you doing with the treatment room? **Check the Chapter 7 Learning Objectives below that you feel you have mastered; leave unchecked those objectives you will need to return to.**

☐ Explain why treatment room preparation is an integral part of providing treatments.

☐ Review the elements of an esthetician's professional appearance.

☐ Outline essential room and station structural features.

☐ Describe the ideal ambience, furniture, and equipment for facials.

☐ Properly manage treatment room supplies and products.

☐ Be able to set up a facial treatment area, such as a facial bar or station.

☐ Prepare the treatment room for services.

☐ Properly clean and disinfect the treatment room.

☐ Perform pre- and post-service procedures to meet safety and health requirements.

GLOSSARY

dispensary dis-PEN-suh-ree	p. 276	room or area used for mixing products and storing supplies
facial station FAY-shul STAY-shun	p. 279	also known as *facial bar*; skin care treatment area within the reception or retail area of the facility, where clients can have express skin care treatments without having to change clothes
implements IM-pluh-mentz	p. 276	tools used by estheticians to perform services; implements can be multiuse or single-use
trolley TROL-ee	p. 270	a rolling cart that holds tools, supplies, and products

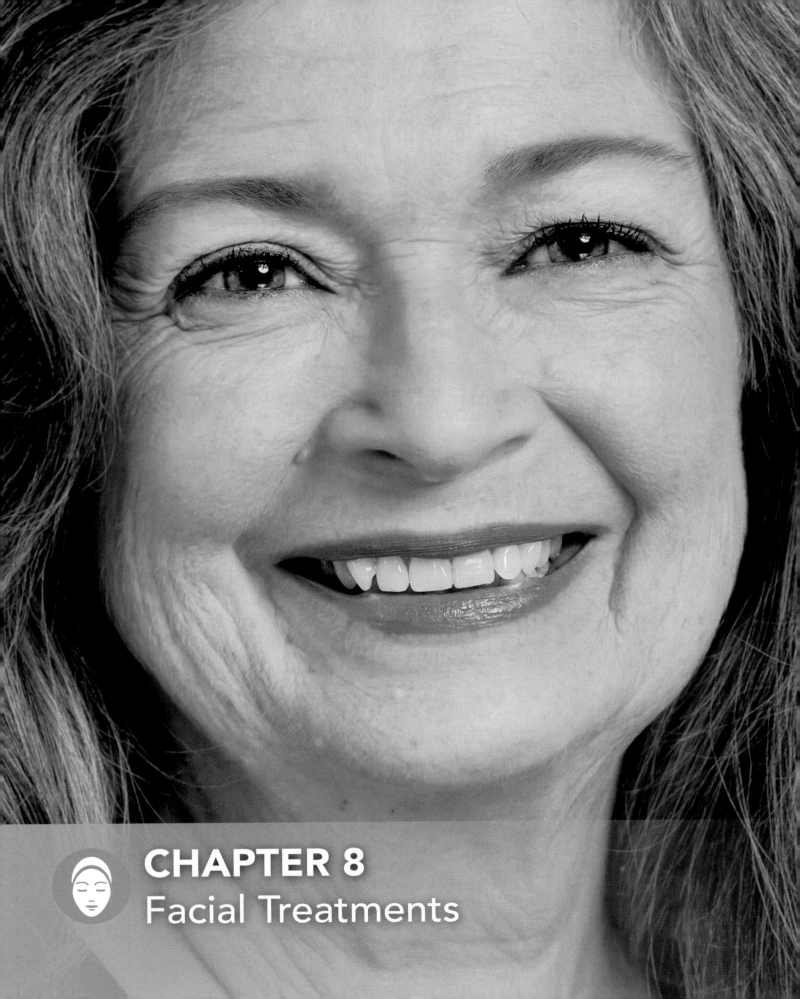

CHAPTER 8
Facial Treatments

"Knowing how to age and not being afraid of aging is very healthy."

– Evelyn Lauder (founder of Clinique)

Learning Objectives

After completing this chapter, you will be able to:

1. Explain the importance of facial treatments as the foundation for all skin care services.
2. Describe the benefits of a facial treatment.
3. List the essential skills needed to successfully perform facials.
4. Perform the facial setup procedures.
5. Explain the key steps of the basic facial treatment.
6. Describe how to consult clients on home care.
7. Discuss variations of the basic facial.
8. Outline the treatment goals for six skin types/conditions (dry, dehydrated, mature, sensitive, hyperpigmentation and oily skin).
9. Describe acne facials.
10. Perform an acne treatment procedure.
11. Discuss men's skin care treatment options.
12. Perform the facial treatment procedures.

Explain the Importance of Facial Treatments

Once considered luxuries, regular facials and skin care maintenance are now regarded as necessities by many for skin heath as well as stress reduction. The skin care field has advanced rapidly in recent years due to the growing interest in health, wellness, and beauty as well as advances in results-driven technology, including advanced treatments, light therapy, and laser technology. Facials offer two benefits at the same time: regular treatments result in noticeable improvements in the skin's texture and appearance while offering a relaxing experience (**Figure 8–1**).

Facial treatments are the core introductory treatments that estheticians perform that lead to other more advanced

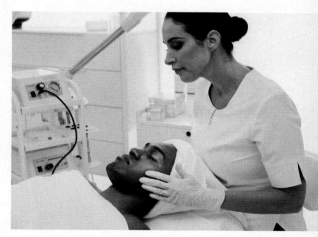

▲ **FIGURE 8–1** Facials offer improvements to the skin and relaxation.

and results-oriented services, which in turn result in repeat appointments and the building of a solid client base.

The basic facial treatment procedure is covered here; however, there are many different types of facials and methods. Once you master the basic routine you can implement new steps and changes in the routine can be based on the client's individual skin needs. The specific steps, products, focus of treatments, and massage methods can all be varied depending on the client's skin concerns.

Estheticians should study and have a thorough understanding of facial treatments because:

- This is a foundational skill for all skin care services. You must be able to provide services that are safe and beneficial for your clients.
- Providing education and consultations on how the skin works, along with the effects of environmental, dietary, aging, and lifestyle choices, are parts of a facial that establish a partnership between the client and the esthetician.
- Facial treatments focus on creating an ongoing program to help reduce the appearance of skin concerns such as oiliness or fine lines and wrinkles, while also engaging the client in a daily maintenance program with long-term benefits to achieve well-balanced skin throughout their life.

Describe the Benefits of a Facial Treatment

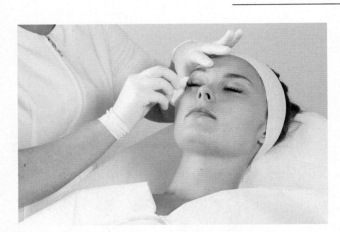

▲ FIGURE 8–2 Cleansing the skin is an important step in the facial treatment.

You were probably attracted to esthetics because you wanted a rewarding and successful career while helping others look and feel their best. After a facial, clients feel rejuvenated when they walk out of your salon or spa.

A facial (FAY-shul) is a professional service designed to improve the appearance of the facial skin (Figure 8–2). This typically includes deep cleansing such as extractions, hydration, massage, mask application or mild peels, possible use of skin treatment machines, and finally the application of serums, moisturizer, and sunscreen.

Facials should be customized for each individual client by choosing the correct products and ensuring the protocol steps implemented are appropriate for that client. A thorough pretreatment skin analysis will provide information on what protocols to use based on the client's individual skin type and concerns.

Facial Treatment Benefits

A skin treatment has many benefits. The market will continue to expand as more people discover these benefits. Having in-depth knowledge of the key elements and benefits of facials gives you the skills and confidence that truly make a difference in treating the client's skin. This also helps you communicate those benefits to your clients—providing education and consultations is also part of a facial.

Facial treatments include the following benefits:

- Deep cleanses
- Exfoliates
- Increases circulation and detoxifies
- Relaxes the senses, nerves, and muscles
- Slows down symptoms of premature aging
- Addresses conditions such as dryness, oiliness, and redness
- Softens the appearance of wrinkles and aging lines
- Helps lessen the appearance of blemishes and minor acne
- Provides access to an esthetician's expertise for at-home skin care maintenance
- Supports skin health and making good lifestyle choices.

 CHECK IN

1. What is a facial treatment?
2. Name six benefits of a facial.
3. As an esthetician, what primary activity can you not perform?

CAUTION!

It is important to know what a facial *cannot* do. An esthetician *cannot* diagnose or treat medical conditions such as rosacea or cystic acne. Facial treatments in conjunction with proper medical care provide a holistic approach to proper skin maintenance.

List the Essential Skills Needed to Successfully Perform Facials

In order to become a successful esthetician, you must master certain skills as well as exemplify certain essential qualities that make a great esthetician—one that is qualified and professional. The following skills are essential to be successful at providing facials. Some of these skills may seem to come more naturally to you, but as you get more experienced, you will improve in all these areas. Pay attention to little details that make the client comfortable. Educated, well-trained estheticians will find many growth-promoting opportunities throughout their careers.

Impeccable Customer Service and Proper Communication Skills

Client-relation skills are an important element of being an esthetician. Knowing how to connect and communicate effectively with clients will determine the success of an esthetician.

Exceptional Skills

Knowledge of skin histology, skin analysis, and skin care products is essential for an esthetician to make informed decisions for the client (**Figure 8–3**). Additionally, knowledge of contraindications, technological advances, and facial equipment is important for the safety of your client. Massage techniques and your touch, pressure, and flow in the facial are valuable parts of your skills.

Mastering Retail Sales Techniques

Retailing and client consultations are another part of the job that requires proper training.

Ongoing Education

Ongoing education on technological advances and facial equipment is important.

- Take classes at a skin care academy or participate in an online webinar on skin care education.
- Stay informed. Subscribe to online news resources to learn about current events; watch interesting, informative television; and read books on a bestseller list.
- Make a commitment to yourself to attend at least one esthetics class or conference every year—this will make a difference in your potential career success.
- Getting degrees at the associate, bachelor, master, and even doctorate levels offers additional options for continuing education.

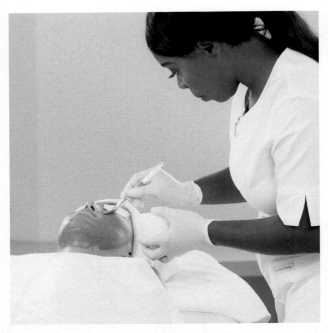

▲ **FIGURE 8–3** A knowledge of skin care products will help you treat your client.

FOCUS ON

Continuing Education

Continuing your education with advanced classes and attendance at conferences and trade shows will keep you informed, excited, and motivated as well as up-to-date on the latest skin care science, knowledge, and techniques. One idea is earning a CIDESCO (Comité International d'Esthétique et de Cosmétologie) diploma. CIDESCO is the world's most prestigious qualification for Aesthetics and Beauty Therapy, and has set international standards since 1957. CIDESCO Section USA provides comprehensive training at national trade shows throughout the year. For information on CIDESCO classes and programs, go to http://cidesco.com/.

Key Elements of Client Interaction

The first step toward a professional approach is your skill in client interaction. This is perhaps the most important aspect of the job. To be successful and to maintain client loyalty, you must know the key factors to a successful client interaction. For the client consultation, these include the following.

FOCUS ON THE CLIENT

- Be genuine in your concern for your client and focus on their needs.
- Give the client your full attention at all times.
- Ask the client what their skin concerns are. Listen carefully before you respond.

CLIENT COMFORT

- Help the client to relax by speaking in a quiet and professional manner.
- Provide a professional atmosphere and work efficiently.
- Make sure the client is comfortable (**Figure 8–4**). Proper treatment tables and chairs are important.
- Always wear disposable gloves.
- Keep your nails smooth and short to avoid scratching the client's skin.
- Remove rings, bracelets, and other jewelry that may injure the client, get in the way, or cause a distraction during the treatment.
- Be aware of your touch and the amount of pressure you apply to the face.

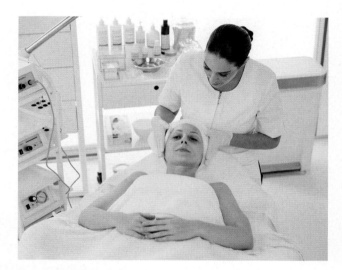

▲ **FIGURE 8–4** Make sure your clients are comfortable.

INFORM THE CLIENT

- Provide a skin analysis and educational consultation.
- Explain the benefits of the products and service you offer, and answer any questions the client may have.

BE DILIGENT, ORGANIZED, AND SKILLFUL

- Maintain neat and clean conditions in the facial work area.
- Arrange supplies in an orderly fashion.
- Keep implements in a closed container when not in use.
- Follow systematic procedures.
- Measure or use premeasured products for consistency and best results.
- Apply and remove products neatly, and avoid getting them in the eyes, mouth, and nostrils.
- Do not let water or products drip down the client's neck or in the eyes or ears.

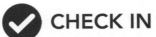 CHECK IN

4. List four essential skills an esthetician needs to master to create and maintain professional success.
5. State five key guidelines to a successful client interaction.

Perform the Facial Setup Procedures

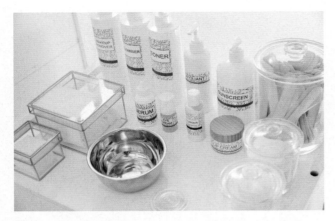

▲ FIGURE 8–5 Have all supplies on hand before the start of the treatment.

Please refer to Chapter 7, The Treatment Room, for room setup and prepare all the supplies needed for a facial treatment. It is important to assemble supplies in an organized, efficient manner and have them on hand before beginning the treatment (**Figure 8–5**).

Use the following resources to prepare for client treatments:

- Review the contraindication information in Chapter 5, Skin Analysis.
- Use the client charts and consultation information in Chapter 5, Skin Analysis.

Meeting and Greeting Clients

One of the most important communications you will have with a client occurs the first time you meet (**Figure 8–6**). Be polite, friendly, and inviting. To develop long-term relationships, you need to give great service every time clients come to see you. The following are essential customer service practices you must perform every time you provide a facial service:

- Always approach a client with a smile.
- Always introduce yourself to new clients and greet returning clients by name. A brief yet warm handshake will make the client feel welcome.
- Set aside a few minutes to take new clients on a quick tour of the facility. This helps clients to feel comfortable and at home.
- Your client is paying for your service; therefore, it is common courtesy to devote the time you are with your client to your client and their needs, not yours. Refrain from discussing your own problems or allowing your mood to intrude on the service. If your difficulties must be dealt with personally, you must reschedule the client rather than risk lessening the value of their treatment.
- Be professional yet genuine. Your clients can sense when you are being genuine and open, and they will have more confidence in you and in your expertise. Your number one objective is to find out and address their skin concerns.

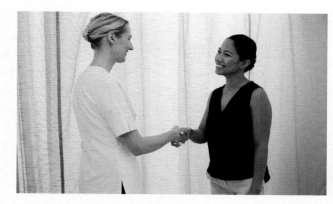

▲ FIGURE 8–6 Be polite, friendly, and inviting while greeting a client.

ACTIVITY

Customer Service

Think of a time when you were treated well as a client and how it made you feel.

Prepare the Client for the Facial Treatment

After warmly greeting the client, assist them in preparing for the facial (**Figure 8–7**).

CHANGING INSTRUCTIONS

The receptionist or esthetician will show the client where to change and store any belongings.

- Clients can change into their robe and/or spa wrap and remove their shoes in a changing room or the treatment room.
- Explain what clothing can be removed: shoes, restrictive pants, and bras.
- Let the client know the neck and shoulders are usually bare for facials.
- Dark fabric will collect lint from sheets, so it is best to remove clothing that will be under the sheets. Let clients decide what clothing they are comfortable removing.
- Instruct the client on how to prepare for the treatment and how to put on the facial wrap. There are many styles of wraps or gowns.

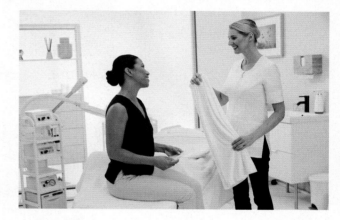

▲ FIGURE 8–7 Assist your client in preparing for the facial.

ASSIST THE CLIENT ONTO THE FACIAL TABLE

- Show the client how to get on the facial table safely and where to position the head.
- Assist the client in getting comfortable.

PERFORM

Procedure 8-1

Pre-Service—Preparing the
Client for Treatment

DRAPE AND ADJUST FOR COMFORT

You will then proceed with draping the client's hair and adjusting the pillow, bolster, and linens (**Figure 8–8**). Detailed instructions on how to drape the client are in Procedure 8–1: Pre-Service—Preparing the Client for Treatment. A client should feel relaxed from the very beginning of the treatment.

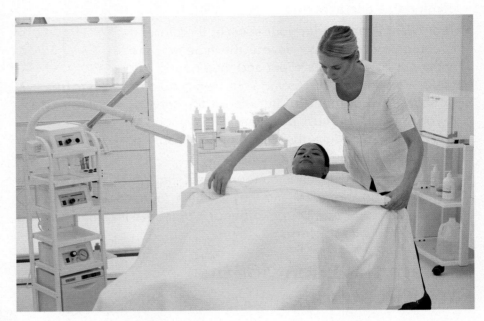

▲ **FIGURE 8–8** Drape your client.

 CHECK IN

6. What are the five essential service practices when greeting clients?
7. What pretreatment activities can an esthetician do to assist the client in preparing for the treatment?
8. What four practices help keep the client and the esthetician on schedule?

Explain The Key Steps of the Basic Facial Treatment

At this point, you've learned how to set up the treatment room, meet and greet the client, and position the client comfortably on the treatment table or chair. You are now ready to familiarize yourself with the remainder of the steps of the facial process before having to perform the procedure at the end of the chapter.

As you practice facials, follow the chart in **Figure 8–9** to memorize the steps. Adapt this basic procedure to fit your local facility and regulations. In general, most basic facials take approximately an hour. Refer to **Table 8–1** on page 306 for timing suggestions. Remember that you are required to wear gloves at all times throughout the facial treatment procedure.

For teaching purposes, the basic facial procedure is divided into the following major steps. (Be guided by your instructor. *Note:* Some facial devices have been added to show you where equipment can be introduced into the basic facial.)

1. Client consultation, including review of contraindications
   - Discussion of the completed client intake form
   - Client signing of consent form; this form must be signed before each treatment
2. Client draping and esthetician hand washing
3. Initial skin analysis and continue the client consultation; treatment plan creation
4. Warm towels (optional) and facial cleansing with appropriate cleanser and toner
5. In-depth skin analysis (refer to Chapter 5, Skin Analysis, and **Table 8–2**)
6. Exfoliation procedure (optional)

*Facial device option: high frequency over gauze (if applicable)

7. Massage (massage and mask steps can be reversed)
8. Softening with steam or warm towels (can also steam performing facial massage or during exfoliation)
9. Extractions and/or deep pore cleansing (if applicable)
10. Mask (clay, hydrating, or any mask type that is appropriate to client's skin type and condition)

*Facial device option: application of galvanic gel and performance of galvanic treatment (if applicable)

11. Toner
12. Serums, eye treatments, and lip treatments
13. Moisturizer
14. Daily sun protection products
15. Service completion, including postconsultation and home care

▲ **FIGURE 8–9** The Facial Procedure At a Glance

▼ **TABLE 8–1 Timing the Facial Procedure**

	Suggested Time (in minutes)	Acne Facial	Express Facial
Setup time (client dresses)	5	5	5
Consultation	3–5	3–5	Brief
Draping	2	2	2
Towels (optional)	2	2	2
Cleansing	3–5	3–5	3–5
Skin analysis	5	5	Brief
Exfoliation	8–10	5	8–10
Steam or towels	5	5	5
Extractions	10	10	Skip
Massage	10	Skip or brief	Skip or brief
Mask	8–10	8–10	Brief
Toner	1	1	1
Moisturizer	1	1	1
Postconsultation	5	5	5
Total time	**~60**	**~50**	**30**

Note: There are many variations to these basic guidelines. Add 30 minutes for cleanup/setup time.

The Initial Consultation and Analysis

The initial consultation and skin analysis determines the products and procedures to be used and gives you time to discuss your recommended treatment as well as begin to discuss the client's home care needs. Many estheticians schedule at least 15 minutes extra for a client's first visit.

Review the client's completed initial consultation form (Figure 5–11 in Chapter 5, Skin Analysis, shows a sample intake form). Information should include important details about the client, including their name, age (optional), occupation, information on their at-home skin care program, medications, medical conditions, diet, and lifestyle habits (**Figure 8–10**).

OBTAIN SIGNED CONSENT
The client will read and sign the consent form, acknowledging that they understand what is being done to them as well as the risks involved in the treatment. Figure 5–12 in Chapter 5, Skin Analysis, shows a sample consent form.

▼ **FIGURE 8–10** Client Intake Forms

Client Intake Form and Medical History

In order to provide you with the most appropriate treatment, we need you to complete the following questionnaire. All information is confidential.

Date ______________________________

Name ______________________________ **Date of birth** *(optional)* ______________

(please print)

Email address ______________________________

Address ______________ ______________ ______________ ______________

Street City State Zip

Phone number (easiest number to reach you) ______________________________

Occupation ______________________________

How were you referred to us? ______________________________

____

Medical History

Are you currently under the care of a physician for any reason? ______________ ☐ Yes ☐ No

If yes, for what? ______________________________

History	Yes	No	Date/List/Comments
List all medications, supplements, and vitamins			
List allergies			
Accutane			
Antibiotics			
Birth control pills			
Hormones			
Aspirin, ibuprofen use			
Retin-A®, Tretinoin			
Metrogel®, MetroCream®			
Glycolic acid on a regular basis			
Antidepressants			
Sun reactions			
Medication allergies			
Food allergies			
Aspirin allergy			
Latex allergy			
Lidocaine allergy			
Hydrocortisone allergy			

(Continued)

(Continued)

History	Yes	No	Date/List/Comments
Diabetes			
Smoking history			
Cold sores, herpes			
Bleeding disorders			
Autoimmune, HIV			
Pregnant or planning to be			
Pacemaker			
Implants of any kind: Dental, breast, facial			
Migraine headaches			
Glaucoma			
Cancer			
Arthritis			
Hepatitis			
Thyroid imbalance			
Seizure disorder			
Active infection			
Radiation in last three months			
Skin Conditions			
Acne			
Melasma			
Tattoos, perm makeup, and microblading			
Vitiligo			
Keloid scarring			
Skin/laser treatments at another office		If so, when?	Results
Botox		If so, when?	Results
Fillers		If so, when?	Results
Hair removal		If so, when?	Results
Chemical peels		If so, when?	Results
Sun exposure/tanning bed in last week? Self tanner?		If so, when?	Results
List Medical Issues Not Listed Above			

(Continued)

(Continued)

Current Skin Care and Lifestyle

1. How do you wash your face? ☐ Soap   ☐ Cleanser
2. If soap, what brand? _____
3. If cleanser, what brand name? _____
4. Do you use a moisturizer? ☐ Yes ☐ No
5. Are you on a special diet? ☐ Yes ☐ No
   If yes, please specify. _____
6. Do you consume water daily? ☐ Yes ☐ No
   If yes, how much? _____
7. Do you drink coffee, tea, or soda daily? ☐ Yes ☐ No
   Coffee ounces ___ Tea ounces ___ Soda ounces ___
8. Do you exercise? ☐ Yes ☐ No
   If yes, how often? _____
9. Have you ever had a facial? ☐ Yes ☐ No
   If yes, when was your last facial? _____
10. Do you give yourself facials at home? ☐ Yes ☐ No
    If yes, how often? _____
11. List additional cosmetics and skin care products you are currently using:

What is the primary reason for your visit today? (Select all that apply in the list below.)
☐ I'm concerned about facial or body hair and would like information on ways to get rid of it.
☐ I'm concerned about fine lines around my eyes.
☐ I'm concerned about scowl lines when I frown.
☐ I'm concerned about pigmentation or age spots.
☐ I'm concerned about broken capillaries on my face or spider veins on my legs.
☐ I'm concerned about skin laxity and sagging.
☐ I'm concerned about the lines around my mouth.
☐ I'd like more defined lips.
☐ Other (please list skin concerns below)

I certify that the preceding medical, personal, and skin history statements are true and correct. I am aware that it is my responsibility to inform the technician of my current medical and health conditions and to update this information at subsequent visits. A current history is essential for the provider to execute appropriate treatment procedures. I have signed the consent form for this procedure. I had the opportunity to ask questions prior to the treatment. I accept arbitration as a means of resolution for practice liability.

_____

Client Signature   Date

Proper Client Draping and Hand Washing

Drape the client properly by adjusting the head drape, pillow, and linens following your instructor's method. Place a towel across the client's chest and a cover over the body as directed. Drape the hair with a towel or headband as necessary. Check to make sure the headband is not too tight and that all of the hair is covered. A bolster placed under the knees (supports the back) and a pillow can be used for the client's comfort as needed. Be sure to follow the protocol outlined in Procedure 8–1: Pre-Service—Preparing the Client for Treatment to ensure proper draping of the client. The proper draping of the client is very important. Wash your hands before analyzing the client's skin (**Figure 8–11**).

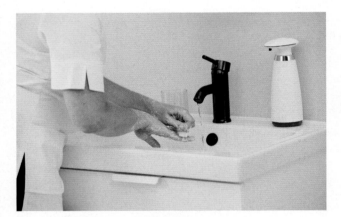

▲ **FIGURE 8–11** Wash your skin before the skin analysis.

PERFORM AN INITIAL SKIN ANALYSIS AND AGREE ON A TREATMENT PLAN

Before cleansing, inspect the skin type and conditions: Is it dry, normal, or oily? Is the skin texture smooth or rough? Are there fine lines or creases? Are there blackheads or acne conditions? Are dilated capillaries visible? Is the skin color even?

You want to see the skin's natural state before cleansing and then again after cleansing, especially if the client is wearing makeup (**Figure 8–12**). Ask the client what their skin concerns are. Listen carefully before you respond. Help the client to relax by speaking in a quiet and professional manner.

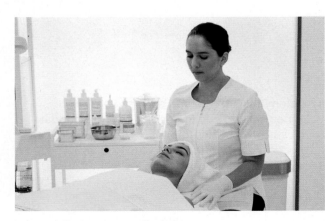

▲ **FIGURE 8–12** Before cleansing, inspect your client's skin.

CREATE A TREATMENT PLAN

Once you have familiarized yourself with the client's skin and their concerns, you need to formulate a clear and precise plan of action. Create a treatment plan to show your client that you are educated and prepared to treat the concerns they may have. Explain the benefits of the products and service you offer and answer any questions the client may have. **Figure 8–13** is a sample plan to develop the treatment you will implement for the client.

Steps	Procedures
Cleansing	☐ Cream ☐ Liquid ☐ Mousse ☐ Gel ☐ Steam hot or cold
Exfoliation	☐ AHA ☐ BHA ☐ Enzymes ☐ Microdermabrasion ☐ Rotary brush
Advanced Protocols	☐ Galvanic ☐ High frequency ☐ Microcurrent
Massage	☐ Oil ☐ Cream ☐ Gel ☐ Serum
Mask(s)	☐ Sheet ☐ Cream ☐ Mud/Clay ☐ Alginate ☐ Mineral

Complete the Facial Cleansing with Appropriate Cleanser and Toner

After the initial dry skin analysis, some estheticians prefer to apply warm towels for a few minutes. Warm towels can be used before cleansing to prepare the client for your touch, to warm and moisten the skin, and to make cleansing more effective and enjoyable.

Always wash your hands before starting any treatment and put on gloves. Cleanse to remove impurities and makeup before the in-depth skin analysis and facial treatment (**Figure 8–14**). Proper cleansing is imperative to the success of your facial treatment, because not all skin types and concerns are the same. There are many different cleansing formulas from rich, creamy cleansers to lightweight foaming cleansers. Based on the skin analysis, choose a cleanser based on the client's skin type and concerns.

- Cream-based cleansers are for dry to more mature skin types.
- Mousse is for combination skin, and gels and liquids are for oilier skin types.

REMOVE EYE AND LIP MAKEUP

Before starting the cleansing procedure, the client's eye and lip color can be removed (**Figure 8–15**). Make sure the client is not wearing contacts. If they wear contacts, they will need to remove them before receiving the treatment. Do not use too much cleanser because it can run into the eyes. Some clients prefer to leave on their eye makeup, which typically is appropriate only if the client is having an express treatment. For a full facial, all makeup should be removed. Clients may have the opportunity to have their makeup reapplied following the full facial if this is a service you offer for an upcharge.

> **CAUTION!**
> If any product gets into the eyes, rinse and flush the eyes immediately with water and cotton. Then resume the procedure.

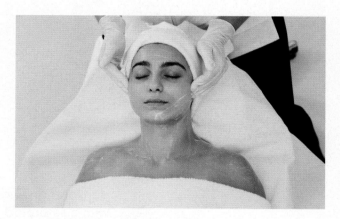

▲ FIGURE 8–14 Cleanse the skin to remove any impurities and makeup.

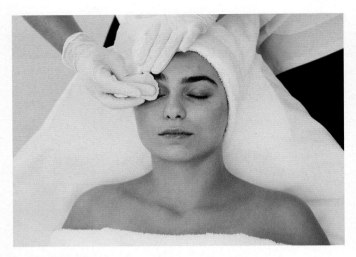

▲ **FIGURE 8–15** Remove eye and lip makeup.

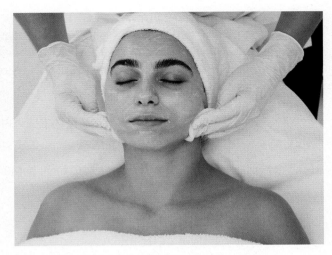

▲ **FIGURE 8–16** Complete the skin cleansing.

CLEANSING

Avoid over-rubbing or overstimulating the skin and thoroughly, but efficiently, complete the cleansing (**Figure 8–16**). If there is makeup residue, do a double cleansing—once before using the towels and once after.

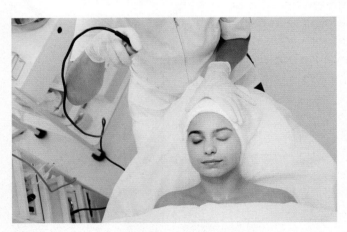

▲ **FIGURE 8–17** Toner can be misted on to the face.

TONERS

Some estheticians use a toner between facial steps to remove any makeup or product residue. Most facial products can be applied with fingertips and removed with esthetics wipes or sponges.

Toners, tonics, and astringents are all referred to as toners for simplicity in this text. Toners finish the cleansing process by removing any residue from the cleanser left on the skin and help restore the skin's pH balance. Astringent formulas can help reduce the appearance of the pores, while toners and tonics can help remove excess cleanser while helping to tone the appearance of the skin. Different formulas can also help skin problems such as dehydration and acne. Toners can be misted onto the face or applied with a saturated cotton pad (**Figure 8–17**).

┌─ PERFORM ─┐
Procedure 8-2
Remove Eye Makeup
and Lipstick

Procedure 8-3
Applying a Cleansing Product

Procedure 8-4
Removing Products

In-Depth Skin Analysis

Analyze the skin after cleansing. Accurate skin analysis is the most crucial step in recommending the most effective professional treatments possible. The examination should be conducted with careful concentration. Complete a thorough analysis with a magnifying lamp, a Wood's lamp, or an electronic imaging system after cleansing (**Figure 8–18**). You should be prepared to recognize and treat any combination of skin conditions.

Check for any other conditions or contraindications prohibiting a facial. A full list of Contraindications for Skin Treatments can be found in Chapter 5, Skin Analysis, on page 178. If you are ever unsure, wait and have the patient obtain clearance from their physician for facial treatments.

As you learned in Chapter 5, Skin Analysis, the four components of skin analysis are look, touch, ask, and listen, and then record your findings (Table 8–2).

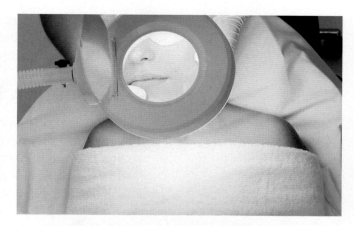
▲ FIGURE 8–18 An accurate skin analysis is crucial.

▼ TABLE 8–2 Skin Analysis Checklist: Look, Touch, Ask, Listen

Analyze the skin using a magnifying lamp. Place eye pads on the eyes. Try not to cover what you need to look at around the eyes. Perform the steps in the following checklist.
☐ Look for any obvious skin conditions and note the skin type.
☐ Touch the skin, noting its elasticity, softness, texture, and skin condition.
☐ Continue the consultation, asking questions while analyzing. Analyze the pore size, hydration level, pigmentation, muscle tone, broken capillaries, facial wrinkles, signs of skin disorders, and so on.
☐ Choose the products.
☐ Note the information on the client's chart (this can be done before, during, or after the facial).

CLIENT CHARTS

During the skin analysis, it is necessary to keep the client's chart on hand to write down any information or changes that have occurred in the client's skin, even if the client is a regular and you are familiar with their skin (**Figure 8–19**). It is very important to keep track of any changes. The client's chart should be filled out and used as a reference each time the client returns. Keep an ongoing file for your client just as a doctor does. All procedures and products used during the consultation or treatment should be recorded for future reference. All products purchased for at-home use should be noted in the client's electronic file or service record card as well.

The esthetician must train their sight and touch to know what to look for during skin analysis. Review the questions to ask during the consultation (see Chapter 5, Skin Analysis, on pages 186–187).

Note: Be sure to ask about the use of Retin-A® and glycolic acid because the skin is more sensitive when such products are used. You may have to avoid mechanical exfoliation,

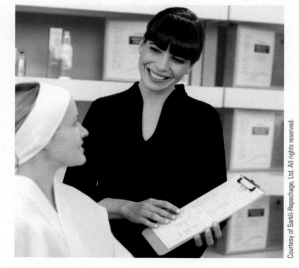

▲ FIGURE 8–19 Use your client chart as a reference.

brushing machines, or chemical peels such as alpha hydroxy acid (AHA) with a pH lower than 4.2, and use only products that are pH balanced and designed to soothe the skin.

Exfoliation Product or Mask

Exfoliation can be achieved by using products such as AHA, BHA, manual scrubs, or enzyme peels, or you can use the brush machine to remove dead skin cells that make the skin feel rough and clog the follicles. Exfoliation makes the skin smoother, helps product penetration by unblocking the surface, and promotes stimulation, which increases the cell turnover rate.

Exfoliation methods include mechanical exfoliants, chemical exfoliants, and electrotherapy. Exfoliation products are discussed in Chapter 6, Skin Care Products: Chemistry, Ingredients, and Selection, and in Chapter 10, Facial Devices and Technology. Here is a quick reminder on types of exfoliation:

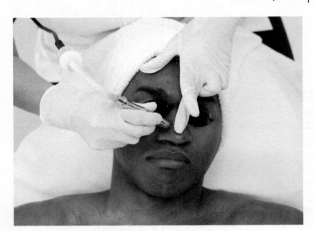

▲ **FIGURE 8–20** Microdermabrasion is an example of mechanical exfoliation.

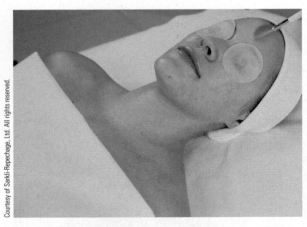

▲ **FIGURE 8–21** Chemical exfoliants can be used to lessen the appearance of wrinkles.

- *Mechanical exfoliation* is the use of the rotary brush or microdermabrasion. When applied to the skin, this will gently remove dead skin cells and aid in a deeper cleansing (**Figure 8–20**). *Granular or manual* exfoliation is the use of a granular product, such as honey and jojoba beads or rice bran wax, to help remove the dead skin and debris by manipulation with the fingertips.

- *Chemical exfoliation* such as an enzyme and alpha hydroxy acids (AHA), beta hydroxy acids (BHA), azelaic acid, or kojic acid can be chosen based on the level of accumulation of dead skin cells and skin sensitivity (**Figure 8–21**). Desincrustation solution can be applied to loosen sebum accumulations in the hair follicles, making extractions easier. The solution softens the sebaceous material (oil, dirt, debris) around the edges of the pores or follicle openings. Desincrustation with a galvanic machine is discussed in Chapter 10, Facial Devices and Technology.

Chemical exfoliants are used to lessen the appearance of wrinkles and skin discoloration. Always apply sun protection with SPF 30 after any chemical exfoliation procedure, and educate your client on post-treatment. Clients must wear SPF 30 sunscreen every day following usage of AHA.

DESINCRUSTATION WITH A GALVANIC MACHINE

Use desincrustation solution or a mask if performing extractions. *Desincrustation* (dis-in-krus-TAY-shun) is the process used to soften and emulsify sebum such as comedones (blackheads) in the follicles.

For blackhead extraction, if the blackheads are very deep and have been lodged in the skin for a while, you will need to further soften the keratinized sebum. For this purpose, a desincrustation solution used in conjunction with a galvanic machine can be very helpful (**Figure 8–22**).

This is a solution that softens the sebaceous material (oil, dirt, and debris) around the edges of the pores or follicle openings. This helps soften the comedones, making extractions easier with minimal trauma to the surrounding tissue.

Steam or Warm Towels

Steam promotes more effective cleansing, as warmth softens the follicles (**Figure 8–23**). Steam should never be used for longer than 10 minutes because it can cause overheating and redness, and may cause irritation. Steam can exacerbate existing conditions so never use steam on clients with sensitive skin, rosacea, or inflamed acne.

Warm towels can be used in place of steam or for product removal during treatments. If using hot towels, always check the towel temperature on the inside of your wrist before applying. Keep towels away from the nostrils.

USE OF THE STEAMER

Steam is typically used before deep pore cleansing. Steaming uses a warm, humid mist to soften skin and allow for easier removal of comedones. The steamer nozzle is placed approximately 18 inches (45 centimeters) away from the client (**Figure 8–24**). Check to make sure the client is comfortable and does not feel claustrophobic. The nozzle can be positioned above or below the client's face. Do not use on inflamed, hypersensitive, or rosacea skin. Refer to Chapter 10, Facial Devices and Technology, for instructions on how to safely and effectively use the steamer.

> ## CAUTION!
> To avoid overstimulation and damage to capillaries, do not use steam or hot towels on rosacea-prone or couperose skin. Use an additional facial mask instead.

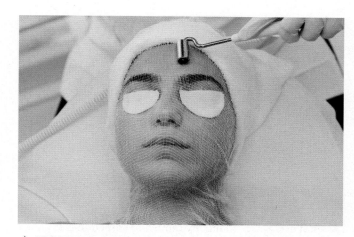

▲ **FIGURE 8–22** Desincrustation with the galvanic machine.

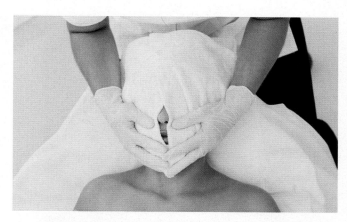

▲ **FIGURE 8–23** Application of a warm towel can soften the follicles.

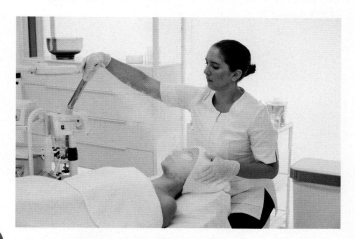

▲ **FIGURE 8–24** Use steam before deep pore cleansing.

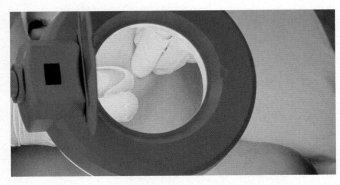

▲ FIGURE 8–25 Manually removing comedones is called extraction.

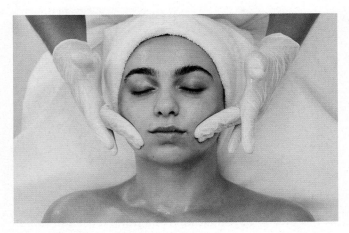

▲ FIGURE 8–26 Massage carries many benefits for the client during the facial.

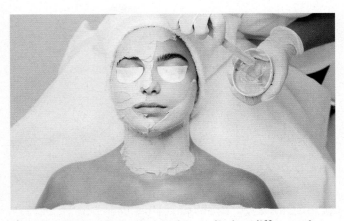

▲ FIGURE 8–27 Masks can be applied at different times during the facial.

Extractions and/or Deep Pore Cleansing

The technique of manually removing comedones from follicles is called **extraction** (EKS-trakt-shun) (**Figure 8–25**). Cleaning out the comedones allows the follicles to contract back to their natural size if skin elasticity is good. Manual extraction is often the only way to expel comedones and clean out the follicles. It may be necessary to gently open papules and pustules with a lancet (when allowed by state regulation) to facilitate easier removal and encourage faster healing. Please refer to your states' regulatory board on use and disposal of lancets during a facial.

Massage

Massage promotes physiological relaxation, stimulates blood circulation, helps muscle tone, cleanses skin of impurities, softens sebum, helps slough off dead skin cells, helps relieve muscle pain, and provides a sense of well-being (**Figure 8–26**). Additionally, the products used for massage have many benefits. Choose the appropriate massage product based on skin type: oil for extremely dry skin, cream for dry to normal skin, or gel for combination to oily skin. Refer to Chapter 9, Facial Massage, for facial massage steps and protocol. The massage can be performed at different times during the treatment, depending on the order of your procedures. Massage products are applied warm, with fingertips or a fan brush.

Treatment Masks

Different forms of mask are used for different effects and skin types. As discussed in Chapter 6, Skin Care Products: Chemistry, Ingredients, and Selection, masks can draw out impurities, clear up blemishes, tighten and tone skin, and hydrate, calm, or rejuvenate the skin (**Figure 8–27**). Types of masks are discussed in greater detail in Chapter 6, such as sheet masks, alginate masks, and modelage masks.

Depending on their function, masks are applied at different times during a treatment—at the beginning, middle or end. If you are drawing impurities out of the skin, it may be beneficial to apply the mask before using steam and doing extractions. If it is a calming, hydrating mask, then it is applied at the end of the facial to calm the skin and leave it hydrated.

Towels or 4" × 4" gauze or cotton pads are used to remove products. Cotton compresses or a "mummy" mask can also be used for removing the mask.

Toners

Toners finish the cleansing process by removing any products left on the skin and help balance the skin's pH (**Figure 8–28**). Different formulas can also help skin problems such as dehydration or acne. Toners, fresheners, and astringents are all referred to as toners for simplicity in this textbook. Toners can be misted onto the face or applied with a saturated cotton pad.

Serums, Eye Treatments, and Lip Treatments

Serums are concentrated ingredients used for specific corrective treatments. Serums and ampoules are applied with fingertips under a mask or moisturizer. They are also used with facial machines in a variety of treatments. Eye and lip creams are usually thicker and are applied with fingertips or cotton swabs (**Figure 8–29**).

Moisturizers

All facials must end with restoring the moisture in the skin. Depending on the formula, moisturizers seal in moisture and help reinforce the barrier layer of the skin (**Figure 8–30**). Moisturizers are emulsions that can be cream, oil, or gel based. Emulsions are created by an emulsifier, an ingredient that brings two incompatible ingredients, such as oil and water, together into one homogenous, uniform blend. They can also hydrate and balance the oil–water moisture content of the skin.

─PERFORM─

Procedure 8-4
Removing Products

Procedure 8-6
Applying and Removing the Cotton Compress

Procedure 8-8
Applying a Sheet Mask

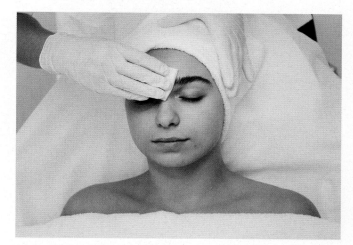

▲ **FIGURE 8–28** Toner finishes the cleansing process.

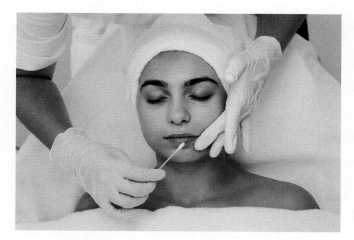

▲ **FIGURE 8–29** Apply lip creams with fingertips or cotton swabs.

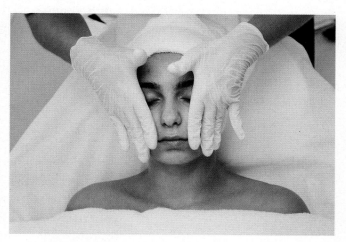

▲ **FIGURE 8–30** Facials must end with restoring moisture to the skin.

Sun Protection Products

The final step of a facial should be the application of a full-spectrum sunscreen. A full-spectrum sunscreen protects the skin from both UVA and UVB rays. Application of sunscreen is especially necessary following the use of any AHA (alpha hydroxy acid) or BHA (beta hydroxyl acid) product or glycolic peel. AHA and BHA may increase skin sensitivity, and clients must be cautioned to use sunscreen and limit sun exposure while using the products and for a week afterward (**Figure 8–31**).

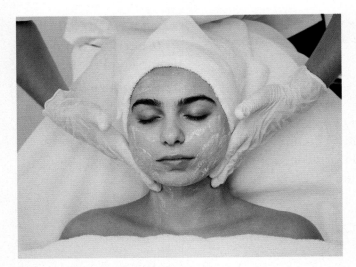

▲ **FIGURE 8–31** Apply sun protection.

Completing the Service

After completing the facial service, remove your gloves, and softly let the client know you are finished. Tell the client to take their time sitting up, offer to assist them in getting off the table, and then do the following before leaving the room so they can change:

1. Explain to the client what to do next—for example, meet you outside in the reception area (**Figure 8–32**). Offer the client some water to rehydrate after the service.

2. The client consultation after the service includes recommending products and booking their next appointment. Show the client which products you recommend, and write them down on a home care instruction sheet for them to keep.

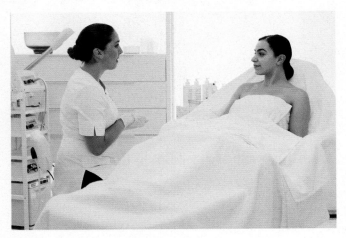

▲ **FIGURE 8–32** Complete the service with a consultation.

3. Explain that you will also record the products you recommend in their file.

4. Recommend that they reschedule once a month for a facial and any other services you believe would benefit them, such as a brow wax or lash tint.

5. Ask them what products they would like to take home with them.

6. Thank them for coming, and let them know you enjoyed meeting them.

┌─────────────────────┐
PERFORM
Procedure 8-9
Post-Service Procedure
└─────────────────────┘

Post-Service Checklist

After the facial, complete the post-service procedures that were thoroughly discussed in Procedure 7–2: Post-Service Procedure—Clean-up and Preparation for the Next Client. A checklist is also available for your use in **Table 8–3**. Be sure to record the client chart notes and write up retail sales. Then prepare the room for the next client, or clean the room in preparation for the end of the day.

Postfacial	Equipment/Room	Supplies	Single-Use Items
☐ Remove your gloves and wash your hands.	☐ Clean the wax machine and turn it off at the end of the day.	☐ Wash and disinfect brushes, spatulas, tweezers, and other multiuse implements used during the process.	☐ Place soiled items such as gloves in a covered waste container.
☐ Say goodbye to the client after the consultation.	☐ Clean and disinfect the steamer. Refill with distilled water.	☐ Clean and disinfect bowls and other multiuse items. Dry and store properly.	☐ Place disposable extraction lancets in a biohazard sharps container.
☐ Rebook the client and make sure they have taken products for at-home use.	☐ Wipe and disinfect the equipment used.	☐ If there is an autoclave on the premises, put multiuse implements such as tweezers in the autoclave for sterilization after every use.	
☐ Make the client chart notes.	☐ Clean all containers and wipe off dirty product containers with a disinfectant.	☐ Remove the dirty linens and remake the table.	
☐ Write up retail sales.	☐ Clean and disinfect all counters, sinks, surfaces, and floor mats.	☐ Turn off the table warmer if used.	
☐ Prepare the room for the next client or carry out end-of-the-day clean-up tasks.		☐ Put the linens, towels, and sheets in the appropriate covered laundry hamper.	
☐ Wear gloves during cleaning procedures.		☐ Change the disinfectant solution to comply with state agency regulations.	
		☐ Remove or change the towels on the workstation tables.	
		☐ Put away the supplies.	

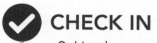

CHECK IN

9. List the steps in a basic facial (excluding facial devices).

┌─ PERFORM ─┐
Procedure 8-5
Performing the Basic Facial

Describe How to Consult Clients on Home Care

Home care is probably the most important factor in a successful skin care program. The key word here is *program*. Clients' participation is essential to achieve results. A program consists of a long-range plan involving home care, salon treatments, and client education.

Every new client should be thoroughly consulted about home care for their skin conditions. After the first treatment, do the following:

- Block out about 15 minutes to explain proper home care for the client. Subsequent visits can be reduced to five-minute intervals.
- Have the client sit in the facial chair, or invite them to move to a well-lit consultation area. A mirror should be provided, so that they can see the conditions you will be discussing **(Figure 8–33)**.

- Explain, in simple terms, the client's skin conditions, informing them of how you propose to treat the conditions. Inform them about how often treatments should be administered in the salon or spa, and very specifically explain what they should be doing at home.
- Set out the products you want the client to purchase and use. Explain each one, and tell them in which order to use them. Make sure to have written instructions for the client to take home.
- It is important to have products available for the client that you believe in and that produce results. Retailing products for clients to use at home is important to the success of your treatments and to your business.

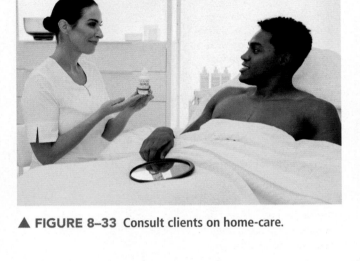
▲ **FIGURE 8–33** Consult clients on home-care.

The Art of Recommendation

Know your client. Do they have lots of time to spend on pampering themselves? Or are they strapped for time? Start by suggesting two basic products such as a cleanser and moisturizer, depending on their main concerns **(Figure 8–34)**. You can always add a new product such as an exfoliator or eye cream to their regimen on their next visit. Focus on providing a product that will deliver results based on their concerns. If you do not coerce them into taking home more products than they want, your client will be more likely to trust your expertise and return for another treatment. They will have used what you did recommend and see the results.

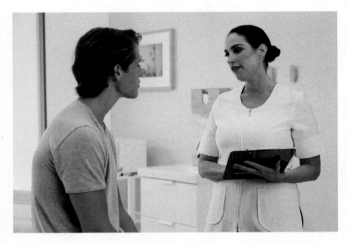
▲ **FIGURE 8–34** Recommend products for your client's home care regimen.

 CHECK IN

10. In your own words, describe how to consult clients on home care.

Discuss Variations of the Basic Facial

Remember that the steps of the facial procedure will vary depending on the focus of the facial. (**Figure 8–35**). Sometimes steam or massage is omitted. Sometimes the massage is the last step after the mask, and sometimes two masks are used. Massage is performed before extractions in the basic facial of this chapter to avoid stimulation that would cause further inflammation. Using massage after extractions could pose possible secondary lesions and clients may experience breakouts.

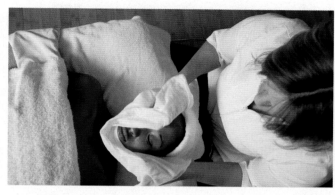

▲ **FIGURE 8–35** Facial treatments have many variations.

Other estheticians may choose to massage after the application of a mask as some of the massage creams and oils used in the industry could lock out further product penetration and benefits from active ingredients.

The procedure used depends on what you are trying to achieve. Are you trying to hydrate and calm the skin, or deep clean and stimulate it? For example, if the client needs hydrating, you may choose to omit the cleansing mask and the extractions. Be guided by your instructor. Do not be too concerned about utilizing different methods or procedures right now. As you continue your practice, you can vary the treatments you offer.

The Express Facial

The main differences between an express facial treatment, also known as mini-facial, and a basic facial are the time and the number of steps and products. An **express facial** (ik-spres FAY-shul) may take

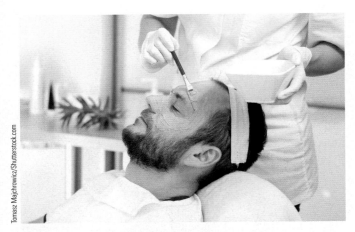

▲ **FIGURE 8–36** An express facial can take 15–30 minutes.

from 15 to 30 minutes and does not include all the steps of a full, 60 to 90-minute facial. Omitted steps may include steaming, massage, or extractions. Cleansing and masking are the most important elements of the express facial because they produce the most visible results in 30 minutes. Express facials may also focus on only one area of the face, such as the eye contour area, or provide a quick exfoliation and hydration (**Figure 8–36**).

The express facial gives clients a treatment that can be completed quickly if they are pressed for time, and can be performed with other services such as waxing, manicure, or pedicure. For men, it can be incorporated into shaving and beard care services. An express facial is also a great way to introduce the client to a beneficial service that may lead to booking for a more in-depth facial series to address specific skin concerns and conditions in an ongoing program.

MINI-PROCEDURE

The Express Facial

1. Provide a brief consultation. Have the client fill out a consultation form and discuss their skin condition and treatment goals. Ask about their current skin care regimen, and any medications or medical conditions that might be contraindicative to certain treatments such as glycolic peels. Find out about their skin care concerns. The client will sign a consent form before treatment begins.
2. Properly drape the client and wash your hands.
3. Analyze the skin with a magnifying lamp.
4. Perform a cleansing to remove makeup. Rinse well with 4" × 4" esthetics wipes moistened with warm water.
5. Perform an exfoliation or facial massage. Remove exfoliant and tone skin.
6. Apply a mask for approximately 10 minutes.
7. Remove the mask.
8. Apply a moisturizer and sunscreen for daytime.
9. Recommend a treatment for the client's next visit.
10. Recommend initial home care products and complete the home care chart.

 CHECK IN

11. How does an express facial differ from the basic facial? For instance, what treatments are typically included in an express facial?

Outline the Treatment Goals for Six Skin Types/Conditions

Skin conditions and products have been covered in Chapters 5 and 6, so review ingredients and the factors that affect the skin's health to choose treatments for each individual client. The following treatments incorporate the same procedures as the basic facial, but certain steps and products are added or omitted, based on the condition and skin type being treated.

Dry Skin

Dry skin is usually the result of underactive sebaceous glands that produce sebum, which softens the skin, creating a natural moisturizing protective barrier. The skin appears coarse, tight, dull in color, and often with visible lines and wrinkles (**Figure 8–37**). It may also become dry from overexposure to sun and wind, harsh soaps, poor diet, lack of fluid intake, medication, and environmental factors and aging. Dry skin can be caused by genetic disposition or as a result of skin aging. As a person advances in years, the body's renewal process slows down, and cells are not replaced as quickly as before. Here is a quick chart to refer to on dry skin characteristics:

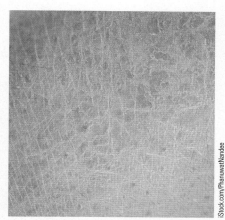

▲ **FIGURE 8–37** Dry skin.

Treatment Goal	☐ Hydrate the skin with rich masks and creamy cleansers as well as a gentle form of exfoliation to remove the dead, dry skin cells and prevent them from accumulating on the surface. Massage can be very effective.

TREATMENTS FOR DRY SKIN

For dry or mature skin, the treatment goals are similar: to hydrate and nourish the skin as well as remove accumulated dead, dry skin cells. Facial treatments and home maintenance can help minimize dryness and stimulate the production of sebum. Massage and exfoliation are beneficial to dry skin. Protecting the barrier function and keeping dry skin well lubricated is important. In general, when performing a facial for dry skin:

- Serums and creams can balance and protect skin with the appropriate products and in the proper amounts.

- Use a gentle enzyme peel, a gentle alpha hydroxy acid peel, or a light microdermabrasion treatment to exfoliate the skin.

- For a mask, peptides, hyaluronic acid or emollient, and natural ingredients such as seaweed or a thermal mask can be used. Be sure to inquire about allergies before use of these products.

- Massage and the galvanic machine can be used to assist in the application of a hydrating serum.

- LED can be used (see Chapter 10 on use of machines).

- A moisturizing cream with an oil base, antioxidants, and a full-spectrum sunscreen finish the treatment.

Dehydrated Skin

Dehydration of the surface is one of the most common skin problems. The major cause of dehydration is evaporation and loss of sebum from the surface of the skin due to the use of harsh, drying soaps and alkalis as well as through drier winter months, heat, and changes in climate. A client's skin may have enough oil, but still feel dry and flaky due to lack of water in the skin (**Figure 8–38**).

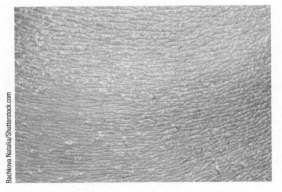

▲ **FIGURE 8–38** Dehydrated skin.

TRANSEPIDERMAL WATER LOSS (TEWL)

The dehydration of the epidermis occurs through a process called *transepidermal water loss (TEWL)*. The deeper tissues of the skin comprise large cells loaded with moisture, with a moisture differential between the lower layers of 80 percent and the upper layers of 15 percent. With such a great difference, there will be a natural tendency for the moisture to move from the lower layers to the upper layers via *osmosis*. This movement is called *transepidermal water loss*.

The surface of the skin naturally contains lipids and sebum that create a natural moisturizing factor (NMF). When the stratum corneum is intact and healthy, it serves as an effective barrier to inhibit evaporation (**Figure 8–39**). If the cells are packed tightly together, the water cannot get through them, but if the cells are loosely packed and flaking, the moisture can easily evaporate. In addition to this, the NMF has the ability to bind moisture into the skin. When the NMF is washed off of the skin with soaps and other alkalis, the cells dry and crack, producing dry skin.

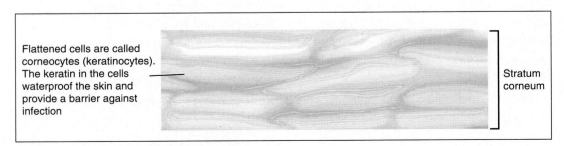

Flattened cells are called corneocytes (keratinocytes). The keratin in the cells waterproof the skin and provide a barrier against infection

Stratum corneum

▲ **FIGURE 8–39** The epidermal barrier structure.

<table>
<tr>
<td>Treatment Goal</td>
<td>
☐ Restore internal skin hydration and retain inner moisture by preventing transepidermal water loss (TEWL).
☐ Concentrate on hydrating and nourishing treatments that deliver the highest amounts of moisture to the skin.
☐ Massage with the use of serums.
</td>
</tr>
</table>

TREATMENTS FOR DEHYDRATED SKIN

It is important to the health of the skin to maintain the natural moisturizing factor and the natural acid mantle. Dehydrated skin is prone to fine lines and wrinkles. It will appear thin and may appear fine in texture but is actually coarse to the touch. If the client's skin seems to be dehydrated from factors that require medical attention (such as diet, lack of fluids, or medication), the esthetician should recommend that the client seek the advice of their physician or dermatologist. In the meantime, facial treatments that can improve the general health of the skin and help it to retain moisture are beneficial.

Superficial dehydration will always lead to superficial lines on the skin's surface which eventually will turn into deeper wrinkles. Therefore, early anti-aging skin care will also greatly benefit this skin type.

Mature or Aging Skin

Anti-aging treatments are an important part of our business. We age from the moment we are born. The speed at which age leaves its signs on our face is influenced not only through (chronological) time, but by genetic encoding and environmental effects (**Figure 8–40**). One part is genetic, the rest is environmental damage, and the main part of this is caused by UV radiation. These topics are also referenced in Chapter 3, Physiology and Histology of the Skin, with additional details to follow.

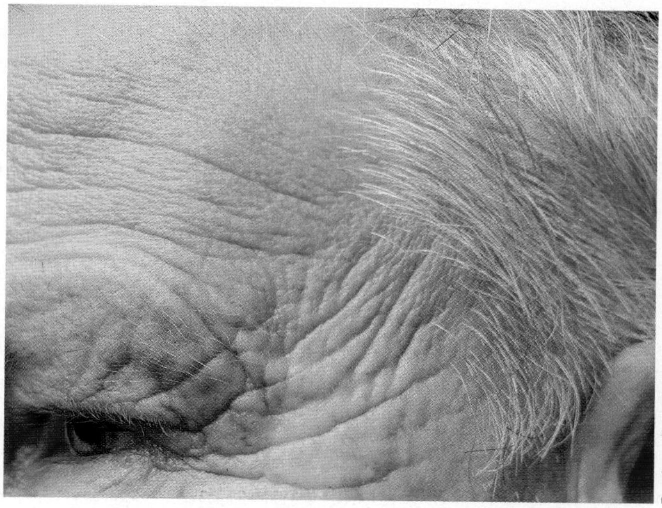

▲ **FIGURE 8–40** Wrinkles develop when the skin loses collagen and elastin.

BIOLOGICAL CHANGES IN AGING SKIN

Aging and sun-damaged skin is different from youthful, healthy skin. The differences are noticeable in loss of moisture, in fine lines and wrinkles, and in the thinning of the epidermis. As skin ages, it undergoes biological changes due to reduction of estrogen, including reduction in collagen and elastin (**Figure 8–41**). With each passing year the average moisture content of the stratum corneum is slightly decreased, manifesting in fine lines. The epidermis thins out and the dermal papilla, which is the anchor of the epidermis, flattens out, resulting in a loose, tissue-like texture. The cell renewal rate slows down, making healing slower. Circulation becomes impaired,

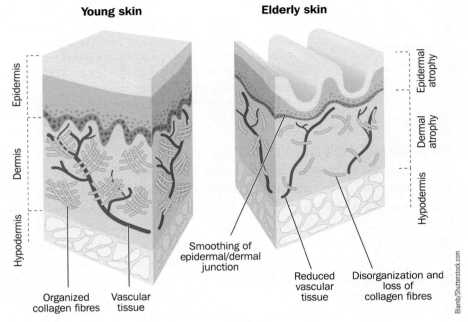

Young skin   Elderly skin

Epidermis

Dermis

Hypodermis

Epidermal atrophy

Dermal atrophy

Hypodermis

Smoothing of epidermal/dermal junction

Reduced vascular tissue

Disorganization and loss of collagen fibres

Organized collagen fibres

Vascular tissue

Blamb/Shutterstock.com

▲ **FIGURE 8–41** As skin ages it undergoes biological changes.

resulting in desquamation becoming uneven, which affects the evenness of skin tone. Likewise, the translucency of the stratum corneum becomes more opaque, resulting in a more yellowish-grey skin tone. A lifetime of repeated movements result in "expression lines" around the eyes and mouth.

As has been pointed out in earlier chapters, other factors, such as pollution, hormones, photoaging from UV light, poor diet, stress, and other factors contribute to the signs of aging.

POLLUTION

Air pollution comprises tiny particles called particulate matter that contain nitrogen dioxide (NO_2) and polycyclic aromatic hydrocarbons (PAH). When they come in contact with the skin, they activate multiple pathways of inflammation.

Some pathways ignite the melanocytes, which create far too much pigment, which manifests in hyperpigmentation. Some excite enzymes that reabsorb damaged collagen. With too much chronic inflammation, the enzymes remove more collagen than your skin can create. This produces skin laxity, causing a cascade that results in fine lines and wrinkles.

POOR DIET

There are many examples of how bad food choices affect the skin. For example, dairy products may contain a hormone called IGF-1 that causes inflammation. Cheese, milk, and other dairy products may also increase the amount of oil that your sebaceous glands secrete. The excess oil is likely to clog pores and lead to acne. Finally, dairy makes it harder for dead skin cells to clear out, which allows for oils to collect and become inflamed. Sugar increases blood sugar levels, which spurs *insulin* (a hormone that helps the body store and use glucose) and *IGF-1* production.

As mentioned before, IGF-1 is a big cause of inflammation. Therefore, the high amount of sugar found in candy, soda, and other sweet treats not only produces a lot of inflammation, but it also reacts with your skin cells and causes dryness, decreased color, and premature wrinkles (**Figure 8–42**). Caffeine is a diuretic, that is, it causes water loss and dehydration.

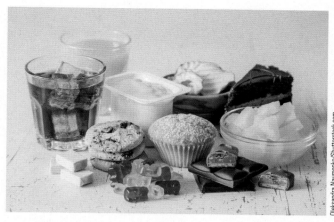

▲ **FIGURE 8–42** A poor diet negatively impacts the skin.

HORMONES

Hormones are chemicals secreted by cells or glands, and they act as messengers that are sent out from one part of the body to signal cells in other parts of the body. Hormones regulate the body's internal environment. As we age the body produces lower levels of hormones, and the ability of hormones to communicate messages decreases.

Effects of imbalanced hormones in skin aging include excess blood glucose, which can damage or destroy collagen, and excessive free radicals, which can cause oxidative damage to the cells as well as hyperpigmentation resulting from changes in estrogen and progesterone. And women are not the only ones who can have signs of skin aging caused by hormonal changes. In men, levels of hormones such as testosterone decrease slowly over time, so that by their late forties to early fifties, men can experience hyperpigmentation, thinning skin, uneven skin texture, and reduced skin firmness. Men may notice that the area of skin around the jawline begins to sag, as well as the area around the mouth, which is the result of a loss of elasticity and underlying fat. They may also experience a noticeable increase in puffiness around the cheeks and eyes.

CAUTION!
Estheticians are not nutritionists and should not encourage clients to remove foods from their diet without the consent of the client's physician.

STRESS

The stress response leads to the secretion of stress hormones (adrenaline, cortisol, and norepinephrine) into the bloodstream to bring about specific physiological changes. Unfortunately, this hyperstimulus effect can impair normal cellular renewal cycles of skin as well. Dermal mast cells (a type of white blood cell) become more reactive, which may lead to the release of a large number of proinflammatory mediators that cause inflammation in your body, resulting in redness of the skin.

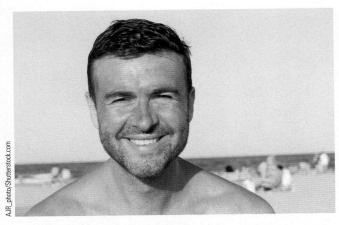

▲ **FIGURE 8–43** Repeated exposure to the sun causes premature aging of the skin.

UV EXPOSURE

As discussed in Chapter 4, Disorders and Diseases of the Skin, repeated exposure to *ultraviolet (UV)* sun can cause premature aging of the skin, and *artificial UV* sources can affect clients in stages throughout their life, as highlighted in the following list (**Figure 8–43**):

- *Group 1*—Classified as mild. Wrinkles do not form during this stage. Clients see mild pigment changes and minimal wrinkles.

- *Group 2*—Classified as moderate. Clients may present with age spots and early signs of parallel smile lines, and they may feel the need to wear foundation to cover facial changes.

- *Group 3*—Classified as advanced. Clients see obvious signs of discoloration, visible capillaries, and visible keratosis, and they may feel the need to wear heavier foundation.

- *Group 4*—Classified as severe. Clients may see yellow-gray skin color and wrinkles throughout.

OTHER EXTERNAL FACTORS

External factors can increase the appearance of aging in the skin. These include:

- Improper or insufficient skin care

- Medications, physiological disease, poor health, and psychological (emotional) problems

- Extreme weight loss can result in loss of muscle tone and lined and sagging skin, which in turn gives the skin an "aged" appearance

- Lifestyle choices such as smoking, and the misuse of alcoholic beverages.

Treatments for Aging and Mature Skin

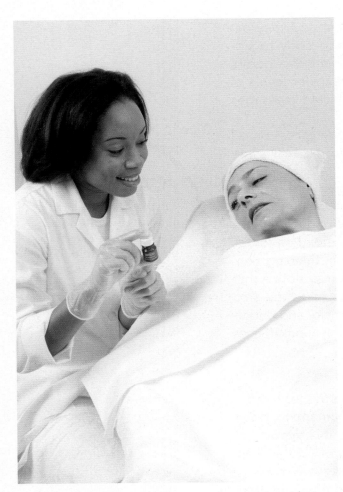

▲ **FIGURE 8–44** There are no miracle treatments that restore aging skin.

The mature client's skin can be improved, but the natural aging process cannot be reversed, nor will the skin be restored to the same vital condition of youth. The client should be advised that treatments can make the skin look and feel better, but there are no miracle treatments that restore aging skin (**Figure 8–44**). Prevention and healthy habits are the key to beautiful skin at any age.

AGING THROUGH THE DECADES

20's
Up to **90%** of the visible skin changes commonly attributed to aging are caused by the **sun** and can be seen as early as in one's twenties.

30's
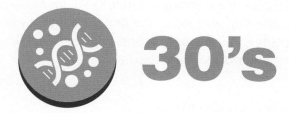

▸ Cell turnover slows down.
▸ Epidermal cells suffer more from environmental damage. Wrinkles still may not be visible.
▸ Dermis begins to lose some volume and bounce.
▸ Collagen fibers aren't as efficiently meshed, elastin coils less tight.

40's
▸ Sebum production reduced.
▸ The stratum corneum is thicker as more dead skin cells linger longer.
▸ Darker pigmentation may appear due to environmental damage.
▸ Expression lines **deepen**.
▸ **Dilated veins** may appear.

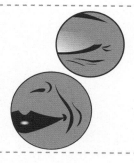

50's
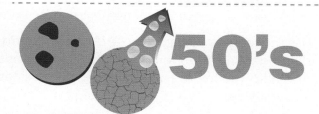

▸ **Age spots** may appear.
▸ Hormonal changes– *decrease* in estrogen, *increase* in androgen– may lead to breakouts.
▸ Sebum production decreases, depriving the skin its natural **moisture**.

60's 70's &BEYOND
▸ Genetic disposition to certain skin type/problems (i.e. bags under the eyes, double chin, pigmentation) reveals itself.
▸ Effects of intrinsic aging vs. environmental aging are now visible.
▸ Less sebum production contributes to skin dryness.
▸ Skin becomes dryer and more fragile.

ELASTICITY OF THE SKIN

Aging skin often lacks elasticity. Elasticity is the skin tissue's ability to return to its normal resting length after a stressor has been removed. One way to test the skin for elasticity is by taking a small section of the facial skin or neck between the thumb and forefinger and giving the skin a slight outward pull. If the elasticity is good, the skin will immediately return to its normal shape when the skin is released. If the skin is slow to resume its normal shape, it is lacking elasticity. Firming ingredients and treatments are beneficial for skin's elasticity.

INGREDIENTS FOR MATURE SKIN

Aging or sun-damaged skin needs antioxidants topically and orally. Antioxidants such as vitamins A, B₃, C, and E; minerals; green tea; and grapeseed extract all help protect the body from free radicals. Other beneficial care for aging skin includes protecting the barrier function of the skin and wearing sunscreen. Additionally, alpha hydroxy acids can help combat the signs of aging and sun damage. Hydrating ingredients such as hyaluronic acid, sodium hyaluronate, sodium PCA, and glycerin all bind water to the skin and retain the moisture that is essential to maturing skin. Peptides, lipids, polyglucans, coenzyme Q10, and liposomes are all beneficial performance ingredients.

Treatment Goal
- ☐ Hydrate and revitalize the skin.
- ☐ Establish regularly scheduled skin evaluations that include skin analysis and review with the client in order to make the appropriate product and treatment adjustments.
- ☐ An ongoing program of anti-aging treatments done in a series.

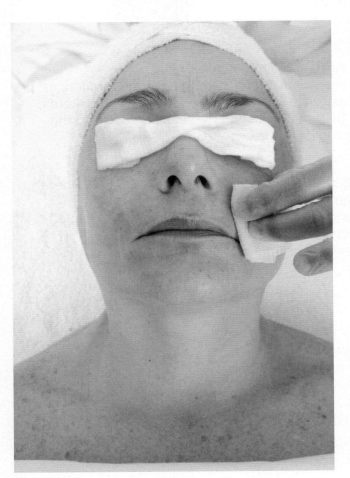

▲ FIGURE 8–45 AHA treatment exfoliating the skin.

MATURE SKIN TREATMENTS

Here are some suggestions for treating mature skin:

- Use procedures similar to those designed for dry skin, adapting the ingredients to include ones that help reduce the appearance of fine lines and wrinkles.

- Extended massage with a moisturizing serum and cream.

- Peptide, collagen, and hydrating masks are all beneficial in a facial treatment for mature skin.

- A thermal mask will force-feed nutrients into the skin and help to soften the appearance of the skin, diminishing the appearance of fine lines and wrinkles.

- Firming products can be effective in visibly tightening the appearance of the skin.

- AHA treatments and products can help exfoliate the skin, creating a more luminescent complexion (**Figure 8–45**).

- Advanced treatments such as light therapy, iontophoresis, and galvanic and microcurrent are effective tools for mature skin. (See Chapter 10, Facial Devices and Technology.)

Sensitive and Sensitized Skin or Rosacea

Our skin, the largest organ in the human body, has a remarkable multifunctional capacity to not only maintain our internal environment but to interact with environmental stimuli such as microbes, chemicals, and other physical elements. Any of these environmental stimuli may evoke a reaction of the skin, leading to dermatitis, an inflammation of the skin.

In addition to redness (erythema), edema (swelling), inflammation, and dryness that is characteristic of dermatitis, sensitive skin also experiences a cascade of free radical activity that causes skin-destructive enzymes to form (**Figure 8–46**). These enzymes attack the skin's integrity, leading to premature aging in the form of wrinkles and loss of elasticity.

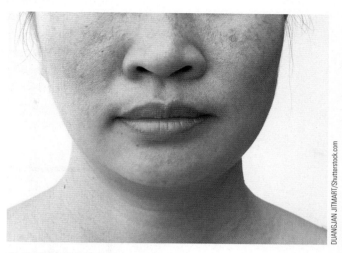

▲ FIGURE 8–46 Sensitive skin.

As learned in Chapter 5, Skin Analysis, *sensitive skin* can be a biologic condition that readily reacts to a variety of factors such as specific chemicals, airborne debris, and/or certain skin care ingredients, resulting in skin that often appears blotchy, broken out, or excessively dry. Dry patches and redness are often present with this type of skin. Skin can easily become red and warm to the touch. This skin type can be confused with rosacea or couperose skin types.

Sensitized skin can result from overaggressive exfoliation, or from exposure to aggressive environmental factors such as cold, wind, low humidity, and air pollution. This skin may become highly sensitive, and needs to be treated as sensitive skin until it returns to its normal state. Avoid inflammatory ingredients until skin has returned to its normal state. Irritants and sensitizing ingredients can be essential oils, exfoliants, fragrances, color agents, and preservatives. All of these may cause skin reactions and irritation.

ROSACEA

Estheticians cannot treat or diagnose any medical condition, and rosacea is considered a medical condition. This condition typically manifests as redness in the central area of the face, including on the cheeks and nose in a butterfly pattern, and it is characterized by flare-ups and remissions (**Figure 8–47**). Over time, this redness can become more persistently visible. Broken blood vessels can also become more apparent. Left untreated, pustules and large, inflamed nodules can result that are often misdiagnosed as acne. After a prolonged period, this condition can result in

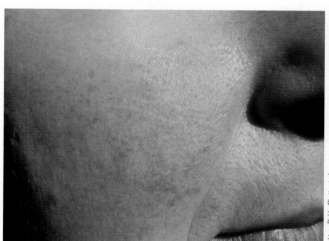

▲ FIGURE 8–47 Estheticians cannot diagnose or treat rosacea.

permanent enlargement of the nasal tissue or rhinophyma, where the tip of the nose becomes enlarged and red. Eyes can also become affected, appearing watery and bloodshot. This skin condition can be exacerbated by factors such as alcohol, spicy foods, and heat, making its symptoms similar to hypersensitive skin. While estheticians cannot treat rosacea, they must know how to properly provide a facial for a client with rosacea. More information on rosacea is in Chapter 4, Disorders and Diseases of the Skin.

CAUTION!

Contraindications for Sensitive or Sensitized Skin, or Rosacea

Individuals with sensitive or sensitized skin, or who have rosacea, should avoid the following:

- Strong exfoliants such as coarse manual materials, microdermabrasion, aggressive AHA or BHA peels, vacuum suction, the brush machine, and any ingredients with a pH of 3.5 or lower
- Steam during treatment
- Stimulating machines or manual massage; a cooling massage device can be used in place of manual facial massage, which can be manipulated to be gentler on the skin
- Drying products with a pH of 8 or higher
- Excessive heat such as hot water, steam, or towels; lukewarm water should be used during facials

---

Treatment Goal	☐ Identify and avoid those stimuli that provoke a sensitive, sensitized, or rosacea response.
	☐ Provide skin with topical application of ingredients that help calm and soothe the appearance of the skin, such as seaweed, silver, quercetin, rutin, olive oil, olive leaf extracts, calamine, calcium carbonate, green tea, and allantoin.
	☐ Help maintain the skin's protective moisture barrier by using fatty acids, ceramides, hyaluronic acid, niacimamide, linoleic acid, squalene, phospholipids, lecithin, evening primrose oil, tocopherol (vitamin E), and ascorbyl palmitate (vitamin C), and low percentages of an AHA such as lactic acid.
	☐ Encourage the client to consult a dermatologist when experiencing severe sensitive skin or rosacea flare-ups.
	☐ For home care, advise these clients to avoid vasodilators that dilate capillaries: heat, the sun, spicy foods, and stimulating products.

TREATMENTS FOR SENSITIVE AND SENSITIZED SKIN OR ROSACEA

Follow the facial procedure and incorporate the following guidelines:

- To lessen the appearance of irritation, a gentle cleanser is the best type of cleanser. Detergent-based cleansers can strip the skin's lipids and barrier protection.

- Cold towels are **vasoconstricting** (vay-zoh-kun-STRIK-ting), which means they constrict capillaries and blood flow.

- An enzyme peel formulated for sensitive skin gently exfoliates the skin.

- A soothing cream or alginate gel mask is great for calming and toning down the appearance of redness. Calamine and calcium carbonate powder mixed with aloe or fresh yogurt are also excellent for sensitive skin.

- Freeze-dried collagen masks are also excellent for redness or sensitive skin.

- Lipids such as olive oil extracts and seaweed help to create a moisture barrier on the surface of the skin.

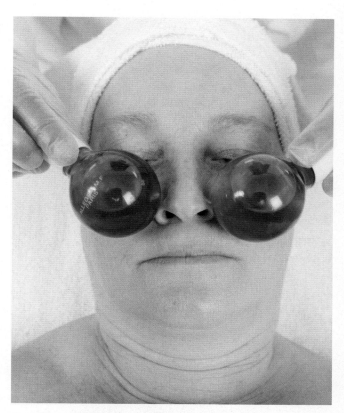

▲ **FIGURE 8–48** Cold globes calm the skin.

- Use a serum and moisturizer with hyaluronic acid or squalene to help soothe the symptoms of sensitive skin.

- Silver ball or cold globes may be used to calm blood flow and reduce redness. They provide a gentle massage with controlled pressure to help both massage skin and apply product (**Figure 8–48**).

Treatments for Hyperpigmentation

Hyperpigmentation is a condition that affects many people. Sun exposure, medication, and chemical reactions cause dark pigmentation areas on the skin that clients often want to diminish (**Figure 8–49**). Advise clients that the best preventative measures are to stay out of the sun and wear protective clothing and sun protection daily.

Follow the facial procedure and incorporate the following guidelines:

- Ingredients that can help brighten the appearance of the skin include kojic acid, alpha arbutin, glycolic acid, mulberry, licorice root, azaleic acid, bearberry, and citrus such as lemon work to help reduce the appearance of dark spots.

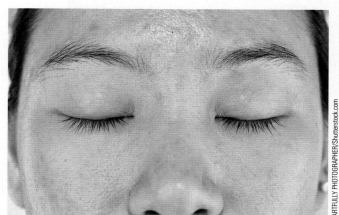

▲ **FIGURE 8–49** Advise clients with hyperpigmentation to avoid the sun.

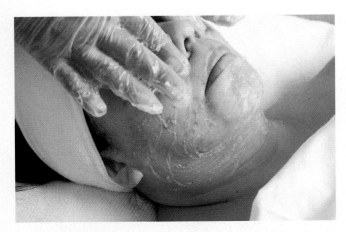

▲ FIGURE 8–50 Exfoliating treatments can help brighten the skin.

- These ingredients can be used in conjunction with exfoliating treatments using AHA, BHA, and other types of exfoliators (**Figure 8–50**).
- Harsh skin-bleaching agents such as hydroquinone (which is banned in several countries) may damage the skin and are controversial.
- Remember that overexfoliating can cause damage and make hyperpigmentation worse— or conversely, cause hypopigmentation. Hypopigmentation results from reducing the appearance of melanin to the extent that lighter skin patches are now evident.

Treatment Goal	☐ Chemical exfoliation and brightening agents can be effective in reducing some hyperpigmented areas.

Treatments for Oily Skin

Oily to combination skin is caused by overactive sebaceous glands and is thicker in texture. The skin has enlarged pores that may be filled with sebum buildup from the environment as well as from the use of comedogenic makeup and other products (**Figure 8–51**). Comedones and whiteheads are present. The skin is sallow in appearance and is more prone to blemishes but is less prone to wrinkles and fine lines because the oil acts as a lubricant and a barrier, helping to keep moisture within the skin from evaporating.

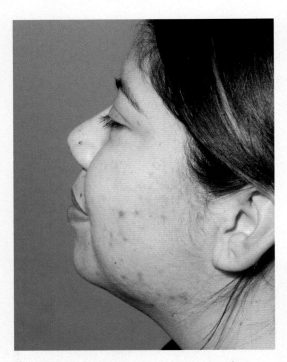

▲ FIGURE 8–51 Enlarged pores may be filled with sebum build up.

Treatment Goal	☐ This type of skin can develop breakouts easily, so it is important to treat the skin with effective deep cleansing and purifying products. ☐ Galvanic current, steam, and extractions can benefit oily skin to keep the pores free of comedones, and exfoliation with oil-controlling ingredients and BHA can lead to a great result as well.

 CHECK IN

12. List a treatment goal that is beneficial for
    a. dry skin; b. dehydrated skin; c. mature skin; d. sensitive skin;
       e. hyperpigmentation; f. oily skin

Describe Acne Facials

Skin with acne has many of the same characteristics as oily skin but hormones, stress, and other biological factors have caused the formation of acne pustules. This is especially common in adolescents but can manifest at any time in a person's life, particularly during perimenopause. The first signs of acne are usually seen during puberty when there is an increase in the androgen hormones, which stimulate the amount of oil produced by the sebaceous glands (**Figure 8–52**). Blackheads, whiteheads, pimples, and pustules are present and easily infected with bacteria.

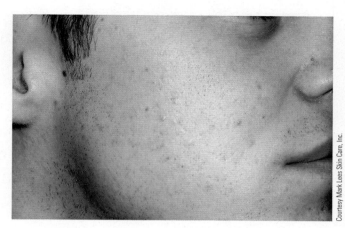

▲ **FIGURE 8–52** Open comedones.

Treatment Goal	☐ Eliminate blackheads from the skin that lead to more breakouts. ☐ Thorough cleansers and deep-cleansing masks that include AHA and BHA are recommended, and the facial treatment should include extractions. ☐ Extractions must be done gently and without pain to the client. ☐ Treatment care and client education regarding acne can be ongoing, and the results are rewarding for clients and the esthetician.

Acne Treatment

Excessive oily and problem skin is one of the leading reasons clients seek out professional help and is one of the most important factors in an esthetician's practice. While estheticians do not diagnose acne, they must be aware of this skin condition and know how to properly provide a facial. Performing consistent effective facial treatments will not only benefit the client's overall appearance but will also help bolster their self-esteem. Both of these results are perhaps the most important achievements to which an esthetician can aspire.

The esthetician can outline an acne treatment plan to balance the skin. Treatments are focused on deep cleansing and extractions. Clients need to understand that they did not get their acne overnight, and it will not go away overnight. Likewise, clients need to be instructed to never pick at their acne pimples. Estheticians should also look for indications of acne excoriee, a condition stemming from habitual, nervous picking of the acne pimples that leads to permanent scarring.

In order to partner with the client on proper care of their skin condition, instruct them on the histology of acne within the skin. Provide simple illustrations on how acne pustules form, such as in **Figure 8–53**.

CAUTION!

Physicians prescribe medications that work to suppress acne flare-ups; however, medications can have adverse side effects and, even with medication, acne can return. Working with problem skin is a continuous process, and clients need to follow regular skin care programs.

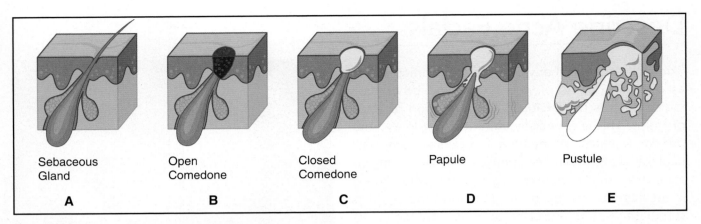

▲ FIGURE 8–53 How acne pustules form.

| Sebaceous Gland | Open Comedone | Closed Comedone | Papule | Pustule |
| A | B | C | D | E |

In this illustration, keratinized (skin cell debris) plugs (A) block sebum from wicking out along the hair shaft. Stagnant sebum (B) is broken down by bacterial enzymes into short-chain fatty acids. An irritated papule (C) is formed. Increased blood flow activates the immune system (D). Finally, white blood cells rush to the area to combat the foreign matter, resulting in infections. Pustules are formed (E).

PRODUCTS AND EQUIPMENT FOR ACNE CARE

Desincrustation, steam, and extractions are all part of an oily and problem skin facial. AHA and BHA exfoliation treatments are also effective. Each client is treated individually according to their needs.

Here are some products recommended for acne:

- *Beta hydroxy acid (salicylic acid)*—These products are found naturally in willow bark extract and are natural keratolytic agents, meaning they are able to dissolve keratin, improving the look and the feel of the skin. This ingredient differs from alpha hydroxy acid in that it is more soluble in oil than water. This means that once the water from the product you are applying evaporates, salicylic acid will seek out oil, in this case sebum, and help to cleanse it further from the skin (**Figure 8–54**). (Check for aspirin allergies before using salicylic acid.)

- *Sulfur masks*—These are effective products that exfoliate skin and dry blemishes (check for sulfur allergies).

- *AHA (glycolic, lactic, malic, citric, and tartaric acids)*—These products are used in different percentages to help dissolve dead skin cells to keep the skin surface exfoliated. Exfoliation also softens acne impactions. In a spa or salon, formulations should never exceed 30 percent and never be lower than a pH of 3.5.

- *Vitamin A or retinol*—Both retinol and retinyl palmitate are forms of vitamin A. This topical vitamin benefits the skin by helping to reduce flaking and restore the appearance of skin suppleness.

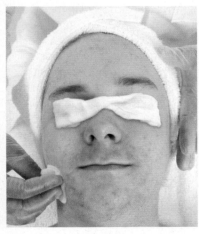

▲ FIGURE 8–54 Beta hydroxy acid (salicylic acid) treatment.

- *Benzoyl peroxide*—This ingredient releases oxygen that kills bacteria as well as helps exfoliate skin.
- *Kojic acid*—This is an ingredient derived from mushrooms that helps to brighten the appearance of the skin.
- *Spot blemish treatments*—These products include ingredients such as beta hydroxyl acid, tea tree oil, and benzoyl peroxide that are applied just on blemishes after cleansing.
- *Increased vitamin C*—This oral vitamin has antioxidant value and healing effects.

Acne Care Tips

Here are some suggestions for clients with acne.

- Eliminate comedogenic products. *Oil-free* does not mean "noncomedogenic." Examine the ingredients on product labels to determine if they are appropriate for problem skin. (Refer to Chapter 6, Skin Care Products: Chemistry, Ingredients, and Selection, for ingredient information.)
- Control oil through proper product usage. Do not irritate the skin with harsh products.
- Exfoliate the skin. Keep the skin clean and exfoliated to keep sebum and cells from building up. Beta or alpha hydroxy acids are beneficial. Do not overuse these products. Once a day is sufficient.
- Protect against environmental aggressors, dirt, grease, UV light, humidity, and pollution.
- Practice stress reduction and good nutrition.
- Have regular facials once a month or as needed.

Home Care for Acne

Proper home care can usually help keep acne under control. However, when clients cannot achieve results with their home care routine, they may seek the aid of an esthetician or a physician (**Figure 8–55**). After the skin is analyzed, suggestions are given to the client specific to their needs. It is important for clients to follow the recommended home care routine as outlined by the esthetician. Treatments must be accompanied by a real commitment from the client to maintain their home care regimen.

It is important to ask clients not to pick at their blemishes. Explain to them that the skin is delicate, and performing self-extractions will cause the infection to go deeper, possibly spread more rapidly, and perhaps cause permanent scarring. You cannot treat infected skin. Advise the client to first see a dermatologist to medically treat the infection.

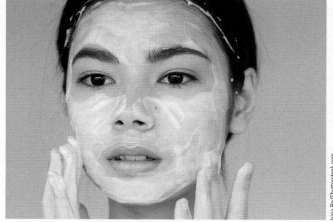

▲ **FIGURE 8–55** Proper home-care is essential for the treatment of acne.

Irina Bg/Shutterstock.com

Home care will include a cleanser, an exfoliant, a mask, a toner, a light-weight hydrator, and a full-spectrum sun protection cream. In addition:

- Make sure recommended ingredients are not irritating or contra-indicated.
- A foaming or gel cleanser with an exfoliant (AHA, salicylic acid, or benzoyl peroxide) is the best choice. Use an astringent with alcohol to prevent infection.
- Apply a light, hydrating, oil-free moisturizer and sunscreen for balance and protection.
- A clay mask is recommended twice per week. A mask with camphor and sulfur also works well for oily skin.
- Other products may include a hydrating, soothing mask to balance the drying products.

All home care includes an analysis of lifestyle to help the client better understand what some of their acne triggers might be. (See Chapter 4, Disorders and Diseases of the Skin.) By understanding the causes, the client is better prepared to follow a home care program.

CAUTION!
Performed incorrectly, extraction can cause excessive skin damage, infection, and scarring.

Extraction Techniques

Practicing proper extraction methodology is one of the most important skills an esthetician must learn. Furthermore, each state in the United States has specific requirements for esthetic training and subsequent licensing, and each state regulates the type of treatment and implements permissible by state law. You must check with your individual state board to thoroughly understand the number of training hours and types of implements allowed in order for you to perform extractions as a licensed esthetician.

IMPORTANCE OF INFECTION CONTROL

Proper infection control is essential when performing extractions, and the process must be correctly executed before, during, and after for each treatment. A sterilizer or autoclave completely kills all microorganisms—including bacteria, viruses, fungi, and bacterial spores—with highly pressurized steam. All reusable implements should be placed in the autoclave between treatments. If you don't have a sterilizer or autoclave, use only disposable implements and dispose of these after every use so there is no risk of cross-contamination (**Figure 8–56**). In addition, a high-frequency machine is a useful and unique tool for acne-prone skin, helping prevent secondary lesions and decreasing the appearance of inflammation.

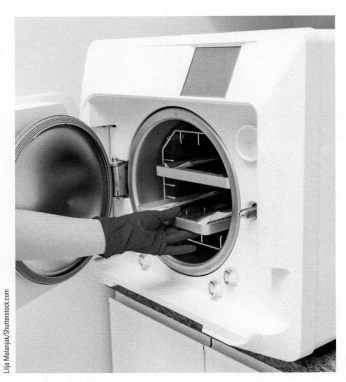

Lilja Malanjak/Shutterstock.com

▲ **FIGURE 8–56** An autoclave completely kills all microorganisms.

EXTRACTION TRAINING

In treating acne or blemished skin, the most important step for the esthetician is the effective cleansing and removal of blemishes. When the follicles are properly cleansed, the client's skin will begin to show marked improvement. It is important to explain to the client that you cannot always remove all blemishes during one treatment.

Training and caution are needed before performing extractions. The skin must be exfoliated and warmed before extractions are performed. It is also imperative that the esthetician wear gloves during extractions and then change the gloves before performing the rest of the facial to prevent the spread of infection. Protective eyewear is also recommended in some instances. Proper extraction procedures are necessary to safely extract oil and debris from the follicles. Do not practice extractions without prior instruction or training. Gloves must be worn at all times.

EXTRACTION METHODS

There are four methods to use for extractions: forefingers wrapped with gauze; cotton swabs; comedone extractors, and lancets (**Figure 8–57**). For the first three methods, press gently around the lesion.

- Manual comedone removal—gauze wrapped around gloved fingers, dampened with astringent—is useful for the majority of extractions.
- Comedone extractors are metal tools used for open comedones and sebaceous filaments.
- Cotton swabs are smaller than fingertips and are especially useful around the nose area.
- Lancets are for the removal of milia or pustules (check with your state board to see if this is permissible). *Important note:* Cysts and nodules must be treated by a dermatologist.

To achieve optimum success when performing extractions, you must put pressure on the skin surrounding the follicular wall so that you can extract the impaction with the least trauma to the surrounding tissue. Understanding the angle of the various follicles in the different locations on the skin will enable you to perform extractions easily and effectively.

TREATMENT FOR MILIA (CLOSED COMEDONES)

As discussed in Chapter 4, Diseases and Disorders of the Skin, milia are small epidermal cysts and are often referred to as *tiny whiteheads*. Milia usually occur around the eyes, upper surface of the cheeks, and forehead. Your clients may have tried to get them cleaned out themselves,

DID YOU KNOW?

All areas of the forehead, the top of the nose, the chin, and the jawline have follicular walls perpendicular to the surface of the skin. The follicles are positioned this way on all flat surfaces. All other areas of the skin, such as the sides of the nose and cheeks, have slanted follicular shafts.

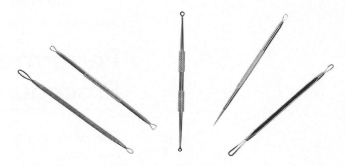

▲ **FIGURE 8–57** A metal comedone extractor is an effective tool for extractions.

─PERFORM─
Procedure 8-7
Performing Extractions

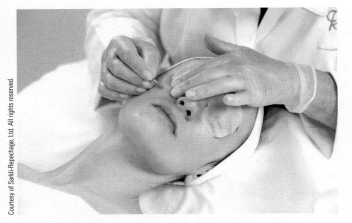

but with no luck. This is because milia are keratinized sebum trapped under the skin surface, and although it looks like it can be extracted easily, you may need the help of a lancet to get the milia out. A lancet is a small, sharp, pointed needle used to make a tiny opening in the epidermis to expose the milia (**Figure 8–58**). Always use a new sterile sealed lancet. Be sure the seal has not been broken. Again, a lancet is permissible only with permission by the state board. Improper lancet use may scar the skin, or may cause infection.

▲ **FIGURE 8–58** A lancet aids in the extraction of milia.

 CHECK IN

13. List four acne care tips you can suggest for clients with acne.
14. Explain the methods that can be used for extractions as permitted in your state.

Perform an Acne Treatment Procedure

The following is a basic outline of a facial that incorporates deep cleansing, comedone extraction, and skin balancing treatments that will help oily, problematic skin get back on track to a beautiful, healthy complexion. Some steps may be omitted or rearranged, depending on the treatment goals and the client's needs.

Products you will need:

- Comedone extractor
- Cotton
- Cotton squares
- Cotton swabs
- Eye pads
- Fresh linens
- Trash can (with closing lid)

- Gauze
- Gloves
- Hand cream
- Lancet (where permissible by state law)
- Makeup remover
- Mixing bowl
- Robe for the client

- Scissors
- Sharps container
- Sink or basin of water
- Spatula
- Unscented tissues

Step 1. Wash hands and put on gloves.

Step 2. Perform deep cleansing.

Cleanse skin using a soap-free formula that deep cleanses without causing dryness, preferably one that contains salicylic acid to gently exfoliate the skin (**Figure 8–59**). Cleansers should also contain soothing ingredients such as seaweed and green, white, and rooibos teas.

Step 3. Analyze the skin.

Use a magnifying lamp to check for open pores, open and closed comedones, pustules, milia, or any redness or irritation. If skin is irritated or sensitive, skip steaming.

Step 4. Steam and apply serum.

Steam the face while applying a gentle skin serum that combines exfoliating ingredients such as alpha and beta hydroxy acids with softening ingredients such as seaweed and natural extracts that help calm the appearance of the skin such as chamomile and lavender. This can be applied in gentle effleurage movements.

Step 5. Proceed with desincrustation.

Soften the outermost layer of the skin before proceeding with extraction. This is because clients are often using dehydrating ingredients such as hydrogen peroxide on their skin at home to treat their acne pimples. The esthetician will most likely find that while the skin is oily, the skin is extremely tight with a lot of dead skin cell accumulation. Even the sebum inside the pores is dried out and dehydrated! You can injure the client's skin at this point if you try to extract a blackhead (open comedone) in this state. The desincrustation solution is the first step in softening the sebum in order to perform a gentle but thorough extraction (**Figure 8–60**).

Step 6. Perform extractions.

The most important skill an esthetician must master is proper extraction. It must be performed in such a way as to not cause further damage to the skin or make the acne worse. Refer to **Procedure 8–7: Performing Extractions** for the full instructions on performing extractions. Choose an extraction method that is permitted by your state (manual comedone removal, comedone extractors, cotton swabs, or lancets are for removal of milia or pustules). Put pressure on the skin surrounding the

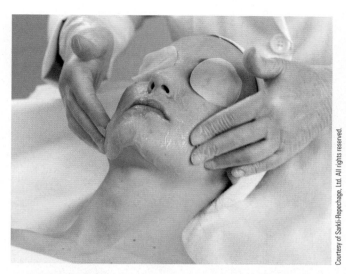

▲ **FIGURE 8–59** Perform deep cleansing of the skin.

DID YOU KNOW?

Remember, the clogging in the sebaceous gland is a keratinaceous plug. Keratin is a hard protein like that found in your hair. We have to soften this keratin before we can do our extraction. It's like opening a bottle with a cork. Before you can remove the contents, you have to remove the cork.

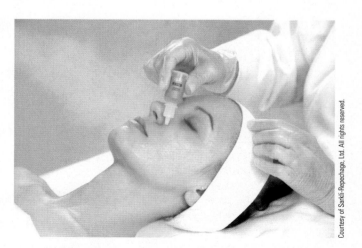

▲ **FIGURE 8–60** Desincrustation is the first step in softening the sebum.

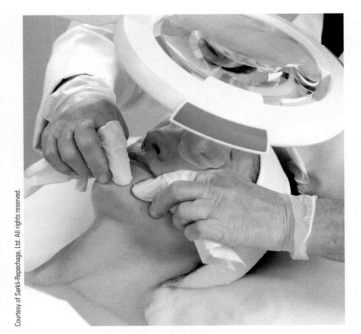

▲ **FIGURE 8–61** Perform extractions.

follicular wall so that you can extract the impaction with the least trauma to the surrounding tissue (**Figure 8–61**).

Step 7. Apply astringent/toner.

Now that extractions have been completed, saturate esthetics wipes with astringent that contains a salicylic acid–tea blend to soothe skin. Applying astringent is critical following extractions to help cleanse the skin, thereby reducing the possibility of secondary infection, and to rehydrate the skin. Do not rub the astringent in, but apply it lightly, paying special attention to the areas where you extracted.

Step 8. Apply a clay-based mask for deep cleansing. Remove with towels.

Follow with a clay-based mask to help deep cleanse the pores while helping to make skin feel soothed (**Figure 8–62**). Look for a mask that contains sea mud, zinc, and kaolin to help promote surface desquamation and help remove excess oils and debris which may contribute to breakouts. There may be some residual blood left on the skin from the extraction process so continue wearing gloves and apply the mask with a spatula. Leave on for seven to ten minutes and remove by applying warm, moist cotton or towels over the entire face, letting the moisture soak in for a moment, then removing the mask using quick, gentle strokes. Remove any residue with astringent and esthetics wipes.

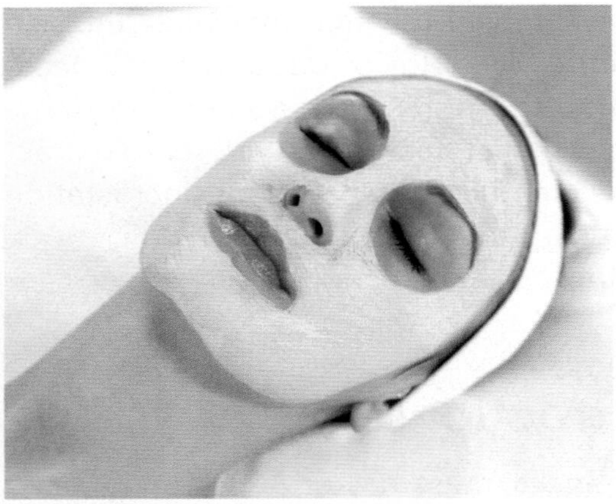

▲ **FIGURE 8–62** Clay-based mask application.

DID YOU KNOW?

Never force extractions

Most clients will tolerate only 10 minutes of extractions. Check to make sure they are comfortable with the procedure if you intend to work longer. Once the skin becomes dry and resistant, it is time to stop the procedure. At the end of your service, book the client's next appointment so that you can continue their extractions during their next treatment.

Step 9. Apply a soothing mask. Remove with wet cotton.

Follow with a soothing mask, such as a calamine mask combined with tea extracts, zinc, and organic buttermilk powder to help reduce the appearance of redness on the skin (**Figure 8–63**). Leave on for

10 minutes and perform a relaxing 10-minute hand massage. Your client will appreciate it after the extractions!

After 10 minutes, remove the mask with wet cotton and clean warm water. Follow up with an astringent that helps tone the skin's appearance. *Note:* A client should never leave the salon with red, irritated skin after a facial treatment.

Step 10. Apply moisturizer.

After masks, we are ready for a moisturizer that does not clog skin while it helps to lessen the appearance of oil. Remember that the client was just deep cleansed and is about to go out into the environment. It is key for the client's skin to be moisturized upon completion of the facial treatment to further reduce dryness and the appearance of irritation. Use a mattifying moisturizer that is formulated with zinc as well as squalane, a moisturizing ingredient found in sebum as essential fatty acids to help restore moisture yet reduce oil and shine.

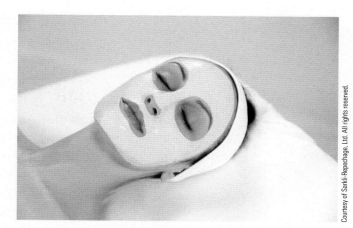

▲ **FIGURE 8–63** Calamine mask application.

Step 11. Perform galvanic or high-frequency treatment.

High-frequency germicidal rays can be applied to the skin for faster healing time of lesions and prevention of secondary infections. (Again, please check with your local and state boards regarding use of galvanic and high-frequency devices.) Contraindications to using high frequency include pregnancy, high blood pressure and/or heart conditions, and patients with a high amount of metal in their mouth from dental procedures. Place your index finger on the electrode and apply to the client's entire face in circular motions, moving over the entire face for a total of three to five minutes (**Figure 8–64**). Remove the index finger when the electrode makes contact with the skin. You can also target specific areas by lifting the electrode on and off the skin. You may also incorporate this step right after extractions.

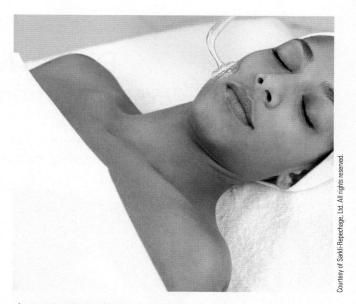

▲ **FIGURE 8–64** High frequency treatment.

Step 12. Finish with the post-treatment consultation.

Education and knowledge are key in helping clients with problem, oily skin. The client should be advised of the importance of in-salon treatments and following a home care program especially designed for them. Additional important points to cover:

- Break bad habits such as picking and squeezing the skin.
- Overcleansing can be detrimental to acne-prone skin. It can further irritate the skin, stripping essential moisture and causing inflammation and additional risk of infection.
- Maintain a healthy diet. New research has found that dairy and fermented or yeast-based foods can exacerbate acne conditions. These include aged cheeses, highly processed milk, wine, beer, champagne, and mushrooms. Skin care experts now recommend probiotics to counteract unhealthy bacteria living in the stomach lining and the resulting inflammation that can increase acne flare-ups.
- Avoid sunbathing, and not just because of the damaging UV light. Once considered part of an acne treatment program, UV light can initially dry up excess sebum and reduce pustules, but can lead to a cascade of reactions that actually increase oil production and sebum buildup on the skin.

 CHECK IN

15. Explain steps to take before extractions.
16. What are the four important points to cover in the post-treatment consultation with a client who has acne?

Discuss Men's Skin Care Treatment Options

As men now are spending more time and money than ever before on improving their appearance as they seek success in both their professional and social lives, estheticians need to educate themselves on the key differences between male and female skin needs. A major skin complaint spa owners hear from their male clientele is razor burn. Men tend to have sensitive skin that they have mistreated for years. The spa is the place to educate them on how to shave properly and to protect their skin before and after shaving.

Traits of Men's Skin

Men often have larger pores and more active sebaceous glands. Their skin tends to be characterized by excess oil and numerous blackheads (**Figure 8–65**). At the same time, male skin often can become dehydrated from harsh soaps and shampoos, as well as from frequent hot showers.

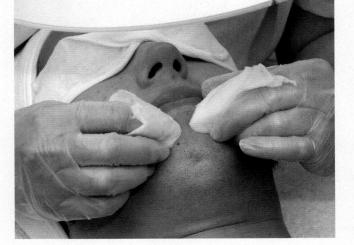
▲ **FIGURE 8–65** Men's skin can be characterized by excess oil and blackheads.

Ironically, their skin can both be excessively oily and have surface dryness. Men need products and treatments that are hydrating but also offer deep pore cleansing and pore refining.

Men also are concerned with aging. They often have hyperpigmentation from years of outdoor activities without wearing sunscreen. They may have crow's feet and dark under-eye circles from long days spent squinting at computer screens. The baby boomer male is being confronted with middle age. In addition, male millennials, now moving into the 25-plus age group, are coming into the workplace with a more evolved approach toward grooming, where it's okay to care about the condition of the skin.

FOCUS ON

Tips for Men's Treatments

- Avoid using perfumed and fragrant products in the facial room. Men already may be feeling a bit apprehensive about having a facial, so keep the service as clean and simple as possible. Cater to specific needs by incorporating grooming services such as trimming or waxing eyebrows, nostril hair, and ear hair.
- Men do not want to walk out of a spa with red, blotchy skin caused by an aggressive extraction session. Additional services to calm skin, apply products, and even concealing makeup should be considered.
- When deciding on a retail line for males, keep in mind the kinds of packaging that many men prefer. It should not be pink or red, but, rather, sleek and simple. Choose products that can be sprayed on quickly, and swap jars for bottles with pumps so they can be easily packed in gym bags and for trips.
- Retail products should be merchandised to emphasize qualities such as nongreasy, rinses off easily, and protects the skin. *Perfume-free, color-free, calming,* and *stress-reducing* are good buzzwords to use when describing offerings that will appeal to men.

Marketing to Men

Men's skin care needs are just as important as women's. It is becoming more common for men to use spa services and to take care of their skin. Estheticians need to take a simple, direct approach when discussing skin care with their male clients (**Figure 8–66**). Men, in general, want to use only a few products on a daily basis.

Male clients are willing to follow suggestions and want a basic, consistent routine. They tend to be loyal customers. Male clients represent a growing percentage of a spa's business. The challenge is to attract male clients so that they will make the initial visit in the first place.

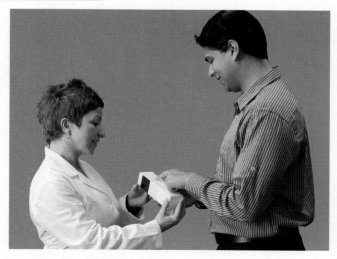

▲ **FIGURE 8–66** Take a direct approach when discussing skin care with male clients.

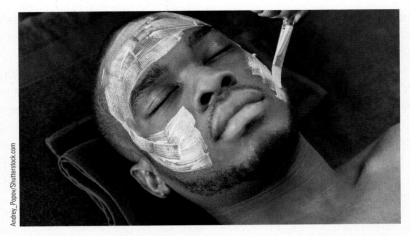

▲ **FIGURE 8–67** The male skin care market continues to grow.

DID YOU KNOW?

Using the term *skin treatment* rather than the term *facial* is a better way to promote men's services.

One way to attract male clientele is to offer special services designed just for them. Make them feel comfortable, and tactfully assure them that it is normal for men to have spa services and practice good skin care habits. Conduct consultations privately, without discussing products and treatments out in the reception area where other clients may be present. Some salons and spas cater to men only. The male market will continue to grow as men feel more comfortable about receiving services (**Figure 8–67**). In fact, there is a rising trend of barbershop services that provide skin care treatments after shaving.

Men's Skin Care Products

To build the market, a salon or spa could carry a specific line of men's skin care products. Most unisex product lines will work as long as the packaging and fragrance are not overly feminine. Men typically have larger sebaceous glands and oilier skin. They also need sun protection. Men may tend to neglect their skin care because it is not considered masculine or a priority. Clients who are especially pleased with visible treatment results are more willing to try a home-maintenance program.

When considering a men's skin care line, keep in mind several key points. Be sure the products are basic and the routines are simple (**Figure 8–68**). Men do not want highly fragranced, feminine products. For instance, lotions need to be light, be without fragrance, be highly absorbent, and have a matte finish. Most men do not like the greasy feeling of some products.

Men prefer simple routines and multipurpose products. They would rather have a moisturizer that they can use day and night, or one that

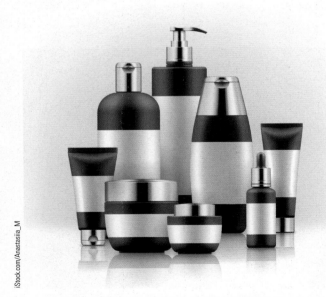

▲ **FIGURE 8–68** Products should be basic with simple routines.

already contains full-spectrum sunscreen. They also like the foaminess of soaps, so a foaming cleanser is a good choice. They can use a toner just like they would an aftershave lotion. They should then apply a light moisturizer with sunscreen. Give male clients specific instructions on how and when to use products.

Keep the following tips in mind when working with male clients:

- Tubes and pumps that are easy to open are more male-friendly than jars are.

- His home care regimen should begin with only two products: a cleanser and a hydrating lotion. If he wants three, add sunscreen.

- As he grows accustomed to the regimen and sees favorable results, he will most likely add to his regimen by purchasing a toner, eye cream, and a mask.

- Educate him on sun protection and skin-cancer facts, even if he chooses not to purchase sunscreen.

- Estheticians can suggest that male clients shave in a downward direction—in the direction of the hair growth pattern—because it is less irritating.

- Once he is accustomed to receiving treatments and using products, your male client will be more likely to use an eye cream if he is taught how. While men may be conscious of lines and wrinkles around their eyes, they seldom request an eye product. Estheticians can point out the benefits of these and other products.

Professional Treatments for Men

Depending on the client's skin conditions, you can offer various treatments. Most men love steam and the brush machine (**Figure 8–69**). Even if a client's skin is slightly sensitive, he will prefer the assertiveness of a brush and foamy cleanser. A firmer touch and deeper massage are also needed on male skin.

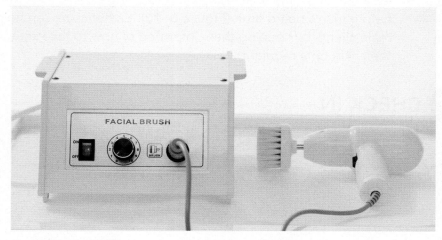

▲ **FIGURE 8–69** The brush machine is a popular treatment for male clients.

There are some other important aspects of men's facials. First, sponges and towels are more appropriate for a man's face. Cotton pads and gauze will grab the beard hair, leaving particles clinging to the face. Shaving before a facial actually makes the skin more sensitive. On freshly shaven skin, exfoliating products or techniques, including strong sensitizing agents such as alpha hydroxy acids and microdermabrasion, may be contraindicated.

Professional movements during a man's facial should flow with the hair growth. For example, most massage movements in the beard area should move downward, not upward. This goes against the typical esthetic procedure of lifting movements up the neck and face. Overall, the beard area tends to be relatively sensitive due to shaving lotions that contain perfume, alcohol, or other similar substances. Shaving itself is also quite abrasive to the skin, so men need more calming and healing products.

FOLLICULITIS

Folliculitis (fah-lik-yuh-LY-tis) is inflammation of the hair follicles. This can be a problem for many men, especially if they have very coarse or curly beard hair. Folliculitis is an infection characterized by inflammation and pus. Improper shaving may also cause **folliculitis barbae** (fah-lik-yuh-LY-tis BAR-bay), where the hair grows slightly under the skin and is trapped there, causing a bacterial infection. The treatment goal for this condition is to alleviate the irritation, dry up and disinfect the pustules, and desensitize the area. A soothing gel mask is probably the most comfortable product for a male client to use in this area.

Pseudofolliculitis (SOO-doe-fah-lik-yuh-LY-tis), also known as *razor bumps*, resembles folliculitis without the infection. This condition also results from improper shaving techniques.

There are products on the market for ingrown hairs that help exfoliate and keep the follicles clean. Exfoliating is necessary to keep the follicles open. A foaming cleanser will also help a man's beard area (**Figure 8–70**). Estheticians can help male clients by keeping them informed of how to take care of their skin on a regular basis.

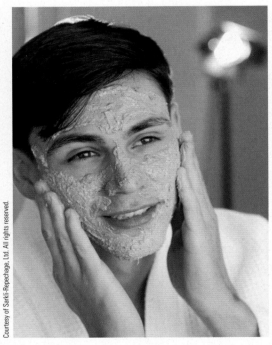

▲ **FIGURE 8–70** A foaming cleanser will more easily cleanse the beard area.

Web Resources

www.cosmeticsandtoiletries.com
www.dayspa.com
www.lneonline.com
www.skininc.com

 CHECK IN

17. What are the key points to consider when choosing skin care products for men?

Procedure 8-1:
Pre-Service—Preparing the Client for Treatment

After the successful completion of this procedure, you will be able to demonstrate a professional client draping.

Equipment, Implements, and Products

Note: Actual products will vary depending on the client's recommended treatment plan. Refer to full list of supplies for a basic facial on page 262.

EQUIPMENT
- ☐ Facial equipment (towel warmer, steamer, magnifying lamp)
- ☐ Covered trash container

IMPLEMENTS
- ☐ 1 Headband/ protective cap
- ☐ 1 Bowl warm water
- ☐ 2 Hand towels
- ☐ 2 Twin-size flat bed sheets
- ☐ 2 Disposable brushes
- ☐ 1 Rubber mixing bowl
- ☐ Blanket
- ☐ Bolster

- ☐ Client charts
- ☐ Gloves
- ☐ Gown or wrap
- ☐ Hair pins
- ☐ Liquid soap (at sink area)
- ☐ Plastic bag for jewelry
- ☐ Pillow and pillowcase
- ☐ Robe
- ☐ Slippers
- ☐ Spatulas

PRODUCTS
- ☐ 1 Cleanser
- ☐ 1 Astringent or toner
- ☐ 1 Moisturizer
- ☐ 1 Serum
- ☐ Mask(s)

Preparation

Perform Procedure 7–1: Pre-Service—Preparing the Treatment Room to set up the treatment room and supplies.

Procedure

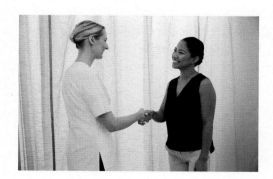

1 Greet the client in the reception area with a warm smile and in a professional manner. Introduce yourself if you've never met, make eye contact, and shake hands. Be sure your handshake is firm and sincere.

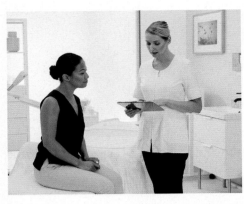

2 Discuss the completed client intake form with the client and confirm their service. Ask about any client concerns and set the expectations for today's service.

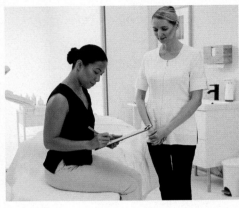

3 Ensure there are no contraindications for the treatment scheduled. Have your client sign a consent form before every service.

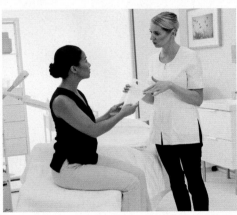

4 Escort the client to the dressing area or the treatment room to change. Inform the client where to place personal items. Ask the client to remove all jewelry and place in a sealable plastic bag to secure items. Due to liability issues do not handle the client's jewelry. Have the client remove contact lenses as well (optional, if wearing them).

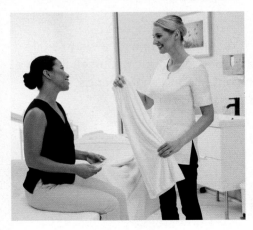

5 Provide them with a robe, spa wrap, and slippers. Explain which clothing may need to be removed and show them how to put on the spa wrap. Indicate where to go once they have changed. Then allow them to undress privately. Always knock before re-entering the room.

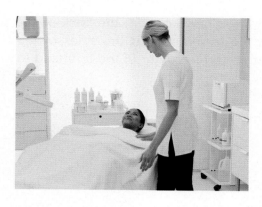

6 Depending on the service to be performed, instruct the client to lie either face down or face up on the treatment table or to take a seat in the treatment chair.

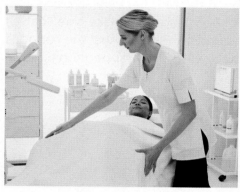

7 Place a bolster under the bottom sheet, below their knees, to relieve pressure on the lower back if they are facing up. (This alleviates pressure on the lower back.) If your client is facing down, place a rolled towel or small bolster under their ankles.

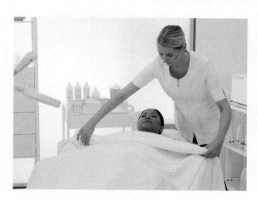

8 Bring the second sheet up and blanket across the décolleté. Then place a hand towel across the chest on top of the covers.

9 Secure a disposable headband, towel, or other head covering around the client's head to protect the hair, making sure all the hair is off the face. To drape the head with a towel, follow steps a, b, and c.

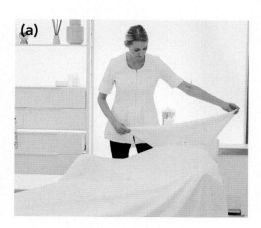
(a)

a. During setup in Procedure 7–1, you placed a hand towel on the headrest. Fold the towel into a triangle from one of the top corners to the opposite lower corner, and place it over the headrest with the fold facing down.

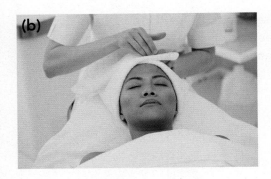

b. When the client is in a reclined position, the back of the head should rest on the towel, so that the sides of the towel can be brought up to the center of the forehead to cover the hairline.

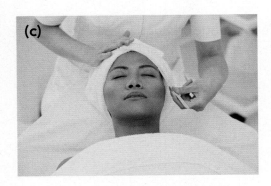

c. Use a disposable headband to hold the towel in place. Use a spatula or the edge of your finger to make sure that all strands of hair are tucked under the towel, that the earlobes are not bent, and that the towel is not wrapped too tightly.

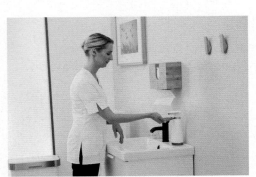

10 Wash your hands with soap and warm water as detailed in Procedure 5–3: Proper Hand Washing located in *Milady Standard Foundations*. Always wash your hands and put on gloves before starting any treatment.

11 Proceed with the next steps in your facial treatment.

Procedure 8-2:
Remove Eye Makeup and Lipstick

Equipment, Implements, and Products

Gather the following supplies and products for this procedure:

IMPLEMENTS
- ☐ Liquid hand soap and hand sanitizer
- ☐ Covered waste container
- ☐ Facial towels
- ☐ Headband and headwrap
- ☐ Clean linens
- ☐ Bolster
- ☐ Plastic sealable bag for personal items

SINGLE-USE ITEMS
- ☐ Gloves
- ☐ Esthetics wipes (4" × 4" or 2" × 2" cotton or gauze pads) or disposable sponges
- ☐ Cotton swabs
- ☐ Spatula
- ☐ Tissues (unscented)

PRODUCTS
- ☐ Eye makeup remover or cleanser
- ☐ Facial cleanser

Eye and Makeup Removal Preparation

Perform Procedure 7–1: Pre-Service—Preparing the Treatment Room and Procedure 8–1: Pre-Service—Preparing the Client for Treatment.

Procedure

A. EYE MAKEUP REMOVAL

Note: If the client is wearing contacts, do not remove the eye makeup. Be especially gentle when cleansing the eyes because the skin around the eyes is very sensitive and can become irritated. Do not get cleanser into the eyes.

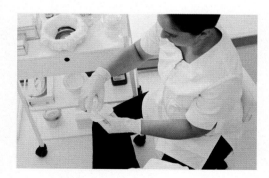

1 Saturate two cotton rounds with a mild cleanser (usually a pH of 7.0–7.2 is recommended) or makeup remover. You also have the choice of using gloved hands to apply the cleanser.

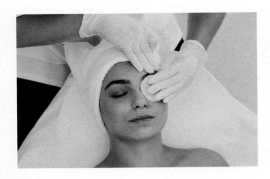

2 Ask the client to close their eyes. Start with the client's left eye. With one hand, gently raise and hold the client's eyebrow. With the cotton pad in your other hand, gently wipe across the top of the eyelid from the nose outward. Use downward movements with the cleansing pad to cleanse the eyelid and lashes. Gently rinse with cotton or gauze pads.

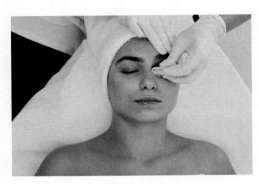

3 While cleansing the eyes, rotate the pad to provide a clean, unused surface. Repeat step 2 as necessary to remove eye makeup.

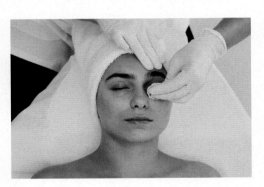

4 Wipe under the eyes, sweeping in toward the nose. Remove any makeup underneath the eyes and along the lash line with a cotton swab or pad. Place the edge of the pad under the lower lashes at the outside corner of the eye, and slide the pad toward the inner corner of the eye. The mascara will gradually work loose and can be wiped clean. Always be gentle around the eyes; never rub or stretch the skin, as it is very delicate and thin.

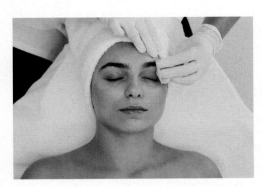

5 Make a complete circular pattern around the eye. Use the pad or a cotton swab to wipe inward under the eye toward the nose and then outward over the top of the eyelid.

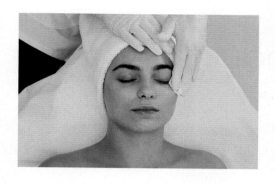

6 Rinse the eye area with a pad or cotton rounds soaked (not dripping) in warm water to remove the eye makeup remover. Make sure the remover is rinsed off thoroughly.

B. LIPSTICK REMOVAL

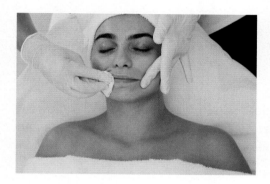

7 To remove the majority of the lipstick, first support the lip and wipe away the lipstick using a dry tissue, then discard the tissue.

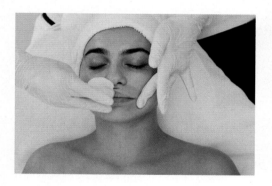

8 Then, apply cleanser to a gauze or cotton pad. With your left hand, hold taut the left side of the client's mouth. Wipe from the corner to the center to prevent the lipstick from being wiped out onto the skin surrounding the mouth.

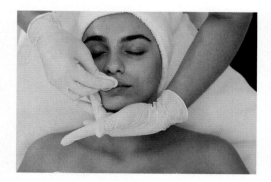

9 Repeat the procedure on the other side until the lips are clean. Proceed with the next step of the basic facial.

Procedure 8-3:
Applying a Cleansing Product

Equipment, Implements, and Products

IMPLEMENTS
- ☐ Hand sanitizer/hand soap
- ☐ Covered waste container
- ☐ Spatula
- ☐ Facial towels
- ☐ Headband and head wrap
- ☐ Clean linens
- ☐ Bolster

SINGLE-USE ITEMS
- ☐ Gloves
- ☐ Plastic resealable bag for personal items

PRODUCTS
- ☐ Eye makeup remover or cleanser
- ☐ Facial cleanser

The following method of application is used when applying cleansers, massage creams, treatment creams, serums, and protective products. If possible, use both hands at the same time for a more even and efficient technique. Use either circular motions or straight, even strokes for cleansing.

Preparation

- Perform Procedure 7–1: Pre-Service—Preparing the Treatment Room and Procedure 8–1: Pre-Service—Preparing the Client for Treatment.

Procedure

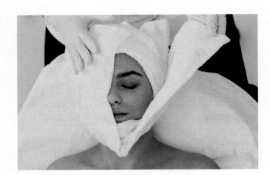

1 Apply warm towels (optional). Check the temperature and apply one towel to the décolleté and one to the face. Leave on for at least 1 minute and then remove.

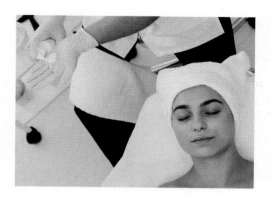

2 Choose a cleanser appropriate to the client's skin type. Use a spatula to remove the product from the container unless using a squirt or pump bottle. Apply approximately one teaspoon of the product to the fingers or palms of the hand and spread evenly between your gloved hands and fingertips.

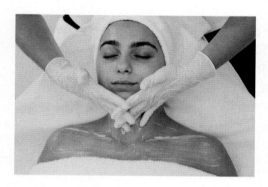

3 Use circular motions to distribute the product onto the fingertips. You are now ready to apply the product to the client's décolleté, neck, and face. Cleanse each area using six passes. If starting on the décolleté, start in the center and work out to the sides moving up to the neck. Be guided by your instructor.

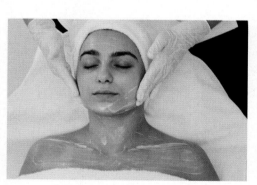

4 Start applying a small amount of the product by placing both hands, palms down, on the neck. Slide hands back toward the ears until the pads of the fingers rest at a point directly beneath the earlobes. While applying the product, it is suggested that hands are not lifted from the client's face until you are finished.

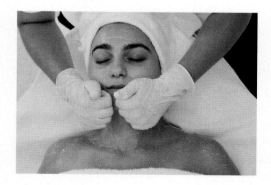

5 Reverse the hands, with the backs of the fingers now resting on the skin, and slide the fingers along the jawline to the chin.

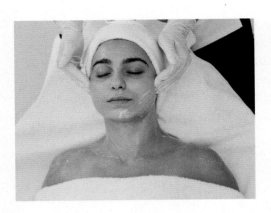

6 Reverse the hands again, and slide the fingers back over the cheeks and center of the face until the pads of the fingers come to rest directly in front of the ears.

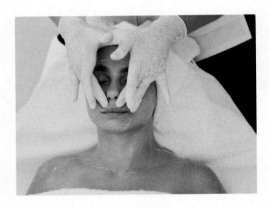

7 Reverse the hands again, and slide the fingers forward over the cheekbones to the nose. Cleanse the upper lip area under the nose with sideways strokes from the center area moving outward. Then slide up to the sides of the nose.

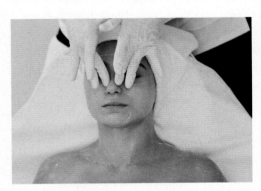

8 With the pads of the middle fingers, make small, circular motions on the top of the nose and on each side of the nose. Avoid pushing the product into the nose.

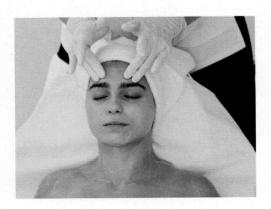

9 Slide the fingers up to the forehead and outward toward the temples, pausing with a slight pressure on the temples. Slide fingers across the forehead using circles or long strokes from side to side. Slowly lift your hands off the client's face.

10 Proceed to Procedure 8–4: Removing Products if the product used needs to be removed, for example, a cleanser or massage cream.

Procedure 8-4:
Removing Products

Implements and Products

☐ Gloves
☐ 4″ × 4″ Esthetics wipes, disposable sponges, or warmed towels from a hot towel cabinet

Removing Products

To remove products, rinse each area at least three to six times. Some estheticians prefer to use wet esthetics wipes when removing product. Others prefer to use towels. Both methods are correct and equally professional, and many estheticians use both methods.

Facial movements are generally done in an upward and outward direction from the center to the edges of the face.

Procedure

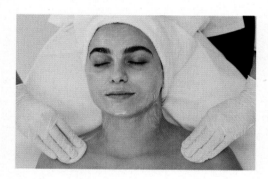

1 Starting at the décolleté, cleanse sideways and up to the neck. When removing the cleanser, mask, or exfoliant, you should make three passes or however many are necessary until no residual makeup shows.

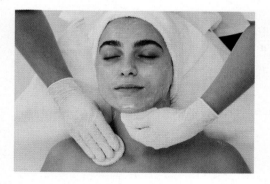

2 Cleanse the neck using upward strokes. To keep the pad from slipping from the hand, pinch the edge of the pad between the thumb and upper part of the forefinger. It is important that most of the surface of the pad remain in contact with the skin. Do not exert pressure on the Adam's apple in the center of the neck.

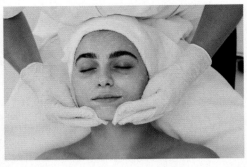

3 Starting directly under the chin, slide along the jawline, stopping directly under the ear. Repeat the movement on the other side of the face. Alternate back and forth three times on each side of the face, or do the movement concurrently by using both hands at the same time.

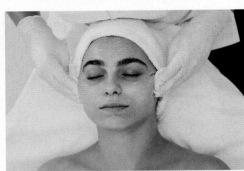

4 Starting at the jawline, use upward movements to cleanse the cheeks.

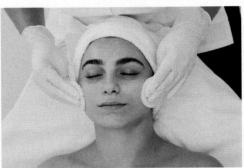

5 Continue the upward movement and cross over the chin to the other cheek if you are using only one hand.

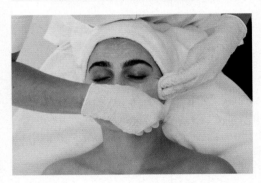

6 Continue the cleansing movement with approximately six strokes on each cheek.

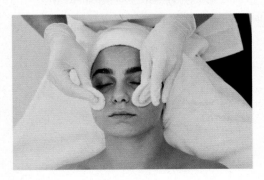

7 Under the eyes, use inward motions to avoid tugging at the eye area.

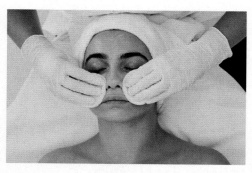

8 Cleanse the area directly underneath the nose by using downward and sideways strokes. Start at the center and work outward toward the corners of the mouth. Rinse at least three times on each side of the face.

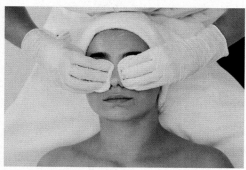

9 Starting on the bridge of the nose, cleanse the sides of the nose and the area directly next to it. Use light, outward movements.

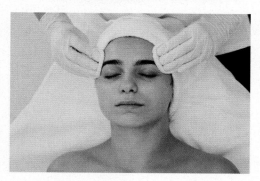

10 Starting at the center of the forehead, move outward to the temples. Apply a slight pressure on the pressure points of the temples. Repeat the movement three times on each side of the forehead.

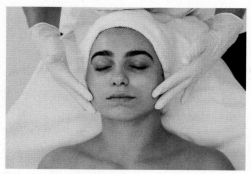

11 Check the face to make sure there is no residue left on the skin. Feather over the areas of the face with the fingertips to check that it is well rinsed. Discard all used supplies in the trash can.

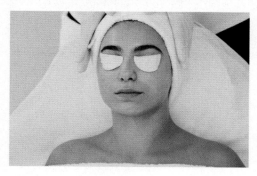

12 Cover the client's eyes with eye pads and prepare to perform the skin analysis.

Procedure 8-5:
Performing the Basic Facial

Equipment, Implements, and Products

EQUIPMENT
- ☐ Facial equipment (towel warmer, steamer, magnifying lamp)
- ☐ Sharps container

SUPPLIES
- ☐ EPA-registered disinfectant
- ☐ Hand sanitizer/ hand soap
- ☐ Covered trash container
- ☐ Bowls (if sink is not available)
- ☐ Spatulas
- ☐ Fan and mask brush (nonporous and must be able to be disinfected, e.g., nonwooden)

IMPLEMENTS
- ☐ Client charts
- ☐ Distilled water for steamer
- ☐ Hand towels
- ☐ Clean linens and blanket
- ☐ Headband/head wrap/or protective cap
- ☐ Client wrap
- ☐ Bolster

SINGLE-USE ITEMS
- ☐ Esthetics wipes (4" × 4" and 2" × 2" gauze or cotton) or disposable sponges
- ☐ Cotton rounds or squares
- ☐ Cotton swabs
- ☐ Paper towels
- ☐ Gloves
- ☐ Tissues (unscented)
- ☐ Distilled water for steamer

PRODUCTS
- ☐ Eye makeup remover
- ☐ Facial cleanser
- ☐ Optional: exfoliant
- ☐ Masks
- ☐ Massage lotion
- ☐ Toner
- ☐ Moisturizer
- ☐ Sunscreen
- ☐ Optional: serums, eye cream, lip balm, extraction supplies

Now that you have practiced the preliminary steps and cleansing, it is time to put it all together in a complete facial. The steps for performing a basic facial treatment are listed here. Facial procedures vary, so be guided by your instructor.

Preparation

- Perform Procedure 7–1: Pre-Service—Preparing the Treatment Room and Procedure 8–1: Pre-Service—Preparing the Client for Treatment.

- Preheat the steamer ahead of time. Check that the water level is at the appropriate fill line.

CAUTION!
Wearing gloves throughout the entire facial service is required by OSHA due to the possibility of bloodborne pathogen exposure. Never remove products from containers with your fingers. Always use a spatula. Do not touch fingertips to lids or openings of containers. Clean and disinfect product containers before and after each service.

Procedure

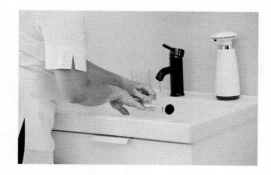

1 **Wash your hands and apply gloves.**

2 **Apply warm towels (optional step).** After checking the temperature, apply one towel to the décolleté and one to the face.

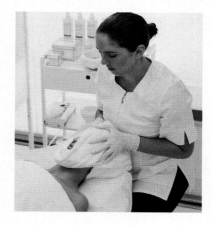

a. Hold the ends of the towels with both hands on either side of the face. Lay the center of the towel on the chin and drape each side across the face with the towel edges draped over to the opposite corner across the forehead.

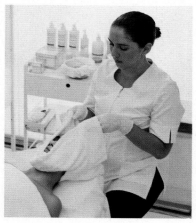

b. To remove, lift each end and remove. For product removal: Use the towels over the hands as mitts. Be guided by your instructor on this method.

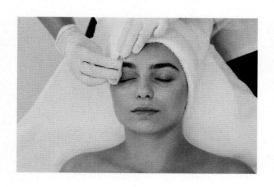

3 **Remove eye makeup and lipstick.** As learned in Procedure 8–2, remember to ask about contact lenses before putting product on the eyes. If the client is wearing contacts, do not remove the eye makeup.

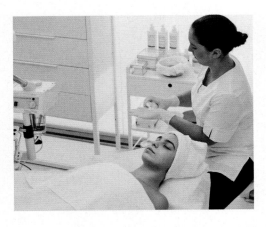

4 **Perform facial cleansing (steps 4 to 10).** Remove about one-half to one teaspoon of cleanser from the container (with a clean spatula if it is not a squirt-top or pump-type lid). Place it on the fingertips or in the palm and then apply a small amount to your gloved fingertips. This conserves the amount of product you use.

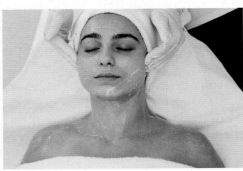

5 Starting at the neck or décolleté and with a sweeping movement, use both hands to spread the cleanser upward and outward on the chin, jaws, cheeks, and temples.

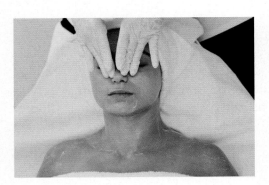

6 Spread the cleanser down the nose and along its sides and bridge. Continue to the upper lip area. Cleanse the upper lip area under the nose with sideways strokes from the center area moving outward.

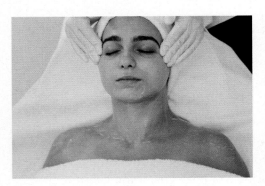

7 Make small, circular movements with the fingertips around the nostrils and sides of the nose. Continue with upward-sweeping movements between the brows and across the forehead to the temples.

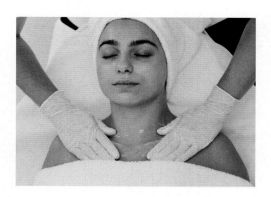

8 Apply more cleanser to the neck and chest with long, outward strokes. Cleanse the area in small, circular motions from the center of the chest and neck toward the outside, moving upward. Try to use both hands at the same time on each side when applying or removing product.

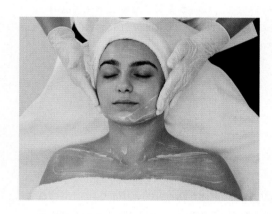

9 Visually divide the face into left and right halves from the center. Continue moving upward with circular motions on the face from the chin and cheeks, and up toward the forehead using both hands, one on each side.

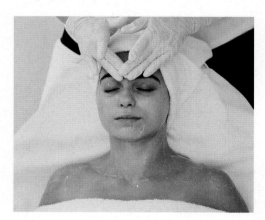

10 Starting at the center of the forehead, continue with the circular pattern out to the temples. Move the fingertips lightly in a circle around the eyes to the temples and then back to the center of the forehead. Lift your hands slowly off of the face when you finish cleansing.

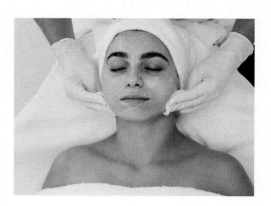

11 **Remove the cleanser.** Start at the neck or forehead and follow the contours of the face. Move up or down the face in a consistent pattern, depending on where you start, according to the instructor's procedures. Remove all the cleanser from one area of the face before proceeding to the next. (Under the nostrils, use downward strokes when applying or removing products to avoid pushing product up the nose. This is uncomfortable and will make the client tense.)

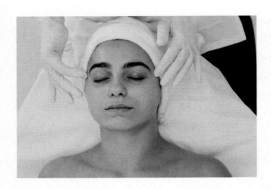

12 **Make sure there is no residue left on the skin.** Blot your hands on a clean towel, and touch the face with dry fingertips to check.

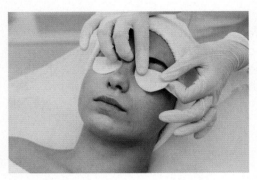

13 **Analyze the skin (steps 13 to 15).** Cover the client's eyes with eye pads. Try not to cover what you need to look at around the eyes.

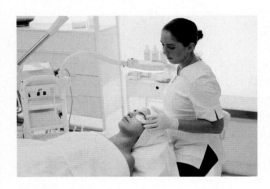

14 Position the magnifying light where you want it before starting the facial, so that you can easily maneuver it over the face. Turn on the lamp away from client before lining it up over the face.

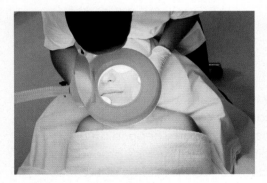

15 Note the skin type and condition, sensitivity, hydration, elasticity, and feel the texture of the skin. Remember to look, touch, ask and listen.

Based on the skin analysis, the remainder of the products will be selected as well as the treatment objectives.

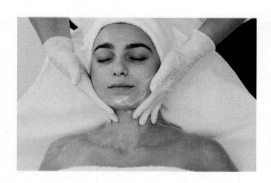

16 Cleanse the face again (optional). Some treatment protocols do not include this second cleansing. Be guided by your instructor.

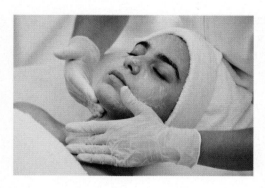

17 Exfoliation (optional). If exfoliation is part of the service, it could be done at this time while steaming. Tone after removing exfoliant to rebalance pH of the skin.

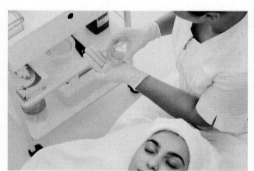

18 Massage the face (steps 18 to 22). Use the facial manipulations described in Chapter 9, Facial Massage. Select a water-soluble massage cream or product appropriate to the client's skin type.

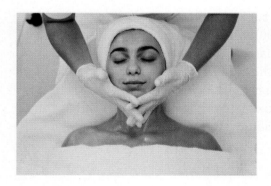

19 Use the same procedure as you did for product application to apply the massage cream to the face, neck, shoulders, and chest. Apply the warmed product in long, slow strokes with fingers or a soft fan brush, moving in a set pattern.

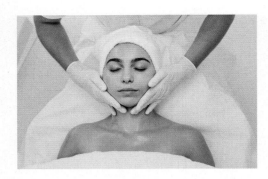

20 Perform the massage as directed.

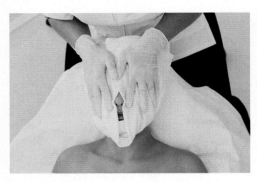

21 Remove the massage medium. Use warm towels or 4″ × 4″ esthetics wipes and follow the same procedure as for removing other products or cleanser.

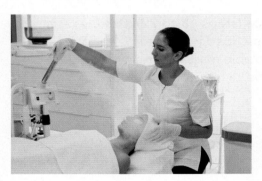

22 **Steam the face using the steamer (steps 22 and 23).** Skip to step 24 if using towels. The steamer should be preheated at the start of the facial. Wait for it to start steaming, and then turn on the second ozone button if applicable while steaming. (Remember that steam should be avoided on sensitive skin types.)

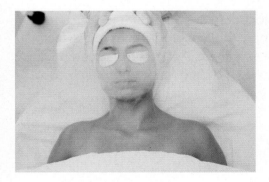

23 Check to make sure the steamer is not too close to the client (it should be approximately 18 inches away) and that it is steaming the face evenly. If you hold your hands close to the sides of the client's face, you can feel if the steam is reaching both sides of the face. Steam for approximately 5 to 10 minutes. Turn off the steamer immediately after use.

CAUTION!

Keep the steamer facing away from the client until it is steaming to avoid potential spitting of water, which may happen if the machine is overfilled or not maintained properly.

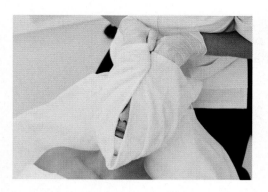

24 **Steam the face using towels.** If using towels in place of steam, remember to test them for the correct temperature. Ask the client if they are comfortable with the temperature. Towels are left on for approximately 2 minutes or until they begin to cool. Steam or warm towels should be used carefully on couperose skin.

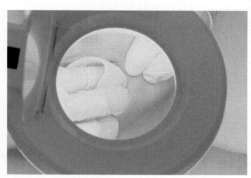

25 **Perform extractions (if needed).** Extractions are done immediately after the steam, while the skin is still warm. Refer to the extractions section of this chapter to incorporate this step into your basic facial procedure if it is applicable to your facility.

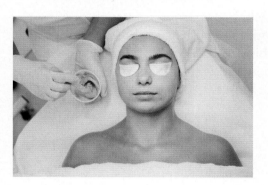

26 **Apply a mask (steps 26 to 29).** Choose a mask formulated for the client's skin condition. Remove the mask from its container, and place it in the palm or a small mixing bowl. (Use a clean spatula or brush, if necessary, to prevent cross-contamination.) Warming the mask is recommended for better results as well as the client's comfort.

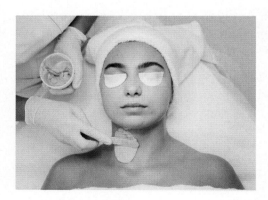

27 Apply the mask with a brush or spatula, usually starting at the neck. Use long, slow strokes from the center of the face, moving outward to the sides.

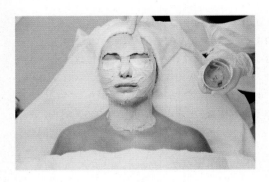

28 Proceed to the jawline and apply the mask on the face from the center outward. Avoid the eye area unless the mask is appropriate for that area.

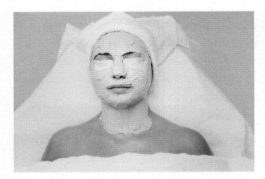

29 Allow the mask to remain on the face for approximately 7 to 10 minutes.

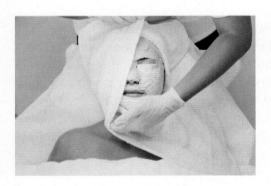

30 **Remove the mask.** Use warm moist towels or 4″ × 4″ esthetics wipes for removal. Cream-based masks can be wiped off, while clay masks can be removed with a mummy-style mask. Some masks may peel off, such as alginate or sheet masks.

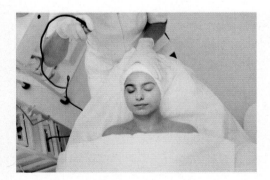

31 **Apply the toner.** Apply the toner product appropriate for the client's skin type.

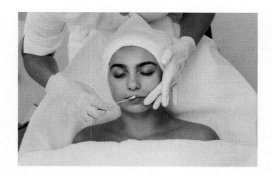

32 **Apply serums, as well as eye and lip treatments.** Serums as well as eye and lip creams are optional for application before the final moisturizer.

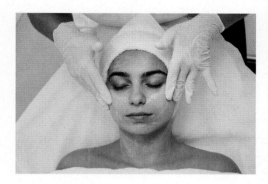

33 Apply a moisturizer (and an additional sunscreen as appropriate).

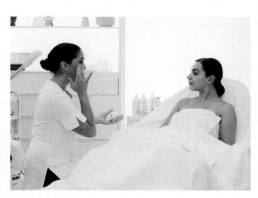

34 **Postconsultation and home care.** End the facial by removing your gloves, and quietly letting the client know you are finished. Give the client instructions for getting dressed. Have the client come out to the reception area when they are ready to discuss the home care products and regimen.

POST-SERVICE

* Complete Procedure 8–9: Post-Service Procedure and Procedure 7–2: Post-Service—Clean-Up and Preparation for the Next Client, including advising the client, promoting products, scheduling a next appointment, thanking the client, and cleaning and setting up the treatment room.

Procedure 8-6:
Applying and Removing the Cotton Compress

Implements and Products

- ☐ 4" × 4" Cotton squares
- ☐ Basin for clean water
- ☐ Product
- ☐ Tissues
- ☐ Toner

Note: This procedure is outdated but some licensing boards may still test on it.

Proper removal of facial masks is critical. By creating a cotton compress, also referred to as a cotton mummy mask, you are continuing the calming and soothing benefits of the facial. The use of disposable cotton will maintain a clean environment.

Procedure

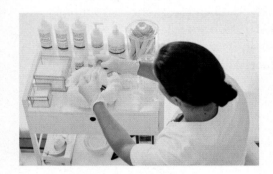

1 After the mask or product has set for the appropriate time, take one cotton 4" × 4" square, open to 4" × 8", and saturate with water.

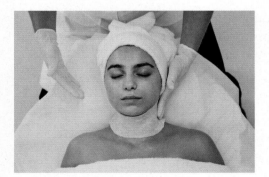

2 After squeezing out excess water, place the cotton lengthwise, first covering the neck.

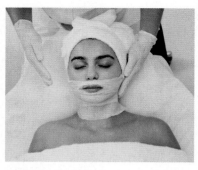

3 Saturate a second piece of cotton with water and make a small opening for the mouth. Place across the chin and mouth from one side of the mandible to the other just below the nose.

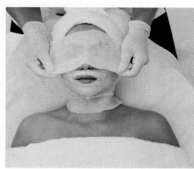

4 When placing the third piece of cotton over the bridge of the nose and across the eyes, be sure to leave the nostrils exposed and airways open.

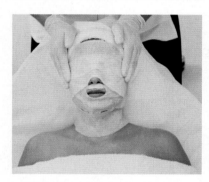

5 Place the fourth piece of wet cotton across the forehead, covering from temple to temple and cheek to cheek from one zygomatic bone to the other. Keep the cotton moist to help "loosen" mask for flawless removal, but not soaking wet to avoid dripping down the client's neck.

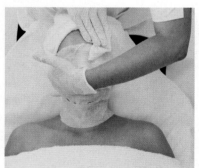

6 To remove the mummy mask, starting at the forehead, use a flat hand to wipe the product from one side of the face to the other. If you are right-handed, remove from left to right; if left-handed, right to left.

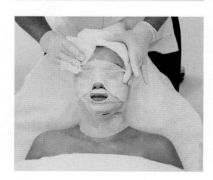

7 Fold the cotton under as you are removing the mask, as this will pick up more of the product and assist in quicker and cleaner removal.

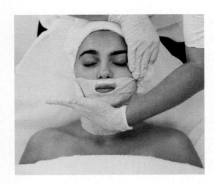

8 Repeat the same movement on the cheek and mandible area. Finish removing from your client's cheek and nose area.

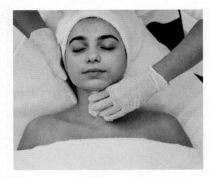

9 Remove the product and cotton from the neck. Use more cotton to remove any remaining residue.

10 Once residue is removed, refresh skin with hydrating mist or the appropriate toner/astringent, and then blot with tissue.

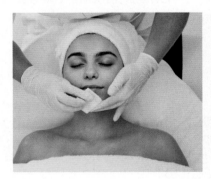 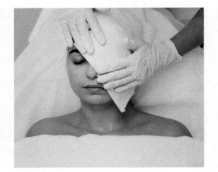

Procedure 8-7:
Performing Extractions

Implements and Products

- ☐ Esthetics wipes (4" × 4" or 2" × 2" gauze or cotton)
- ☐ Gloves
- ☐ Astringent
- ☐ Other appropriate facial supplies, products, and equipment
- ☐ Access to water or basin of water

- ☐ Cotton swabs
- ☐ Lancet
- ☐ Sharps container

Extractions are performed during a treatment only after the skin has been cleansed and prepared for comedone removal. This preparation can include exfoliation, desincrustation, and steaming. These methods help loosen the kertinaceous plugs within the follicle to help make the extractions easier. Never perform extractions for more than 10 minutes. It will make the client too uncomfortable and could be too aggressive to the skin.

Preparing Premade Pads

- If you are using 4"×4" or 2"×2" premade pads, apply astringent to pads (without oversaturating them) and wrap around your fingers. Always wear gloves during extractions and during the entire facial treatment.

Preparing for Extractions

Extractions must be performed in such a way as to not cause further damage to the skin or make the acne worse.

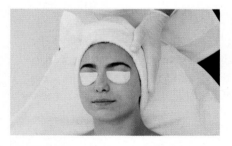

1 Wash hands and put on a new pair of gloves. Gloves are critical here because this is an invasive procedure.

2 Place eye pads over the client's eyes.

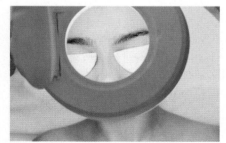

3 Position the magnifying lamp over the client's face. Always look through a magnifying lamp when performing extractions. This will protect you from any debris that come from the clogged pore. Again, advanced acne such as cysts and nodules should be treated only by a dermatologist.

4 Proceed with manual comedone removal, using the cotton swab technique, comedone extractor, or a lancet as permitted by your state board regulations.

A. MANUALLY REMOVING COMEDONES

Prepare the client's skin. Extractions are performed during a treatment after the skin is warmed and prepared/softened with product.

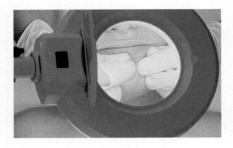

1 Wrap your fingers with cotton or gauze slightly moistened with a few drops of astringent at the tips.

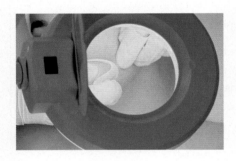

2 For proper removal of comedones, use the side of your fingertips to exert firm pressure on the skin surrounding the blackhead or comedone, applying slight pressure from side to side, alternating angles to gently lift the comedone from the follicle opening. Comedone extractors can also be used for this (be guided by your instructor). Do not squeeze with your nail, only the side of your finger.

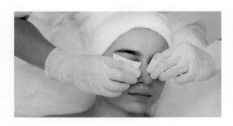

3 **Start at the chin.** On a flat area, press down, under, in, and up. Work around the plug, pressing down, in, and up. Bring fingers in toward each other around the follicle without pinching. Place the comedone on a tissue and proceed to other areas.

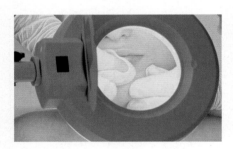

4 **Nose.** Slide fingers down each side of the nose, holding the nostril tissue firmly, but do not press down too firmly on the nose. The fingers on top do the sliding, while the other one holds close to the bottom of the follicle. Do not cut off the air flow to the nostrils.

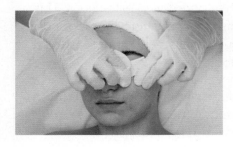

5 **Cheeks.** Slide fingers together down the cheek, holding each section of the skin as you go. The lower hand holds and the other hand slides toward the lower hand.

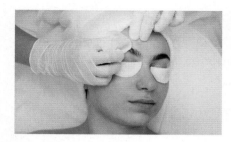

6 **Forehead; upper cheekbones.** Extract as on the chin: press down, in, and up.

7 Dispose of gloves and supplies properly. Change gloves to continue the facial treatment.

B. USING THE COTTON SWAB TECHNIQUE

An alternative to comedone removal is with cotton swabs.

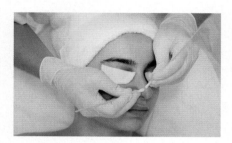

1 Hold the cotton swabs with your index finger and thumb and gently press down on both sides of the follicle.

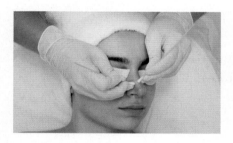

2 If the contents do not expel right away, move the swabs from side to side and the debris will gently lift up. Do not apply too much pressure, as it can bruise the client's skin. In both cases, if the contents are still not expelling, simply leave the comedone for the next treatment, and proceed to the next area of concern.

C. COMEDONE EXTRACTOR

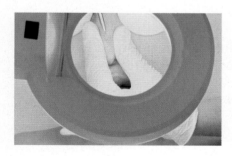

1 To use the comedone extractor, place the loop over the lesion so that the lesion is inside the loop.

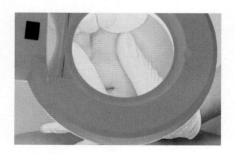

2 Press gently next to the lesion to push it up and out. Be aware that the pressure exerted can traumatize tissues. The follicle walls can rupture, spilling sebum and bacteria into the dermis. This debris can cause infection and irritation that leads to the start of even more blemishes.

D. EXTRACTING WITH LANCETS

Please check with your regulatory agency to see if you are permitted to use lancets in your state.

When a lesion is sealed over, as in old blackheads and closed comedones, a small-gauge needle or lancet is used for extraction.

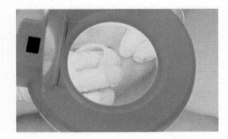

1 Wrap the index fingers with cotton or use sterile cotton swabs.

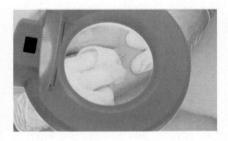

2 Hold the lancet parallel to the surface of the skin or at a 35-degee angle and gently pierce the skin horizontally to release sebum. If you prick into the skin in a downward motion, you can cause scarring.

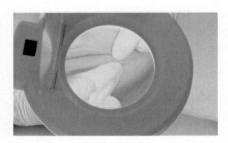

3 After piercing the skin horizontally, gently press down on both sides of the milia and remove it.

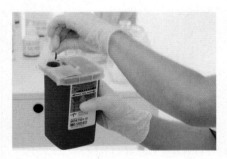

4 Dispose of the lancet in the biohazard containers also known as sharps boxes. Do not reuse the lancet.

Procedure 8-8:
Applying a Sheet Mask

Implements and Products

☐ Gloves
☐ Serums appropriate for client's skin (optional)
☐ Sheet mask
☐ Other appropriate facial supplies, products, and equipment

Procedure

When you have reached the masking step in the facial treatment, you will perform the following steps:

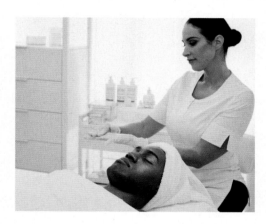

1 Apply the serum of your choice. (This is optional, as you may choose to just apply the sheet mask directly to the face.)

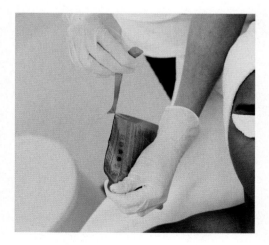

2 With a new pair of gloves, open the sheet mask packet and place the open packet on your station.

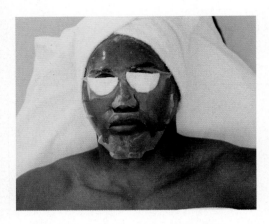

3 Beginning at the chin, remove the backing on the sheet mask. Apply the sheet mask in a uniform format, smoothing the mask onto the face such that the mask is optionally positioned to ensure all areas of the face are benefiting from the sheet mask.

4 Process the mask according to the manufacturer's recommended processing time.

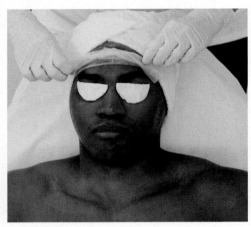

5 Remove the mask and proceed with the next steps in your facial treatment.

Procedure 8-9:
Post-Service Procedure

A. ADVISING CLIENTS AND PROMOTING PRODUCTS

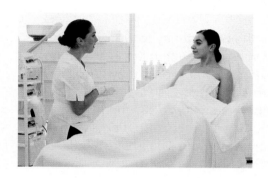

1 Before the client leaves your treatment area, ask them how they feel and if they enjoyed the service. Explain the conditions of their skin and your ideas about how to improve them. Be sure to ask if they have any questions or anything else they'd like to discuss. Be receptive and listen. Never be defensive. Determine a plan for future visits. Give the client ideas to think over for the next visit.

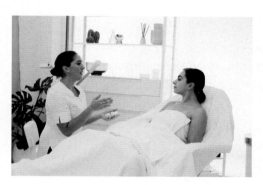

2 Advise the client about proper home care and explain how the recommended professional products will help to improve any skin conditions that are present. This is the time to discuss your retail product recommendations. Explain that these products are important and how to use them.

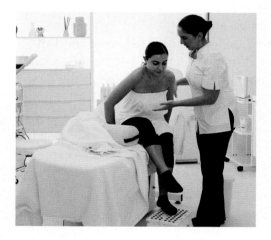

Schedule Next Appointment and Thank Client

3 Escort the client to the reception desk and write up a service ticket for the client that includes the service provided, recommended home care, and the next visit/service that needs to be scheduled. Place all recommended home care products on the counter for the client. Review the service ticket and the product recommendations with your client.

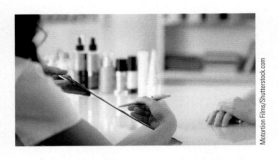

4 After the client has paid for their service and home care products, ask if you can schedule their next appointment. Set up the date, time, and type of service for this next appointment, write the information on your business card, and give the card to the client.

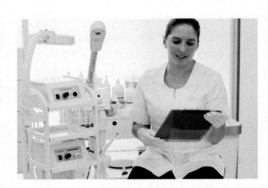

5 Thank the client for the opportunity to work with them. Express an interest in working with them in the future. Invite the client to contact you should they have any questions or concerns about the service provided. If the client seems apprehensive, offer to call them in a day or two in order to check in with them about any issues they may have. Genuinely wish them well, shake hands, and wish them a great day.

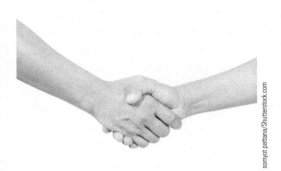

6 Be sure to record service information, observations, and product recommendations on the client record, and be sure you return it to the proper place for filing.

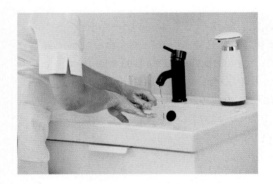

7 Continue with setting up for the next service or end-of-day checklist as outlined in Procedure 7–2: Post-Service— Clean-Up and Preparation for the Next Client.

COMPETENCY PROGRESS

How are you doing with facial treatments? **Check the Chapter 8 Learning Objectives below that you feel you have mastered; leave unchecked those objectives you will need to return to:**

☐ Explain the importance of facial treatments as the foundation for all skin care services.

☐ Describe the benefits of a facial treatment.

☐ List the essential skills needed to successfully perform facials.

☐ Perform the facial setup procedures.

☐ Explain the key steps of the basic facial treatment.

☐ Describe how to consult clients on home care.

☐ Discuss variations of the basic facial.

☐ Outline the treatment goals for six skin types/conditions (dry, dehydrated, mature, sensitive, hyperpigmentation and oily skin).

☐ Describe acne facials.

☐ Perform an acne treatment procedure.

☐ Discuss men's skin care treatment options.

☐ Perform the facial treatment procedures.

GLOSSARY

desincrustation dis-in-krus-TAY-shun	pg. 314	process used to soften and emulsify sebum and comedones (blackheads) in the follicles.
express facial ik-spres FAY-shul	pg. 321	a professional service designed to improve the appearance of the skin that takes less than 30 minutes
extraction EKS-trakt-shun	pg. 316	manual removal of impurities and comedones
facial FAY-shul	pg. 298	professional service designed to improve and rejuvenate the skin
vasoconstricting vay-zoh-kun-STRIK-ting	pg. 333	refers to something that causes vascular constriction of capillaries and reduced blood flow

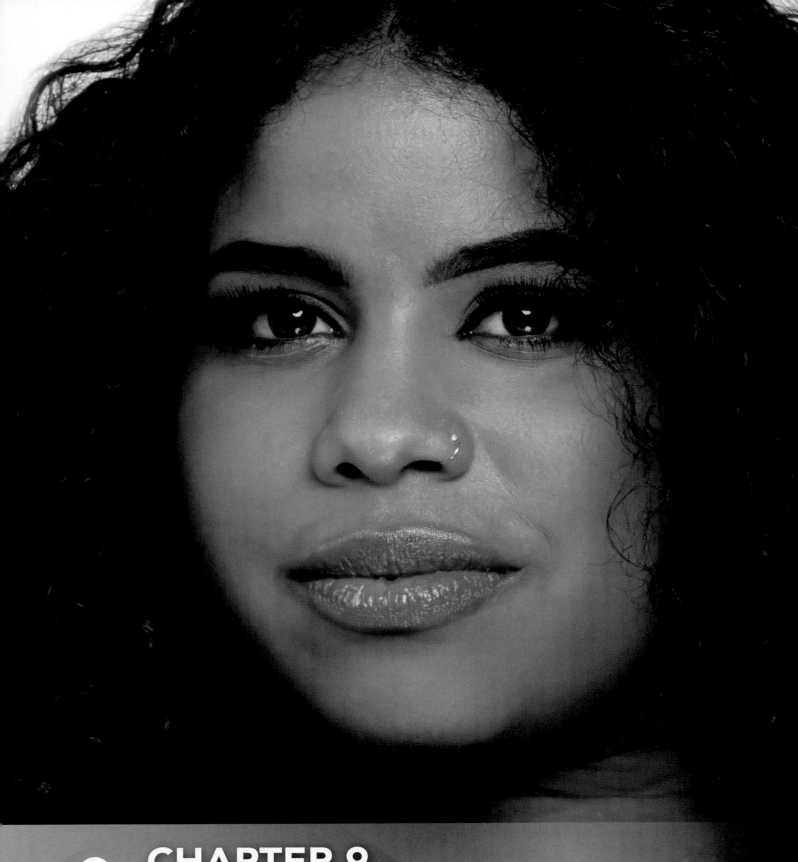

CHAPTER 9
Facial Massage

"If the path be beautiful, let us not ask where it leads."

–Anatole France

Learning Objectives

After completing this chapter, you will be able to:

1. Explain the importance of facial massage as an esthetics service.
2. Describe the benefits of massage.
3. Discuss facial massage contraindications.
4. Describe the five types of massage movements used by estheticians.
5. Explain how to incorporate massage during the facial treatment.
6. Perform a basic facial massage.

Explain the Importance of Facial Massage as an Esthetics Service

Massage is a key step and relaxing part of the facial that keeps clients coming back. A thorough knowledge of muscles, nerves, connective tissues, and blood vessels is vital to performing a correct massage. Massage (muh-SAHZH) is a manual or mechanical manipulation achieved by rubbing, kneading, or other methods that stimulate metabolism and circulation (Figure 9–1). It has many mental and physical benefits. When the body senses touch, reflex receptors respond by increasing blood and lymph flow. The central nervous system is affected, resulting in a state of relaxation. Massage also assists in product absorption and relieves pain.

Estheticians should have a thorough understanding of facial massage because:

- Learning and practicing your technique will allow you to provide your clients with superior results and create a loyal clientele.
- You must be able to explain the physiological and psychological benefits of facial massage to the client.

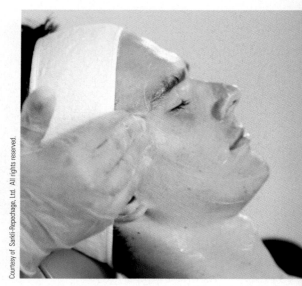

▲ Figure 9–1 Massage is a manual or mechanical manipulation resulting in a state of relaxation.

- Knowing the proper techniques and the contraindications for facial massage is important for client safety.
- This is another foundational service that enhances product effectiveness. Facial massage provides relaxation, and increases circulation to assist with oxygenating the skin and bringing vital nutrients to the epidermis while assisting in the removal of waste.

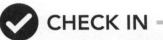 **CHECK IN**

1. What is the definition of massage?

ACTIVITY

Key Contributors in Massage History

Massage is one of the oldest therapeutic methods, dating back thousands of years (**Figure 9–2**). The ancient cultures of China, Japan, Egypt, India, Greece, and Rome all utilized massage as a form of medicine.

Research additional facts about these historical figures and their role in massage to share with the class:

- Pehr Henrik Ling of Sweden
- Olof Rudbeck
- Johann Georg Metzger
- George Henry Taylor
- Dr. Lucien Jacquet

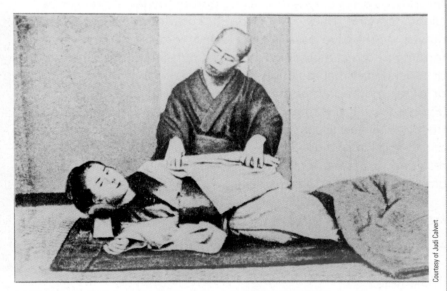

Courtesy of Judi Calvert

▲ **Figure 9–2** A massage practitioner in Japan (ca. 1880).

Describe the Benefits of Massage

Massage during facials benefits the client in many ways. A variety of techniques can be used to give the best massage for each client's individual needs. Be mindful of the results you are trying to achieve when giving a facial massage. Massage should never be given too long or too deeply. Always be mindful of the client's comfort and adjust your pressure accordingly. Stimulating muscle and nerve motor points will both contract muscles and relax the client. In fact, one study found significantly decreased levels of cortisol, the chemical your body releases when you are stressed, with an average decrease of 31 percent. Massage also has been noted to increase levels of dopamine and serotonin, neurotransmitters that are responsible for feelings of happiness and self-worth. Following massage, an average increase of 28 percent was noted for serotonin and an average increase of 31 percent was noted for dopamine.[1] Most new clients are surprised at how relaxing a facial can be, and they enjoy the benefits of skin rejuvenation as well as an overall feeling of well-being (**Figure 9–3**).

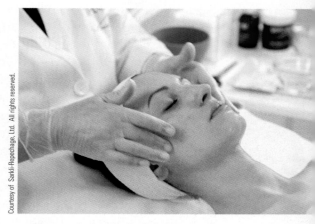

▲ **Figure 9–3** The facial massage has numerous benefits.

The following are benefits of facial massage:

- Relaxes the client, especially the facial muscles
- Stimulates blood and lymph circulation
- Improves overall metabolism and activates sluggish skin
- Helps muscle tone
- Helps cleanse the skin of impurities and softens sebum
- Helps slough off dead skin cells
- Reduces puffiness and sinus congestion
- Helps product absorption
- Relieves muscle tension and pain
- Provides a sense of well-being.

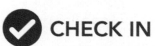 CHECK IN

2. What are at least five benefits of massage?

---

[1] Hernandez-Reif, M., Diego, M., Schanberg, S., & Kuhn, C. (2005, October). Cortisol decreases and serotonin and dopamine increase following massage therapy. *International Journal of Neuroscience*, *115*(10), 1397–1413. Available at https://www.ncbi.nlm.nih.gov/pubmed/16162447.

Discuss Facial Massage Contraindications

Certain health problems and skin conditions contraindicate a massage. Before performing a service that includes a facial massage, consult the client's intake form. During the consultation, acknowledge and discuss any medical conditions that may contraindicate a facial massage (**Figure 9–4**).

If your client expresses a concern about having a facial massage and has a relevant medical condition, advise them to speak with a physician before having the service. When in doubt, do not include massage as part of your service. If you cannot perform a massage, you can alter your service by substituting another step or leaving a mask on longer. Light acupressure massage is also a good alternative to the stronger European-style massage.

Facial massage contraindications, such as product allergies, are the same as facial contraindications discussed in Chapter 8, Facial Treatments. Contraindications include:

- Contagious diseases
- Inflamed acne (do not massage any area that has pustular breakouts)
- Sunburn, windburn, irritation, severe redness
- Sensitive skin (or skin severely sensitized by use of acne drugs, or other topical peeling agents)
- Open lesions, cuts, sores, abrasions
- Skin disorders
- Severe, uncontrolled hypertension
- Uncontrolled diabetes.

If your client has sensitive or redness-prone skin, avoid using vigorous or strong massage techniques.

Traditionally contraindicated, it is now acceptable for many clients who have high blood pressure (hypertension), diabetes, cancer, or a circulatory condition to have facial massage without concern, especially if their condition is being treated and carefully looked after by a physician.

Know Your Scope of Practice

An esthetician's massage services are commonly limited to certain areas of the body: the face, neck, shoulders, and décolleté, depending on your state's scope of practice. Therapeutic massage, such as deep tissue massage and manual lymph drainage, should be performed only by licensed massage therapists who specialize in these areas.

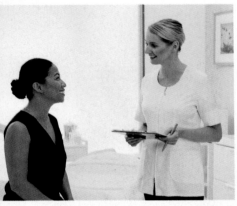

▲ **Figure 9–4** Consult the client's intake form before performing a facial massage.

CAUTION!

Those receiving cancer treatment should not receive massage unless it is from an oncology-trained esthetician. The movement of lymph through the body could cause complications for the client.

Although skin treatments such as back facials and body treatments are part of esthetics services, massage is not performed when working on these treatment areas—only the application of products.

 CHECK IN

3. What are five facial massage contraindications?
4. At what time during the facial can you discuss possible contraindications to facial massage?
5. On which areas of the body are estheticians typically allowed to perform a massage?
6. How do you find out what the licensing regulations for massage are in your state?

Describe the Five Types of Massage Movements Used by Estheticians

Administering classic massage movements includes five forms of hand manipulation: effleurage, pétrissage, tapotement, friction, and vibration. Massage should involve a rhythmic movement to the skin and tissues and as such, usually requires a massage medium that will allow enough slip to complete the massage comfortably and successfully.

Effleurage

Effleurage (EF-loo-rahzh) is a soft, continuous stroking movement applied with the fingers (digital) and palms (palmar) in a slow and rhythmic manner (**Figure 9–5**). The gliding movement is soothing and relaxing. The fingers are used on smaller surfaces such as the forehead and face. The palms are used on larger surfaces such as the shoulders. Effleurage is often used to begin and end massage sessions. It is used on the forehead, face, scalp, shoulders, neck, chest, arms, and hands.

To correctly position the fingers for stroking, slightly curve the fingers with just the cushions of the fingertips touching the skin. Do not use the ends of the fingertips because fingertips cannot control pressure and may scratch the client. To correctly position the palms for stroking, hold the whole hand loosely. Keep the wrist and fingers flexible, and curve the fingers to conform to the shape of the area being massaged.

Effleurage, the most important of the five movements, is used in conjunction with other types of massage. Once you begin effleurage, your hands should never leave the face or other body part being massaged.

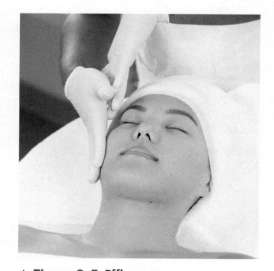

▲ Figure 9–5 Effleurage.

Pétrissage

Pétrissage (PEH-treh-sahzh) is a compression technique that includes kneading, squeezing, and pinching. This affects the deeper muscle tissue of the face. These movements stimulate the underlying tissues (**Figure 9–6**). The skin and flesh are grasped between the thumb and forefinger. As the tissues are lifted from their underlying structures, they are squeezed, rolled, or pinched with a light, firm pressure. Pétrissage is performed on the fleshier parts of the face, shoulders and arms. The pressure should be light but firm and the movements should be rhythmic. Pétrissage can stimulate circulation, and thus improve the skin's appearance and tone.

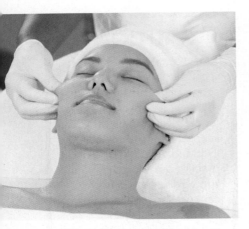
▲ Figure 9–6 Pétrissage.

Tapotement

Tapotement (tah-POT-ment), also known as *percussion*, is a percussive stroke in which the fingertips strike the skin in rapid succession or fast tapping movements (**Figure 9–7**). This technique improves circulation by stimulating the diffusion of the capillary network. It helps nourish the skin by releasing nutrients. This technique also purifies the system by releasing carbon dioxide and other waste material.

Tapotement is the most stimulating of the forms of massage and should be applied carefully and with discretion. It is good for toning and is beneficial to sluggish skin. Only light digital tapping should be used on the face. The fingertips are brought down against the skin in rapid succession. This movement is sometimes referred to as *a piano movement.*

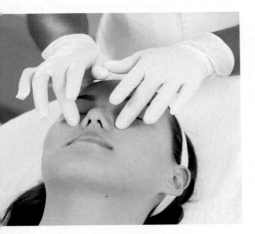
▲ Figure 9–7 Tapotement.

Friction

Friction (FRIK-shun) is an invigorating rubbing technique that stimulates the circulation and glandular activity of the skin. It can be performed in a circular manner or a criss-cross manner with the fingers working in opposition to each other. Pressure is maintained on the skin while the fingers or palms are moved over the underlying structures (**Figure 9–8**). Circular friction movements are usually used on the scalp, arms, and hands. Lighter circular friction movements are used on the face and neck.

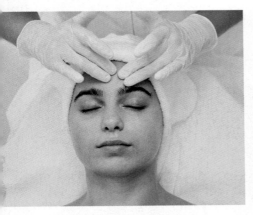
▲ Figure 9–8 Friction.

Vibration

Vibration (vy-BRAY-shun) is a rapid shaking movement in which the esthetician typically uses their body and shoulders—not just the fingertips—to create the movement. It is accomplished by rapid muscular contractions in the arms (**Figure 9–9**). The balls of the fingertips are pressed firmly on the point of application. Vibration is a highly stimulating movement, but it should be used sparingly and never for more than a few seconds on any one spot.

Alternative Massage Techniques

Different types of massage are based on body structure and energy flow within the body. Most massage techniques are based on classical, or Swedish, massage movements. There are many additional advanced techniques that stimulate and detoxify the body. These advanced massage techniques require additional training. A combination of techniques can be used in various treatments. Some of these are discussed more thoroughly in Chapter 13, Advanced Topics and Treatments.

- *Acupressure* is massage technique derived from Chinese medicine and consists of applying pressure to specific points of the face and body (acupressure points) to release muscle tension, restore balance, and stimulate *chi* (CHEE) (life force; energy). These points follow the same pattern of meridians in the body as acupuncture does.

- *Shiatsu* (shee-AH-tsoo) is a form of acupressure and is the Japanese technique of using acupressure massage points to relax and balance the body. Many of the motor points on the face and neck are acupressure points (**Figure 9–10**). Every muscle has a motor point that

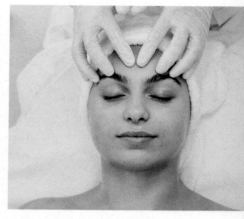

▲ **Figure 9–9** Vibration.

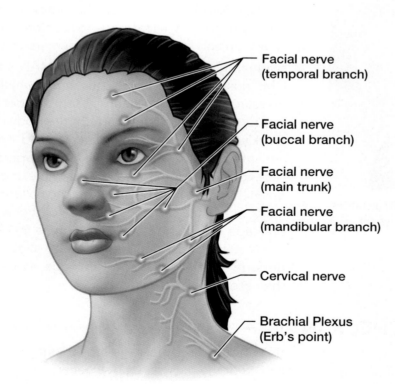

Facial nerve (temporal branch)

Facial nerve (buccal branch)

Facial nerve (main trunk)

Facial nerve (mandibular branch)

Cervical nerve

Brachial Plexus (Erb's point)

▲ **Figure 9–10 Motor nerve points of the face.**

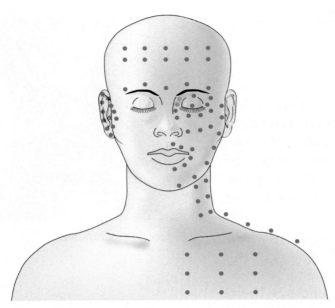

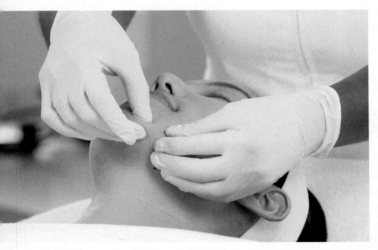

▲ Figure 9–11 Pressure point massage is very relaxing and therapeutic.

▲ Figure 9–12 Manual lymph drainage (MLD) increases the movement of lymph into and through the lymph system.

is a specific spot on the skin over the muscle where pressure or stimulation will cause contraction of that muscle, nerve stimulation, and overall relaxation. The standard pressure point technique is to pause briefly for a few seconds over the motor points using light pressure. This technique is also used on the scalp.

- *Pressure point massage* is similar to acupressure. On each point, the movement is repeated three to six times. Pause for three to six seconds on each point, moving from point to point from the top to the bottom of the face, using light inward pressure at each point and then lifting the pressure to slide to the next point. Training is necessary to perform this massage correctly. Techniques and patterns vary with different methods (**Figure 9–11**). Pressure point massage is a form of acupressure, but the technique can be incorporated into treatments without being a true acupressure massage. There are other types of pressure point massage that do not follow the body's specific acupressure meridians, such as massage on motor points.

- *Aromatherapy massage* uses essential oils mixed with an emulsion or oil and applied to the skin during massage movements. These oils are often used during the facial massage to promote mental relaxation and to treat the skin in numerous ways.

- **Manual lymph drainage (MLD)** (MAN-yoo-ul LIMF drayn-IHJE) massage uses gentle, rhythmic pressure on the lymphatic system to detoxify and remove waste materials from the body more quickly. It reduces swelling and is used before and after surgery for pre- and post operative care. It is a very light touch. For example, moving down the side of the neck toward the collar-bone helps drain fluid from the face to the lymph drainage channel in that area (**Figure 9–12**). In some states, master estheticians are allowed to perform manual lymphatic drainage as part of their scope of practice.

 CHECK IN

7. List the five main types of basic massage movements.
8. Briefly describe each of the massage movements.
9. Define acupressure.
10. What is manual lymph drainage?

Explain How to Incorporate Massage During the Facial Treatment

This chapter contains general guidelines that vary according to each specialized treatment. When massage is performed in the facial depends on many factors. A facial massage routine will change depending on the training or protocols established by the facility or product manufacturer. A facial massage is performed for approximately 10 to 20 minutes during a facial. Some treatments incorporate more massage, and others do not include massage at all. Massage techniques also depend on the client's skin analysis and what you are focusing on in the treatment.

Learn the Technical Skills

A professional facial massage is one of the major differences between a professional treatment in a spa and a home care regimen. When performed correctly, massage is relaxing and beneficial to the client (**Figure 9–13**). The key is that the massage is performed correctly. Here are important tips and techniques to know when you are performing a facial massage (further explanation follows):

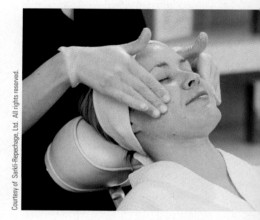

▲ **Figure 9–13** Mental focus is important when giving a massage.

- When performing massage, hand movements need to flow and be consistent, gliding easily from one area to the next.
- Mental focus is important when giving a massage. Do not let mental distractions reduce your focus on the massage and your clients.
- It is helpful to explain to clients what you are trying to achieve with your facial massage techniques.
- Communicate with clients, and adjust your touch according to their preferences.
- Educate your clients so they understand that excessive or deep massage is too rough for facial skin. Too much pressure on the face can weaken elastin fibers and break down elasticity.
- Massage pressure, massage type, and the duration will vary according to skin type
- An even tempo, or rhythmic flow, promotes relaxation. The sequence of massage movements is designed for a smooth and graceful flow from one movement into another.
- Massage may be started on the chin, décolleté, or forehead.
- Do not remove your hands once you have made contact with the skin.
- Always massage from muscle insertion to origin of the muscle to avoid damage to muscular tissues. Massage movements usually are performed upward and outward on the face and neck.

Maintain Hand Mobility

An esthetician's hands need to be flexible and have a controlled and firm touch. Hands should be soft with short, smooth, well-filed nails. Hand mobility is important in maintaining a smooth rhythm and regulating the massage pressure. Both the left and right hands need to be synchronized, using equal pressure on both sides. The correct balance comes with practice and being attentive to your touch.

Hand exercises can help strengthen hands and prevent repetitive motion problems, such as carpal tunnel syndrome (**Figure 9–14**). Estheticians are susceptible to problems because of repetitive movements, muscle and tendon strain, and fatigue due to improper or poor posture. (Refer to Chapter 7, The Treatment Room, for hand-strengthening exercises.)

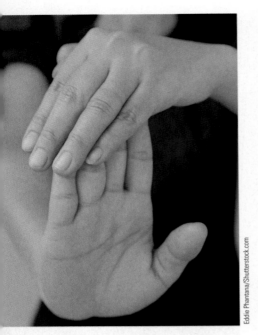

▲ **Figure 9–14** Hand exercises are key to prevent fatigue and help strengthen hands.

Use Proper Massage Products

When choosing a massage product, be sure that the product not only provides a smooth glide on the face, neck, and chest, but that the formula works with the client's skin type. A serum or gel-based massage product provides gentle friction and the ideal glide to leave all skin types relaxed and hydrated (**Figure 9–15**). Rich herbal cream-based products provide the ideal glide to perform facial massages for drier skin types, while the scents of the herbal extracts, which can include Roman chamomile, rose, and lavender, can be soothing and calming. Be sure to check your client's intake form for allergies before selecting a massage product.

Relax

Talking eliminates the relaxation therapy of the massage. If the client is talking, invite them to relax and enjoy the massage and don't continue the conversation. Speak in a quiet voice and only when necessary during the facial.

Put aside all distractions during a service. An esthetician's mood and mental disposition will affect the service and the client. Take a minute to clear your mind and forget about everything except giving a relaxing service. Many estheticians close their eyes and take a few deep breaths before working on a client. The close contact in a massage is very personal and intimate. It is a service that can be calming to the esthetician as well as the client.

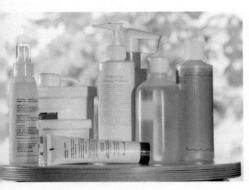

▲ **Figure 9–15** Choose a massage medium that suits your client's skin type and needs.

Choose Your Starting Point

Starting points can vary. Massage may be started on the chin, décolleté, or forehead. Different massage movements may be used on the various parts of the face, chest, and shoulders. Most movements are repeated three to six times before moving on to the next one. Use both hands at the same time or alternate hands with a flowing rhythm, depending on the steps. Slide the hands back down to each starting point to repeat the movements in each step.

Maintain Contact

The sequence of massage movements is designed for a smooth and graceful flow from one movement into another. To keep the relaxing flow and connection, do not remove your hands from the client once you have made contact with the skin to begin the facial massage. Maintaining contact gives the client a sense of physical continuity that is very soothing and calming (**Figure 9–16**). Should it become necessary to lift the hands from the client's face (if you need to apply more product, for example), slow down the movements and then gently replace them with feather-like movements (which are often called *feathering*). When coming back to the face, gently make contact on the side of the face or top of the head to avoid startling the client. To aid in relaxation, choose instrumental music with a slow, even tempo.

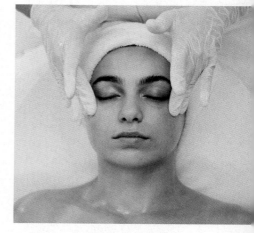

▲ **Figure 9–16** Refrain from removing your hands from the client's face once the massage has started.

Massage from Insertion to Origin

Always massage from muscle *insertion* to *origin* (**Figure 9–17**). Know the correct direction to massage to avoid breaking down tissue and potentially causing premature aging.

- The *insertion* is the portion of the muscle at the more movable attachment (where it is attached to another muscle or to a movable bone or joint).

- The *origin* is the portion of the muscle at the fixed attachment (where it is attached to an immovable section of the skeleton).

    To avoid undue pressure and stress, it is important to massage the muscles using outward strokes. This is because inward strokes can weaken the skin, causing premature folds and wrinkles. With outward strokes, the skin is not pulled and muscles are not weakened.

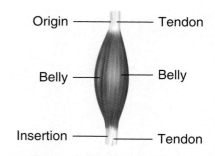

▲ **Figure 9–17** Massage from muscle insertion to origin.

Check Pressure

It is important to adjust your pressure as necessary. Check in with the client about their comfort. Ask about the pressure of your touch and whether it should be more or less firm. Remember that the facial massage should be lighter than a body massage and let the client know that the skin on the face should be treated more carefully. We are not massage therapists, so it is important to educate clients about the reasons that we do not perform stronger deeper tissue massage on the face, so they are not disappointed if they expected a stronger touch. A light firm touch, when performed well, is more relaxing than a heavier one.

Sharpen Your Professionalism

If a client seems dissatisfied with a facial treatment, it could be due to the following reasons:

- Offensive breath or body odor
- Rough, cold hands or ragged nails that may have scratched the client's skin
- Allowing cream or other facial products to get into the client's eyes, mouth, nostrils, or hairline
- Applying too much massage oil or cream
- Towels that are too hot or too cold
- Talking too much
- Manipulating the skin roughly or in the wrong direction
- Being disorganized and interrupting the facial to get supplies
- Sloppy product application or movements
- Noise or distractions during the service.

 CHECK IN

11. In what direction do you massage on the muscles?
12. Why should you always have at least one hand on the client after you begin a facial massage?
13. How many times should you repeat the massage movements?

Perform a Basic Facial Massage

It is recommended that you first practice the facial massage steps on a mannequin before doing the massage. By this point in your training, you will already have experience with setup procedures, client consultation, and infection control procedures.

DID YOU KNOW?

For your male clients, use downward movements in the area of beard growth. It feels uncomfortable when you massage against hair growth. Pressure point massage in the beard area works well.

Massage is the most relaxing part of the facial and has many benefits. Various massage techniques can be incorporated into facial treatments. Appropriate massage movements are based on the anatomy of the facial structure, nerves, and muscles (**Figure 9–18**). Using the proper techniques is important. It is also necessary to know the contraindications for massage. Once the basic massage flows smoothly, other movements can be added to the routine. Many estheticians find that giving a facial massage is also relaxing to them and one of the most enjoyable parts of their job.

┌─────────────────────────┐
│ ──────PERFORM────── │
│ **Procedure 9-1** │
│ Basic Facial Massage │
└─────────────────────────┘

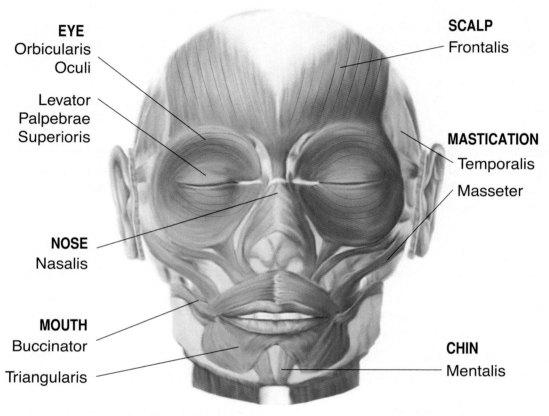

EYE
Orbicularis Oculi

Levator Palpebrae Superioris

NOSE
Nasalis

MOUTH
Buccinator

Triangularis

SCALP
Frontalis

MASTICATION
Temporalis
Masseter

CHIN
Mentalis

▲ **Figure 9–18 Facial structure and muscles.**

ACTIVITY

Review Massage Movements

To help you remember your massage steps and feel comfortable practicing massage try these helpful tips.

1. Write the massage steps out and refer to them often while learning the massage and its movements.
2. Practice the facial massage steps on a facial mannequin or mannequin head.
3. Review video tutorials to help master your massage techniques.

Procedure 9-1:
Perform a Basic Facial Massage

MATERIALS
- ☐ 4" × 4" esthetic wipes
- ☐ Gloves
- ☐ Lotion, cream, serum, oil or gel specific to the skin type
- ☐ Soft fan brush (optional)
- ☐ Towels for hot towel cabinet

PREPARATION
- ☐ Perform Procedure 7–1: Pre-service—Preparing the Treatment Room.
- ☐ Perform Procedure 8–1: Pre-service—Preparing the Client for Treatment.

By this point in your studies, you will already have experience with setup procedures, client consultation, and infection control procedures. Massage is not intended to be used on every client in the same way, and should be customized to suit their needs. For example, someone with sensitive skin should not receive friction or tapotement movements.

Setup

The following procedure is a standard facial massage. Consider the following reminders before getting started:

- Select a product that is appropriate for the client's skin type, such as lotion, serum, cream, or gel. Start out with a light touch, gradually using firmer pressure where applicable.
- The number of movements to perform for each step may vary. In this massage routine, it is recommended to repeat each of the movements (each pass) consecutively three to six times to maintain consistency.
- Each instructor may have developed their own routine. Follow your instructor's lead.
- Blood returning to the heart from the head, face, and neck flows down the jugular veins on each side of the neck. All massage movements on the side of the neck are done with a downward (never upward) motion. Always slide gently upward in the center of the neck and circle out and then down on the sides.
- To keep the relaxing flow and connection, do not remove your hands from the client's face once you have started the massage. Choose spa music with a slow, even tempo.

DID YOU KNOW?

Whatever movements you use, be consistent in the number of passes you make for each step. If you repeat a step three times or six times, repeat all your steps the same number of times. Always perform the same routine on both the left and right sides of the area being massaged.

Application of Facial Massage Product

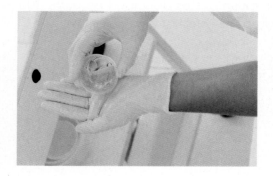

1 **Dispense the massage product.** Safely dispense the correct product for the client's skin type and needs into a container. One teaspoon (5 millimeters or 5 to 10 grams) should be enough product for the facial area, neck, and décolleté.

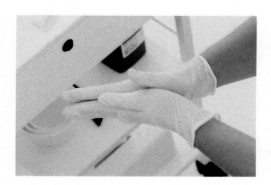

2 **Put on gloves and prepare massage product.** Put on well-fitting gloves to perform the facial massage properly. Ensure the massage cream is evenly distributed on both gloved hands. You are now ready to apply the product to the client's décolleté (includes the upper chest area, neck, and cleavage) and face.

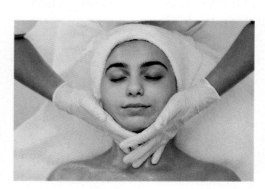

3 **Use effleurage to apply product evenly to the décolleté, neck and face.** While applying the product, it is suggested that hands not be lifted from the client until you are finished. Start applying a small amount of the product by placing both hands, palms down, on the décolleté. Slide hands across the décolleté toward the shoulders, back to the center of the décolleté, up the neck to the face, out to the cheeks; then glide inward, up the nose, and end the application by tapering the movement off until the fingers are gradually lifted from the forehead, a process also referred to as *feathering*.

Facial Massage Routine

Optional: Begin massage with décolleté, shoulder, and neck manipulations as discussed on page 408 and then proceed to step 1 below or perform only the massage steps as listed below.

1 **Start with hands on the décolleté.** Using your full hands, including the palms, move slowly up the sides of the neck and face to the forehead. Beginning on the forehead, slide to each of the next steps without breaking contact or lifting fingers off the face.

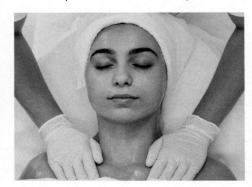 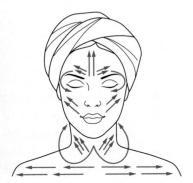

2 **Effleurage strokes on the forehead.** With the middle and ring fingers of each hand, start upward strokes in the middle of the forehead, starting at the brow line and moving upward toward the hairline. Move toward the right temple and back to the center of the forehead. Now move toward the left temple and back to the center of the forehead. Repeat three to six times.

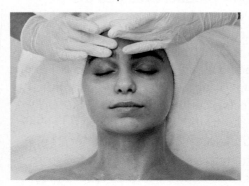 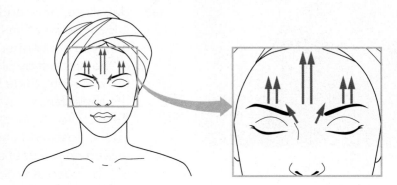

3 **Circular friction on the forehead.** With the middle or index finger of each hand, start a circular movement in the middle of the forehead along the brow line. Continue this circular movement while working toward the temples. Each time the fingers reach the temples, pause for a moment and apply slight pressure to the temples. Make sure the pressure is acceptable to your client. Bring the fingers back to the center of the forehead at a point between the brow line and the hairline. Move up on the forehead toward the hairline for the final movements. Repeat three to six times.

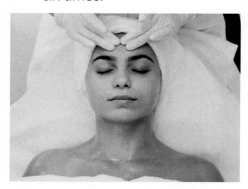 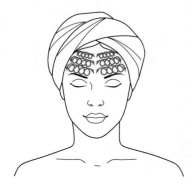

4 **Friction using crisscross strokes on the forehead.** With the middle and ring fingers of each hand, start a criss-cross stroking movement at the middle of the forehead, starting at the brow line and moving upward toward the hairline. Move toward the right temple and back to the center of the forehead. Now move toward the left temple and back to the center of the forehead. Repeat three to six times.

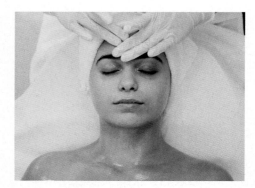 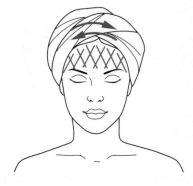

5 **Friction near the brows.** Place the ring fingers under the inside corners of the eyebrows and the middle fingers over the brows. Slide the fingers to the outer corner of each eye, lifting the brow at the same time. This movement continues with the next step.

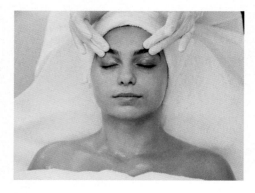 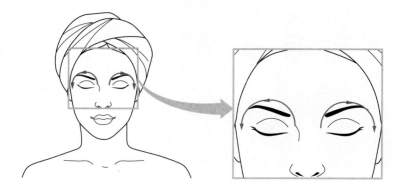

6 **Circular friction around the eye area and zygomatic.** Start a circular movement with the middle and ring fingers at the inside corner of each eye. Continue the circular movement on the zygomatic bone (cheekbone) to the point under the center of the eye, and then slide the fingers back to the starting point. Repeat three to six times. The left hand moves clockwise, and the right hand moves counter-clockwise.

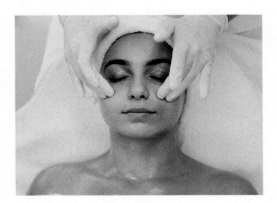
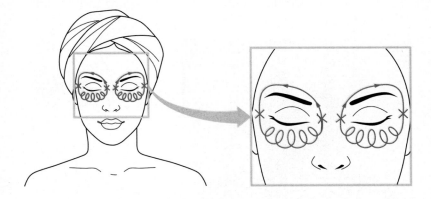

7 **Tapotement around the eyes.** Start a light tapping movement with the pads of the fingers. Tap lightly around the eyes as if gently playing a piano. Continue tapping, moving from the temple to under the eye, toward the nose, up and over the brow, and outward back to the temple. Do not tap the eyelids directly over the eyeball. Repeat the movements three to six times.

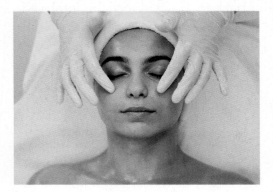
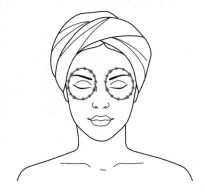

8 **Circular friction across the cheeks to the temples and back.** With the middle, index, or ring finger of each hand, start a circular movement down the nose and continue across the cheeks to the temples. Slide the fingers under the eyes and back to the bridge of the nose. Repeat the movements three to six times.

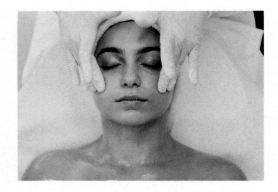
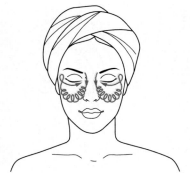

9 **Pétrissage motion on the chin.** With the middle and ring fingers of each hand, slide the fingers from the bridge of the nose, over the brow (lifting the brow), and down to the chin. Start a firm circular movement on the chin with the thumbs. Change to the middle fingers at the corners of the mouth. Rotate the fingers five times, and slide the fingers up the sides of the nose and over the brow, and then stop for a moment at the temples. Apply slight pressure on the temples. Slide the fingers down to the chin, and repeat the movements three to six times. The downward movement on the side of the face should have a very light touch to avoid dragging the skin downward.

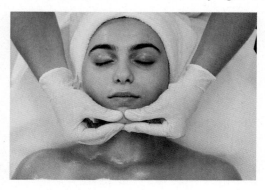 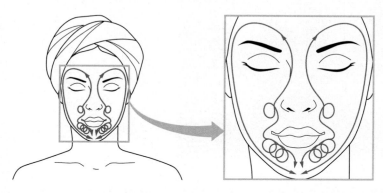

10 **Perform tapotement or pétrissage on the cheeks.**

a. If using pétrissage, grasp the skin between the thumb and forefinger of the index finger, gently lift and pinch the fleshy areas of the cheeks with light but firm pressure. Remember to use this type of pétrissage movement only on the fleshy areas of the face. Work in a circle around the cheeks. Repeat the movements three to six times.

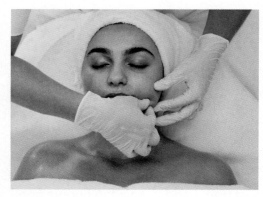 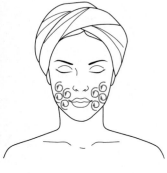

b. If using tapotement, start a light tapping motion (piano playing) on the cheeks, working in a circle around the cheeks. Repeat three to six times.

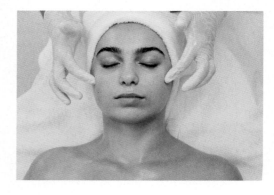 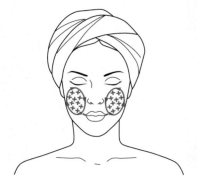

11 **Circular friction or rubbing motion.** Slide to the center of the chin. Using the middle and ring fingers of each hand, start a circular movement at the center of the chin and move up to the earlobes. Slide the middle fingers to the corners of the mouth and then continue the circular movements to the middle of the ears. Return the middle fingers to the nose and continue the circular movements outward across the cheeks to the top of the ear. Repeat each of the three passes three to six times. Slide down to the mouth.

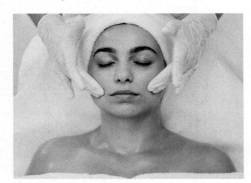 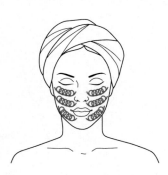

12 **Friction using scissoring movement.** Place the index finger above the mouth and middle finger below the mouth. Start the "scissor" movement, gliding from the center of the mouth and upward over the zygomatic bone (cheekbone), and stopping at the top of the zygomatic. Alternate the movement from one side of the face to the other, using the right hand on the right side of the face and then the left hand on the left side. As one hand reaches the zygomatic bone (cheekbone), start the other at the center of the mouth. Repeat the movements three to six times.

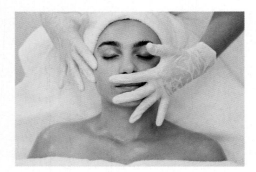 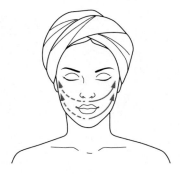

13 **Circle around the mouth and chin.** With the middle fingers of both hands, draw the fingers from the center of the upper lip around the mouth and under the lower lip, and then continue a circle under the chin. Repeat the movements three to six times.

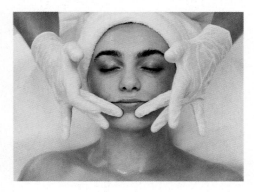 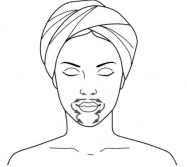

14 **Friction using scissor movement.** With the index finger above the chin and jawline (the middle, ring, and little fingers should be under the chin and jaw), start a scissor movement from the center of the chin and then slide the fingers along the jawline to the earlobe. Alternate one hand after the other, using the right hand on the right side of the face and the left hand on the left side of the face. Repeat three to six times on each side of the face. Slide down to the neck.

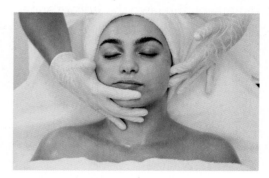 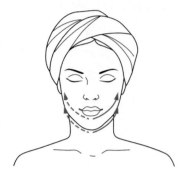

15 **Effleurage near the neck.** Using both hands, apply light upward strokes over the front of the neck. Circle down and then back up, using firmer downward pressure on the outer sides of the neck. Repeat the movements three to six times. Do not press down on the center of the neck.

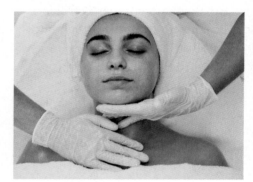 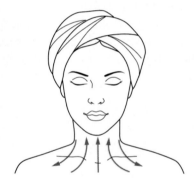

16 **Tapotement on the underside of the chin.** With the middle and ring fingers of the right hand, give two quick taps under the chin, followed with one quick tap with the middle and ring fingers of the left hand. The taps should be done in a continuous movement, keeping a steady rhythm. The taps should be done with a light touch, but with enough pressure so that a soft tapping sound can be heard. Continue the tapping movement while moving the hands slightly to the right and then to the left, so as to cover the complete underside of the chin. Without stopping or breaking the rhythm of the tapping, move to the right cheek.

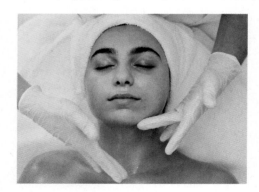 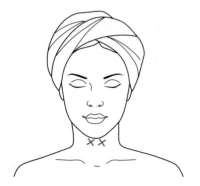

17 **Tapotement and lifting movement on the cheeks.** Continue the tapping on the right cheek in the same manner as under the chin, except the tapping with the left hand will have a lifting movement. The rhythm will be tap, tap, lift, tap, tap, lift, tap, tap, lift. Repeat this rhythmic movement three to six times. Without stopping the tapping movement, move the fingers back under the chin and over the left cheek, repeating the tapping and lifting movements. Move up and out of the area in a consistent pattern. Avoid tapping directly on the jawbone because this will feel unpleasant to the client.

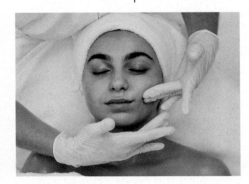 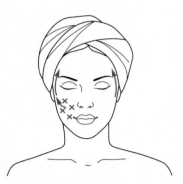

18 **Tapotement stroking movement near corners of the mouth.** Without stopping the tapping movement, move the hands over to the corners of the mouth. Break into an upward stroking movement with the first three fingers of each hand. One finger follows the other as each finger lifts the corner of the mouth. Use both hands at the same time or alternate each hand—as one hand ends the movement, the other starts. Repeat the stroking movement three to six times.

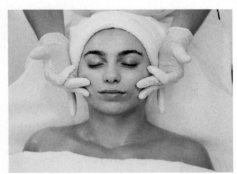 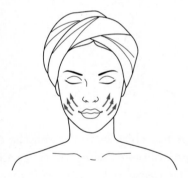

19 **Effleurage stroking movement near outside corner of eyes.** Without stopping the stroking movement, move up to the outside corner of the left eye and continue the stroking upward movement. Continue the stroking movement across the forehead to the outside corner of the right eye. Continue this stroking movement back and forth three to six times in each direction.

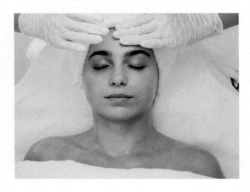 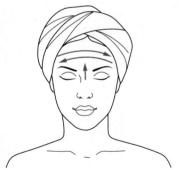

20 **Effleurage stroking movement across the forehead and complete routine.** Continue the stroking movement back and forth across the forehead, gradually slowing the movement. Let the movements grow slower and slower as the touch becomes lighter and lighter. Taper the movement off until the fingers are gradually lifted from the forehead.

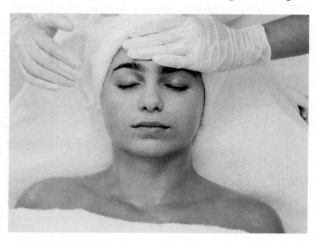 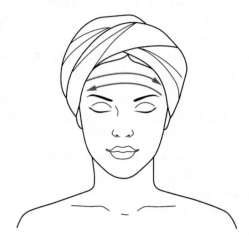

21 Remove the massage medium. Use warm towels or 4" × 4" esthetics wipes and follow the same procedure for removing other products or cleansers. Continue with the facial service.

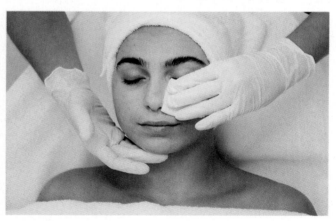 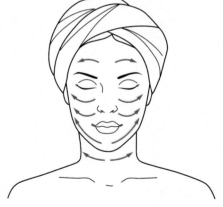

Post-Service

• Complete Procedure 7-2: Post-Service Procedure.

Décolleté, Shoulder, and Neck Manipulations (Optional)

Estheticians may decide to include only a face and neck massage in their facial. If their goal is to include an extended massage in their facial treatment, they may choose to include the décolleté, shoulder, neck, and face area. As you increase the areas massaged in your facial, you will need to abbreviate other facial steps to accommodate the additional time spent on the massage segments, or increase the total time of the facial treatment itself.

Some prefer to treat these areas first before starting the standard facial massage. There are variations on this standard technique. Apply massage cream and perform the following manipulations:

- *Décolleté and upper back movement*—Use a rotary circular movement outward across the décolleté to the shoulders, and then inward across the shoulders down to the back. Slide your fingers up to the sides of the base of the neck. Rotate three times.

- *Shoulders and upper back movement*—Rotate on top of the shoulders three times. Glide your fingers in toward the spine and then to the base of the neck. Apply circular movement up and behind the ear and then slide your fingers to the front of the earlobe. Rotate three times. Slide down the neck to the shoulders and repeat three times.

- *Shoulder massage*—Use your thumbs and bent index fingers to grasp the tissue on top of the shoulders in a kneading-type movement. Rotate six times. Slide up to the neck and continue with the massage.

COMPETENCY PROGRESS

How are you doing with facial massage? **Check the Chapter 9 Learning Objectives below that you feel you have mastered; leave unchecked those objectives you will need to return to:**

- ☐ Explain the importance of facial massage as an esthetics service.
- ☐ Describe the benefits of massage.
- ☐ Discuss facial massage contraindications.
- ☐ Describe the five types of massage movements used by estheticians.
- ☐ Explain how to incorporate massage during the facial treatment.
- ☐ Perform a basic facial massage.

GLOSSARY

effleurage EF-loo-rahzh	p. 389	light, continuous stroking movement applied with the fingers (digital) or the palms (palmar) in a slow, rhythmic manner
friction FRIK-shun	p. 390	invigorating rubbing technique requiring pressure on the skin with the fingers or palm while moving them under an underlying structure
manual lymph drainage MAN-yoo-ul LIMF drayn-IHJE	p. 392	abbreviated *MLD*; gentle, rhythmic pressure on the lymphatic system to detoxify and remove waste materials from the body more quickly; reduces swelling and is used before and after surgery for pre- and postoperative care
massage muh-SAHZH	p. 385	manual or mechanical manipulation of the body achieved by rubbing, gently pinching, kneading, tapping, and performing other movements to increase metabolism and circulation, promote absorption, and relieve pain
pétrissage PEH-treh-sahzh	p. 390	kneading movement that stimulates the underlying tissues; performed by lifting, squeezing, and pressing the tissue with a light, firm pressure
tapotement tah-POT-ment	p. 390	also known as *percussion*; movements consisting of short, quick tapping and slapping, movements
vibration vy-BRAY-shun	p. 390	in massage, the rapid shaking movement in which the esthetician uses the body and shoulders, not just the fingertips, to create the movement

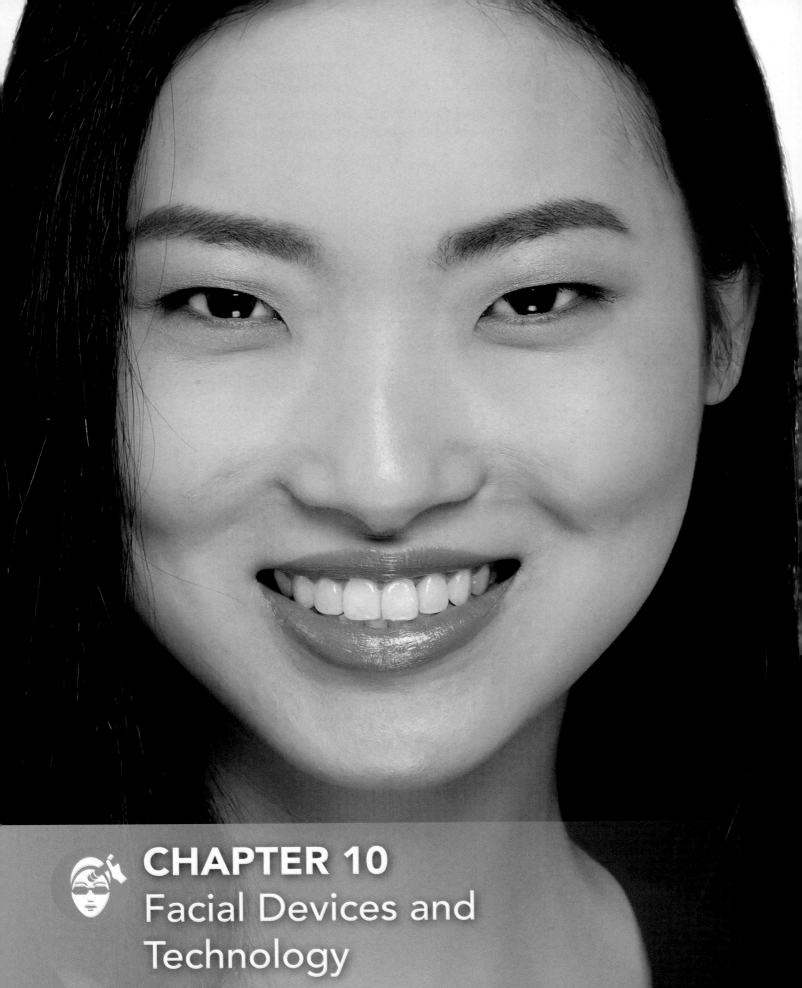

CHAPTER 10
Facial Devices and Technology

"Beauty begins the moment you decide to be yourself."

—Coco Chanel

Learning Objectives

After completing this chapter, you will be able to:

1. Explain the importance of the use of facial devices and technology.
2. Identify the basic concepts of electrotherapy.
3. Explain the benefits of the hot towel cabinet.
4. Discuss the magnifying lamp and its uses.
5. Discuss the Wood's lamp and its uses.
6. Demonstrate how to safely and effectively use the rotary brush.
7. Demonstrate how to safely and effectively use the steamer.
8. Demonstrate how to safely and effectively use the vacuum machine.
9. Demonstrate how to safely and effectively use galvanic current.
10. Demonstrate how to safely and effectively use the high-frequency machine.
11. Demonstrate how to safely and effectively use spray machines.
12. State the benefits and use of paraffin wax.
13. State the benefits and use of electric mitts and boots.
14. Identify why you should make informed decisions when purchasing equipment as a licensed esthetician.

Explain the Importance of the Use of Facial Devices and Technology

There are a variety of useful machines and devices that will enhance the esthetician's services. Each machine or device has a specific benefit for the skin and makes clients feel as though they are receiving a specialized service. In this chapter you will learn how these tools are integrated into facial treatments. Although facial treatments can be performed effectively without electrical devices, optimal outcomes can be achieved more readily with facial devices and technology.

Estheticians should study and have a thorough understanding of facial devices and technology because:

- They need to operate machines and devices safely, provide the best results for their clients, and enhance their service menu.
- It is vital to understand how to safely use each machine and device and the potential contraindications in using the machine or device.
- There are a variety of useful machines and devices and new high-performance tools that will enhance the esthetician's services and it is important to be able to explain the benefits of each machine or device.
- To maintain professional credibility, estheticians must continue to be educated about the latest methods in skin care as new machines and technology emerge each year.
- Investing in high-quality machines and devices will increase both credibility and potential business revenue.

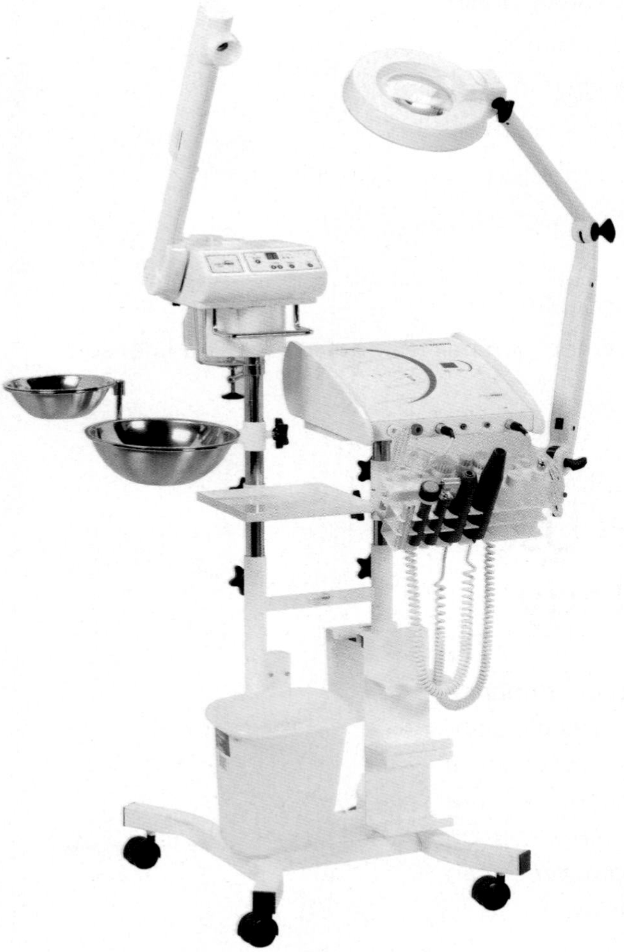

▲ FIGURE 10–1 Multifunctional machines are a popular option when trying to save space.

Identify the Basic Concepts of Electrotherapy

Electrotherapy is the use of electrical devices for therapeutic benefits. Electrical devices enhance facial treatments by making it easier to give a skin analysis, by helping to achieve better product penetration, or by exfoliating the skin. These tools are especially effective for more challenging skin conditions such as aging or sun-damaged skin. Machines and devices can be purchased separately or as multifunctional units with many of the modalities (machines) all part of one unit (**Figure 10–1**).

Estheticians must continue to be educated about the latest methods in skin care, while being cautious of expensive, trendy machines. Lasers, light therapy, microdermabrasion, and microcurrent are some of the advanced machines discussed later in Chapter 13, Advanced Topics and Treatments. It is important to be familiar with machines and devices even if you choose not to work with them, as it is important to be able to educate your clients on the benefits provided. Today's clients are well educated and have greater access to information, and they will expect you to be knowledgeable about all skin care topics, trends, and tools. To maintain professional credibility, it is important that you are aware of current technology.

General Contraindications for Electrotherapy

There are several contraindications for electrotherapy. These include the standard facial contraindications discussed in previous chapters. (See Chapter 5, Skin Analysis.)

To prevent physical harm, some electrotherapy machines should never be used on:

1. Clients with heart conditions, pacemakers, metal implants, or braces
2. Clients who are pregnant
3. Clients with epilepsy or seizure disorders
4. Clients who are afraid of electric current
5. Clients with open or broken skin

If you ever have any doubts about whether a client can have electrotherapy safely, request that the client get a note from their physician approving electrotherapy treatment. Ensure the client removes jewelry and piercings before using electrical devices such as the galvanic machine. Use all machines as directed by the manufacturer because similar machines may have different mechanisms and work differently. Most machines discussed in this chapter are used for approximately 5 to 10 minutes while being integrated into the facial treatment.

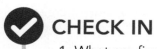 CHECK IN

1. What are five contraindications for electrotherapy?

Explain the Benefits of the Hot Towel Cabinet

Towel warmers, also called *hot towel cabinets* or *hot cabbies*, are used to heat towels or products used in treatments and are commonly used in the treatment room (**Figure 10–2**).

When to Use a Hot Towel Cabinet

Hot towels can be used for both face and body treatments. Cotton pads, 4″ × 4″ esthetic wipes, and products can be warmed in a towel warmer or specialized product warmer. Some towel warmers are equipped with ultraviolet lamps. Ultraviolet lamps in towel warmers may reduce bacteria but are not effective for disinfection.

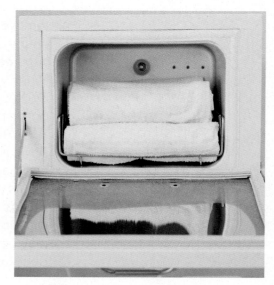

▲ **FIGURE 10–2 Hot towel cabinet.**

Effects of Warm Towels from a Hot Towel Cabinet

Clients who do not have contraindications would benefit from the warm, soothing, softening action provided by steamed towels, which can be used in the following ways:

- For removing facial masks and products such as massage creams
- For softening the skin before performing extractions.

Contraindications and Best Practices for Warm Towels from a Hot Towel Cabinet

Hot towels should not be used on clients who have:

- Extremely fragile or extremely sensitive skin
- Uncontrolled or advanced rosacea
- Open wounds or contraindicated skin conditions such as excessive acne lesions.

Before placing the warm towel on the skin be sure to adhere to the following guidelines:

- Always test the temperature of the towel or product on your wrist prior to use.
- Towels should never be too warm or left on the skin too long because they can damage capillaries, cause overstimulation, and increase redness or irritation.
- Plastic melts in hot towel warmers; therefore, use heat-resistant dishes to warm products.

It is important to understand that while working on a client, anytime you enter the hot towel cabinet to retrieve an item, you must first remove your gloves, or you will contaminate the cabinet door and entire contents of the hot towel cabinet. Once you remove the item you need, put on a new pair of gloves prior to returning to work on the client. Avoiding cross-contamination during any service is required by OSHA, as is the use of gloves, because you can be exposed to blood-borne pathogens the minute you begin any service.

With advances in many products, ingredients, and advanced devices, you may find your treatment more geared toward a clinical approach when addressing product removal. These types of treatments primarily use 4" × 4" esthetic wipes for removal versus hot towels. As you increase exfoliation or stimulation of the skin, as occurs with some advanced services, you will find that the use of hot towels may be contraindicated. Examples of such services are some advanced peels as well as in-depth microdermabrasion treatments.

OSHA ALERT

OSHA requires that you use gloves whenever you may be exposed to bloodborne pathogens. In reality, you have an exposure risk whenever you work on a client. Gloves should be worn at all times.

PREPARATION OF THE HOT TOWEL CABINET

Always follow the manufacturer's instructions, as there may be subtle differences in each devices' use and optimum effectiveness. In general, these are the steps you should perform to prepare the hot towel cabinet:

1. Put on gloves, fold a towel in half, and roll the towel up.
2. Add warm water, squeeze excess water from the towel, insert the towel in the hot towel cabinet, and turn on the cabinet to heat the towel.
3. Load the cabinet until you have the desired number of towels for your treatment or plan ahead for your full client schedule.

Safety and Maintenance of the Hot Towel Cabinet

When you are ready to use the heated steam towel from the hot towel cabinet:

- Put on a new pair of gloves and remove the towel.
- Test the temperature of the towel on the inside of the wrist over the gloved hand. If the towel is too warm, open it slightly and allow the towel to slightly cool and then retest the temperature of the towel.
- Open the towel and apply the towel to the client's face, never covering the nose and mouth areas. While the towel is on the client's face, you may apply gentle pressure to the towel to provide further relaxation.

To remove the towel gently begin at the top and work your way down, lifting the towel off the face. If using the towel for product removal you will use the ends of the towel to methodically remove the product, working from the top of the face down and circling back to address any remaining product once the towel has been removed.

It is important to keep the hot towel cabinet clean and free from mold or mildew. At the end of the day:

- Clean the inside and outside of the cabinet with an EPA-registered disinfectant.
- Empty, clean, and disinfect the water catchment tray underneath the cabinet.
- Leave the door open at night to allow the cabinet and rubber seals to dry thoroughly.

 CHECK IN

> 2. Why is it important to enter the hot towel cabinet with clean gloves?

Discuss the Magnifying Lamp and Its Uses

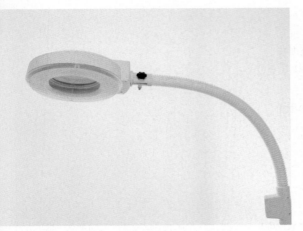

▲ **FIGURE 10–3 Magnifying lamp.**

The magnifying lamp (also referred to as a *loupe*; pronounced "loop") magnifies the face to help the esthetician treat and analyze the skin (**Figure 10–3**).

- The lamp uses a cool fluorescent light bulb.
- The magnifying lamp has various powers of magnification known as *diopters*. One diopter is equivalent to 10 times the magnification. Most lamps in the industry come in values of 3, 5, or 10 diopters, which means 30 times the power magnification, 50 times the power magnification, or 100 times the power magnification, respectively.
- Five diopters are the most common magnification.
- A good-quality light should have a clear lens and be free of distortion. Since you are using this light often, any distortion will add strain to your eyes and make it more difficult to see the skin.

Some skin analysis devices include hand-held magnification tools, head visors, and cameras that view the skin at up to 200 × magnification and may include components that can assess the skin's hydration level. These devices are especially useful to track treatment progress in medical esthetics or when performing advanced treatments such as peels or microdermabrasion.

When to Use the Magnifying Lamp

You should use the magnifying lamp:

- During skin analysis to determine the correct facial treatment
- During extractions
- As a source of additional lighting when needed for a treatment.

Best Practices for the Magnifying Lamp

Lamps are designed to sit on a floor base or attach directly to a facial cart. The base that a magnifying lamp sits on may be sold separately from the lamp itself. Carts are not as mobile, so floor stands are preferred. It is worth getting a quality lamp that has good knobs that stay tight instead of one that hinges, as it will last longer due to all the constant adjustments that are used in positioning the lamp correctly for each client and treatment.

- Always use eye pads when the lamp is positioned directly over the client.

- It is important to loosen the adjustment knobs before moving the lamp arms up or down. Follow the manufacturer's recommendations for adjusting the knobs to ensure the longevity of the device. If you force the lamp into positions without loosening the knobs first, you will wear out the hinge of the light and then it will not stay in position.

- To avoid overreaching and hurting your back or wrists, you may need to stand up to move and adjust the lamp.

- It is recommended not to adjust the hinge over the client's face or body.

Safety and Maintenance of the Magnifying Lamp

Magnifying lamps can last many years if they are well constructed and maintained. Conversely, if they are abused and roughly handled, their longevity is compromised. If problems do occur, they typically involve the adjustment arm. The spring on the arm can wear out and may break if not used with care. Some less expensive magnifying lights have hinges rather than knobs that adjust, but these usually wear out faster. Periodically check the screws around the light to ensure that they are not loose. The arm and bolt underneath the base may also need tightening. A simple toolbox with screwdrivers and wrenches is handy to have in the facility.

- To clean the lens, turn off the lamp, let it cool, and then spray it with a disinfectant and wipe with a soft cloth. Avoid using paper products because paper towels and tissues will scratch the lens.

- Clean and disinfect the entire lamp, including the base, after each use.

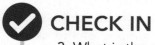 **CHECK IN**

3. What is the most common diopter for a magnifying lamp?

Discuss the Wood's Lamp and Its Uses

The **Wood's lamp** (WOODZ LAMP), developed by American physicist Robert Williams Wood, is a filtered black light that is used to illuminate fungi, bacterial disorders, pigmentation problems, and other skin problems (**Figure 10–4**).

Skin scopes are similar to Wood's lamps. These larger skin analysis tools use a UV light with an interior mirror. A client can look at their face on one side of the scope while the esthetician looks

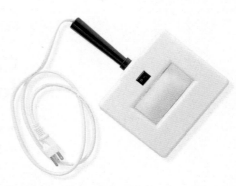

▲ **FIGURE 10–4** Wood's lamp.

through the scope and examines the skin from the other side. These scanners use a magnifying lamp and black light to analyze skin features such as hydration and pigmentation.

When to Use the Wood's Lamp

The Wood's lamp allows the esthetician to conduct a more in-depth skin analysis, illuminating skin problems that are ordinarily invisible to the naked eye. Under the lamp, different conditions show up in various shades of color. For instance, the thicker the skin, the whiter the fluorescence will be.

Table 10–1 provides some examples of skin conditions and how they appear under the Wood's lamp.

▼ TABLE 10–1 Wood's Lamp Reference Chart

Skin Condition	Appearance Under Wood's Lamp
Thick corneum layer	White fluorescence
Horny layer of dead skin cells	White spots
Normal, healthy skin	Blue-white
Thin or dehydrated skin	Light violet/purple
Acne or bacteria	Yellow or orange
Oily areas of the face/comedones	Yellow or sometimes pink or orange
Hyperpigmentation or sun damage	Brown
Hypopigmentation	Blue-white or yellow-green

Not all pigmentation that shows up under the Wood's lamp can be completely lightened with regular exfoliation treatments. Pigmentation located at the dermal epidermal junction can only be addressed at the medical level. Only pigmentation on the surface of the skin can be potentially lightened by exfoliation treatments and lightening products. It is also important to let clients know that addressing pigmentation is an ongoing challenge, for example, with pigmentation associated with sun damage. Pigmentation can reappear if the skin is in contact with the initial stimuli of heat or UV rays.

Contraindications and Best Practices for the Wood's Lamp

- When using the Wood's lamp, the room must be totally dark.
- Place small eye pads on the client, making sure the area around the eye is still visible.
- The bulbs can get hot, so be careful not to touch the skin or have the lamp turned on too long.

Safety and Maintenance of the Wood's Lamp

Treat the Wood's lamp carefully, as you would a magnifying lamp. Follow the manufacturer's directions for cleaning. To protect the bulbs, store the cooled lamp in a safe place where it is protected from breakage. A small covered plastic tub and protective wrapping are helpful in storing the glass parts of various tools and machines.

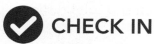 **CHECK IN**

4. What skin conditions does a Wood's lamp reveal?

ACTIVITY

Test It Out!

With a partner in class, use a Wood's lamp and Table 10–1 to identify skin conditions your classmate may have. Record your findings and communicate them to your partner.

Demonstrate How to Safely and Effectively Use the Rotary Brush

The main purpose of the **rotary brush** (ROH-tuh-ree BRUSH), also known as a facial brush, is to lightly exfoliate the skin (**Figure 10–5**). The brush can be rotated at different speeds and directions. Some brushes are simple rotary; some come with additional options such as ultrasonic technology that provides additional deep-cleansing results. Brushes come in smaller sizes for the face and larger sizes for other areas of the body, such as the back, and they have two or three small brushes with different textures ranging from soft to firm. In recent years more advanced technology such as the ultrasonic spatula, used for deep cleansing, has replaced the rotary brush.

When to Use the Rotary Brush

Integrating the rotary brush into your service can help you achieve various goals:

- Use the brush when your goal is to lightly exfoliate the skin without the use of chemicals such as enzymes or peels.
- Use the brush during the second cleansing step in a facial to save time.

Effects of the Rotary Brush

The effects of using a rotary brush include:

- The rotary brush provides light exfoliation of the client's skin.
- Cleansing brushes can stimulate the skin and help soften excess oil, dirt, and cell buildup.

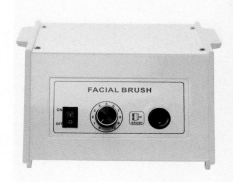

▲ **FIGURE 10–5** Rotary brush.

Contraindications and Best Practices for the Rotary Brush

To prevent harm to your client, it is important to be aware of contra-indications and best practices when using the rotary brush.

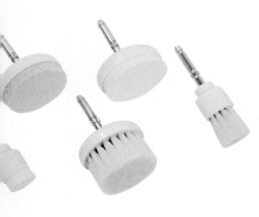

- To avoid damaging or further irritating the skin, do not use brushes on acne, couperose, fragile, or inflamed skin.
- Moisten the brush before each use to soften the bristles.
- More sensitive skin requires a slow, steady rotation and soft brushes with fewer passes.
- Thicker, oily skin can tolerate a faster speed and firmer brushes with more passes.
- Fewer passes produce less exfoliation.
- The brush should not be overused, or it will cause irritations and sensitivity.
- Apply gentle pressure.

Safety and Maintenance of the Rotary Brush

It is important to note that only brush heads that can be fully immersed in a disinfectant of appropriate strength should be used. Some brushes with natural bristles may deteriorate and are prohibited from use due to the inability to clean and disinfect them. Rotary brush machines come with detachable brushes for cleaning. Here are some guidelines for maintaining the brushes:

- Remove the brushes after each use and wash them thoroughly with soap and water.
- Thoroughly clean the hand piece, cords and the machine with disinfectant.
- After manual cleansing, immerse the brushes in a disinfectant for the time recommended in the manufacturer's instructions.
  - It is important to clean, rinse, dry, and store the brushes so that they do not lose their shape when drying. If the bristles become bent or lose their shape, they will not rotate properly.
  - Although they can be stored temporarily in a dry ultraviolet sanitizer, the brushes will break down if left in the ultraviolet sanitizer too long. When they are completely dry, transfer them to a closed container.

The Rotary Brush

1. Insert the appropriate size of brush into the hand-held device.
2. Apply cleanser or water to the skin. Do not let water or cleanser drip down the face or into the eyes. Use a piece of cotton or 4" × 4" gauze to catch any excess water.
3. Use the brush up to three passes on each area, or for approximately three to five seconds, unless directed otherwise. (Limit the number of passes according to the sensitivity of the client's skin or area you are working on.)
4. Keep the brush moving across the face at all times, with light pressure and in a circular pattern, ensuring the bristles remain straight and uncompressed throughout the process.
5. Apply water to the bristles as needed, adjust the speed, and begin a horizontal pattern across the forehead. Do not allow the brush to drag the skin. The brush should be damp, but not to the point it is dripping on the client. Wipe excess water on a 4" × 4" pad or towel if necessary.
6. Continue the sequence down to the cheeks, nose, upper lip, chin, jaw, and neck areas.
7. Lift the brush from the skin and turn off the machine, disengaging the attachment.

 CHECK IN

5. Name one of the effects of a rotary brush.

Demonstrate How to Safely and Effectively Use the Steamer

Many estheticians consider the steamer to be the most important machine used in esthetics. Professional steamers come in various sizes and models. Use only distilled water in the steamer, because the mineral and calcium deposits in tap water can damage the machinery. The steamer takes approximately 5 to 10 minutes to heat up. Do not direct the arm of the steamer toward the client's face until mist begins to flow. The mist/vapor is directed onto the skin's surface by a nozzle at the end of the steamer's arm. Steamers may have a place for an aromatherapy ring on the inside of the nozzle head, and they may have a special feature for using essential oils. A quality steamer will last for years; inexpensive models break down quickly. It is worth the extra money to buy a good-quality steamer that will last and be reliable (**Figure 10–6**).

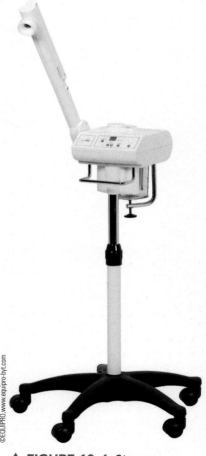

©EQUIPRO,www.equipro-byt.com

▲ **FIGURE 10–6** Steamer.

When to Use the Steamer

Integrating the steamer into your service can help to soften the skin.

- The steamer is typically used during the second cleanse in a facial.
- It can be used prior to extractions to soften the skin, but this effect is only temporary.
- It can be used to soften a facial mask and facilitate its removal.

Effects of the Steamer

There are many benefits of using a steamer during a service.

- Steam helps to stimulate circulation, as well as soften sebum, dead cells, and other debris. The warmth relaxes the skin and tissues, making it easier for the esthetician to extract comedones.
- Steam can also be beneficial for the sinuses and congestion.
- Steamers with ozone (O_3) may have an antiseptic effect on the skin that is beneficial for acne and problematic skin.

STEAMERS WITH OZONE

Ordinary oxygen in the atmosphere consists of two oxygen atoms (O_2). Ozone consists of three oxygen atoms (O_3). Ozone is what is created after a lightning storm and has a distinct smell. Ozone also has antiseptic qualities. These molecules have the power to kill bacteria and other microorganisms; that being stated, ozone is also a strong oxidizer that creates free radicals. The third atom can detach from the O_3 molecule and reattach to other molecules.

Some steamers have ozone mechanisms. High-frequency machines also create ozone. According to the EPA, exposure to ozone affects the respiratory system, can irritate the eyes, and may cause shortness of breath and coughing. OSHA standards for normal exposure should not exceed 0.1 part per million (ppm). Ozone air purifiers are ineffectual and may exceed safe levels of O_3. Check the ozone output for machines before purchasing or using one to make sure it is under the maximum exposure limits.

Contraindications and Best Practices for the Steamer

It is important to be aware of the contraindications and best practices for the steamer to prevent harming your client.

- Do not use too much steam on couperose or inflamed skin, because it dilates the capillaries and follicles, causing more redness and irritation.
- Avoid placing the steamer arm too close to the face.

- To avoid burning yourself, never touch the glass jar on the steamer when it is hot—it takes a long time to cool down. Ask your instructor for a demonstration on how to safely remove, clean, and replace the glass jar.

- Do not leave the room while steaming the client in case the steamer starts spraying water—this may burn the client.

- Do not overfill the steamer because the steamer may spray excess water and burn the client.

- Clean the steamer regularly to avoid mineral buildup that causes water to spray and burn the client. Do not let the water level run low in the steamer, as the glass may break in steamers that do not have an automatic shutoff safety mechanism. If the steamer is positioned with the steam directed from below the nose and is too close for the client, try steaming from above the head. Reposition it a few times if necessary to get an even placement of steam across the face.

- Do not add cold water to the steamer until it has cooled off so as not to break the glass jar.

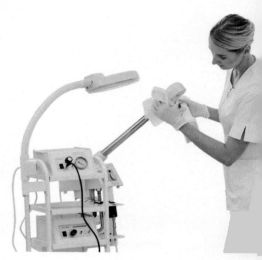

Safety and Maintenance of the Steamer

To ensure proper usage, always read and follow the manufacturer's directions for the steamer. Following these guidelines will keep your machine in peak working condition for years.

- After each use, wipe down the outside of the steamer with a disinfectant.

- At night when the glass jar is completely cooled, unscrew and empty the jar to let it dry. Make sure that the rubber seal along the rim of the jar is clean.

- Refill the steamer machine with fresh distilled water each morning. Do not overfill.

- Before each treatment turn the steamer on to give it a chance to warm up. This will save valuable time when treating each client.

- Water used inside the steamer should be as free of chemicals and minerals as possible; therefore, it is always recommended that distilled, not tap, water be used. Most tap water contains chlorine, other chemicals, and mineral deposits.

- Do not leave water in the steamer overnight or on weekends. If the steamer is not emptied regularly, deposits can collect on the heater element. Empty the jar and lightly clean with vinegar and then with soap and water. Allow the coils to dry.

- Neglected steamers tend to spit hot water due to the buildup of mineral deposits that occur with daily use. Mineral deposits may appear as a white or yellow crusty film on the heating element. The hot water can land on the client's face and may cause a serious burn.

- Some steamer models have solid tanks, preventing you from seeing the element; therefore, they need to be cleaned at least two times a month. Use a cleaning solution of plain vinegar and water.

- Never put essential oils or herbs directly into the water. Essential oils are highly active. When dropped directly into a closed jar with boiling water, they can cause excessive spitting of water or, even worse, clog the steamer or cause the glass to break from pressure. Some steamers are equipped with a wick-type apparatus that fits at the mouth of the nozzle. A couple of drops of essential oil can be placed here before the steamer is preheated. The steam picks up the aroma as it vaporizes out into the room.

- Other steamer models make use of a special container for herbs. These specialized steamers are normally more expensive; however, they provide the esthetician with the added benefit of incorporating therapeutic herbs into the steaming process. You can also put a few drops of essential oil on your hands or a cotton pad or swab and hold it close to the steam for aromatherapy.

- Do not leave the room when preheating the steamer, or you may forget about it and run the water down too low and shatter the glass. Water levels must be kept above the safety line marked above the element on the glass jar. Not all steamers have automatic shutoffs.

- Some machines may have automatic regulators that detect the water level. When it becomes too low or empty, a safety switch is triggered, turning off the machine.

- Some machines have timers that shut off after the set time. Timers are useful but some may tick and then ding when the timer goes off, which can be a loud and distracting noise. Try before you buy.

- Always keep a spare glass jar and rubber seal handy.

——PERFORM——
Procedure 10-1
Use and Care
for the Steamer

CHECK IN

6. List the benefits of using a steamer.

Demonstrate How to Safely and Effectively Use the Vacuum Machine

The **vacuum machine** (VAK-yoom muh-sheen), also known as the *suction machine*, is used in a facial when the esthetician's goal is to remove impurities, stimulate the skin, or perform a machine-aided facial lymphatic massage. The machine uses glass and metal suction cups that come in different sizes and shapes, depending on their use.

The movement of these cups across the face and neck mimics the contractions naturally made by the lymph vessels and artificially aids in the movement of lymphatic fluid (**Figure 10–7**).

When to Use the Vacuum Machine

Determining when to use the vacuum machine during a service is the first step in using one.

- This machine can be used after desincrustation and before extractions.
- It can also be used in place of massage.

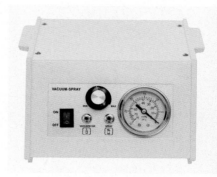

▲ **FIGURE 10–7** Vacuum machine.

Effects of the Vacuum Machine

The vacuum machine serves two main functions:

- To suction dirt and impurities from the skin
- To stimulate the dermal layer as well as lymphatic and blood circulation.

Contraindications and Best Practices for the Vacuum Machine

It is important to be aware of the contraindications and best practices for the vacuum machine to prevent harming your client.

- A vacuum machine should not be used on couperose skin with distended or dilated capillaries or on open lesions. To avoid harming the client's skin, do not use suction on inflamed, rosacea, or couperose skin.
- Never suction liquids or oils into the suction device.
- Avoid using strong suction because it may cause tissue damage or bruising. Holding the skin taut with the proper settings will allow you to avoid damaging the skin.

Safety and Maintenance for the Vacuum Machine

To clean and maintain the vacuum machine, follow these guidelines.

- Clean all glass devices with soap and water and soak them in a disinfectant of appropriate strength.
- Follow the manufacturer's directions to clean the hand pieces and hoses.
- Normally a filter is located at the end of the hose where the hose attaches to an orifice connected to the machine. The filter may have to be changed frequently, depending on use.
- Store the tips wrapped in cloth in a covered storage area to protect against breakage.

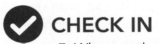

CHECK IN

7. What are the two effects of the vacuum device?

Demonstrate How to Safely and Effectively Use Galvanic Current

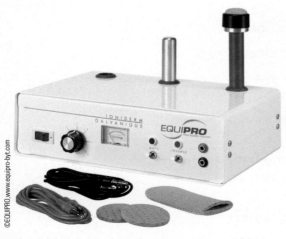

©EQUIPRO,www.equipro-byt.com

▲ **FIGURE 10–8** Galvanic current machine.

Galvanic current is used to create two significant reactions in esthetics: chemical **desincrustation** (des-in-krus-TAY-shun) and ionic **iontophoresis** (eye-ahn-toh-foh-REE-sus). The galvanic machine converts the alternating current received from an electrical outlet into a direct current. Electrons are then allowed to flow continuously in the same direction. This creates a relaxation response that can be regulated to target specific nerve endings in the epidermis. The machine can leave a metallic taste in the mouth, which is normal (**Figure 10–8**).

When to Use Galvanic Current

Galvanic current is used when the esthetician's goal is to prepare the skin for extractions or assist in delivering targeted products to the skin. It can be used in a facial after the exfoliation step and prior to the extraction steps and can be used prior to masking to deliver ingredients or during the final stages of a facial.

Effects of Using the Galvanic Machine

There are two main benefits that occur when using the galvanic machine.

- Desincrustation causes an alkaline reaction to soften the follicles for deep cleansing.
- Iontophoresis is used for introducing a water-soluble product into the skin.

DESINCRUSTATION

Desincrustation uses galvanic current to create a chemical reaction in the skin that emulsifies sebum and debris in the follicle.

To perform desincrustation a negative pH/alkaline-based, electro-negative solution is placed onto the skin's surface. The solution is formulated to remain on the surface of the skin rather than being absorbed. When the esthetician is conducting desincrustation, the client holds the positive electrode, set on the positive polarity. The esthetician uses the negative electrode, set on negative polarity, on the face. This creates a chemical reaction that transforms the sebum of the skin into soap—a process known as **saponification** (sah-pahn-ih-fih-KAY-shun). Soap is made from fat and lye (sodium hydroxide). When the electrical current interacts with the salts (sodium chloride) in the skin, it creates the chemical known as sodium hydroxide—or lye. This soapy substance helps dissolve excess oil, clogged follicles, comedones, and other debris on the skin, while softening it at the same time.

Various types of electrodes are available for the galvanic machine. The most common are the flat electrode and the roller. To make proper contact, each electrode must be covered with cotton, and the client must hold the electrode whose charge (either positive or negative) is the opposite of the electrode on the skin.

Baking soda in water can be used as a desincrustation fluid for anaphoresis. Most water-based serums can be used as iontophoresis products for cataphoresis.

Effects of Desincrustation Desincrustation is beneficial for oily or acne skin because it helps soften and relax the debris in the follicle before extractions.

Best Practices and Safety Considerations for Desincrustation Keep even contact with the skin once the galvanic machine is on. Electricity is flowing through the electrode and when it is lifted even slightly the client may feel a mild tingling or shock. To avoid this sensation, turn off the machine first and then remove the electrode from the skin. Clients should be advised of the possibility of these sensations prior to starting the treatment.

> **CAUTION!**
> Do not use negative galvanic current on skin with broken capillaries or pustular acne conditions, or on a client with high blood pressure or metal implants.

IONTOPHORESIS

Iontophoresis is the process of using electric current to introduce water-soluble solutions into the skin. This process allows estheticians to transfer, or penetrate, ions of an applied solution into the deeper layers of the skin. **Ions** (EYE-ahns) are atoms or molecules that carry an electrical charge. Current flows through conductive solutions from both the positive and negative polarities. This process is known as **ionization** (eye-ahn-ih-ZAY-shun), the separating of a substance into ions.

Theoretically, iontophoresis is based on universal laws of attraction. For example, negative attracts positive, and vice versa. Similar to a magnetic response, iontophoresis creates an exchange of negative and positive ions or charges.

The process of ionic penetration takes two forms: **cataphoresis** (kat-uh-fuh-REE-sus), which refers to the infusion of a positive product, and **anaphoresis** (an-uh-for-EES-sus), which refers to the infusion of a negative product, such as a desincrustation fluid.

Effects of Iontophoresis Several possible skin reactions and effects can occur during ionization (**Table 10–2**).

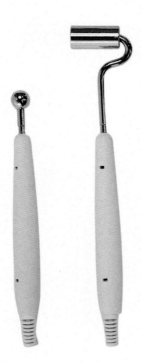

▼ **TABLE 10–2** Effects from the Galvanic Current: Iontophoresis

EFFECTS FROM THE GALVANIC CURRENT: IONTOPHORESIS	
NEGATIVE POLE (CATHODE): ANAPHORESIS	**POSITIVE POLE (ANODE): CATAPHORESIS**
Negative Solutions	**Positive Solutions**
Causes an alkaline reaction	Causes an acidic reaction
Softens and relaxes tissue	Tightens the skin
Stimulates nerve endings	Calms or soothes nerve endings
Increases blood circulation	Decreases blood circulation

Best Practices and Safety Considerations for Iontophoresis Keep even contact with the skin once the galvanic machine is on. Electricity is flowing through the electrode and when it is lifted even slightly the client may feel a mild tingling or shock. To avoid this sensation, turn off the machine first and then remove the electrode from the skin. The electrode should be continuously moving at all times.

Some machines have a switch on the panel that controls the positive and negative modes so that you do not have to manually switch the red and black wires but instead move only the switch.

Polarity of Solutions You need to always check the labeling of the product to identify the polarity of the ampoule (AM-pyool) or solution. Slightly acidic pH products are considered positive and are mostly used for iontophoresis. If the product were positive, the client and esthetician would use the opposite electrodes. The technician holds the positive and the client holds the negative. Alkaline (or base) pH products are considered negative and are used for desincrustation. If the product is negative, the esthetician infuses the solution with the electrode set at negative and the esthetician holds the negative electrode. The client holds the positive electrode (**Figure 10–9**). Some manufacturers may include ingredients in the same vial that are simultaneously positive and negative. In that case, the product should be ionized for three to five minutes on negative followed by three to five minutes on positive. If neither a negative nor a positive polarity is indicated for an ampoule, as a general rule the esthetician should first use the negative pole and then the positive pole. This way you are stimulating and softening the skin first and preparing it for the treatment with anaphoresis, and then ending with the product penetration, skin tightening, and soothing with cataphoresis.

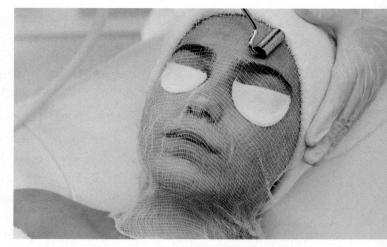

▲ **FIGURE 10–9** Galvanic current can stimulate and soften the skin.

- The molecular weight of a product is also a factor in permeability. Smaller molecules have greater penetration ability, while larger molecules cannot penetrate the skin.

- Water-based products will penetrate better than oil-based products.

Contraindications and Best Practices for the Galvanic Machine

To avoid potential health complications, do not use galvanic current on clients with the following conditions:

- Metal implants or a pacemaker
- Braces
- Heart conditions, including MVP, also known as mitral valve prolapse
- Epilepsy
- Pregnancy
- High blood pressure, fever, or any infection
- Diminished nerve sensibility due to diseases such as diabetes
- Open or broken skin (e.g., wounds, new scars) or inflamed pustular acne
- Couperose skin or rosacea
- Chronic migraine headaches
- Apprehension about the use of electrical appliances.

Safety and Maintenance of the Galvanic Machine

Before attempting to clean the electrodes, always read and follow the manufacturer's directions for cleaning and disinfecting the equipment.

- Detach the electrode cord from the electrode.
- Remove any cotton from the electrode and discard.
- Wash the electrode in warm soapy water to remove any organic material, rinse, and dry. Soak the electrode in disinfectant for the manufacturer's directed time, rinse, dry, and store in a nonairtight container.
- Never place the metal electrode in an autoclave, unless directed by the manufacturer. Carefully spray and wipe the electrode attachment cord, hand piece, and machine with a disinfectant.

─PERFORM─

Procedure 10-2

Perform Desincrustation and Iontophoresis Using the Galvanic Machine

 CHECK IN

8. List and define the two main reactions of the galvanic current.
9. What are the contraindications for using a galvanic machine?
10. What are the effects on the skin from anaphoresis?
11. How does the negative pole of the galvanic current affect the skin?
12. Define cataphoresis.

Demonstrate How to Safely and Effectively Use the High-Frequency Machine

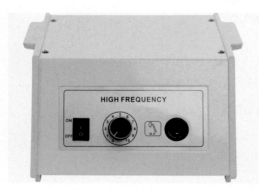

▲ **FIGURE 10–10** High-frequency machine.

The **high-frequency machine** (HY-FREE-kwen-see muh-SHEEN) is an apparatus that utilizes an alternating or **sinusoidal current** (sy-nuh-SOYD-ul KUR-unt)—which is a smooth, repetitive alternating current—and produces a heat effect. The high-frequency oscillating current passes through a device that allows for the selection of a *Tesla* pulse current. This current can produce a frequency of 60,000 to 200,000 hertz, depending on how it is regulated. The frequency indicates the repetition of the current per second (**Figure 10–10**). Because high-frequency current is capable of changing polarity thousands of times per second, it basically has no polarity and in effect does not produce chemical changes. This makes product penetration physically impossible. Product penetration is achieved instead by using the galvanic current.

The rapid oscillation created by the high-frequency machine vibrates water molecules in the skin. This can produce a mild to strong heat effect. It is important to note that esthetic high-frequency devices have a mild effect. An example of a stronger heat reaction is seen in **thermolysis** (thur-MAHL-uh-sus), which is used for electrolysis (permanent hair removal). The high-frequency machine creates noise, and the ozone has a distinctive smell to it. Let clients know what to expect when using high-frequency machines and that this is normal.

Electrodes

Several types of direct or indirect electrodes are available with high frequency. Each of these electrodes has unique benefits and features that produce specific physiological reactions in esthetic treatments. If you use the high-frequency machine, you will need to be trained in the procedure and on how to use the different electrodes.

During the manufacturing process, most of the air is removed from high-frequency electrodes, creating a vacuum in the tube. The air is replaced, mainly with neon gas. However, some electrodes may also contain argon gas. As electricity passes through these gases, they emit visible shades of light. Neon gas produces a pink, orange, or red light and is typically used for sensitive skin and aging skin. Argon or rarified gas produces blue or violet light and is typically used for normal to oily skin and acne prone skin. Sometimes these lights are inaccurately called *infrared* or *ultraviolet* because of their colors; however, there are no infrared or ultraviolet rays in high frequency.

In addition to different forms of gas, the electrodes come in different shapes and sizes to accommodate the treatment area.

TYPES AND GENERAL APPLICATION OF ELECTRODES

There are many types of electrodes that can be used in a high-frequency machine treatment. Refer to **Table 10–3** for a breakdown of various types and their applications.

When to Use High Frequency

The high-frequency machine is a useful and versatile esthetic tool.

- It may be applied after extractions or used over a product but will not penetrate a product as iontophoresis would.
- The machine also creates ozone, which has a germicidal action on the skin.

▼ **TABLE 10–3 High-Frequency Electrode Reference Table**

Electrode	General Application
Small mushroom	1. Place the electrode into the hand-held device. Twist it gently into place. 2. Adjust the rheostat to the proper setting if the machine is not automatic. 3. Place an index finger on the glass electrode to ground it until it touches the client's skin, then remove. 4. Glide the electrode over the gauze in circular movements (across the forehead area) and then to the nose, cheeks, and chin areas. 5. To remove from the skin, place an index finger on the electrode to ground it and then remove it. Turn the power switch off and disengage the electrode. Remove the gauze.
Large mushroom	1. The large mushroom is used in the same way as the small mushroom. 2. Another effective way to use this apparatus is to open a piece of cotton gauze and glide the mushroom electrode over the gauze which is placed on the client's face. This produces a small spray of sparks onto the skin. This treatment is ideal for acne or problematic skin. 3. Facial finish: High frequency may be used at the end of a treatment over cream. Place cotton gauze between the cream on the client's skin and the electrode. Glide in circular motions over the entire area. Remove the gauze.
Indirect **(spiral)**	Indirect electrodes are used indirectly to stimulate the skin during massage. This treatment is ideal for sallow and aging skin. 1. Apply cream to the client's face. (Do not apply gauze.) 2. Give the wire glass electrode to the client, who then holds it with both hands. 3. Place the fingers of one hand on the forehead. 4. With the opposite hand, turn the high frequency on and move to a low setting. 5. Using both hands, perform a piano finger motion, gently tapping the skin. Move around in a systematic manner over the entire face. 6. To discontinue, remove one hand from the skin, turn the power switch off, and disengage the electrode. 7. In order to keep the current flowing do not lose contact with the skin during this procedure.
Sparking (glass tip)	A glass tip electrode is used to direct sparking to a specific area such as an acne lesion. It helps disinfect and heal the lesion. Sparking is visible and creates an interesting zapping noise. 1. Place the electrode into the hand-held device. 2. Place the glass electrode over the lesion area, removing your finger so that the electrode is not grounded prior to placing on the face so that the area is sparked for a few seconds. Touch the electrode to the blemish for a few seconds and remove. Repeat this a few times. 3. Remove the electrode from the skin by placing the finger once more on the glass. Turn the power switch off and disengage the electrode.
Comb (rake)	To apply the comb electrode, follow the directions for the mushroom electrode. It is mainly used in a scalp treatment.

Effects of High Frequency

The high-frequency machine benefits the skin in the following ways:

- It has an antiseptic and healing effect on the skin.
- It stimulates circulation.
- It helps oxygenate the skin.
- It increases cell metabolism.
- It helps coagulate and heal any open lesion after extraction by sparking it with the mushroom electrode.
- It generates a warm feeling that has a relaxing effect on the skin.

Contraindications and Best Practices for High-Frequency Machines

Be sure to know all the contraindications of using a high-frequency machine before implementing it in treatments.

High frequency should not be used on clients with the following conditions or devices:

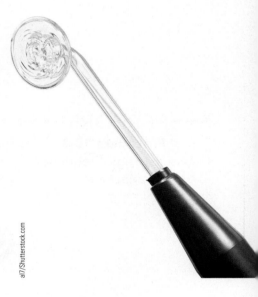

al7/Shutterstock.com

- Couperose skin
- Inflamed areas
- Pacemakers
- Metal implants
- Heart problems
- High blood pressure
- Braces
- Epilepsy
- Pregnancy
- Body piercings from the waist up; the client should avoid any contact with metal—such as chair arms, jewelry, and metal bobby pins—during the treatment; a burn may occur if such contact is made.

Adhere to the following guidelines.

- To avoid being burned, the client should avoid contact with metal during electrical machine treatments.
- Clients should remove all jewelry and piercings prior to the treatment.
- The technician should ground their finger on the electrode prior to applying it to the client and prior to removing it from the client.
- The electrode should be continuously moving at all times.
- Electrodes should be gently removed from the hand piece to avoid snapping the electrode.

Safety and Maintenance for High-Frequency Machines

Follow these maintenance guidelines for high-frequency machines.

- After each use, clean the glass electrode by wiping it with a solution of soap and water.
- Do not use alcohol on electrodes.
- Do not immerse the electrodes directly in water. Place only the glass end (not the metal) into a disinfectant solution for manufacturer's recommended time. Wipe the entire electrode with a disinfectant-saturated paper towel.
- Rinse the electrodes. Do not get the metal end wet. Dry with a clean towel and store in a nonairtight closed container. Do not place electrodes in an ultraviolet machine or in an autoclave.
- Unless they break or are damaged, most electrodes do not need replacing, but keep in mind that the electrodes are very fragile. Take extra care to wrap them in a soft material and then store them in a drawer where they will not be knocked around or damaged. Some of the newer machines offer inserts for storing the electrodes right on the machine. Be sure to cover the electrodes so they remain clean and undamaged.
- The high-frequency coil should be replaced after a few years of use if it is losing power.
- Clean the handpiece, cords, and machine with disinfectant.
- Check with the manufacturer for additional service requirements.

---PERFORM---
Procedure 10-3
Use the High-Frequency Machine

✔ **CHECK IN**
13. What is high frequency used for?

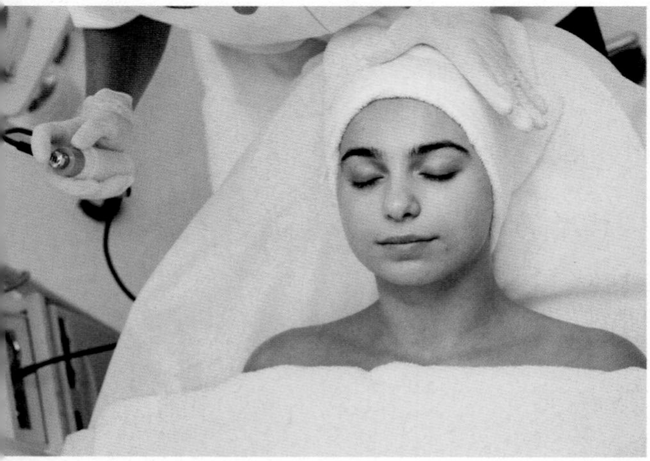

▲ **FIGURE 10–11** A spray machine can be used to apply toner.

Demonstrate How to Safely and Effectively Use Spray Machines

Spray mists are beneficial in calming and hydrating the skin (**Figure 10–11**). The spray machine (SPRAY muh-SHEEN) is part of the vacuum machine and is attached via a hose that is connected to a small plastic bottle with a spray nozzle.

When to Use a Spray Machine

This bottle with the spray nozzle can be filled with a freshener solution or toner (one part toner, two parts distilled water) to gently mist the client's face after cleansing or another treatment step, such as massage.

Effects of Using the Spray Machine

The spray machine affects the skin by adding moisture during or after a treatment and is used to calm and hydrate the skin.

Contraindications and Best Practices for the Spray Machine

- Do not use on clients who have respiratory issues where the spray may cause breathing irritation.
- Do not allow the spray to drip into a client's eyes, ears, or mouth or run down their neck. Use eye pads for a safety precaution if using the mist extensively.
- Do not leave toners and other liquids in the spray bottle for extended periods of time or overnight. This may cause the plastic to break down.
- Do not use the spray machine in a room that is not well ventilated.

Safety and Maintenance for the Spray Machine

Here are some general guidelines for spray machine maintenance.

- After use, clean the spray bottle, cords and machine with disinfectant and follow the cleaning directions supplied by the manufacturer. Flush with distilled water regularly.
- Mineral buildup in the nozzle of the sprayer should be cleaned monthly or more often.

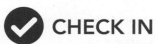

┌─ PERFORM ─┐
Procedure 10-4
Use the Spray Machine
└──────────┘

CHECK IN

14. What are the effects of the spray machine?

State the Benefits and Use of Paraffin Wax

The paraffin wax heaters that allow for direct immersion of a client's hand or foot in a paraffin bath should not be used due to concerns of cross-contamination. However, modern methods have developed. One method uses a machine that heats up a plastic sleeve filled with paraffin for single-use disposable application. Another technique developed to prevent contamination of the wax is the use of a disposable brush to apply the wax to your client. (**Figure 10–12**).

When to Use Paraffin Wax

The warm paraffin mask is used for hydrating dry skin and is generally applied over a hydrating body lotion to the hands and feet.

Effects of Using Paraffin Wax

Paraffin wax allows the esthetician to provide a treatment that offers quick results, but it lasts only for a limited period of time.

Contraindications and Best Practices for Paraffin Wax

Clients who have compromised skin or skin conditions or general health conditions that are not cleared for use of heat-based modalities are not cleared for paraffin wax treatments.

Safety and Maintenance

Paraffin wax heaters stay warm at a safe, low level of heat. They must be replenished as you discard the used wax. These heaters tend to take a long time to heat up in the morning. Always use a professional wax bath machine that emits low heat. A substitute heater, such as an electric cooking pot, regulates heat differently and is not recommended. The use of a machine that heats up a plastic sleeve filled with paraffin for single-use disposable applications for the hands and feet prevents cross-contamination. After use, clean machine with disinfectant and follow the cleaning directions supplied by the manufacturer.

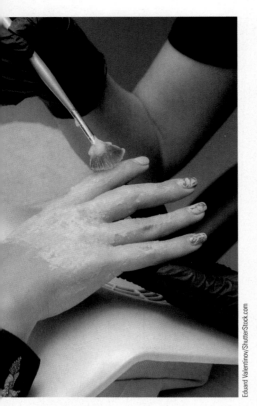

▲ **FIGURE 10–12** New paraffin wax techniques have been developed using a disposable brush for application to avoid cross-contamination.

Eduard Valentinov/ShutterStock.com

 CHECK IN

15. What method of applying paraffin wax is best for preventing cross-contamination?

State the Benefits and Use of Electric Mitts and Boots

Electric boots and mitts are similar to electric heating pads and have adjustable settings. Although not commonly used, it is important to understand their function and benefits for a client (**Figure 10–13**).

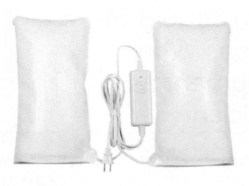
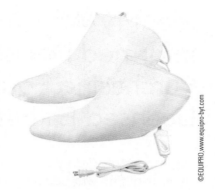

▲ FIGURE 10–13 Electric mitts and boots.

When to Use Electric Mitts and Boots

- Boots and mitts heat the hands and feet to increase circulation and to promote overall relaxation.
- Often promoted as an add-on to a service, boots and mitts actually perform an important function. The heat helps lotion penetrate, and it soothes aching feet and hands.

Effects of Electric Mitts and Boots

Due to the application of heat, electric mitts and boots increase penetration of lotions and creams applied to the skin.

Contraindications and Best Practices for Electric Mitts and Boots

- To use electric mitts and boots, put lotion on the client's hands and/or feet and cover with plastic single-use liners before inserting into the warmers.
- Warm the mitts and/or boots for approximately 10 minutes.
- Make sure the warmers do not get too hot. If the client feels sweaty, then the lotion cannot penetrate.

Safety and Maintenance of Electric Mitts and Boots

- To clean the electric mitts and boots, wipe them with a disinfectant after each use.

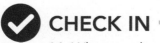 CHECK IN
16. What are the effects of electric mitts and boots?

It may be more affordable to purchase individual machines rather than the all-in-one machines that have the different modalities together on one unit. If anything needs to be repaired, you do not have to ship—or be left without— all your machines.

Choosing a Machine

Choose two machines that interest you. Think about what would be important in purchasing these machines. What should you look for when purchasing a machine? Compare at least three different manufacturers, the selling points of each machine, the prices, and the quality. Which machines will assist you in expanding your business in the future? Which machines would you purchase? Why?

Identify Why You Should Make Informed Decisions When Purchasing Equipment as a Licensed Esthetician

It is important to do your research before purchasing equipment. Regulations define what devices can be used within an esthetician's scope of practice. Another purchasing consideration is insurance coverage for the devices to protect you and your clients. Make sure the manufacturer's claims are accurate and there is clinical evidence to support the claims. It is advisable to go slowly when considering purchasing expensive machines. Warranties and training provided from the manufacturer and distributor are two important considerations when purchasing equipment. Education and training are required for many high-tech machines.

Advances in science and technology have generated many new high-performance tools that enhance the esthetician's work. Estheticians must continue their education to keep abreast of the latest developments in therapeutic skin care. In this chapter, we have presented an overview of specialized tools and equipment designed to help the esthetician obtain the best results possible in skin care treatments. While some machines are not used on a regular basis, it is good to be familiar with them. See Chapter 13, Advanced Topics and Treatments, for additional information on the more advanced equipment.

Study and review the suggested guidelines for operating machinery and practice your skills until you are comfortable working with the equipment. Always be conscientious about safety issues and contraindications when using machines. Clients want instant results, so make sure you can deliver what you promise. Invest in high-quality machines, and your investment will increase your credibility and revenue as an esthetician. What machines would you like to incorporate into your services? High-tech equipment just may be the wave of the future.

 CHECK IN

17. Why is it important to research insurance coverage before purchasing a device?

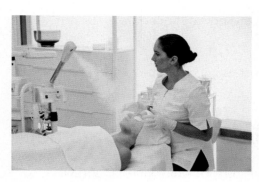

12 Keep the steam approximately 15 to 18 inches (37.5 to 45 centimeters) from the face. Place the steamer farther away, if necessary, so that it is warm but not too hot on the face. If placed too close, steam can cause overheating of the skin, possible irritation, or burning.

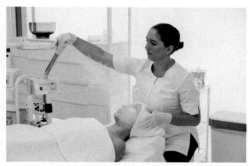

13 Always check the client's comfort level and ensure even distribution of the steam on the face. If the steamer is positioned with the steam directed from below the nose and is too close for the client, try steaming from above the head. Reposition it as needed to get an even placement of steam across the face.

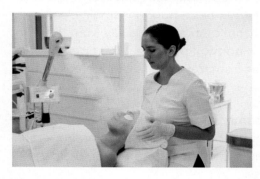

14 Never leave the client unattended while steaming as the water can spray out and burn the client. Do not oversteam the skin. Steaming should last 5 to 10 minutes but should be adjusted for less time if needed.

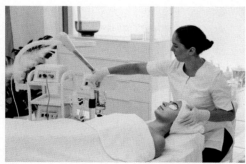

15 When you are ready to discontinue the steam, move the steamer away from the client then turn off the steamer.

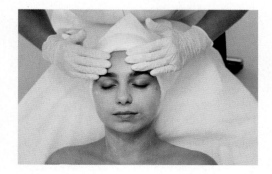

16 Continue with the next step in the facial or close out this procedure.

17 Remove eye pads or goggles, apply moisturizer and sun protection.

18 Perform Procedure 8–9: Post-Service Procedure.

19 Perform Procedure 7–2: Post-Service Clean-Up and Preparation for the Next Client

B: Cleaning and Disinfecting the Steamer

20 Add 2 tablespoons (10 milliliters) of white vinegar and fill jar to the top fill line with water.

21 Turn on the steamer and let it heat to steaming. Do not turn on the ozone.

22 Let the machine steam for 20 minutes or until the water level is low, but make sure it stays above the bottom low-level line to avoid jar breakage.

23 Turn off the steamer and let the vinegar solution rest in the unit for 15 minutes. Because vinegar has a pungent smell, clean the steamer in your utility room or in an area away from the treatment rooms. Open a window, if possible, when performing maintenance to keep fumes from traveling to other areas of the salon.

24 After it cools, drain the steamer jar completely and then refill with water. Let the steamer heat to steaming again and operate for approximately 10 minutes. If there is still an odor, drain the unit and repeat the process.

CAUTION!

Do not allow the caustic vinegar and water solution to sit on the heating coil without steaming immediately. If left overnight, it will corrode the copper coils.

NOTE

There is usually a reset button on steamers for additional safety in the event the steamer runs out of water. If the steamer is not running, check the reset button before you call for help. The reset button is ordinarily found on the back of the machine.

Procedure 10-2:
Perform Desincrustation and Iontophoresis Using The Galvanic Machine

Implements and Materials

- [ ] Standard treatment table setup with linens
- [ ] Galvanic machine and attachments
- [ ] Moistened 4" × 4" esthetics wipes
- [ ] Gloves

- [ ] Hand sanitizer
- [ ] 2" × 2" Esthetics wipes,
- [ ] Cotton rounds
- [ ] Cleanser
- [ ] Toner
- [ ] Water
- [ ] Desincrustation fluid

- [ ] Ampoule or serum
- [ ] Precut gauze face mask or gauze pads
- [ ] Moisturizer
- [ ] Sun protection
- [ ] Disinfectant solution and paper towels for clean-up

Procedure

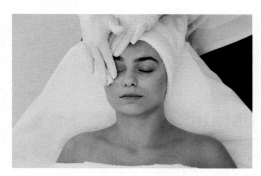

1 Perform Procedure 7-1: Pre-Service Preparing the Treatment Room.

2 Perform Procedure 8–1: Pre-Service Prepare the Client for Treatment.

3 Apply a makeup-remover to an esthetics wipe or cotton round and remove makeup.

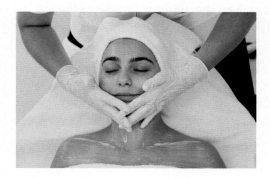

4 Apply a cleanser to the skin.

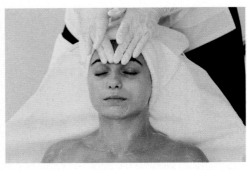

5 Massage the cleanser into the skin to loosen makeup.

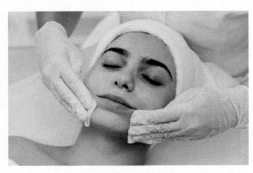

6 Remove the cleanser from the skin.

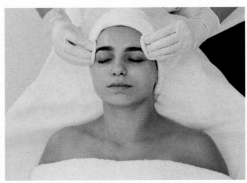

7 Using 2″ × 2″ esthetics wipes or cotton rounds moistened with toner, remove any residue.

Part 1: Desincrustation

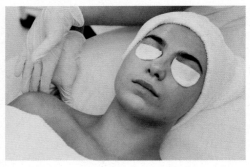

8 Cover the entire positive electrode that makes contact with the client with a piece of dampened cotton around the electrode. Give this to the client to hold or place behind the client's shoulder. This electrode is connected to the positive wire.

9 Apply desincrustation fluid to the entire face and then apply the precut gauze face mask over the face.

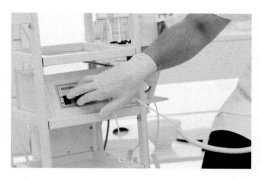

10 Apply the electrode to the client's forehead. Make sure the electrode is directly on the skin before turning on the galvanic current.

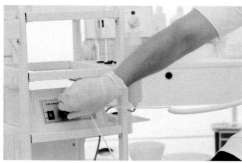

11 Turn the switch to negative and set at the appropriate level for the client.

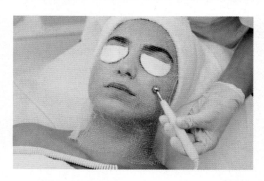

12 Gently rotate the electrode while gliding it over the client's face. Do not lift the electrode or break contact once the machine is on the skin, or it will be uncomfortable for the client. Keep the electrode as flat as possible and parallel to the skin's surface at all times.

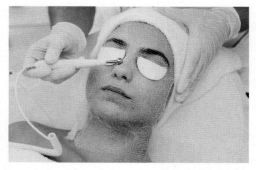

13 Continue in the T-zone area down the nose and into the chin area (or into any area that is oily or needs desincrustation). Best practice is to use desincrustation only in congested areas that need it and avoid areas with dry skin conditions.

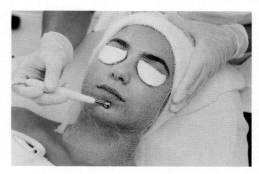

14 Keep the electrode constantly moving to avoid overstimulating an area. Keep the skin moist. Add water to face if it gets too dry to glide over the skin.

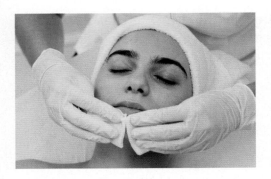

15 When you are finished, turn off the machine first and then remove the electrode. Rinse the skin thoroughly with moistened esthetics wipes.

16 Continue with the next step; iontophoresis.

Part 2: Iontophoresis

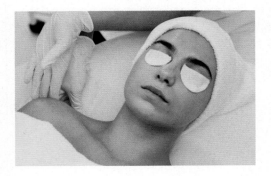

17 Cover the entire positive electrode that makes contact with the client with a piece of dampened cotton around the electrode. Give this to the client to hold or place behind the client's shoulder. This electrode is connected to the positive wire.

18 Apply ampoule or serum to the entire face and then apply the precut gauze face mask over the face.

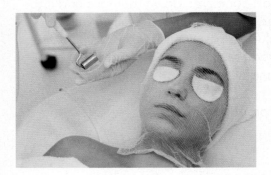

19 Dip the electrode into water or a conductive gel solution. Apply the electrode to the client's forehead. Make sure the electrode is directly on the skin before turning on the galvanic current.

> ## CAUTION!
> No metallic electrode should ever be placed directly on the skin. Gels can be used with metallic electrodes as long as the skin is completely covered with the gel and gauze. Pieces of gauze can be moved around the face and held on each section as needed.

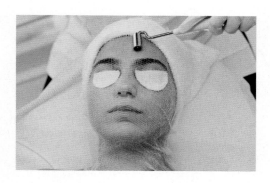

20 You have the option of switching positive and negative poles when infusing solutions. Consult the product manufacturer's instructions when doing so.

21 Beginning on the forehead, gently rotate the electrode while gliding it over the client's forehead. Do not lift the electrode or break contact once the machine is on the skin, or it will be uncomfortable to the client. Keep the electrode as flat as possible and parallel to the skin's surface at all times.

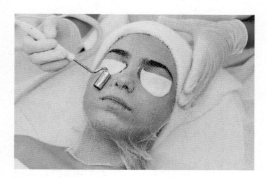

22 Continue to the cheeks and the rest of the face.

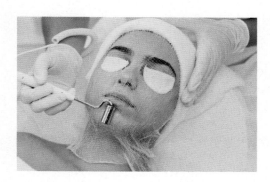

23 Keep the electrode constantly moving to avoid overstimulating an area. Keep the skin moist and the pads wet. Add water to the pad or face if it gets too dry to glide over the skin.

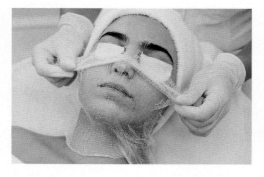

24 When you are finished, turn off the machine first and then remove the electrode. Remove the gauze and rinse the skin thoroughly.

NOTE

Some product companies do not recommend rinsing the serums or ampoule posttreatment.

25 Perform Procedure 8–9: Post-Service Procedure.

26 Perform Procedure 7–2: Post-Service—Clean-Up and Preparation for the Next Client.

Procedure 10-3:
Use the High-Frequency Machine

Implements and Materials

- ☐ Standard treatment table setup with linens
- ☐ High-frequency machine and attachments
- ☐ Precut gauze face mask or gauze pads
- ☐ Massage cream, if performing as part of a massage, with the spiral electrode
- ☐ Moistened 4″ × 4″ esthetics wipes
- ☐ Gloves
- ☐ Hand sanitizer
- ☐ 2″ × 2″ Esthetic wipes or cotton rounds
- ☐ Cleanser
- ☐ Toner
- ☐ Moisturizer
- ☐ Sun protection
- ☐ Disinfectant solution and paper towels for clean-up

Procedure

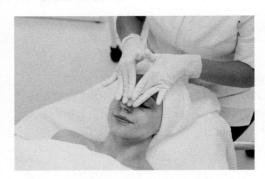

1 Perform Procedure 7–1: Pre-Service—Preparing the Treatment Room.

2 Perform Procedure 8–1: Pre-Service—Prepare the Client for Treatment.

3 Apply and massage a cleanser suitable to remove makeup into the skin with your gloved hands.

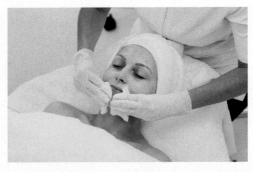

4 Remove the cleanser using 4″ × 4″ esthetic wipes or chosen material.

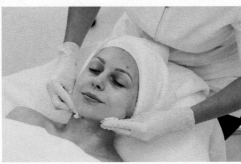

5 Using 2″ × 2″ esthetic wipes or cotton rounds moistened with toner, remove any residue.

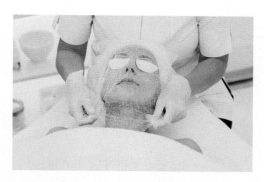

6 Apply the precut gauze face mask over the face, unless the electrode application listed later in this procedure does not require the gauze.

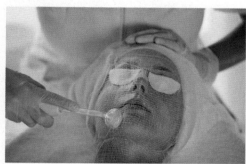

7 Continue as noted with the appropriate electrode selection as detailed in Table 10–3 and proceed with the indicated steps listed for the specific electrode.

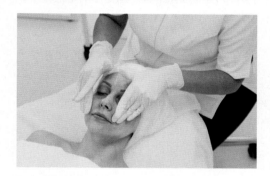

8 Continue with the next step in the facial or close out this procedure with steps 11 through 13.

9 Apply moisturizer and sun protection.

10 Perform Procedure 8–9: Post-Service Procedure.

11 Perform Procedure 7–2: Post-Service—Clean-Up and Preparation for the Next Client.

Procedure 10-4:
Use the Spray Machine

Implements and Materials

- ☐ Standard treatment table setup with linens
- ☐ Spray machine
- ☐ Moistened 4" × 4" esthetics wipes
- ☐ Gloves

- ☐ Hand sanitizer
- ☐ 2" × 2" Esthetics wipes or cotton rounds
- ☐ Towel to place under client's chin while spraying mist
- ☐ Cleanser to remove makeup

- ☐ Mist solution: freshener solution or toner (one part toner, two parts distilled water)
- ☐ Moisturizer and sun protection
- ☐ Disinfectant solution and paper towels for clean-up

Procedure

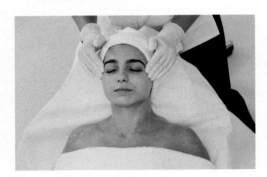

1 Perform Procedure 7–1: Pre-Service—Preparing the Treatment Room.

2 Perform Procedure 8-1 Pre-Service—Prepare the Client for Treatment.

3 Apply and massage a cleanser suitable to remove makeup into the skin with your gloved hands.

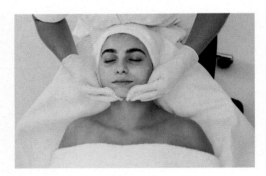

4 Remove the cleanser from the skin using 4" × 4" esthetic wipes or chosen material.

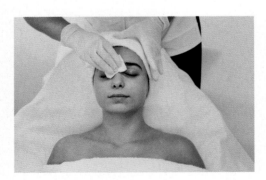

5 Using 2" × 2" esthetic wipes or cotton rounds moistened with toner, remove any residue.

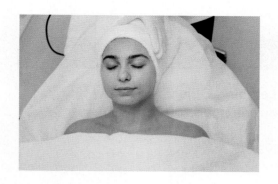

6 If using the spray machine on a high setting you can place a towel under the client's chin to stop the mist from dripping down the neck. Turn on the power and adjust the velocity of the spray. Remind the client to keep the eyes and mouth closed during the misting.

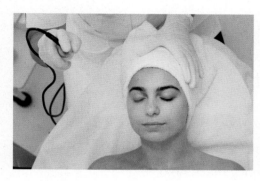

7 Hold the spray approximately 12 to 15 inches (30 to 37.5 centimeters) away from the face and mist for approximately 5 to 20 seconds. If necessary, pause and make sure the client can take a breath between the misting.

8 Turn off the power.

9 Perform Procedure 8–9: Post-Service Procedure.

10 Perform Procedure 7–2: Post-Service—Clean-Up and Preparation for the Next Client.

COMPETENCY PROGRESS

How are you doing with facial devices? **Check the Chapter 10 Learning Objectives below that you feel you have mastered; leave unchecked those objectives you will need to return to:**

- ☐ Explain the importance of the use of facial devices and technology.
- ☐ Identify the basic concepts of electrotherapy.
- ☐ Explain the benefits of the hot towel cabinet.
- ☐ Discuss the magnifying lamp and its uses.
- ☐ Discuss the Wood's lamp and its uses.
- ☐ Demonstrate how to safely and effectively use the rotary brush.
- ☐ Demonstrate how to safely and effectively use the steamer.
- ☐ Demonstrate how to safely and effectively use the vacuum machine.
- ☐ Demonstrate how to safely and effectively use galvanic current.
- ☐ Demonstrate how to safely and effectively use the high-frequency machine.
- ☐ Demonstrate how to safely and effectively use spray machines.
- ☐ State the benefits and use of paraffin wax.
- ☐ State the benefits and use of electric mitts and boots.
- ☐ Identify why you should make informed decisions when purchasing equipment as a licensed esthetician.

CHAPTER GLOSSARY

anaphoresis an-uh-for-EES-sus	p. 428	process of infusing an alkaline (negative) product into the tissues from the negative pole toward the positive pole
cataphoresis kat-uh-fuh-REE-sus	p. 428	process of forcing an acidic (positive) product into deeper tissues using galvanic current from the positive pole toward the negative pole; tightens and calms the skin
desincrustation des-in-krus-TAY-shun	p. 426	process used to soften and emulsify sebum and blackheads in the follicles
high-frequency machine HY-FREE-kwen-see muh-SHEEN	p. 430	apparatus that utilizes alternating, or sinusoidal, current to produce a mild to strong heat effect; sometimes called *tesla high-frequency or violet ray*
ions EYE-ahns	p. 428	atoms or molecules that carry an electrical charge
ionization eye-ahn-ih-ZAY-shun	p. 428	the separation of an atom or molecule into positive or negative ions
iontophoresis eye-ahn-toh-foh-REE-sus	p. 426	process of infusing water-soluble products into the skin with the use of electric current, such as the use of positive and negative poles of a galvanic machine or a microcurrent device

rotary brush ROH-tuh-ree BRUSH	p. 419	machine used to lightly exfoliate and stimulate the skin; also helps soften excess oil, dirt, and cell buildup
saponification sah-pahn-ih-fih-KAY-shun	p. 427	chemical reaction during desincrustation during which the current transforms the sebum into soap
sinusoidal current sy-nuh-SOYD-ul KUR-unt	p. 430	a smooth, repetitive alternating current; the most commonly used alternating current waveform, used in the high-frequency machine; can produce heat
spray machine SPRAY muh-SHEEN	p. 434	spray misting device
thermolysis thur-MAHL-uh-sus	p. 431	heat effect; a modality of electrolysis utilizing alternating current (AC); used for permanent hair removal
vacuum machine VAK-yoom muh-sheen	p. 424	also known as *suction machine*; device that vacuums/suctions the skin to remove impurities and stimulate circulation

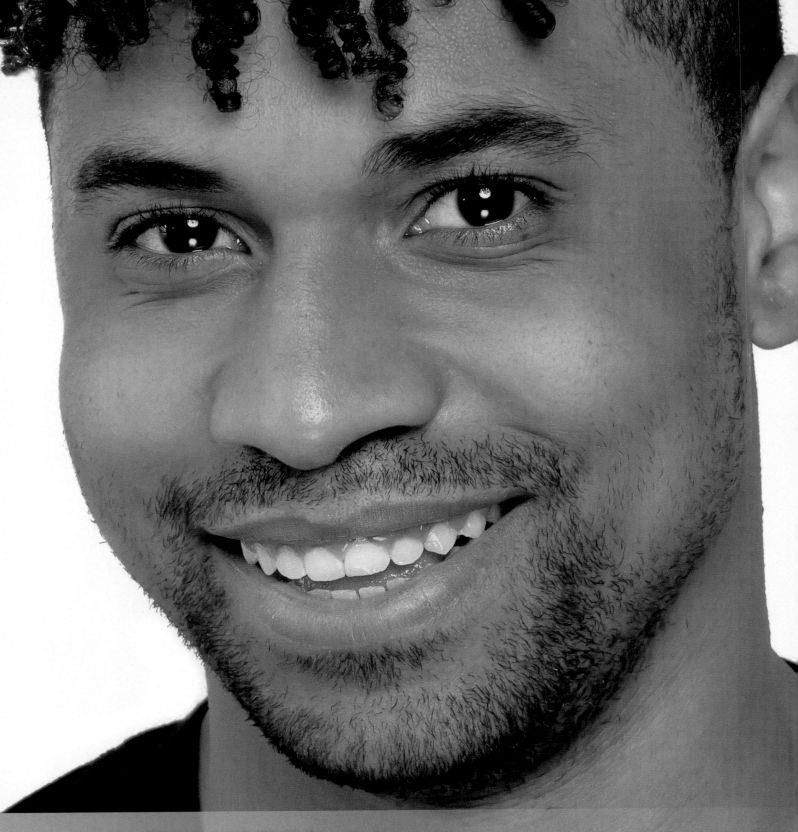

CHAPTER 11
Hair Removal

"People rarely succeed unless they have fun in what they're doing."

—Dale Carnegie

Learning Objectives

After completing this chapter, you will be able to:

1. Explain the importance of hair removal.
2. Describe the structure of hair.
3. Explain the hair growth cycle.
4. Identify the causes of excessive hair growth.
5. Compare temporary and permanent hair removal and reduction methods.
6. Explain when to use hard and soft wax methods of hair removal.
7. Provide a thorough client consultation for hair removal services.
8. List items needed in a wax treatment room.
9. Demonstrate waxing head to toe with soft and hard waxes.

Explain the Importance of Hair Removal

Consumers in the United States spend millions of dollars per year on hair removal products and services.

Today hair removal methods range from procedures such as waxing and tweezing, to more advanced techniques that require special training, like electrolysis, laser, and intense pulsed light (IPL). Face and body hair removal has become increasingly popular as evolving technology makes it easier to perform with more effective results for both men and women for esthetic purposes or sport performance.

Estheticians should study and have a thorough understanding of hair removal because:

- The growing popularity of hair removal makes up a large part of a salon's business (**Figure 11–1**) and is one of the most lucrative services offered.

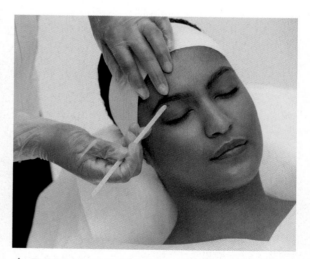

▲ **FIGURE 11–1** Hair removal makes up a large part of an esthetician's business.

- Waxing is the most common method of hair removal in salons, making it an important service to learn, become proficient in, and provide.
- Understanding the benefits, the risks, and how to perform various techniques is vital to an esthetician's success in this profitable market.
- Knowing what methods are used, room preparation, safety, and infection control procedures are an important part of hair removal procedures.

Describe the Structure of Hair

The scientific study of hair and its diseases is called **trichology** (tri-KAHL-uh-jee). The average human is born with skin that houses approximately 5 million pilosebaceous units capable of producing hair. It is important to understand all aspects of hair, including its structure, its appendages, and the types of hair found on the body. This will help you to suggest and provide the best hair removal services to your client.

The Hair Follicle and Its Appendages

A **hair follicle** (HAYR FAHL-ih-kul) is a mass of epidermal cells forming a small tube, or canal (**Figure 11–2**). Follicles extend deep into the dermis. The *pilosebaceous unit* (py-luh-seh-BAY-shus YOO-knit) contains the hair follicle and its appendages, which include the hair root, hair bulb, hair papilla, hair shaft, and the arrector pili muscle and sebaceous glands.

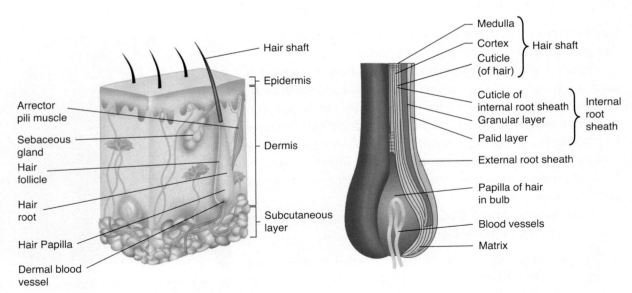

▲ **FIGURE 11–2** The structure and appendages of hair.

FOLLICULAR CANAL

The *follicular canal* is lined with epidermal tissue. These epidermal cells produce the follicle and hair matrix. The matrix is where cell mitosis (division) happens.

HAIR ROOT

The **hair root** (HAYR ROOT) anchors hair to the skin cells and is part of the hair located at the bottom of the follicle below the surface of the skin. The root is part of the hair that lies within the follicle at its base, where the hair grows.

HAIR BULB

The **hair bulb** (HAYR BULB) is a thick, club-shaped structure made from epithelial cells that surround the papilla. This forms the lower part, or base, of the hair follicle. This is where hair grows from cell division. The lower part of the bulb fits over and covers the papilla. The hair bulb contains the dividing cells of the hair matrix that produces the hair and both the external root sheath (epidermal tissue) and internal root sheath lining the follicle. The external root sheath is made of horny epidermal tissue. The internal sheath is the innermost layer of the follicle, closest to the hair. The internal sheath is the thick layer of cells you see attached to the base of a hair when epilating it.

HAIR PAPILLA

The **hair papilla** (plural: papillae) (HAYR pah-PIL-uh), is a cone-shaped elevation of connective tissue that contains the capillaries and nerves located at the base of the follicle that fits into the bulb. Hair papillae are necessary for hair growth and nourishment of the follicle. The blood vessels bring nutrients to the base of the bulb, causing it to grow and form new hair. Sensory nerves surround the base of the follicle.

HAIR SHAFT

The **hair shaft** (HAYR SHAFT) is defined as the part of the hair located above the surface of the skin. As cell division within the hair matrix occurs, the hair grows and gets longer. Keratinization is complete by the time these cells approach the skin's surface where the hair shaft protrudes from the skin. This is similar to skin-cell division and migration. Basal cells in the hair matrix divide and form the three main layers of the hair shaft: the cuticle, cortex, and medulla. The cuticle is the outermost layer, the cortex is the middle, and the medulla is the center, or innermost, layer of the hair shaft. The two outer layers of the shaft are hard keratin and the inner layer is soft keratin.

SEBACEOUS GLAND

The **sebaceous gland** secretes the waxy substance called sebum, which lubricates the skin and hair. This helps keeps skin supple and waterproof and protects against external factors.

ARRECTOR PILI MUSCLE

The *arrector pili muscle* contracts when affected by cold or other stimuli. It pulls on the follicle and forces the hair to stand erect, causing goosebumps. This reaction is also thought to keep skin warmer by creating an air pocket under the upright hairs. The muscle contraction also helps disperse the protective lipids from the sebaceous gland to the skin and hair.

List the Types of Hair

There are three major types of hair to be found on the human body: lanugo, vellus hair, and terminal hair.

LANUGO

Lanugo (luh-NOO-goh) is soft downy hair found on a fetus. The lanugo hair sheds after birth and is replaced with either vellus or terminal hair.

VELLUS HAIR

Vellus hair (VEL-lus HAYR) is found in areas that are not covered by the larger coarse terminal hairs. For example, vellus hair usually grows on women's cheeks (also known as peach fuzz). Removing vellus hair, especially against the hair growth, can result in the follicles producing new terminal hairs, so it is not recommended to tweeze, shave, or wax these fine hairs.

TERMINAL HAIR

Terminal hair (TUR-meh-null HAYR) is the longer, coarse hair found on the head, brows, lashes, genitals, arms, and legs. With hormone changes during puberty, follicles are naturally regulated to switch from producing vellus hairs to producing terminal hairs in these areas.

 CHECK IN

1. What are hair papillae necessary for?
2. What is a benefit of the arrector pili muscle?
3. What is the difference between lanugo and vellus hair?
4. What is the main catalyst for vellus hairs transitioning to terminal hairs?

Explain the Hair Growth Cycle

Hair growth is a result of the activity of cells found in the basal layer. These cells are found within the hair bulb. Hair growth occurs in three stages: anagen, catagen, and telogen (**Figure 11–3**). These stages vary

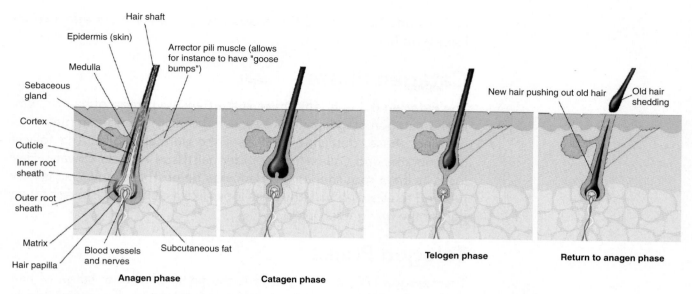

Anagen phase

Catagen phase

Telogen phase

Return to anagen phase

Hair shaft

Epidermis (skin)

Arrector pili muscle (allows for instance to have "goose bumps")

Medulla

Sebaceous gland

Cortex

Cuticle

Inner root sheath

Outer root sheath

Matrix

Hair papilla

Blood vessels and nerves

Subcutaneous fat

New hair pushing out old hair

Old hair shedding

▲ **FIGURE 11–3** Hair growth occurs in three stages known as anagen, catagen, and telogen.

in duration on different parts of the body, for example, scalp hair has a longer anagen phase, so the hair on the scalp can grow down to the knees in some cases. Conversely, eyelashes have a relatively short duration of the anagen phase before shedding and being replaced, which is why we do not need to get our eyelashes trimmed. These cycles can also be determined and affected by many factors including age, genetics, hormones, and a person's health and prescription drugs. Use the acronym ACT to remember the growth stage sequence. Hair follicles in any given part of the body will be in different phases at any given time.

Anagen Phase

The **anagen** (AN-uh-jen) phase is the growth stage during which new hair is produced. New keratinized cells are manufactured in the hair follicle during the anagen stage. Activity is greater in the hair bulb, which pushes down into the dermis and swells with cell mitosis in the matrix. Stem cells at the junction between the arrector pili muscle and the follicle grow downward and stimulate cell mitosis in the matrix. New cells form hair and root sheaths while the older part of the hair is pushed upward. Once hair has reached its full length, it can remain there for weeks or years, depending on its location on the body. Hair on the scalp remains in the anagen phase for years. Other areas, like eyelashes, have a short anagen phase. The length of the anagen phase determines the length of the hair. This stage is the most important stage for estheticians in effective hair removal, as removing hairs during the anagen stage will be more effective for long-term hair reduction.

Catagen Phase

The **catagen** (KAT-uh-jen) phase is the transition stage of hair growth. In the catagen stage, mitosis ceases. The hair, having completed its growing phase, detaches itself from the dermal papilla. The follicle degenerates and collapses as epidermal tissue retracts upward. Hair loses its inner root sheath and becomes dryer. The mature hair is now referred to as a *club hair* (the base looks like a club). This is the shortest part of the hair growth cycle.

Telogen Phase

The **telogen** (TEL-uh-jen) phase is the final, or resting, stage of hair growth. During the telogen stage, the club hair moves up the follicle and is ready to shed. The hair is at its full size and length and is erect in the follicle. It is clearly visible above the skin's surface unless it has already shed. The hair bulb is not active, and the hair is released and is attached only by epidermal cells. Hair may sit in the follicle until it is pushed out by a new anagen hair or falls out on its own. In some cases the hair may share the follicle with a new anagen hair, giving the appearance of two hairs coming from a single follicle. The empty and dormant follicle is latent until the cycle begins again with a new anagen phase.

 CHECK IN

5. What is the most effective stage for hair removal?
6. What makes scalp hair grow longer than eyelashes?

Identify the Causes of Excessive Hair Growth

The amount of hair an individual has differs from person to person. What would be normal hair growth in one person might be extreme in another. Hair growth, in terms of density on the scalp, face, and body, is determined by genetics and ethnicity as well as health and hormonal influences. It is important to recognize the differences when assessing the client for hair removal services.

Hypertrichosis versus Hirsutism

Hypertrichosis (hy-pur-trih-KOH-sis) is an excessive growth of terminal hair in areas of the body that normally grow only vellus hair (lower back, eyelids, abdomen), and not necessarily in the adult male, hair growth patterns (**Figure 11–4**). This type of hair growth is genetically and ethnically inherited but can also occur due to natural life occurrences (e.g., puberty, pregnancy, and menopause), certain medical procedures and treatments (e.g., cancer), or reactions to certain medications (e.g., steroids). It is not stimulated by male androgens, and while there may not be a cure to address the cause of the superfluous hair, it may be treated esthetically.

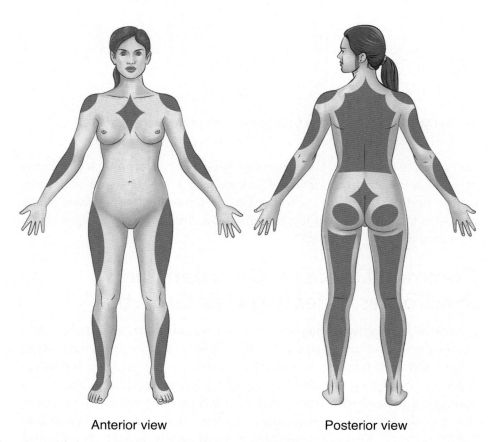

Anterior view   Posterior view

▲ **FIGURE 11–4 Areas of the body prone to hypertrichosis.**

Hirsutism (HUR-suh-tiz-um) is excessive hair growth on the face, chest, underarms, and groin, especially in women. It is caused by excessive male androgens in the blood (**Figure 11–5**). This hormone imbalance may be caused by stimulation of male androgens at puberty, medications, illness, and stress. It can be resolved by eliminating the

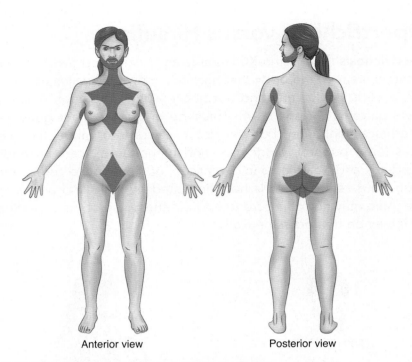

Anterior view   Posterior view

▲ FIGURE 11–5 Areas of the body prone to hirsutism.

cause of the condition. Excessive hair growth on a female face or body may be attributed to hormonal imbalances and excessive androgen production secreted from the ovaries or adrenal glands. Menopause may also cause excessive facial hair. These changes may dissipate with time and medical attention.

Common Diseases, Disorders, and Syndromes Affecting Hair Growth

Excessive hair growth may indicate a medical issue, and there are a number of documented diseases, disorders, and syndromes that, when diagnosed and treated, can reduce the problem of hirsutism. A disease is pathological, like conditions caused by viruses and bacteria, with a series of signs and symptoms. A disorder is an abnormality of function, like a birth defect or genetically inherited malfunction. A **syndrome** (SIN-drom) is a group of symptoms that, when combined, characterize a disease or disorder.

DISEASES AFFECTING HAIR GROWTH
Medical conditions related to excessive androgen production that affect hair growth are acromegaly (ak-roh-MEG-uh-lee) and Cushing syndrome.

DISORDERS AFFECTING HAIR GROWTH
Adrenogenital (uh-dree-nuh-GEN-uh-tul) syndrome is a malfunction of the adrenal cortex that causes an overproduction of androgens.

SYNDROMES AFFECTING HAIR GROWTH

The most notable and prevalent syndrome relating to hair growth is polycystic ovarian syndrome (PCOS), formally known as Stein–Levanthal (STYN LEV-un-tahl) syndrome. An individual with this syndrome would present with hirsutism, irregular menses, ovarian cysts, and obesity. Another notable syndrome is Achard–Thiers (AR-churd TEERS) syndrome, which is a combination of Cushing and adrenogenital syndromes.

FOCUS ON

Common and Current Medicines Affecting Hair Growth

Medications Causing Hirsutism	Medications Causing Hypertrichosis
• Anabolic steroids	• Clomid (clomiphene citrate)
• Brevicon (norethindrone and ethinyl estradiol)	• Cortisone (cortone acetate)
	• Dilantin (phenytoin)
• Ciclosporin (axorid)	• Loestrin (norethindrone acetate, ethinyl estradiol, ferrous fumarate)
• Restasis (cyclosporin)	
• Danazol (danocrine)	
• Prednisone (corticosteroid)	• Rogaine (minoxidil)
• Provera (medroxyprogesterone acetate)	• Proglycem (diazoxide)
	• Provera (medroxyprogesterone acetate)
• Premarin (conjugated estrogens)	
• Tagamet (cimetidine)	
• Tamoxin (tamoxifen citrate)	

 CHECK IN

7. What disease, disorder, or syndrome most commonly causes hirsutism?
8. Between hirsutism and hypertrichosis, which is attributed to genetics and not male androgens?

Compare Temporary and Permanent Hair Removal and Reduction Methods

Methods of hair removal fall into two general categories: temporary and permanent, including permanent *reduction*. Temporary hair removal involves repeat treatments as hair grows. With permanent hair removal, the papilla is destroyed, making regrowth impossible. Spa and salon techniques are generally limited to temporary methods such as waxing, sugaring, and threading and some may offer electrolysis as a permanent method of hair removal. Some states allow laser and IPL hair removal that offer permanent reduction. Medical spas, or medi-spas, with physicians on staff offer laser and IPL hair removal, but rarely temporary methods.

Temporary Methods, Home and Professional

Temporary methods of hair removal include depilation and epilation. Depilation (DEP-uh-lay-shun) is a process of removing hair at or near the level of the skin. Both shaving and chemical depilation are included in this category (Figure 11–6). Another temporary method of hair removal is epilation (ep-uh-LAY-shun), the process of removing hair from the bottom of the follicle by breaking contact between the bulb and the papilla. The hair is pulled out of the follicle. Tweezing, waxing, sugaring, and threading are all methods of epilation.

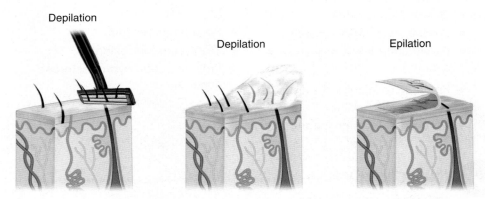

▲ FIGURE 11–6 The effects on the follicle from different types of hair removal.

TWEEZING AND "ELECTRONIC TWEEZING"

The method of using tweezers to pull hair out by the root one at a time is called tweezing. Eyebrows can be shaped and contoured by tweezing. Tweezing is also used on remaining hairs after waxing. If clients are sensitive to waxing, tweezing is a slower, but effective, alternative for removing the dark, coarse hair on the face.

Another less common tweezing method used is the electronically charged tweezers. The tweezers are used to grasp a single hair and transmit radio-frequency energy down the hair shaft into the follicle area. The idea is that the papilla is desiccated and eventually destroyed; however, the efficacy of this method is controversial as the hair is not a good conductor of heat or radio frequency. Electronic tweezers are not a method of permanent hair removal and the process is slow. Separate licensing may be required to perform electronic tweezing in some states.

Tweezing Pros:
- Minimal cost after purchase of good pair of tweezers
- Convenient to use

Tweezing Cons:
- Can be uncomfortable, even painful
- Eyeglasses impede tweezing
- Poor vision makes it difficult
- Time consuming and laborious for clearing dense growth
- Only feasible in small areas
- Hairs broken with tweezing can create bumps and pimples

┌─ PERFORM ─┐
Procedure 11-1
Perform Eyebrow
Tweezing

SHAVING

With shaving, as with any depilation method, the hair is removed down to the skin's surface. It may appear that hair is growing in thicker and darker after shaving but that is because the fine tip of the shaft is removed, and the thicker part of the shaft is visible as it protrudes. The protruding cut hair feels coarse to touch. Shaving the terminal hair on a woman's face could be problematic as vellus hair would also be removed and repetitive shaving stimulates terminal regrowth, especially with the onset of menopause. Additional problems are the potential for PFB, or pseudofolliculitis barbae (SOO-do-fah-lik-yuh-LY-tis BAH-bay)—which is a term for razor bumps, rash, and ingrown hairs—and *folliculitis,* which is an infection of the hair follicles. Both these problems can be corrected by using clean razors, not shaving so close that the cut hair drops underneath the skin, and not changing the direction of shaving.

Shaving Pros:
- Inexpensive
- Convenient
- Fast
- Painless

Shaving Cons:
- Causes stubble hair growth in one to four days
- Vellus hair also removed when terminal hair on the face shaved
- May cause folliculitis, PFB, and ingrown hairs
- May cut skin

CHEMICAL DEPILATORY

A **depilatory** (dih-PIL-uh-tohr-ee) is a chemical substance spread on the skin to dissolve the hair at the surface of the skin and just below the stratum corneum. On contact, the hair expands and the disulfide bonds of the hair (protein and cystine) break, and the hair can be wiped or washed away. The active ingredients are alkaline such as sodium hydroxide, potassium hydroxide, thioglycolic acid, or calcium thioglycolate. Although depilatories are not commonly used, you should be familiar with them in case your clients have used them or are using them. If the depilatory is left on longer than recommended, perhaps to try to dissolve coarse terminal hair on the face, dermatitis could result, so as with any home care method, it is important to follow the manufacturer's recommendations and instructions.

Depilatory Pros:

• Relatively inexpensive, though costlier than shaving
• Can be conveniently applied in privacy of own home
• Regrowth is slower and softer than that of shaving

Depilatory Cons:

• Results not as long-lasting as waxing
• Strong odor during chemical processing
• Can cause irritation and later reactions such as contact dermatitis because the skin's natural protective barrier is compromised as the depilatory is removed
• Should not be used on nonintact skin

THREADING

Threading is an ancient method of epilation that began in the Middle East and is now rapidly spreading throughout the Western world. **Threading** (THRED-ing), also known as *banding*, works by using cotton thread that is looped and twisted in the middle then quickly and selectively guided along the surface of the skin, snagging the unwanted hairs in the twisted portion of the thread and epilating them (**Figure 11–7**). Its effect is tantamount to mass rapid tweezing.

Threading can be accomplished using a two-handed technique or a hand and the mouth. The two-handed technique uses a closed loop and cat's cradle technique where each end is looped around the thumbs and forefingers. The thumb and forefinger of each hand alternately open and close, moving the twist forward and backward. The hand and mouth technique, which should not be performed as a professional service, loops the thread around the thumb and forefinger of one hand. The other thumb and forefinger grip a loose end, and the other loose end is placed in the practitioner's mouth and gripped by the teeth. The

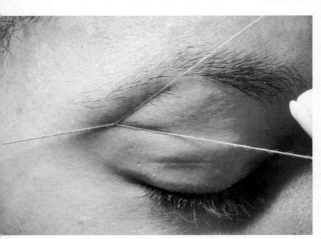

▲ **FIGURE 11–7 Example of threading.**

practitioner uses their head to maneuver the piece of thread. Licensing and regulations for threading may vary from state to state.

Threading Pros:

- Fast, inexpensive method of hair removal
- Requires minimal products and supplies
- The thread is discarded after use, so it is hygienic
- It can be performed on clients whose skin cannot tolerate waxing

Threading Cons:

- It can be painful as hairs are snagged in clusters
- It should not be performed on vellus facial hair as it distorts the follicles, stimulating them to produce terminal hair over time
- It may cause some redness and irritation
- Can cut hairs, causing bumps and breakouts

SUGARING

Sugaring is another ancient method of hair removal, dating back to the ancient Egyptians. It is an alternative for those who have sensitive skin or who react to waxing with bumps and redness. The original recipe is a mixture of sugar, lemon juice, and water, heated to form syrup, which is then molded into a ball and pressed onto the skin and quickly stripped away. The sugar can be used over and over on the same client until the hair left in the product interferes with the process. Then it is discarded.

Sugaring (SHUH-gar-ing) is similar to waxing methods except that it uses a thick, sugar-based paste and is especially appropriate for more sensitive skin types. One advantage with sugar waxing is the hair can be removed even if it is only 1/16 to 1/8 inch (1.5 to 3 millimeters) long, without adhering to the skin. It can be removed in the direction of the hair growth, which is less irritating than waxing. It can be used for some who have certain wax contraindications.

Sugar mixtures are now manufactured in large quantities and sold in small containers ready to be placed in a heater. The sugar mixture melts at a very low temperature. It is hygienic because it is used on a specific client and then discarded. True sugar products should be natural and resin free. Additives in the formula will change the results and effects on the skin.

Sugaring uses both directions of applying and removing the product: with the hair growth and against the hair growth. The application and removal depend on the product and the manufacturer's instructions. There are two types of sugaring methods:

- Hand applied
- Spatula applied

Hand method. With the hand method, the product is held in the hand and applied against the hair growth and removed in the direction of the hair growth. (**Figure 11–8**). The application is similar to

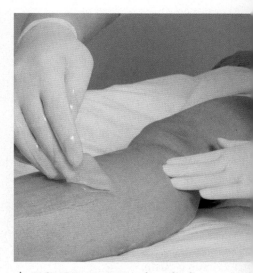

▲ **FIGURE 11–8** Hand applied sugar paste.

hard wax. The hand-applied method is performed at body temperature (98° F/37°C).

Hand-Applied Sugaring Pros:

- There is no risk of burning because it is applied at body temperature
- There is minimal risk of bruising as it does not adhere to skin and pull during removal
- Sugar paste manufacturers consider that the lower temperature and minimal adhesion to skin make it possible to apply over varicose and spider veins, dry psoriasis, and dry itch eczema. Caution and good judgment should be used
- The same area can be gone over more than once during the service without the risk of causing irritation and trauma
- It is considered safe to use on people with diabetes; however, a physician's approval should be obtained, and a medical release signed
- Hair length need be only ⅟₁₆ inch long for removal of virgin (previously untreated) hair
- No hair follicle distortion or breakage of hair because it is removed in direction of growth
- Regrowth hair is lighter, softer, and less dense
- Easy clean-up for the client
- Naturally antiseptic properties inhibit bacterial growth
- Hygienic as the sugar paste is not reused on other clients
- Easy clean-up of equipment, room, and treatment table, as it is water-soluble
- Inexpensive if homemade

Hand-Applied Sugaring Cons:

- Slower and more time consuming to perform than soft wax, especially on larger areas
- Some minimal discomfort similar to, but not as uncomfortable as, waxing
- Not suitable for precise hair removal in areas such as eyebrows
- Folliculitis and ingrown hairs possible, although considerably less with this method than with both the spatula-applied method and waxing

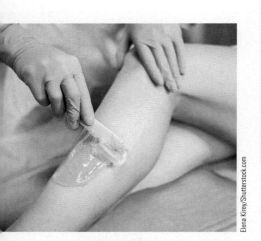

▲ FIGURE 11–9 Spatula applied sugar paste.

Spatula-applied sugaring method. The product is applied with a spatula in the direction of hair growth and removed against the hair growth with muslin or pellon strips (**Figure 11–9**). The spatula-applied method is warmed according to manufacturers' instructions, as it may be affected by additives like resins.

Spatula-Applied Sugaring Pros (if sugar paste has no added resins):

- Reduced risk of burning because it is applied at a cooler temperature than hot wax
- Faster service than the hand-applied method as larger applications are made
- Minimal discomfort and trauma to the skin
- Safe for dry psoriasis and dry itch eczema
- The same area can be gone over more than once without the risk of causing irritation and trauma
- The hair length need be only ¹⁄₁₆ inch in length for removal of virgin (previously untreated) hair
- Regrowth hair is lighter, softer, and less dense
- Easy clean-up for the client
- Naturally antiseptic properties inhibit bacterial growth
- Hygienic as the sugar paste is not reused on other clients
- Easy clean-up of the equipment, walls, floors, and treatment table, as the sugar is water soluble (if resin free)

Spatula-Applied Sugaring Cons (if sugar paste contains resins):

- Risk of burning if the sugar paste is not tested for appropriate safe-to-use temperature prior to the application
- Some discomfort similar to waxing
- Folliculitis and ingrown hairs possible
- Possible distortion of hair follicles

WAXING

Waxing is the primary hair removal method used by estheticians. Wax is a commonly used epilator, applied in either soft or hard form. Both products are made primarily of resins and beeswax (**Figure 11–10**). Honey wax is the most common, to which **gum rosin** (GUM ROZ-in) is added. Wax is applied evenly over the hair and then removed. Hard wax is thicker than soft wax and does not require fabric strips for removal. The recommended time between waxing appointments is generally four to six weeks, dependent on the anagen and telogen phases for the area being waxed, and the percentage of hairs in the anagen phase. Waxing is addressed more fully later in the chapter.

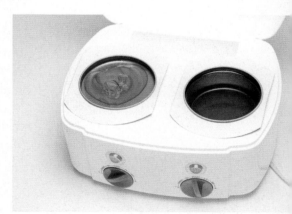

▲ **FIGURE 11–10** Wax is applied in either soft or hard form.

Waxing Pros:

- Relatively fast and efficient way to temporarily remove unwanted hair
- Wax kits and products available for home use
- Estheticians, with training and practice, can become "speed" waxing technicians, cutting the typical service time in half and increasing profits

- Shorter waxing time means minimal discomfort to the client
- Hair can take six to eight weeks to return
- Regrowth is often softer to the touch
- Some clients report reduction in hair growth after multiple wax services

Waxing Cons:

- Several contraindications to waxing, especially with soft wax
- Rosins in wax adhere to the skin and are a cause of irritation
- Risk of irritation and burning due to overheating the wax
- Risk of lifting the epidermal layer of skin if the wax is too cool and goes on too thickly
- Can be messy until one is skilled with the use of waxing
- Hair length of ½ inch for coarse and ¼ inch for fine hair is required for removal
- Irregular regrowth can occur after multiple waxing treatments, especially when the hair is removed in the direction opposite of hair growth
- Poor technique can leave behind up to 30 percent breakage that will be felt within a few days

Permanent Hair Removal and Reduction

The methods of permanent hair removal and reduction are **electrolysis** (ee-lek-TRAHL-ih-sis), **laser hair removal** (LAY-zur HAYR ree-MOOV-uhl), and *intense pulsed light (IPL)*. Electrolysis is the only proven method of hair removal recognized and given the designation permanent hair *removal* by the U.S. Food and Drug Administration (FDA) and the American Medical Association (AMA), as it is an effective method on all hair and skin types.

Laser and IPL have been given the designation of permanent hair *reduction,* as the effectiveness of both of these methods is dependent on the levels of pigment (melanin) in the hair and skin. With laser hair removal, a laser beam is pulsed on the skin using one wavelength at a time, which impairs hair growth; it is an intense pulse of electromagnetic radiation.

ELECTROLYSIS

There are three main modalities that fall under the classification of electrolysis: thermolysis, galvanic electrolysis, and the **blend** (BLEND) (a combination of the two methods applied alternately or simultaneously) (**Figure 11–11**). **Thermolysis** (thur-MAHL-uh-sus) uses alternating current (AC) that is applied and emitted from the probe, inserted into the follicle of the hair to be eliminated, to destroy the dermal papilla. **Galvanic electrolysis** (gal-VAN-ik ee-lek-TRAHL-ih-sis) utilizes direct

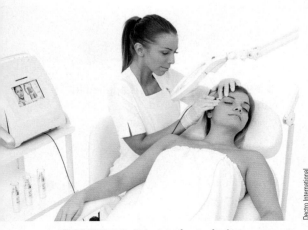

Dectro International

▲ **FIGURE 11–11** An electrolysis treatment.

current (DC) from the probe, which creates a chemical reaction of sodium hydroxide (NaOH), also known as lye, to cause decomposition of the follicle. Electrolysis should be practiced only by a professional certified and licensed (if the state requires it) in the field of electrology. If the state does not license this profession, an electrologist should become a Certified Professional Electrologist (CPE) via the American Electrology Association (AEA) or a Clinical Medical Electrolysis (CME) from the Society of Clinical and Medical Hair Removal (SCMHR), which is also the association that supports laser/IPL professionals. Talk with your instructor for additional information about classes and licensing in electrolysis.

Electrolysis Pros:
- The only method of permanent hair removal recognized by the FDA
- Can be performed successfully on all types and color of hair
- Can be used effectively on all skin types (dry, oily, mature) and with all races
- Can remove hairs with great precision, one at a time, making it a great choice for shaping the perfect eyebrow

Electrolysis Cons:
- Requires the cessation of other forms of hair removal on the areas to be treated, except for trimming or shaving
- More costly than tweezing
- Can cause discomfort for some people
- Success depends on a commitment to regularly scheduled appointments
- Treatments can cause redness, bumps, and swelling
- Makeup should not be worn on treated area for 24 hours after treatment
- Extensive electrolysis may take months, even years, to complete
- Higher Fitzpatrick skin types can develop postinflammatory hyperpigmentation if appropriate aftercare of sunblock is not applied

LASER AND INTENSE PULSED LIGHT

Both laser and intense pulsed light offer permanent hair *reduction*. While these methods are sometimes called permanent, the hair bulb must be destroyed completely or there may be some regrowth. Food and Drug Administration (FDA) guidelines require that these procedures be defined only as *permanent hair reduction*.

The word *laser* is an acronym for "light amplification by stimulated emission of radiation." Lasers use intense pulses of electromagnetic radiation that in the case of hair removal are attracted to, and heat up, pigment, that is, melanin (**Figure 11–12**). The best candidates are those with dark hair and minimal pigment in the skin; conversely, those with grey hair are the least favorable candidates as the hair would not

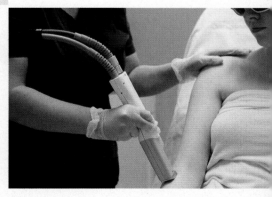

▲ **FIGURE 11–12** Lasers use intense pulses of electromagnetic radiation to target pigment.

respond because the laser is designed to target pigment. Fitzpatrick IV through VI would be less favorable candidates in comparison to Fitzpatrick I through III because the former have increased pigment in the skin and therefore a greater risk of burning and hyperpigmentation.

Different from a traditional laser, *intense pulsed light (IPL)* produces a quick flash of light. These short, powerful pulses shatter their target without allowing heat to build up and burn the surrounding skin.

Both laser and IPL are normally performed in a medical setting or under medical supervision, although local regulatory agencies regulate who can use these devices.

Laser/IPL Pros:

- Both methods offer a fast, long-lasting hair reduction treatment
- Treatment may produce some permanent results in hair reduction
- Large body areas can be treated with greater speed because multiple hairs are treated at once, unlike the hair-by-hair method of electrolysis
- No risk of disease transmission from blood
- Not considered as uncomfortable as electrolysis, though this is subjective
- Regrowth is often finer in texture and lighter in color

Laser/IPL Cons:

- Costly treatment requiring an average of three to six or more treatments
- Issues of long-term safety and effectiveness
- Not effective on light and nonpigmented hair such as blonde, red, or grey/white
- Depending on the specific laser, generally not an effective method on dark or tanned skin
- Safety concerns for the eyes and the need for protective eyewear
- Uncomfortable for some people
- No guarantee of satisfaction
- Inadequate and inconsistent state regulatory controls and guidelines

 CHECK IN

9. What are the main active ingredients in depilatories?
10. What is another name for threading?
11. What is the biggest benefit of cleaning up after hand-applied sugaring?
12. What is the minimal length of hair that can be removed with sugaring?
13. Which modality of electrolysis utilizes direct current?
14. What is a main benefit of electrolysis?
15. What is a downside to electrolysis?
16. Name a safety concern for laser/IPL.

Explain When to Use Hard and Soft Wax Methods of Hair Removal

Waxing services are one of the most popular services in salons and spas, and still the most common form of hair removal. There are two types of waxes:

- Hard wax, where no strip is used for removal
- Soft wax, which uses a strip for removal

Both waxes have different qualities that make them a preferred choice for different kinds of hair removal services. Estheticians generally use soft wax in larger areas, such as the back and legs, and hard wax in smaller areas, such as the eyebrows, axillae, and bikini area. Wax formulas are made from rosins (derived from pine tree resin), beeswax, paraffin, honey, and other waxes and substances. They may also include additives such as azulene or chamomile for sensitive skin or tea tree oil for its soothing and antiseptic benefits.

Wax product consistencies vary, as do melting points. It is important to keep the wax at the temperature recommended by the manufacturer so that it works effectively and optimally. Leaving the wax unit on overnight or overheating the wax diminishes its effectiveness and may cause injury.

Both hard wax and soft wax regrowth is softer and there is no stubbly feeling. Regrowth generally takes six to eight weeks after waxing.

CAUTION!

Gloves must be worn for *all* waxing services!

Hard Wax Essentials

Hard waxes are available in blocks, disks, pellets, or beads (**Figure 11–13**). Generally, the harder the wax, the more heat is required to melt it. They are based on a resin called **rosin** (ROZ-in) that is often combined with beeswax as well as **candelilla** (can-dih-LIH-lah) and **carnauba** (car-NOO-bah) waxes to modify the melting point and provide increased strength. The used wax is discarded after each service.

Hard waxes are gentle enough for facial area, yet strong enough to be used on hard-to-remove, coarse hair and areas where hair growth converges from multiple directions. Some like to use it on the bikini and underarm areas. Hard wax is thicker than soft wax.

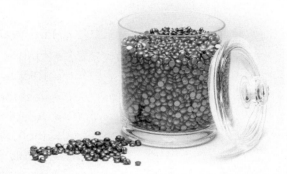

▲ **FIGURE 11–13** Hard waxes come available in blocks, disks, pellets, or beads as featured.

PRETREATMENT FOR HARD WAX

Cleanse and prepare the client's skin with products recommended by the manufacturer of the wax, as they are formulated for optimal results. With cotton and cleanser or makeup remover, remove all traces of makeup on the area to be waxed, as makeup can be an irritant and can prevent the wax from adhering. For larger areas of the body, such as arms, legs, and back, a spray cleanser containing the wax manufacturer's recommended product, or a general antiseptic product such as witch-hazel, is faster and more economical. This wax method generally requires a thin application of prewax oil to protect the skin. It should absorb and not leave an oily film.

HARD WAX TECHNIQUE

Hard waxes are applied with an applicator at a 45-degree angle directly to the skin in a thick, wet appearing layer that hardens as it cools (**Figure 11–14**). It is first applied against the hair growth, then back over in the direction of hair growth in a figure eight pattern, like frosting a cake. This is done to ensure that each strand of hair is completely coated, as hard wax is not as thin as soft wax and does not run under the hair as soft wax does. As the wax hardens it tightens, grips the hair, and lifts off the skin. The esthetician then grips the wax at one end and pulls it while it still feels tacky. The gripping is helped by creating a tab of slightly thicker wax at the end where the pull originates.

Hard wax can be removed in the direction of hair growth; thus, the follicle is not distorted. It can also be removed against or sideways to the direction of hair growth. It is especially effective in areas where hair grows in multiple directions or on thin or fragile skin; therefore, application and removal depend on the area to be waxed and how coarse the hair is, as well as the individual manufacturer's instructions for their brand of hard wax. Hard wax can be applied to an area a second time during the service.

HARD WAX: POSTTREATMENT CARE

It is uncomfortable to remove remaining pieces of hard wax by picking them off. They should be removed with a posttreatment oil. Products containing chamomile, tea tree oil, or aloe vera can provide soothing aftercare.

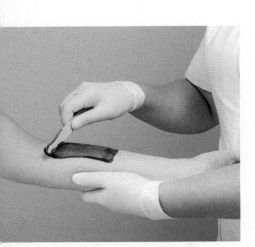

▲ FIGURE 11–14 A hard wax application.

Hard Wax Dos:
- Follow the manufacturer's recommendations for heating the wax.
- Regularly stir the wax and refresh with pellets or beads if necessary.
- Test the wax prior to use on the client.
- Apply the wax in a figure eight movement, under and against then over and with hair growth.
- Apply the wax with clean borders to avoid leaving wax behind after the removal pull.
- Apply the wax to the thickness of a nickel with no visible hair beneath it.
- Form a slightly thicker tab at the end for gripping during removal.
- Discard used wax.
- Check for contraindications with the client and obtain a signed release.

Hard Wax Don'ts:

- Do not overheat the wax or leave the heat on overnight.
- Do not apply wax to a client without testing the temperature for safety.
- Do not double dip a spatula.
- Do not reuse the wax.
- Do not apply wax inside the ear canal or nostrils.

Soft Wax Essentials

Soft wax is the most common method of hair removal. There are multiple brands with various additives for the face and other body areas and levels of sensitivity, but they are predominately made of rosins that adhere to the skin. Professional soft waxes have a lower melting point and come in cans, although some come in plastic bottles for single client use with roller heads for application in place of a spatula. Soft wax has the consistency of honey when melted and ready for use. Soft wax, when applied in a timely manner, runs down and around the hair while also adhering to the skin, and must be removed immediately with a piece of muslin or pellon, while still warm (**Figure 11–15**).

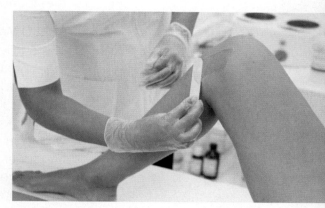

▲ **FIGURE 11–15** A soft wax application.

PRETREATMENT FOR SOFT WAX

Cleanse and prepare the client's skin with the manufacturer's recommended products. If there is no makeup to be removed, a product such as witch-hazel can be used. If waxing the face, a thin film of tea tree oil can be applied to protect the skin and minimize redness, followed by a dusting of baby powder, to ensure the area is dry and oil free.

SOFT WAX TECHNIQUE

Soft wax should be tested for correct and safe temperature and consistency before being applied to the client. Using an appropriate size applicator for the area, apply a thin coating of wax in the direction of hair growth, by swiftly gliding the edge of applicator at a 45-degree angle across the area, allowing the wax to slide off the applicator as it moves across. Quickly place the appropriate size muslin or pellon strip over the area. Make sure there is a wax-free portion at the pulling end of the strip to grip it for removal. Rub firmly over the strip two to three times in the direction of growth. Place one hand firmly on the skin at the pulling end while using the other hand to grab the strip and swiftly pull it, close and parallel to the skin, back against the direction of hair growth. Immediately after the pull apply gentle pressure to the area. Removing soft wax in the incorrect direction can have serious consequences, as will waxing over an area a second time during the same appointment.

CAUTION!

Some regions may prohibit the use of roll-on wax due to concerns with cross-contamination in the wax and proper disinfection of the applicators. Bottles of wax with roller applications must be single use. They are used on a client, and then the roller must be disinfected prior to its use on a subsequent client. Make certain to check with your state regulatory board and OSHA to be in compliance.

BLENDING

Blending is a technique that utilizes the wax that has built up on the muslin or pellon strip to remove the more obvious hairs, while leaving shorter hairs behind. It produces a gradual demarcation between completely hairless and some hair.

POSTTREATMENT CARE FOR SOFT WAX

Residual stickiness should be removed with a soothing wax removal lotion. Puffiness (mainly on the upper lip) can be treated with aloe, ice in a bag, or cold stones immediately following the service. Hives can also occur and can be avoided subsequently if the client takes an over-the-counter antihistamine.

SPEED WAXING

The quick application and removal of soft wax is known as *speed waxing*. Speed is more comfortable for the client. Faster procedures save time, lead to more revenue, and ensure more satisfied clients. To prepare the limbs it is faster and more pleasant for the client if you work simultaneously by spraying the cleaning solution on both limbs then wiping in sequence down the limbs with both hands, finishing at the fingers or toes. To prepare the underside of the client's legs, the legs should be bent with the knees up so that your hands can easily reach without inconveniencing the client. Wipe any excess moisture off with two paper towels, one in each hand.

Soft Wax Dos:

- Follow the manufacturer's directions for heating the wax to the correct and optimal temperature.
- Test the wax prior to applying to the client.
- Check for contraindications.
- Obtain a signed release.
- Wear gloves.
- Apply the wax in the direction of hair growth.
- Apply the wax thinly to prevent injury.
- Remove the wax (strip) against the direction of hair growth.

Soft Wax Don'ts:

- Do not provide service without a consultation and obtaining a signed release.
- Do not apply the wax without testing first for temperature.
- Do not apply the wax thickly; it will injure the client.
- Do not double dip the spatula.
- Do not let the soft wax cool before pulling. It will bruise or lift skin.
- Don't go over a waxed area a second time in the same service, as it could burn, lift, or otherwise damage the skin.

Selecting the Right Wax for the Best Service

Knowing the pros and cons of hard and soft wax helps determine the most suitable wax for the client and the area to be treated (Refer to Table 11–1).

▼ **TABLE 11–1** Hard Wax versus Soft Wax

Facts about Hard Wax	Facts about Soft Wax
Hard wax, when removed in the direction of the hair growth, does not distort follicles.	Soft wax is removed against the direction of hair growth and distorts hair growth. Regrowth stands to attention rather than lying flat.
Hard wax does not adhere to the skin and therefore causes less irritation.	Soft wax adheres to the skin and can cause redness and irritation.
Hard wax is effective where the hair grows in multiple directions such as in the axilla region.	Where hair grows in multiple directions, soft wax has to be applied in small sections.
Hard wax is preferred for the labia during a Brazilian bikini wax.	Soft wax cannot be removed against the hair growth on the labia, making it a poor choice for a Brazilian bikini wax.
With hard wax the area can be waxed a second time during the service, provided there is no irritation.	With soft wax the area cannot be waxed a second time during the service.
Hard wax may be used with caution on individuals who use glycolic or other alpha hydroxy acid (AHA) skin care.	Soft wax cannot be used on individuals using glycolic acid or AHAs.
Eyebrows may be waxed with hard wax if topical prescriptions such as Retin-A® or Differin® are being used by the client but have not been applied directly to the eye area.	Soft wax cannot be used anywhere on the face if prescriptions such as Retin-A® or Differin® are being used by the client.
Hard waxing is a slow and laborious method and takes considerably longer than soft waxing, especially on large body areas like legs and back.	Soft wax is a considerably faster method of waxing than hard waxing and the preferred choice for larger body areas.
With hard wax, the hair cannot be blended.	Soft wax already present on the strip is perfect for blending, especially around the shoulder between a waxed back and nonwaxed chest.
If hot wax is left to get old in the wax heater and new wax is not added periodically, the old wax heater becomes brittle when used and loses its removal properties.	Soft wax does not need to be refreshed to maintain its removal properties.

FACIAL WAXING DURING FACIALS

Eyebrow or upper lip waxing can be performed during a facial, but it should be done after the cleansing, *gentle* exfoliation, steam, and extractions and before the mask. Waxing should not be performed if any aggressive exfoliation has taken place, or over an area where extractions were performed. The mask should be soothing. If the

New wax formulas continue to appear on the market. Some take hold, while others dwindle into obscurity. One current wax formulation that is gaining popularity is flex-wax. It coats the hair like a soft wax, being applied in the direction of the hair growth, but is removed against the hair growth without a strip, like hard wax, after being allowed to set for 30 seconds until it becomes tacky. In testing it has been found to also be effective when applied like hard wax, under and against hair growth and back over in the direction of growth and removed with the growth, thus not unnecessarily distorting hair follicles.

indicated mask therapy is *not* going to be soothing, then a soothing lotion and cool damp cotton should be applied to the waxed area and the area should be avoided with the mask.

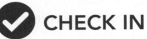 CHECK IN

17. What are two benefits to speed waxing?
18. What are two downsides of waxing?

Provide a Thorough Client Consultation for Hair Removal Services

A successful hair removal service is achieved with a detailed consultation, a prepared room, and following all protocols for cleanliness, precare, the service, and postcare.

Complete the Client Consultation Forms

A client intake form should be completed by each new client and kept in the client's file folder (**Figure 11–16**). Ask the client to complete a questionnaire that discloses all products and medications being used, both topical (applied to the skin) and oral (taken by mouth), along with known skin disorders or allergies. Allergies or sensitivities must be noted and documented. Changes in medications, facial treatments, and skin care can occur between clients' visits; therefore, clients should read, update, and sign a release form at the start of each appointment (**Figure 11–17**). Clients should also be given postcare instructions and precautions at this time and again after each waxing service.

THE INTAKE/CLIENT ASSESSMENT FORM
Intake or client assessment forms can be long and in depth for certain procedures requiring a medical history or for new clients who may become regular clients. A longer intake form is not required to be filled out for each and every wax appointment, but regular clients should be asked, prior to each appointment, if there are any changes to their health or skin care regimen. There should always be a place on the intake form or record card for consent to receive the service and acknowledgment that it is the client's responsibility to inform the esthetician of any changes that could affect the outcome of the procedure.

THE WAX RELEASE FORM
In place of the longer intake form or client record, a simpler wax release form should be signed prior to each wax appointment, particularly for any facial waxing service, as clients may have changes to their prescriptions

CLIENT ASSESSMENT FORM

(Sample form)

(assessment should be performed/reviewed prior to each treatment)

Name _____ Date _____

Phone _____ Address _____

E-mail _____

Have you been waxed before?   Yes ____ No ____

The following are potential contraindications for waxing:

Any chemical exfoliation treatment such as a glycolic acid peel or
any other AHA treatment? (wait at least two weeks before waxing):   Yes ____ No ____ If yes, when: _____

Applied any topical products containing AHAs (glycolic or lactic acid),
BHAs (salicylic acid), or lightening or bleaching gels? (wait at least
48 hours; a week is better)   Yes ____ No ____

Have you had microdermabrasion, laser resurfacing, light therapy, or
injectable treatments? (wait 4 weeks or longer—treatment dependent)   Yes ____ No ____ If yes, when: _____

Are you taking acne drugs and/or using exfoliating topical products
such as Retin-A® or other vitamin A products ? (wait at least
3 months or longer—drug dependent)   Yes ____ No ____ If yes, what type: _____

Exposure to continuous sun, or shaved, scrubbed, or experienced
any recent peeling or irritation in the last 48 hours?   Yes ____ No ____

Skin treatments: _____Date(s): _____

Currently using, or has used, the following topical products on face and neck:

_____

Medical conditions: _____

Currently taking, or has taken, the following medications: _____

Pregnant or lactating?   Yes ____ No ____

Seen or seeing dermatologist?   Yes ____ No ____ Date:_____

Name of doctor: _____

Allergies to products or medications: _____

History of fever blisters or cold sores?   Yes ____ No ____

Tanning regime or use of tanning booths? _____ Frequency: _____

Client initials: _____

WAX TREATMENT RECORD

(esthetician to fill out chart notes on back of assessment form for each service)

Client Name: _____

Date	Esthetician	Wax Service	Notes
9/8	Teresa	Brow with soft wax	*New client: shaping for more arch, close-set eyes* *Tweezed chin* *No redness*

▲ **FIGURE 11–16** The client wax intake form.

Wax Release Form
(Sample form)

Name _____ Date _____

Phone _____ Address _____

E-mail _____

I understand that topical creams, medical conditions, and medications can affect the results of waxing. I understand that I cannot be waxed if I have certain contraindications such as taking topical acne drugs or if I am using Retin-A® (or other peeling agents) topical prescription products.

I understand that I am accepting full responsibility for skin reactions if I do not inform my technician of contraindications prior to waxing.

Certain medications, products, and treatments used prior to waxing may result in irritation, skin peeling, blotchiness, pigmentation, and sensitivity.

I understand that some redness and/or sensitivity may result. I agree to avoid sun exposure, excessive heat (saunas, hot tubs), and all active products for the next 48 hours or as instructed by the technician.

The hair removal process has been explained and I have had an opportunity to ask questions and receive satisfactory answers.

I consent to be waxed and will not hold the salon or technician responsible for any adverse reactions from treatments or products.

Name (print) _____ Signature _____

Parent or Guardian if under 18 years of age:

Name _____ Signature _____

Initial below for each visit:

Date: _____ Client initials: _____ Date: _____ Client initials: _____

Date: _____ Client initials: _____ Date: _____ Client initials: _____

Date: _____ Client initials: _____ Date: _____ Client initials: _____

▲ **FIGURE 11–17** The wax release form.

or skin care. This can alert the esthetician and client to anything that might contraindicate the service, or negatively affect the outcome. The wax release form should list the contraindications and potential risks to the wax service and have a place for the client's signature. By signing the form, the client assumes the responsibility of informing the esthetician of any changes in health or skin care and an awareness of the risks that go with waxing. For the client and also the esthetician, the wax release form serves as a protection against a formal complaint.

INFORMED CONSENT FOR MINORS
Minors, that is, individuals younger than 18, should be accompanied by a parent, guardian, or other caregiver who has written authorization from the parent or guardian. The responsible adult should sign the release giving permission for wax services and be present for those services.

POSTWAX INSTRUCTIONS AND PRECAUTIONS

Following waxing, clients should avoid sun exposure and tanning booths, exfoliation, creams with fragrance or other ingredients that may be irritating, and excessive heat (e.g., hot tubs, saunas) for at least 24 to 48 hours and if any redness or irritation is present.

Discuss the Client's Indications and Contraindications

Indications are outward signs that the desired service would be successful and beneficial. In relation to waxing indications include:

- Hair to be waxed should be a minimum of ¼ inch long if it is virgin hair, meaning previously untreated hair, or fine regrowth.
- Hair should be ½ inch long if it is shaven and coarse, which is approximately 10 to 14 days' growth post-shaving.
- If possible, the client should lift ingrown hairs four days to a week prior to the service, leaving the hair in the follicle and allowing the follicle to heal and normalize.
- Working the area of the body with a loofah or using an exfoliating body scrub prior to waxing is recommended, but not on the day of the service.
- The client should avoid tanning (sun or booths) for 24 hours before and after the area is depilated.

A contraindication is a symptom or condition that makes a service or procedure unadvisable or that it should proceed with utmost caution. See **Table 11–2** for waxing contraindications.

Consider the Needs of the Transgender Client

Male-to-female gender reassignment is of professional interest to estheticians, as their professional services in hair removal are often called for.

The stages that a patient must go through to complete gender reassignment from male to female are as follows:

1. Emotional and psychological counseling: Patients may be advised to dress as women for increasing amounts of time. At this early stage of transition, they may seek temporary services listed here, so they feel more feminine in women's clothing. They may not elect to do much to the face at this time, other than be clean shaven, as they may need to return to their male persona for work.

2. Hormone replacement therapy (HRT): Once the decision is made to go ahead with a permanent form of gender reassignment, a careful program of HRT is given to counter the male hormones with female hormones. At this stage of transition, the patient also often undergoes laser treatment and/or electrolysis to the face and other body areas, including the penile shaft. Many patients also request more dramatic and obvious beauty services.

Contraindications for Waxing Procedures

- Leg waxing should not be performed on clients who have varicose veins.
- Body waxing should not be performed on clients with phlebitis, skin disorders, epilepsy, diabetes, hemophilia, or other contraindicated medical conditions.
- Facial waxing should not be performed on clients who have any of the contraindications listed in the remainder of this table, until physicians' approval is obtained.

Recent Treatments or Product Use

- Recent chemical exfoliation using glycolic acid, salicylic acid, or other acid-based products
- Recent microdermabrasion or injectables (Botox® or other dermal fillers)
- Recent cosmetic or reconstructive surgery, laser treatments, or IPL treatments
- Recent use of exfoliating topical medication, including Adapalene®, Retin-A®,
- Renova®, Tazorac®, Differin®, Azelex®, vitamin A, or other topical peeling agents
- Recent use of hydroquinone for skin lightening
- Recent use of topical or oral cortisone medication

Medical Conditions or Medications

- Acne medications such as tetracycline and accutane (physician guidance required)
- Recent use of blood-thinning medications (e.g., Coumadin®, Lovenox® [warfarin, heprin])
- Circulatory disorders (e.g., phlebitis, thrombosis)
- Chemotherapy or radiation
- Epilepsy, diabetes, hemophilia
- Autoimmune disorders (e.g., HIV/AIDS, lupus)

Skin Conditions

- Acute acne vulgaris
- Rosacea or very sensitive skin
- Sunburn, inflammation, bruising
- History of fever blisters or cold sores (herpes simplex)
- Presence of pustules or papules on area to be waxed

Other Contraindications

- Scar tissue, moles, skin tags, warts
- Skin disorders (e.g., eczema, seborrhea, psoriasis)
- Thin, fragile skin
- Lack of skin sensation

Other Considerations

- Avoid the inside of the nose, ears, over the eyelids, and over the areola and nipples.
- Pregnant women in their last trimester should not get a waxing service if they have to lie flat for more than 20 minutes.
- Check for product allergies to wax ingredients.
- Contraindicated products and treatments should be stopped one month to six weeks prior to waxing or according to a physician's recommendations. It can take up to three months or longer before the skin is ready to be waxed following the use of harsher products and treatments. These are only guidelines and a client's medical information needs to be carefully reviewed.

3. Reassignment surgeries: There are three main types of surgery that the transgender male-to-female patient may undergo: (1) facial feminization surgery, which may include facial plastic surgery and breast augmentation; (2) genital surgery; and (3) voice feminization surgery, in which adjustments are made to their vocal cords.

MOST COMMON SERVICES

The most common services for the male-to-female transgender client will vary depending on what phase of the transition they are in. In the early stages, phase 1 of the preceding list, many will book arm and leg waxing, simple manicures and pedicures, minimal eyebrow trimming, facials, makeup applications and lessons, and fitting for wigs.

During phase 2 of the preceding list patients often undergo electrolysis; laser hair removal; more dramatic facial peels; more dramatic shaping of the eyebrows with either tweezing, waxing, or electrolysis; and more feminine hair and nail services. In phase 3 of the preceding list, there is a continuation of the services of phase 2.

List Items Needed in a Wax Treatment Room

The waxing room and equipment should be immaculately clean, warm, and comfortable. Optimally there should be a sink. The music can be livelier than the music that is played during more relaxing treatments like massages and facials.

Wax Equipment

Furniture should be ergonomically designed so that both the esthetician and client are comfortable.

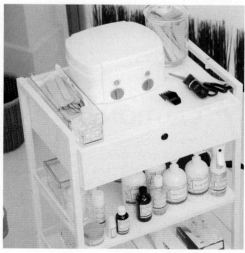

▲ **FIGURE 11–18** A well-stocked wax cart.

- The waxing table should be adjustable to different heights and able to adapt from flat to a semi-reclining chair position for face waxing. If this is not possible, it should be the best height for the esthetician to provide lengthy services, without straining.

- A stool may be necessary to help the client onto and off of the table.

- A multitiered rolling cart for holding waxing pots and supplies (**Figure 11–18**) can be moved near the client, keeping tools and supplies close at hand.

- Set up an assortment of covered containers for applicators, cotton, and gauze squares.

- Prepare a covered holding tray and disinfection solution daily.

- A covered container stores clean and disinfected items like tweezers and scissors.

- A covered waste container is necessary for the proper disposal of all used supplies.
- An assortment of towels and linens in a cabinet allows for easy access.

WAX TREATMENT ESSENTIALS

- Wax heaters, one containing hard wax and the other soft wax
- Tweezers, slanted and pointed, made of surgical steel able to withstand disinfection
- Scissors for trimming eyebrows (must be able to withstand disinfection)
- Scissors for cutting wax strips
- Metal spatulas that can be disinfected (a sufficient number to ensure double dipping is not necessary)

SINGLE-USE ITEMS

- Bikini bottoms
- Cotton rounds
- Facial tissues
- Gauze
- Headbands, hair clips, or bobby pins
- Paper drapes
- Paper towels
- Single-use wooden wax applicators: large (tongue depressor), medium (popsicle sticks), or small
- Treatment table paper rolls
- Gloves, nonlatex
- Wax strips of pellon (fiber) or muslin (cotton), which comes in rolls 3 inches wide or as precut packets for the body (3" × 9") and eyebrow and upper lip (1" × 3").

CONSUMABLES

- **Precare:** Hand soap, wax manufacturer's recommended products, and/or cleansers/makeup remover, antiseptic lotions such as witch hazel, tea tree oil, and baby powder, numbing/topical anesthetic products, and desensitizing spray.
- **Postcare:** Petroleum jelly for removing wax from eyelashes or other hair. Wax-removing lotion for skin, calming products such as aloe vera gel, salicylic lotion, arnica, and azulene. Baking soda for soothing compress solution. Eyebrow pencils in assorted colors, sharpener, eyebrow brushes.

DID YOU KNOW?

You can cut 9 of 1" × 3" brow or lip strips from a 9" × 3" body strip.

CAUTION!

Desensitizing spray products must never be sprayed on the face; rather, spray onto a cotton round and apply to the face.

HYGIENE AND INFECTION CONTROL

Following protocols and maintaining high standards of hygiene, cleanliness, and infection control reduce the risk of cross-contamination from esthetician to client, from client to esthetician, from client to client, and from esthetician to esthetician.

- Keep applicators, strips, gauze, and cotton supplies in covered containers when not in use.
- Clean tongs can be used to retrieve items after starting a service
- Gloves must be worn for all services and for cleaning and processing equipment.
- Tweezers and any other multiuse items should be thoroughly cleansed, dried, and placed into a wet disinfectant following the manufacturer's instructions.
- After cleaning, place the used instruments into an EPA-registered disinfectant solution that is designated to kill all microbes, including staphylococcus, tuberculosis, pseudomonas (a pathogen), fungus, and the HIV virus.
- Stainless steel instruments can also be processed and sterilized in an autoclave.
- A metal spatula is exclusively used on a single client, any remaining wax is discarded, and the container is disinfected and refilled or replaced.
- Multiple metal spatulas can be removed without double dipping, and then processed after the service.
- Double dipping is never acceptable.

TABLE AND CHAIR PROTECTION

Any part of the table that will come in contact with clients' skin or scalp must have protection, either paper that is disposed of immediately after the service or linens that are placed in a closed laundry hamper immediately after use and replaced with each client.

Place a clean sheet or sheet of paper on the entire waxing table for each new client for body waxing. If the client is receiving face waxing, place protective paper sufficient for under the head, neck, and shoulders.

DRAPING AND DISPOSABLE PROTECTION

Clients have differing views on modesty. The standard should be to keep areas covered that are not being waxed, uncovered immediately prior to waxing, then recovered after waxing. Disposable paper drapes serve this purpose well. Until the esthetician can perform waxing services neatly and cleanly, towels and linens should be avoided in favor of disposable drapes (**Figure 11–19**). Wax is damaging to linens and towels, as it does not easily wash away. Disposable bikini bottoms for bikini waxing not only provide modesty

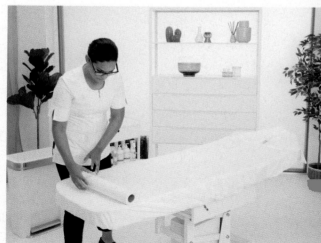

▲ **FIGURE 11–19** Disposable drapes are ideal for protecting linens from wax drips.

but also protect sensitive areas. Disposable headbands protect unruly or flyaway hair from getting in the way of face wax.

LEARN HAND WASHING AND INFECTION CONTROL MEASURES

- Estheticians' hands must be thoroughly washed before and after contact with the client.
- Do not put contaminated hands or gloves into clean containers.
- Use clean gloves or disinfected tongs to open and reach into a drawer if more supplies are needed.
- Hand washing in front of the client inspires confidence.

UNDERSTANDING GLOVE USE

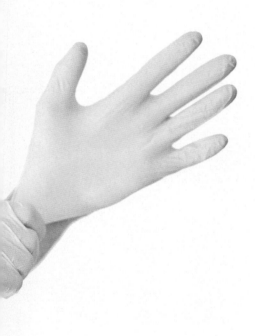

Always wear gloves. Hair removal causes trauma to the follicle. When the hair is forcefully removed from the follicle, blood spots may occur, and blood and fluids may rise to the surface of the skin. This is normal— this is the blood that has been nourishing the hair papilla.

Use vinyl or nitrile gloves, not latex. Latex breaks down easily, via a process known as wicking, which occurs when the gloves come in contact with wax and certain products that act as surfactants, creating minute holes that allow pathogens to pass through. Change your gloves if they become excessively sticky during a waxing service.

DO NOT DOUBLE DIP

Do not double dip the spatula or applicator unless you are disposing of the entire pot of wax after treating that individual client. Otherwise, use a new spatula each time to dip into the pot of wax.

DISPOSAL OF CONTAMINATED WASTE ITEMS

All blood-stained, bodily fluid–contaminated cotton, gauze, and other materials should be immediately discarded by double bagging or placed in a biohazard waste container and disposed of properly.

MASTERING CLEAN-UP

Clients should be booked so as to allow enough time to "turn the room over" in between, making it clean, tidy, and presentable. The following steps are necessary in this process:

- Throw away disposable drapes and other disposable items.
- Clean and disinfect the treatment table and work area.
- Change table linens.
- Change wax heater collars if overly soiled with wax drips.
- Place tools in a disinfectant holding tray.
- Use a wax removal solution to wipe away wax from all surfaces, including the floor.
- Retrieve new clean items and have them at the ready for the next service.
- Retrieve paperwork, including the client's intake form and wax release form.

UfaBizPhoto/Shutterstock.com

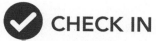
19. List three important infection control methods.
20. What is the best way to remove wax from eyelashes?

Demonstrate Waxing Head to Toe with Soft and Hard Waxes

While waxing with either soft or hard wax can be accomplished on virtually any part of the face or body (with the exception of a man's beard, nostrils, ears, and eyelids), there are preferred wax choices for differing areas and situations. Both will be addressed, with the emphasis on the preferred method.

General Waxing Dos and Don'ts

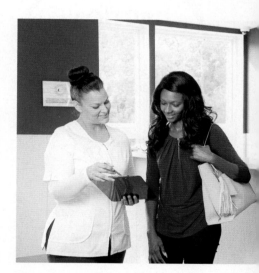

General Waxing Dos

- Complete a client consultation card and have the client read and sign a release form.
- Check for allergies, particularly beeswax, performing a patch test in a nonconspicuous area if necessary.
- Wear single-use gloves to prevent contact with any possible bloodborne pathogens.
- Make sure hair is at least ¼ inch (0.6 centimeters) to ½ inch (1.25 centimeters) long for waxing.
- Trim hair before waxing if it is longer than ¾ inch (2 centimeters).
- Perform a temperature safety test on the inside of your wrist before applying wax to the client.
- Avoid creating messy threads of wax by scraping the underside of the spatula or applicator after dipping.
- Avoid wax threads or drops falling on the client's eyes or lashes.
- The client's eyes should be closed for face waxing.
- Protect scalp hair with a headband for face waxing.
- Protect clothes to avoid wax drips near the area you are waxing.
- Select the best choice of wax with the appropriate pre- and posttreatment.
- Always apply gentle pressure (fingers for small areas or the entire hand for larger body areas) immediately after removal.
- Redness and swelling sometimes occur with sensitive skin. Apply aloe gel, or cortisone cream, or a compress of gauze soaked in baking soda to calm and soothe the skin after waxing.
- Always provide posttreatment instructions.

General Waxing Don'ts

- Do not apply wax without first checking the temperature.
- Do not reapply soft wax to an area already waxed in the same session.
- Do not touch the client without washing your hands.
- Do not double dip.
- Do not remove vellus hair; doing so may cause the hair to lose its softness and uniformity.
- Do not apply wax over warts, moles, abrasions, or irritated or inflamed skin.
- Never wax over curves or two different planes in one application.
- Do not wax male mustache or beard hair or sideburns as it is terminal, coarse and grows deep into the skin.

Face Waxing on Women and Men

The following section covers information on waxing the eyebrows, lips, chin, and sides of the face.

WAXING THE EYEBROWS

Eyebrows enhance and provide expression to the face. They provide a natural frame for the eyes. Incorrectly shaped eyebrows can give the entire face an odd appearance, and correctly shaped eyebrows can enhance natural beauty and attractiveness. Correctly shaping eyebrows is an art combined with following a few simple rules. The start of the brow is the corner nearest the nose, with an ascent to the point of the arch, followed by the descent to the end of the brow on the outer edge. The start, arch, and endpoint are all determined with the placement of an applicator using the guide illustrated (**Figure 11–20a**). Some clients have wider nostrils than others, which could affect the start line. An alternative guideline is to rest the applicator alongside the nose, just above the nostril, for a more accurate start point (**Figure 11-20b**).

An initial eyebrow shaping appointment will require more time than follow-up maintenance visits. Discuss in detail with the client what your professional knowledge and experience tell you should be achieved with the shape, while listening and being sensitive to the client's opinion. Giving the client a hand mirror and using the handle of the eyebrow brush, show the client where the arch is, and if it is misplaced, where it should be. Some eyebrows require minimal shaping, whereas others may need a complete reshaping that requires not only removal of unwanted eyebrow hair but applying eyebrow pencil to fill in where hair should be allowed to grow back. Clients can be instructed to apply the eyebrow pencil while waiting for incorrectly removed hairs to grow back in. Brush the eyebrow and determine exactly what you want to accomplish and convey that to the client, making sure they are in complete agreement before you proceed and apply any wax. Waxing above the eyebrows, especially on the descent, can diminish the hair growth that may be wanted in years to come as eyebrows thin and eyes droop.

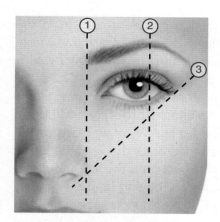

▲ FIGURE 11–20a Brow shaping guidelines.

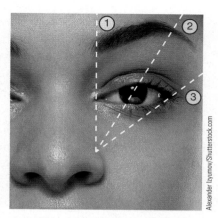

▲ FIGURE 11–20b Alternate brow shaping guidelines.

After any eyebrow wax, hairs that were too short, and so not removed, may be tweezed. This brings those hairs into the same forced telogen cycle as the waxed hairs. After completing the eyebrow wax apply after-care with a soothing antiseptic lotion to the area and massage both eyebrows simultaneously, finishing with gentle pressure at the temple.

Performing a Men's Eyebrow Wax with Soft Wax

Male clients generally just want a unibrow and any heaviness under the brow removed, but without emphasizing an arch. The start point should be slightly further in towards the center from the corner of the eye, unlike the start point for women. To avoid waxing a totally clean line that can look strange on a male client, be conservative with the amount of hair to be removed, allowing for intermittent tweezing along the brow line for a more natural look.

Waxing the Lip

With any face waxing but especially lip waxing, ask a new client if it is for a special occasion and let them know that there could be redness and puffiness and sometimes pimples following the waxing. Hard wax is a good choice for this area, or a cream wax or a soft wax designed for more sensitive skin, reducing the occurrence of redness.

The upper lip is divided, under the nose, into two equal sections for hair removal. The hair grows down and outward at a slight angle, following the lip line. Under the nose it grows straight down. Under the nose it is impossible to pull the hair against its growth to remove those hairs; the hair, which is usually fine in texture, is easily removed when pulling across the lip line sideways to the growth with the rest of the hair on that half of the upper lip. If the hair is coarse, hard wax may be the better choice (**Figure 11–21**).

---PERFORM---
Procedure 11-2
Eyebrow Wax with Hard Wax

---PERFORM---
Procedure 11-3
Eyebrow Wax with Soft Wax

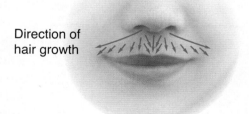

Direction of hair growth

▲ FIGURE 11–21 The hair on the upper lip grows down and outward at a slight angle, following the lip line.

┌─ PERFORM ─┐
Procedure 11-4
Lip Wax with Hard Wax
└───────────┘

┌─ PERFORM ─┐
Procedure 11-5
Lip Wax with Soft Wax
└───────────┘

Clients may choose to have superfluous hair removed from the lower lip. Because the hair of the lower lip grows downward away from the lip, soft wax can be used effectively in this area, or hard wax is acceptable if that's what is being used on the upper lip.

There are often nuisance hairs that stand up and bother clients along the immediate lip line—the **vermillion border** (ver-MILL-yun bore-dur)—and the outside corner of the lip line. Wax as close to the border as possible without getting wax on the fragile tissue of the lip, as it can be easily lifted and torn. Any wax that gets onto the lips should be removed with either petroleum jelly or a wax removing lotion. Finish by applying the aftercare lotion, massaging both sides simultaneously with fingertips, with gentle pressure on the outer edges of the lip. Offer the client some ice in a baggie if the area remains sensitive or feels puffy.

Waxing the Chin

A chin wax is often considered to include not only the chin but also the area just under the jaw. Waxing should not be considered the primary choice of hair removal for the chin if the client has never removed the hair with wax before, and if there are just a few sporadic hairs. Multiple waxings with soft wax against the growth cause the regrowth on the chin to grow back in an irregular fashion, standing up and looking wispy.

Along with removing unwanted hair, waxing also removes nonbothersome vellus hair, leading to even more irregular regrowth. The chin has no specific boundaries. The more it is waxed, the more it will need to be waxed, spreading the problem along the jaw, up the sides of the face, and down the throat. As the facial hair is stripped away in one area, the hair adjacent to it appears more obvious and apparent. Before long the client has to deal with excessive irregular hair growth that has to grow in before it can next be waxed, resulting in ingrown hairs, folliculitis, and the risk of injury to the skin as it matures. The client will not be able to utilize many of the antiacne or antiaging treatments available.

If there is an abundance of superfluous hair, laser or IPL may be preferred. If there are only a few terminal hairs surrounded by vellus hair, electrolysis may be the better choice. If that is not an option, then using hard wax and removing the hair in the direction it grows is preferred.

Waxing should not be performed on terminal, beard-type, deep, coarse hair on the face.

┌─ PERFORM ─┐
Procedure 11-6
Chin Wax with Hard Wax
└───────────┘

Waxing the chin is performed by standing at the head of the table rather than facing the client, allowing for an easier, less restricted, and smoother removal process. The section under the jaw and the throat are waxed first. Ask the client to tilt their head back as far as possible to help stretch the skin. Separating the throat area from the chin avoids going over any curves. To do so will cause bruising. After the throat and under the jawline are waxed, continue to the chin. The chin should be waxed in small sections.

Waxing the Sides of the Face

Waxing the sides of the face can create problems for your client in the future (**Figure 11–22**). If they have not had the sides of their face waxed before then educate and inform them of the consequences down the road. Fine nonpigmented vellus hair is normal and acceptable. However, bright lights and high-magnification mirrors often make hair growth appear more superfluous than it really is. Have the client look in a regular hand-held mirror held at just short of arms-length away and in normal lighting. If the hair is not visible, it should not be considered a problem, and it may not warrant the disturbance of removal and problems for the client in the future, causing them to regret choosing to wax.

Multiple wax treatments with soft wax cause distorted hair follicles and irregular hair growth. Vellus hair that had shallow follicles closer to the epidermis may gradually grow deeper into the dermis, which has a rich blood supply. When the client experiences hormonal changes the hairs transition to become terminal in their growth pattern. As the client's skin matures, it becomes more fragile and wax treatments could cause an adverse reaction. The client is left in a quandary, needing to choose other methods such as laser, or if the hair is strong but gray, electrolysis.

If the area is to be waxed, hard wax removed in the direction of growth is the better option, thus not distorting the affected follicles. Sugaring is also an option if the hair is not too strong. Hard wax will also grip the stronger hairs of the sideburn without much skin irritation.

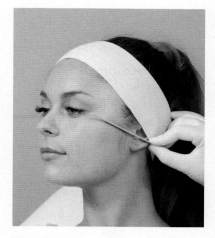

▲ **FIGURE 11–22** Isolation of hair on side of the face.

CAUTION!

Do not wax the axilla if the client has had a mastectomy or has mastitis.

Waxing the Underarm (Axilla)

Axilla (ag-ZIL-uh) is the correct professional and anatomical term, although *underarm* is an appropriate term to use with clients. The axilla is the region between the arm and the thoracic wall. There is often asymmetry to the hair growth of the axilla. One side may have more directions of hair growth than the other. The different directions of growth converge in the center and for this reason, hard wax is a preferred method of hair removal. The hair may be coarse, especially if it has been shaved, which also makes hard wax an optimal choice. The sudoriferous (soo-duh-RIF-fer-us), or sweat, glands soften the skin, so if you do not choose hard wax then consider a cream or honey wax for sensitive skin.

Clearly ascertain the directions of growth, and which section is going to be waxed first. The initial section to be waxed should be toward the outside edge, and removal should proceed in sections to the center (**Figure 11–23**).

After completing the removal on one side, apply a soothing lotion to the area to prevent the skin from sticking while working on the second side. If the underarm is particularly tender, a cool cotton compress of cold water and baking soda can be applied to the area while the other side is being waxed.

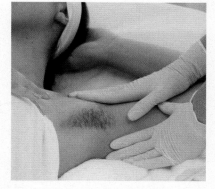

▲ **FIGURE 11–23** Determine the directions of hair growth before applying wax.

┌─ **PERFORM** ─┐
Procedure 11-7
Axilla Waxing with
Hard Wax

Waxing the Arm and Hand

─PERFORM─
Procedure 11-8
Axilla Waxing with
Soft Wax

─PERFORM─
Procedure 11-9
Arm and Hand Waxing
with Hard Wax

─PERFORM─
Procedure 11-10
Arm and Hand Waxing
with Soft Wax

Soft wax is the fastest, most effective way to remove hair on the arms. However, removing hair against the growth will cause the hair to grow back in an unruly fashion, sticking up. Hard wax or sugaring and removing with the growth will prevent this, although both of those methods are much slower than using soft wax. If the hair growth is strong or already unruly, then soft wax is the better choice. If the hair is fine and virginal, meaning it has not been removed before, it may be worth taking the time to remove the hair with hard wax or sugar paste, removing it with the growth and thus not distorting the hair follicles. This is especially important if the hair removal is a one-time service for a special occasion.

WAXING THE UPPER ARM
Most often the upper arm has just a few hairs right above the elbow. These can often be removed with blending, using the wax that is already on the strip. If the hair of the upper arm is obvious it will require complete removal.

Waxing the Upper Body on Women and Men

While it is not common for women to receive chest or back waxing, there are some women who request these services. Usually it is in small patches such as the diamond shape of hair at the base of the spine or hair growing and converging in the cleavage between the breasts.

Conversely, many men—whether due to personal preferences or athletic performance—request waxing services so that they can be as free of hair as possible in certain body areas. Therefore, the following descriptions are relevant for both male and female clients.

Waxing body hair may involve trimming the hair to ½ inch. If using an electric trimmer, cover the wax pot or trim the hair well away from the wax to prevent fly-away hair from contaminating it.

Waxing the Chest

Although the female areola should not be waxed, hairs surrounding the areola can be waxed away. They grow in a circular direction, surrounding the areola, from the outside toward the cleavage. Occasionally random hairs deviate from this direction of growth, especially if they have been tweezed. Chest hair generally grows upward in the décolleté, and across the chest and over the breast from the outside toward the center. Then it gradually transitions to growing downward in the center (**Figure 11–24**).

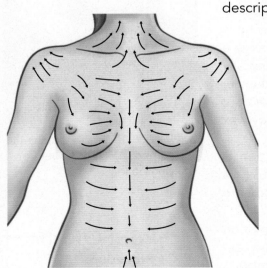

▲ **FIGURE 11–24** Diagram of chest showing direction of hair growth.

Before waxing a man's chest, with shirt removed, discuss what areas he would like waxed. Men sometimes book this service wanting abdominal hair or hair in front of the shoulders removed, right up to but not including the chest area. A clear understanding is important before beginning.

┌──────PERFORM──────┐   ┌──────PERFORM──────┐
│   **Procedure 11-11** │   │   **Procedure 11-12** │
│   Men's Chest Waxing   │   │   Men's Chest Waxing   │
│   with Hard Wax   │   │   with Soft Wax   │
└────────────────────┘   └────────────────────┘

Waxing the Back

When men book a back wax, they generally want all the hair removed from just below the waistband upward. If the client is wearing a business suit and will be returning to work, suggest that he remove his pants along with the upper clothing. Provide a hanger to hang them up and a towel or drape to place around his waist. Leave the room while he gets ready. If the client does not need to remove his pants, have him at least remove the belt from his pants for comfort and undo the top button to facilitate placing paper towels along the top edge of his pants.

Unless you have a long reach, stand on the same side that the wax is going to be applied first, changing sides after that half is completed. The hair grows from the outside toward the center (**Figure 11–25**). If standing on one side for the entire service, complete the side furthest away first. This prevents back strain from fatigue.

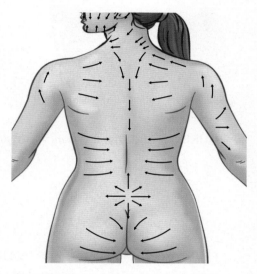

▲ **FIGURE 11–25** Diagram of back showing direction of hair growth.

Waxing the Lower Body on Women and Men

Waxing of the lower body includes the bikini area, abdomen, and upper and lower legs.

┌──────PERFORM──────┐   ┌──────PERFORM──────┐
│   **Procedure 11-13** │   │   **Procedure 11-14** │
│   Men's Back Waxing   │   │   Men's Back Waxing   │
│   with Hard Wax   │   │   with Soft Wax   │
└────────────────────┘   └────────────────────┘

BIKINI WAXING

Bikini waxing can be categorized in three ways: American (or standard), French, and Brazilian (**Figure 11–26**). The waxing method used depends on the client's preference and the extent of hair to be removed. While soft wax is appropriate for the outer regions, areas where there are different hair growth directions, coarse hair, and delicate skin, hard wax is preferred. Blood spots are normal when waxing the bikini area, so inform the client that this is both normal and acceptable.

Styles for bikini waxing. The standard *American* bikini wax is the removal of all hair that protrudes from a standard bikini bottom.

The *French* bikini wax (named for hair protruding from French thong underwear) leaves hair on the front pubis area—everything else is removed. The shape of the hair left and amount of hair to be removed should be clearly ascertained from the client prior to starting the waxing procedure.

With *Brazilian* waxing, all of the hair in the bikini area is removed, including on the pubis, genital area, and perineum.

Importance of communication prior to bikini waxing services (for the extent of the wax). Good communication with the client is paramount to be sure that both parties understand what hair is to be removed and what should remain. A client may want hair removed from the labia and perineum and request a Brazilian wax, but in fact she wants to keep some hair on the pubis.

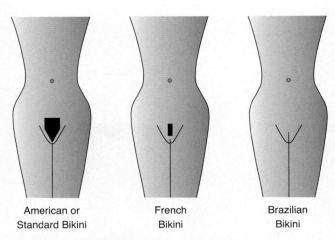

American or Standard Bikini   French Bikini   Brazilian Bikini

▲ **FIGURE 11–26** Different bikini wax styles.

```
┌──────PERFORM──────┐     ┌──────PERFORM──────┐
│  Procedure 11-15  │     │  Procedure 11-16  │
│ American Bikini Wax│     │ American Bikini Wax│
│   with Hard Wax   │     │   with Soft Wax   │
└───────────────────┘     └───────────────────┘
```

WAXING THE LEG

Waxing half a leg can vary considerably between an upper leg and a lower leg. The hair of the upper leg may be less dense in its growth when compared to the lower leg, but a larger surface area still has to be covered, taking more time and using more wax than the lower leg (**Figures 11–27** and **11–28**).

```
┌──────PERFORM──────┐
│  Procedure 11-17  │
│Leg Waxing with Soft Wax│
└───────────────────┘
```

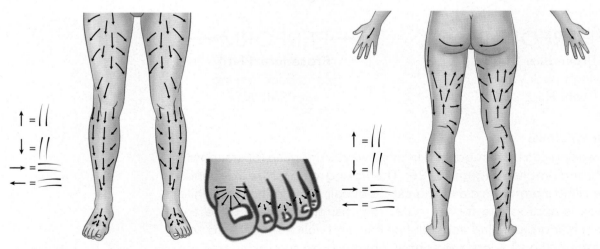

▲ **FIGURE 11–27** Diagram of hair growth direction on front of the leg.

▲ **FIGURE 11–28** Diagram of hair growth directions on the back of the leg.

Procedures: 11-1 to 11-17

Equipment, Materials, and Implements

Gather the following supplies and products as required for hair removal procedures.

EQUIPMENT AND SUPPLIES

- ☐ Assortment of covered containers for applicators, cotton, gauze squares
- ☐ Assortment of towels and linens
- ☐ Client charts
- ☐ Clothes hangers
- ☐ Covered holding tray for disinfectant solution
- ☐ Covered steel container for processed items like tweezers and scissors (optional)
- ☐ Covered trash container
- ☐ Disinfectant
- ☐ Eyebrow pencils in assorted colors
- ☐ Hand soap
- ☐ Hand sanitizer or antibacterial soap
- ☐ Multitiered rolling cart
- ☐ Pencil sharpener
- ☐ Reusable spatulas that can be disinfected, and enough of them to not double dip
- ☐ Scissors, that can be disinfected, for trimming eyebrows
- ☐ Scissors for cutting wax strips
- ☐ Stool
- ☐ Tweezers, slanted and pointed, made of surgical steel able to withstand disinfection
- ☐ Waxing table
- ☐ Wax heaters, one containing hard wax and the other soft wax

SINGLE-USE ITEMS

- ☐ Bikini bottoms
- ☐ Cotton rounds or squares
- ☐ Cotton swabs
- ☐ Eyebrow brushes
- ☐ Gauze
- ☐ Headbands
- ☐ Hair clips, disposable metal or washable plastic
- ☐ Paper drapes
- ☐ Paper towels
- ☐ Trash bag
- ☐ Tissues (unscented)
- ☐ Treatment table paper rolls
- ☐ Vinyl or nitrile gloves
- ☐ Wax removal strips of pellon (fiber) or muslin (cotton), which come in rolls 3 inches wide or precut packets: for body 3" × 9" (7.5 cm × 22.86 cm) and eyebrow and upper lip size 1" × 3"
- ☐ Wooden wax applicators: large (tongue depressor), medium (popsicle sticks), or small

PRODUCTS

- ☐ Antiseptic lotions (witch hazel, tea tree oil, baby powder, numbing/topical anesthetic products)
- ☐ Baking soda for compress solution
- ☐ Cleansers/makeup remover
- ☐ Desensitizing spray products (topical numbing solution)
- ☐ Petroleum jelly for removing wax from eyelashes or hair
- ☐ Wax manufacturers' recommended products
- ☐ Wax removing lotion for skin; calming products like aloe vera gel, salicylic lotion, arnica, azulene

Procedure 11-1:
Perform Eyebrow Tweezing

Time for this service: 10 minutes; 15 minutes for complete reshaping

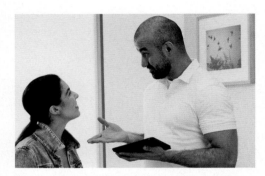

1 Discuss with the client the desired and appropriate shape.

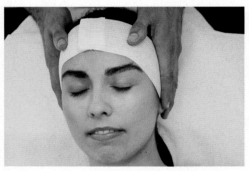

2 The head of the table should have protective paper for under the head, neck, and shoulders. The client should be in a semireclined position on the table, with the scalp hair protected and off the face. Wash and dry your hands then put on gloves.

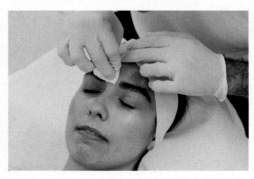

3 Cleanse and prepare the skin, using a makeup remover to remove makeup if present, otherwise using a mild antiseptic.

4 With a disposable brush measure the start point, endpoint, and correct arch location.

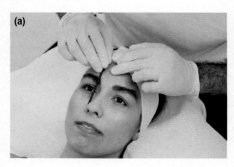 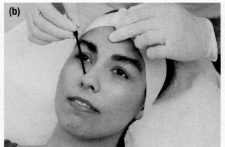 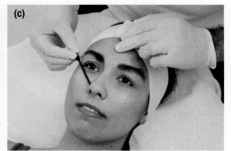

(a) (b) (c)

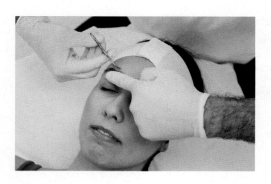

5 Brush the brows upward and isolate longer hairs that require trimming. Trim longer hairs with small round-tipped scissors to be uniform with the natural brow line. Brush along the top of the brow line and decide which hairs need to be removed.

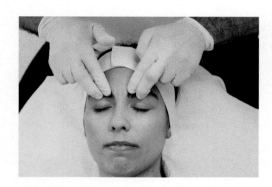

6 Standing or sitting behind the client and using the middle finger and forefinger, apply gentle friction to the brow area to warm the area, open the pores, and minimize discomfort during tweezing.

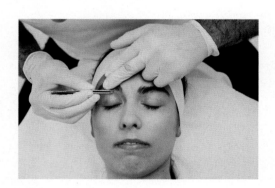

7 Using the forefinger and middle finger of the hand not holding the tweezers, hold the skin of the brow taut. Remove unwanted hairs underneath the brow closer to the nose, working to the outer edge using a quick smooth motion, grasping the hair as close to the skin as possible without pinching it, and tweezing the hair in its direction of growth rather than pulling straight up.

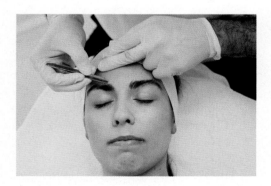

8 Brush the hair downward and remove hairs above the brow as necessary for the predetermined shape. After completing the brow, repeat the procedure on the second brow.

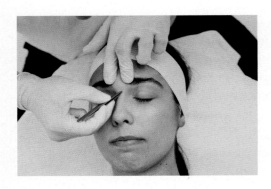

9 Proceed to the **glabella** (glow-BELL-ah), the area between the brows, where some hairs grow upward and some downward.

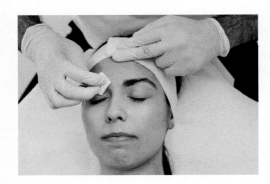

10 Wipe the treated area with a soothing, nonirritating antiseptic lotion to close the follicles and reduce the risk of infection.

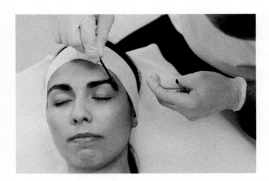

11 Finish by brushing the eyebrows in line.

Procedure 11-2:
Perform an Eyebrow Wax with Hard Wax

Time for this service: 20 minutes; 30 minutes for complete reshaping

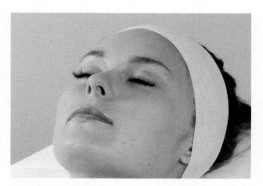

1 The head of the table should have protective paper for under the head, neck, and shoulders. The client should be in a semireclined position on the table, with hair and clothing protected. Wash and dry your hands then put on gloves.

2 The area to be waxed should be cleansed of makeup, facial oils, and pollutants.

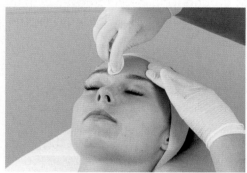

3 Pretreatment should be in accordance with the wax manufacturer's recommendations, which may mean, with hard wax, its complementary prewax oil.

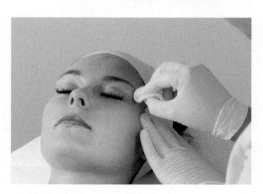

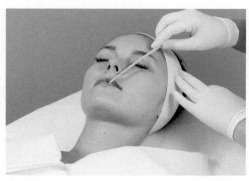

4 Having agreed on the desired shape during the consultation, brush the eyebrows using a disposable brush. Measure the eyebrows for the start point, endpoint, and point of arch.

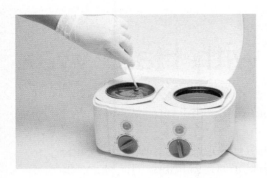

5 Dip the small applicator into the wax and scrape the underside, to avoid threads.

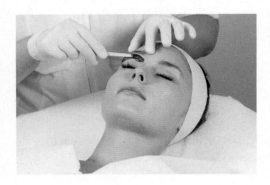

6 Standing behind the client, with a small spatula, apply the wax to the entire area under the brow, first against the direction of hair growth, and back over the same area in the direction of growth. Two or three applications may be necessary so that neither the hair nor the skin is visible through the wax. The strip of wax should have a clean, even edge all the way around for a clean removal, with a thicker tab at the outer edge where it will be lifted for the removal.

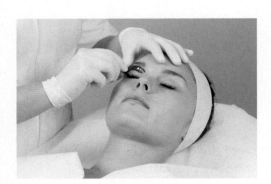

7 Within 30 seconds, when the wax looks opaque and maintains a fingerprint it is ready to lift off. Flick up the grasping edge of the wax on the outer edge of the eyebrow and with a thumb, hold the skin taut at the outer edge. Grasp the wax and pull quickly against the direction of growth as close to the skin as possible.

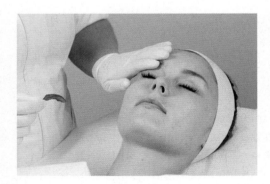

8 Immediately apply pressure to the area. Once you have become proficient in the use of hard wax, the wax can be applied to the second eyebrow while you are waiting for the wax on the first eyebrow to set.

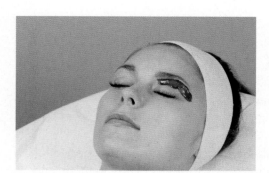

9 Repeat on the other eyebrow.

10 When applying wax to the glabella, the area between the eyebrows, the procedure is the same—apply the wax first against the growth then back on top in the direction of growth and remove against the growth. Although there may be growth upward at the top of the glabella and downward at the top of the nose, hard wax can remove both directions in a single application and removal.

Note: If needed, tweeze above each brow to remove any stray hairs. If needed, trim any extra-long stray hairs using rounded brow scissors.

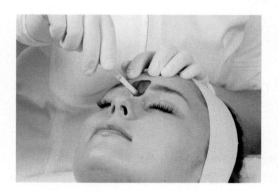
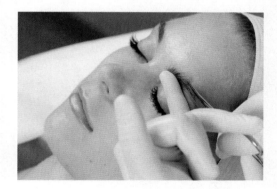

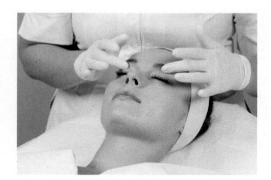

11 Finish with aftercare by massaging both eyebrows simultaneously with a soothing lotion and brushing the eyebrows.

Procedure 11-3:
Perform an Eyebrow Wax with Soft Wax

Time for this service: 15 minutes; 30 minutes for an eyebrow reshaping

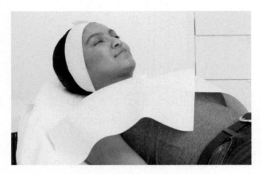

1 The head of the table should have protective paper for under the head, neck, and shoulders. The client should be in a semireclined position on the table, with hair and clothing protected. Wash and dry your hands then put on gloves.

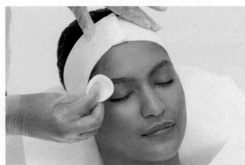

2 The area to be waxed should be cleansed of makeup, facial oils, and pollutants.

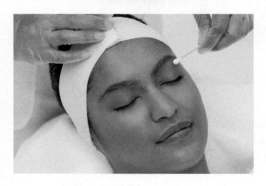

3 Pretreat the area to be waxed with the wax manufacturer's recommended products for soft wax or a thin film of tea tree oil followed by an application of baby powder.

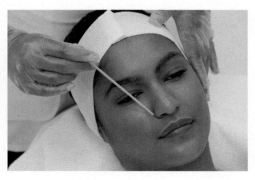

4 Having agreed on the desired shape during the consultation, brush the eyebrows using a disposable brush. Measure the eyebrows for the start point, endpoint, and point of arch.

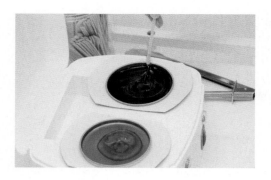

5 Dip the small applicator into the wax and scrape the underside, to avoid threads.

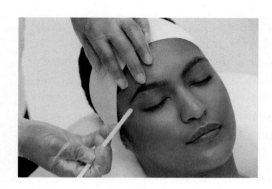

6 Standing behind the client, glide the applicator at a 45-degree angle along the underside from the nose point to the outer edge, following the desired line for hair to be removed. For extensive reshaping of considerable hair, a tiny amount of wax on the applicator can be used to separate and pull hairs down and away from the brow line. This can be done facing the client, although the actual waxing is better achieved by standing behind the client.

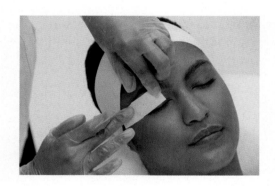

7 Then place the 1" × 3" strip over the wax, leaving a free edge at the endpoint to grasp. Give two or three quick strokes over the strip, also in the direction of hair growth.

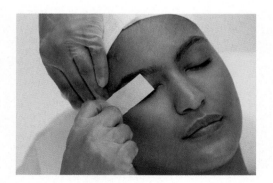

8 Place the forefinger and middle finger at the endpoint, holding the skin taut, and pull the strip quickly back against the hair growth, as close to the skin as possible.

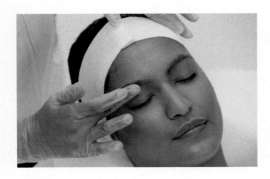

9 Quickly apply gentle pressure with the fingers that held the skin taut.

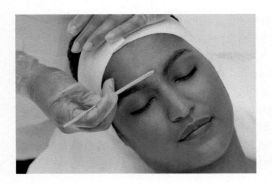

10 Repeat on the other eyebrow, and then the glabella. Following the rules for soft wax application and removal, the hairs higher up, growing upward, need to be treated separately from those at the top of the nose that grow downward. *Note:* If needed, tweeze above each brow to remove any stray hairs and trim any extra-long stray hairs using rounded brow scissors.

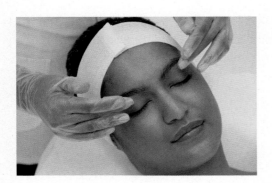

11 Finish with aftercare by massaging both eyebrows simultaneously with a soothing lotion and brushing the eyebrows.

Procedure 11-4:
Perform a Lip Wax with Hard Wax

Time for this service: 15 minutes

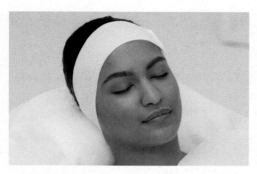

1 Complete draping and pretreatment preparations as outlined in Procedure 11–2.

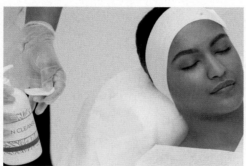

2 The area to be waxed should be cleansed of makeup, facial oils, and pollutants.

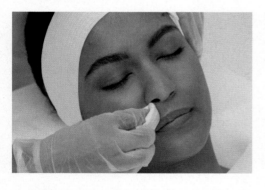

3 Pretreatment should be in accordance with the wax manufacturer's recommendations, which may mean, with hard wax, its complementary prewax oil.

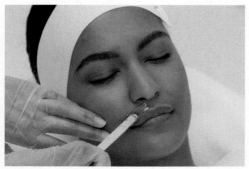

4 Standing behind the client and using a medium-sized applicator, apply the wax to half of the upper lip, gliding up under the hair, against the growth, from the outer edge to the halfway point, under the septum of the nose, then back down in a figure eight motion. The hair may be removed either with the hair growth (if you don't want to distort the hair follicles) or against the hair growth. A thicker tab of wax should be formed at the end where the pull will originate.

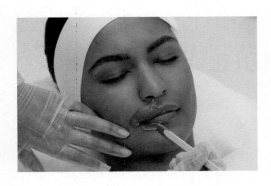

5 If also waxing the lower lip, for expediency, wax can be applied to half of the lower lip while the first application is setting.

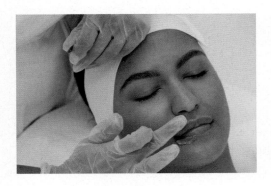

6 When the wax has lost its stickiness and wet shine, grasp the tab and remove the wax close and parallel to the skin. Then apply immediate pressure.

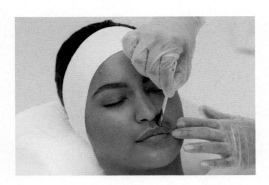

7 Repeat on the opposite side of the upper lip (and lower if called for).

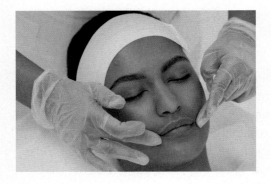

8 Finish by using both hands to massage with a soothing aftercare lotion.

Procedure 11-5:
Perform a Lip Wax with Soft Wax

Time for this service: 10 minutes

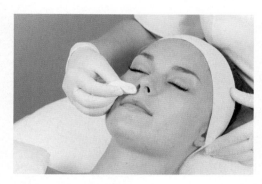

1 Complete draping and pretreatment preparations as outlined in Procedure 11–3. The area to be waxed should be cleansed of makeup, facial oils, and pollutants.

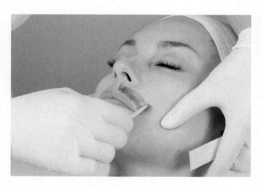

2 Pretreatment should be in accordance with the wax manufacturer's recommendations.

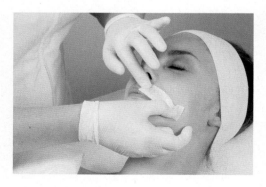

3 Standing behind the client and using a medium-sized applicator, start under the septum of the nose and apply a thin layer of wax in a downward, outward direction. It is important to make sure that the area under the nostril is covered and that no hairs are missed on the edge of the nostril as well as the hair along the edge of the vermillion border, all while avoiding the lip.

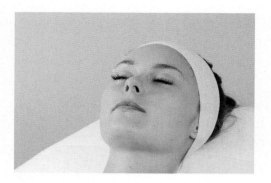

4 Immediately after the wax is applied, place the 1" × 3" strip over it, leaving enough of a free edge on the outside to grasp. Give the strip two firm rubs in the direction of growth.

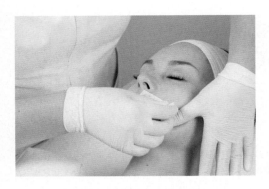

5 With your fingers holding the same outer edge of the lip taut and stable, grasp the strip and pull it quickly across the lip area in the direction opposite of growth, as close to the skin as possible, following through with a quick sweeping movement.

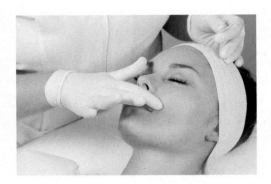

6 Quickly apply pressure to the area with the hand that held the skin taut, to ease the smarting sensation common with this type of waxing in this area.

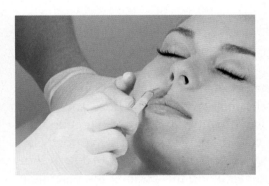

7 Proceed to the other side of the lip.

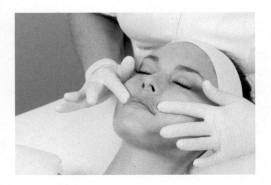

8 Finish with an application of soothing lotion.

Procedure 11-6:
Perform a Chin Wax with Hard Wax

Time for this service: 15 minutes

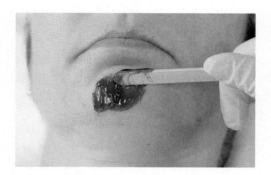

1 Complete draping and pretreatment preparations as outlined in Procedure 11–2.

2 Decide how many sections of wax have to be applied to remove the hair under the jaw and down the throat based on sections of approximately no more than 2" x 3" and divide the area accordingly. Hair on the throat grows up toward the chin and from the center outward along the jawline. On the chin hair grows downward.

3 Standing behind the client, by the top of their head, apply the wax with a medium spatula to the first section. For expediency wax can then be applied to another section as long as it is not immediately adjacent to the first application.

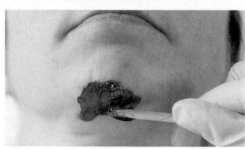

4 Holding the skin taut, remove one or more sections in the direction of the hair growth and apply pressure immediately after the pull.

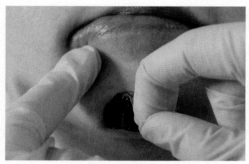

5 Apply the wax in small sections below the curve of the jawline.

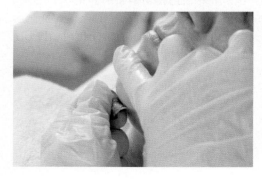

6 Remove the wax. Due to the contours of the chin, this area should be waxed in small sections.

7 If there is hair along the jawbone, it can be removed in a sideways fashion, similar to a lip wax, preventing the chance of follicle distortion.

8 Finish with aftercare as previously instructed.

Procedure 11-7:
Perform Waxing of the Axilla with Hard Wax

Time for this service: Approximately 20 minutes

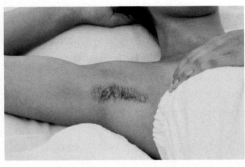

1 Complete the draping and pretreatment preparations, having the client lie flat on the table. If the axilla is deep, place a rolled-up towel bolster under the back directly under the axilla to be waxed.

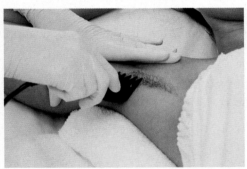

2 If the hair is long so that it curls over, it should be buzzed or trimmed to ½ inch in length. This will make the service more comfortable and easier to evaluate the different directions of hair growth.

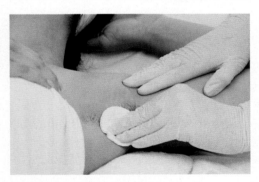

3 Make sure both axilla are thoroughly cleansed of perspiration and deodorant and are dry.

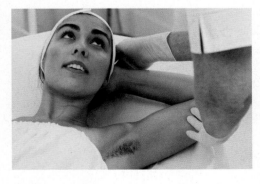

4 Have the client raise the arm above the shoulder, placing the hand behind the head. They should then reach across the body with the other hand and move the breast tissue down and away.

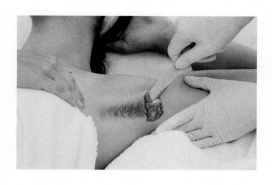

5 Apply the wax against the growth, getting underneath all the hairs growing in different directions first before going back over the top, forming a thicker tab at the end where the pull will originate.

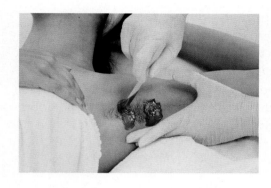

6 If three different applications are necessary, a second application can be done while the first is hardening, as long as it is not directly adjacent to the previous wax application and enough space is left in between for the third application.

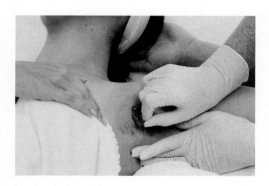

7 Have the client turn their face away from the axilla to avoid any chance of being hit during the swift removal of the wax.

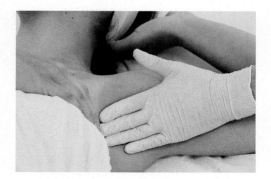

8 Apply immediate pressure to the area after each removal pull, to ease any discomfort.

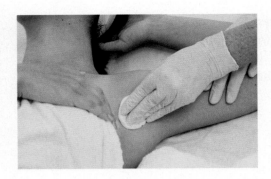

9 Apply aftercare of soothing lotion to the completed side before moving to the next side.

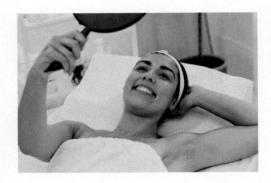

10 Complete the opposite side and finish with aftercare. Reassure the client that any blood spots are due to the fact that the hair was removed at the papilla, this is a sign of a successful epilation, and they will soon reabsorb into the skin. Ask the client to refrain from using deodorant on the area for at least 24 to 48 hours and until all signs of redness and irritation pass.

Procedure 11-8:
Perform Axilla Waxing with Soft Wax

Time for this service: Approximately 15 minutes

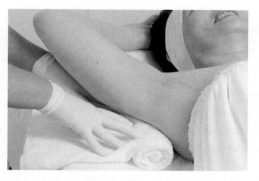

1 Complete preparation, draping and positioning of client, and bolstering. To do this, have the client lie flat on the table. If the axilla is deep, place a rolled-up towel bolster under the back directly under the axilla to be waxed. Have the client raise the arm above the shoulder, placing the hand behind the head.

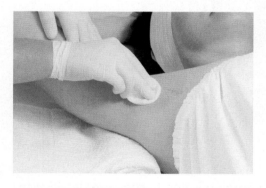

2 If the hair is long so that it curls over, it should be buzzed or trimmed to ½ inch in length. This will make it more comfortable and easier to evaluate the different directions of hair growth.

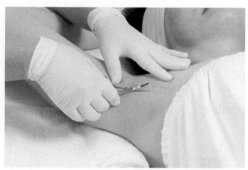

3 Clean the axilla on both sides thoroughly, removing any trace of perspiration and deodorant and pat dry.

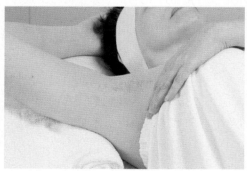

4 Ask the client to reach across their body and move the breast tissue down and away.

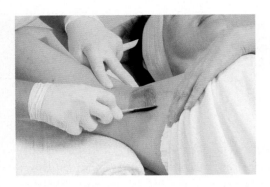

5 With the edge of a large applicator, apply wax at a 45-degree angle in the direction of hair growth, where possible. If there are different directions within the same cluster, there could be breakage and some hairs left behind. As the same patch cannot be waxed a second time during that service, the remaining hair needs to be tweezed.

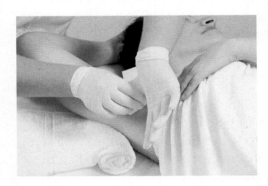

6 Using a 3″ × 9″ wax removal strip, place the strip of wax and rub two times in the direction of growth. Instruct the client to turn their head away to avoid being hit and pull against the hair growth and close to the skin.

7 Each application should proceed by clearing the outer edges working toward the center until the hair has been removed.

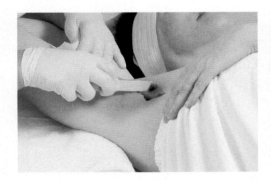
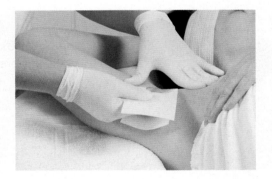

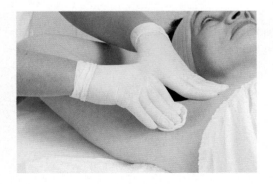

8 Apply aftercare of soothing lotion to the completed side before moving to the next side.

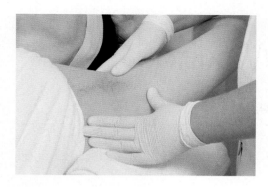

9 Evaluate the directions of growth on the second axilla as they may well be different than the first, This is more pertinent to soft waxing than hard waxing.

10 Complete the wax application and removal on the opposite side and finish with aftercare as instructed in Procedure 11–8, step 8. As the same patch cannot be waxed a second time during that service, the remaining hair needs to be tweezed.

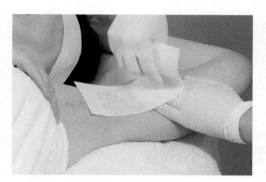

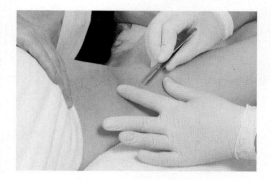

Procedure 11-9:
Perform Arm and Hand Waxing with Hard Wax

Time for this service: Lower arm wax should take approximately 20 minutes; whole arm including hands, 30 to 40 minutes.

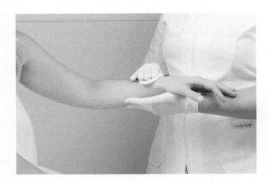

1 Have the client sit on the side of the table and remove clothing from arms, exposing the area to be waxed.

Complete draping by offering a disposable plastic apron or placing a drape across the client's lap and apply the pretreatment for hard wax.

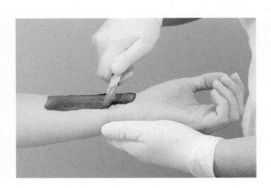

2 The first arm to be waxed is outstretched with the palm facing up. Start by waxing the inside lower half of the arm where there is less hair downward toward the wrist following the application rules for hard wax.

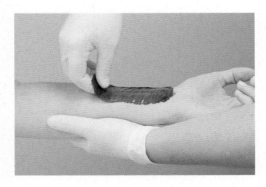

3 The removal pull can be in the direction of growth if the goal is to not distort the hair follicles.

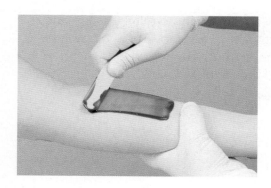

4 The next section to wax should be just above the previous section.

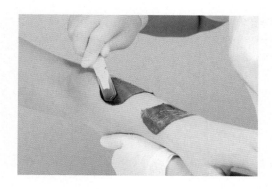

5 After completing the inner arm have the client turn their still outstretched arm, so the palm faces down. Then hold the arm firmly in place and, starting at the wrist, apply the wax across the top of the arm from the inside (thumb side) to the outside (little finger side), leaving the width of a strip between each application all the way up the forearm to the elbow.

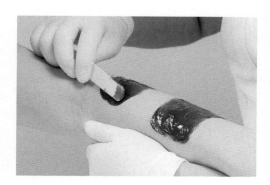

6 After removing the wax go back and wax those in-between sections.

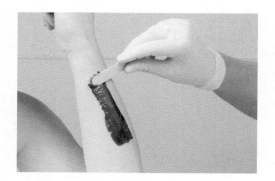

7 Next have the client hold their arm straight up, bent at the elbow, to wax the side that follows down from the little finger. This can be done in two sections starting near the elbow, working up toward the wrist. The hair grows down toward the elbow. Remove the wax.

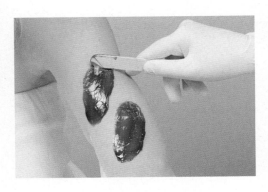

8 For the upper arm, ask the client to relax the arm and allow the forearm to rest on the lap. Apply the wax in alternating sections, starting toward the elbow and working up toward the shoulder.

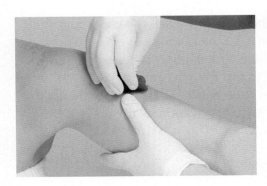

9 After removing those sections of hard wax, apply the wax to the remaining in-between sections. Remove the wax. If waxing only the arm, apply aftercare.

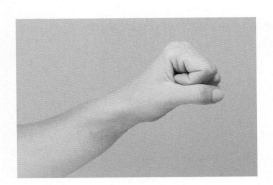

10 To continue to the hand wax, ask the client to form a fist by tucking the fingers under, as this tightens the skin.

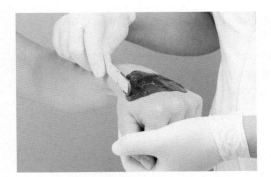

11 Apply the wax, down toward the fingers, angling out slightly toward the little finger. The entire top of the hand can be done at once.

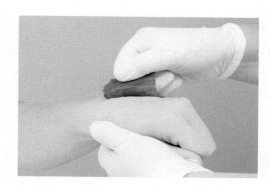

12 To remove the wax, since the client's hand is "floating" without solid support, it is important to have a good grip on the hand for the removal pull.

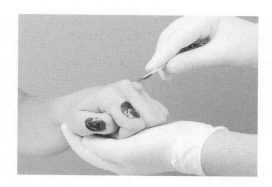

13 If the fingers need waxing, as the hair grows in a horseshoe shape, the hard wax can be applied in circular patches on each finger starting with the thumb across to the little finger.

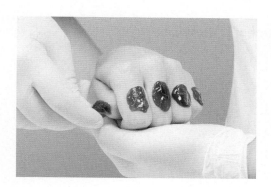

14 Once each finger application is completed, you will be ready to remove the wax in the same order.

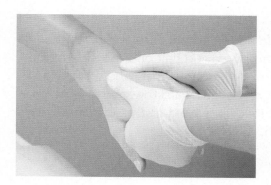

15 Apply aftercare by grasping the hand and applying the soothing lotion in long strokes up to the elbow and back down to the hand followed by a hand and finger massage. Proceed to the second arm.

Procedure 11-10:
Perform Arm and Hand Waxing with Soft Wax

Time for this service: Lower arm wax should take approximately 20 minutes; whole arm including hands, 30 minutes.

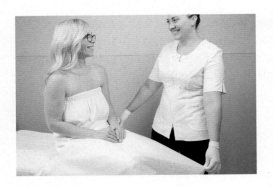

1 Have the client sit on the side of the table and remove clothing from arms, exposing the area to be waxed.

Complete draping by offering a disposable plastic apron or placing a drape across the client's lap.

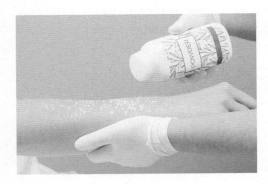

2 Apply the pretreatment for soft wax.

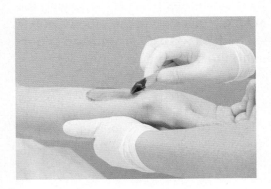

3 With the client holding the arm outstretched with the palm facing up, start by waxing hair on the inside of the lower half of the arm, toward the wrist, where there is less hair. The hair grows downward toward the wrist, so the wax is applied following the growth and is removed against the growth.

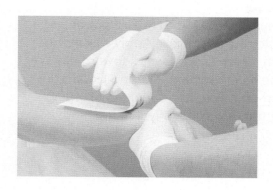

4 Apply the wax strip and rub firmly two times in the direction of hair growth. Hold the skin taut and remove the wax strip in one quick pull. The next section to wax should be just above the previous section.

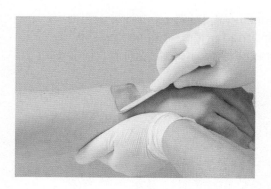

5 Next the client should turn their still outstretched arm so the palm faces down. Then hold the arm firmly in place and start at the wrist, applying the wax the width of the strip across the top of the arm from the inside (thumb side) to the outside (little finger side). Follow the rules of application and removal.

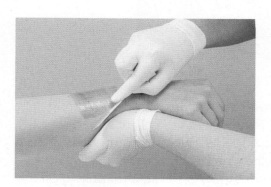

6 Continue in strip-size sections all the way up the forearm to the elbow.

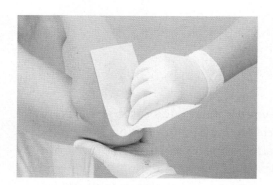

7 Next have the client hold the arm straight up, bent at the elbow, and apply the wax to the side that follows down from the little finger. This can be done in two sections. The hair grows down toward the elbow.

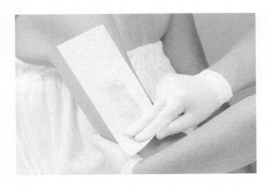

8 For the upper arm, ask the client to relax the arm and allow the forearm to rest on the lap. Apply wax in the direction of growth, which is downward, toward the elbow. Remove the hair in sections starting toward the elbow and working up toward the shoulder, blending if necessary at the top. If waxing only the arm, apply aftercare.

9 To continue to the hand wax, ask the client to form a fist by tucking the fingers under, as this tightens the skin. Apply the wax with the growth, down toward the fingers, angling out slightly toward the little finger. The entire top of the hand can be done at once, not including the fingers.

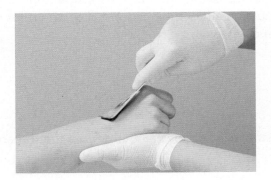
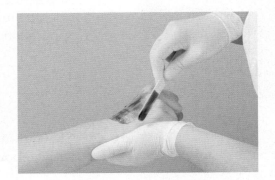

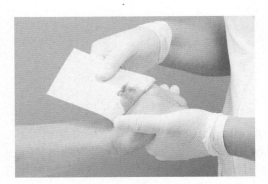

10 Apply the strip over the entire area and rub firmly in the direction of growth. As the client's hand is "floating" without solid support, it is important to have a good grip on the hand when you pull quickly back against the growth. Apply pressure after pulling off the wax strip.

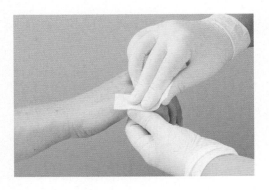

11 If the fingers have hair that needs to be removed and it is minimal and soft, it can often be removed with the wax that is already on the strip. The hair grows toward the middle knuckle, so take one finger at a time, press the wax onto the hair, rub in the direction of growth, and quickly pull off against the growth.

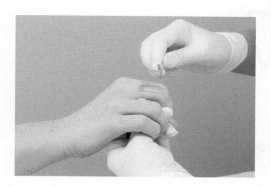

12 If the finger hair cannot be removed by pressing the wax-saturated strip, complete the process by starting at the thumb and applying wax to each finger, then quickly going back and removing it.

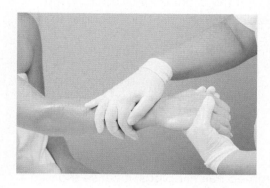

13 Apply aftercare by grasping the hand and applying the soothing lotion in long strokes up to the elbow and back down to the hand followed by a hand and finger massage. Proceed to the second arm.

Procedure 11-11:
Perform a Men's Chest Waxing with Hard Wax

Time for this service: Approximately 30 to 45 minutes, depending on the amount of hair to be removed

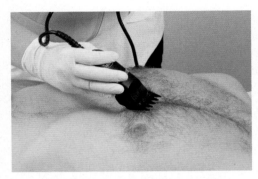

1 Complete draping with the client undressed from the waist up and fully reclined. Trim hair that is longer than ½ inch.

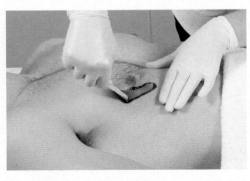

2 Brush away the trimmed hair clippings, cleanse the skin and apply the pretreatment for hard wax.

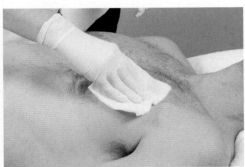

3 Using a large applicator, apply the wax on the furthest lower outer edge of the area of the chest where there is minimal hair.

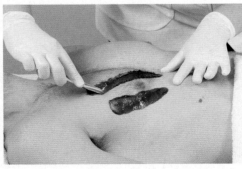

4 For expediency, a second wax application can be done while waiting for the previous one to set, as long as it is not immediately adjacent.

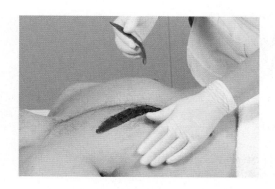

5 Remove the wax. Apply gentle pressure immediately after each pull in this sensitive area.

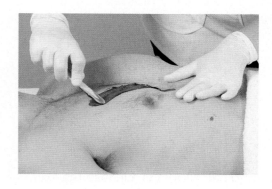

6 Move in sections upward and inward. As you get to the denser areas be mindful of changes in the direction of hair growth and make sure that the hair is well coated in wax.

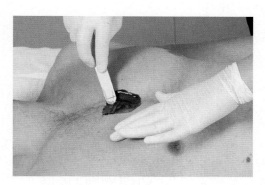

7 After completing the furthest side, continue in the same manner on the nearest side, beginning at the lower outer edge with less hair.

8 Next turn your attention to the hair growing in a different direction in the center, again starting where there is less hair, usually lower on the chest, and moving toward more dense hair, usually in the center and higher up on the chest.

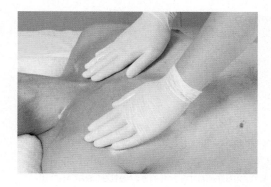

9 After hair removal is complete, finish by applying and massaging a soothing wax removal lotion to the area and checking for blood spots before the client dresses. Remind the client that blood spots are normal where hair is coarse and grows deep and that they are a sign of a successful epilation, not a cause for concern.

Procedure 11-12:
Perform a Men's Chest Waxing with Soft Wax

Time for this service: Approximately 30 to 45 minutes, depending on the amount of hair to be removed

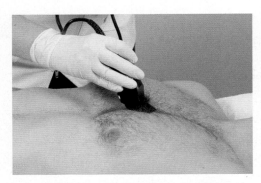

1 Complete draping with the client undressed from the waist up and fully reclined. Trim hair that is longer than ½ inch.

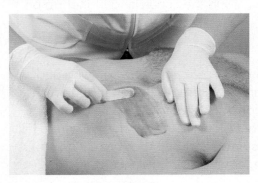

2 Brush away the trimmed hair clippings, cleanse the skin, and apply the pretreatment for soft wax.

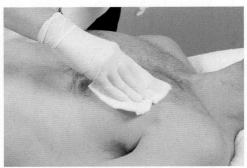

3 Using a large applicator, apply the wax on the furthest lower outer edge of the area of the chest where there is minimal hair. The application should be no larger than the 3" × 9" removal strip.

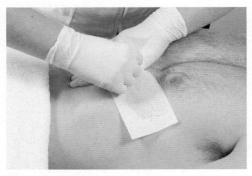

4 Rub the strip in the direction of the hair growth and remove the strip against the growth and parallel to the skin. Apply gentle pressure immediately after each pull in this sensitive area.

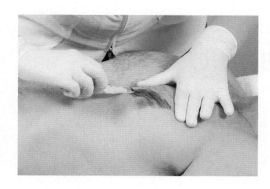

5 Move in sections upward and inward. As you get to the denser areas be mindful of changes in the direction of growth.

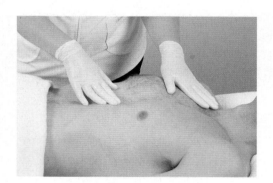

6 After completing the furthest side, continue in the same manner on the nearest side, beginning at the lower outer edge with less hair.

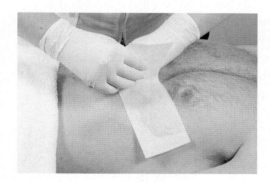

7 Next remove the hair growing in a different direction in the center, starting where there is less hair, usually lower on the chest, and moving toward more dense hair, usually in the center and higher up on the chest. Wax this area in smaller sections, paying attention to the most dominant direction of growth or switch to hard wax in those areas.

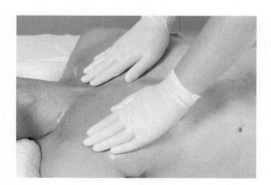

8 After hair removal is complete, finish by applying and massaging a soothing wax removal lotion to the area and checking for blood spots before the client dresses. Remind the client that blood spots are normal where hair is coarse and grows deep and that they are a sign of a successful epilation, not a cause for concern.

Procedure 11-13:
Perform a Men's Back Waxing with Hard Wax

Time for this service: Approximately 30 to 45 minutes, depending on the amount of hair

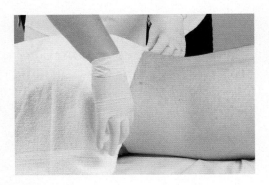

1 Complete draping with the client undressed from the waist up and fully reclined face down. The face should be in a face cradle with a disposable cover or with the forehead resting on the hands with the elbows sticking out. For comfort, you could place a bolster or rolled towel under their feet.

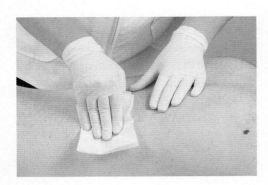

2 Cleanse and complete the pretreatment preparations for hard wax. While cleansing, familiarize yourself with the directions of hair growth on the client's back, the length of hair, and inspect the back for skin tags, moles, and lesions.

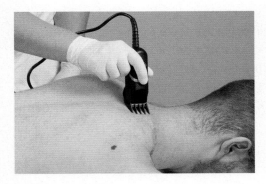

3 If the hair is longer than ½ inch, it should be trimmed. Afterwards, wipe away the trimmed hair with an esthetics wipe, and then apply a dusting of powder, or pretreatment recommended by the hard wax manufacturer.

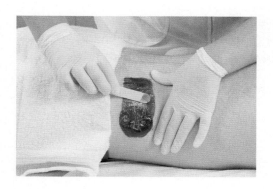

4 Using a large applicator, first apply the wax on the outer edge of the torso, just above the waistline where there is minimal hair. Apply the wax in a manageable strip of approximately 2″ × 5″, using the application rules for hard wax.

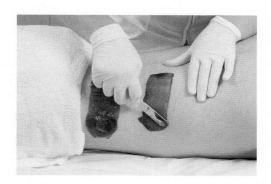

5 For expediency, while the wax is setting another application can be made, not immediately adjacent to the first application but one section over.

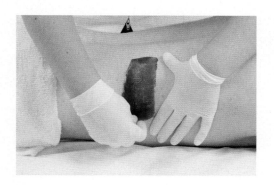

6 Remove the sections following the rules for hard wax removal. Immediately apply gentle pressure to the area.

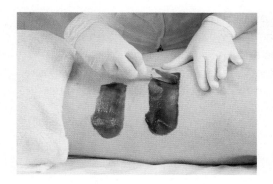

7 Go back to the in-between section for the third application. Then while it sets, apply the fourth application to the area immediately adjacent to the second application, and so on.

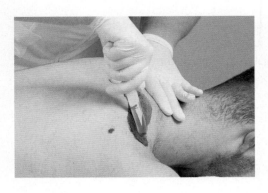

8 Continue in this manner until the side is cleared, following the waxing rules and directional changes. Include the back of the shoulder, if requested.

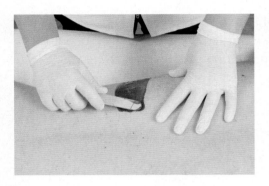

9 Repeat on the opposite side.

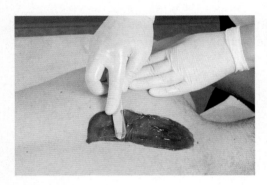

10 Next wax the hairs growing down the center of the back, over the spine.

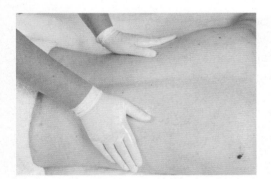

11 Apply aftercare of antiseptic lotion to the area that was waxed to remove wax residue, using effleurage massage strokes and being careful not to extend beyond the treated areas, as there may be a few more hairs to remove at the top with the client sitting up.

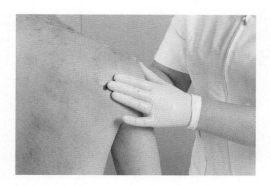

12 The client should sit up, facing you with their arms at their side and a drape on their lap so the rest of the shoulder area can be waxed. These sections are smaller, so wax one surface at a time to avoid waxing over a curve.

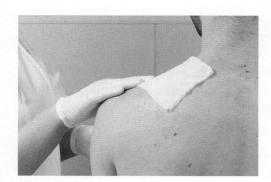

13 Make sure both sides are balanced and even. Waxing the front is considered a separate service (part of the chest wax). Apply aftercare to the remaining areas.

14 After wax residue is removed, apply a cool compress soaked in a baking soda solution for a few minutes. Remind the client that it is not unusual for hives to develop in the waxed area and they will settle down within an hour or so. Applying a salicylic acid product to the area can help reduce redness and bumps. As the client cannot see the back, let the client know when the blood spots have diminished before getting dressed.

Procedure 11-14:
Perform a Men's Back Waxing with Soft Wax

Time for this service: Approximately 30 to 45 minutes, depending on the amount of hair, and whether soft wax and speed waxing is used.

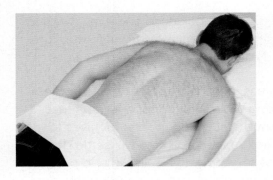

1 Complete draping with the client undressed from the waist up and fully reclined face down. The face should be in a face cradle with a disposable cover or with the forehead resting on the hands with the elbows sticking out. Waistband and undergarments should be protected with disposable towels.

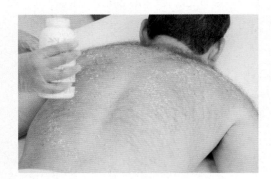

2 Cleanse and complete the pretreatment preparations for soft wax. While cleansing, familiarize yourself with the directions of hair growth on the client's back, the length of hair, and inspect the back for skin tags, moles, and lesions.

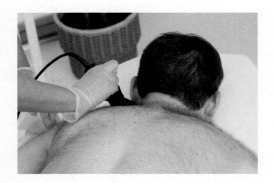

3 If the hair is longer than ½ inch, it should be trimmed. Afterwards, wipe away the trimmed hair with an esthetics wipe, and then apply a dusting of powder.

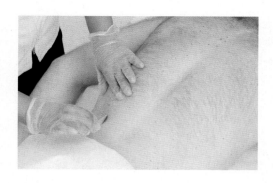

4 Begin the hair removal at the area just above the waistline of the pants using a large spatula. The first application of wax should begin from the outside edge of the torso where hair growth is minimal.

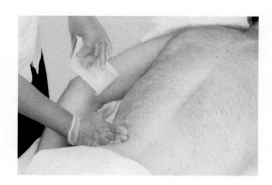

5 Follow the standard rules for soft wax application and removal. Grasp the strip, hold skin taut, and quickly pull parallel against the hair growth. Apply gentle pressure immediately after wax removal to ease any discomfort.

6 The next application should be immediately above the previous one (Photo A).

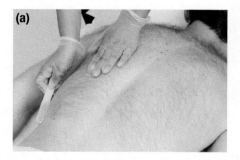

(a)

If the length of the strip will be too long to do all at once, then apply a second strip next to the first. Remove the outside strip first, then the center (refer to Photo B and C for example).

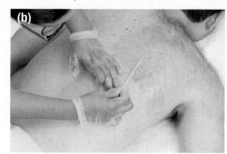

(b)

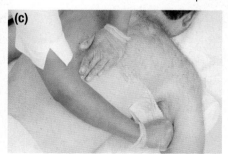

(c)

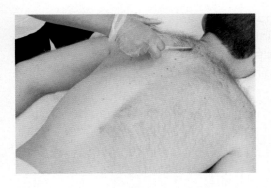

7 Repeat this process until you reach the top (towards the shoulders) as this is where you'll notice a change in hair direction. It begins to turn downward in the center along the spine.

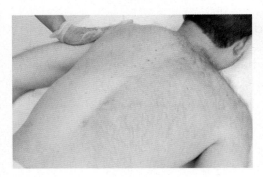

8 Complete the removal on that side by following the waxing rules and directional changes. Include the back of the sholder, if requested.

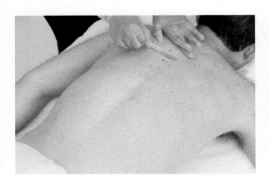

9 Repeat on opposite side followed by the hairs growing down the center, over the spine.

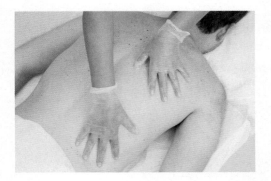

10 Apply plenty of soothing antiseptic lotion to the area that was waxed to remove the wax residue, being careful not to extend beyond the treated areas, as there may be a few more strips to do with the client sitting up.

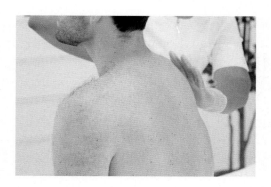

11 The client should now sit up, facing you with his arms at his side and a drape on his lap so the rest of the shoulder area can be waxed.

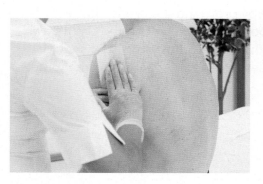

12 The shoulders are waxed one surface area at a time. Do not attempt to round a curve with the strip. The hair on the shoulder usually grows inward to the center of the shoulder from the back, and inward toward the center from the front.

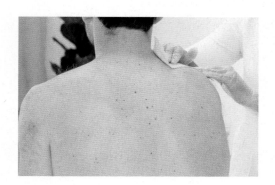

13 Finish by blending toward the front and top of the arms, using existing wax on the strip and making sure both sides are balanced and even. Waxing the front is considered a separate service (part of the chest wax) but blending a little with wax already on the strip is acceptable.

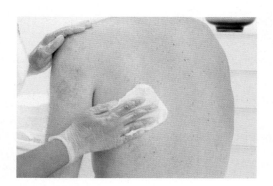

14 After all wax residue is removed, you can apply a cool compress soaked in a baking soda solution for a few minutes. Applying a salicylic acid product to the area will help reduce redness and bumps. Inform the client when the blood spots have diminished before getting dressed.

Procedure 11-15:
Perform an American Bikini Wax with Hard Wax

Time for this service: Approximately 30 to 40 minutes, depending on the amount of hair to be removed

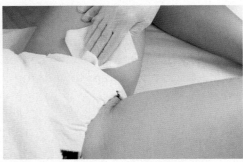

1 Complete draping by providing the client with disposable bikini bottoms or protecting the client's own undergarments with paper drapes. The client should lay face up flat or semireclined. Cleanse the area to be waxed.

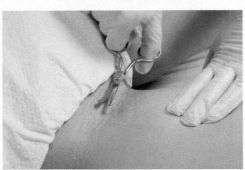

2 With an applicator select the hair to be removed, forming clean, even margins on both sides and keeping hair not to be removed securely tucked away and protected from the wax.

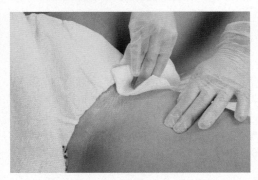

3 If the hair is longer than ½ inch, it should be trimmed.

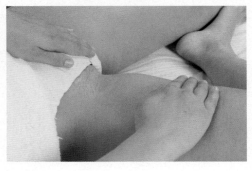

4 Apply the pretreatment for hard wax.

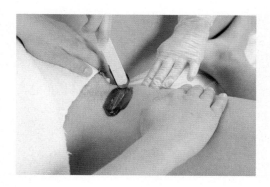

5 Ask the client to place the sole of the other foot to the level of the knee on the straight leg. The client should place one hand firmly on the paper or disposable panties on the pubis, fingers straight down. The other hand is placed on the outer edge of the thigh of the bent leg to help pull the skin taut. The hands and bent leg are reversed for waxing the opposite side.

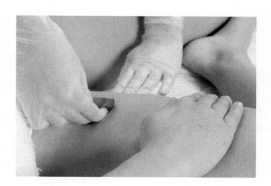

6 With a large applicator, apply the wax following the panty line up to the femoral ridge in a wax strip 2 inches wide and 4 to 5 inches long. Follow the rules for hard wax application, leaving a thicker tab at the end nearest the femoral ridge to grasp for the removal pull. If this area of hair is wide, it may take two parallel applications, so begin on the outer edge and work inward.

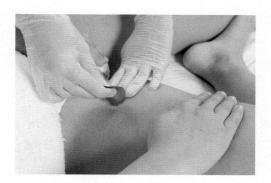

7 Remove the wax, following the rules for hard wax removal and immediately applying pressure to the area after the removal pull.

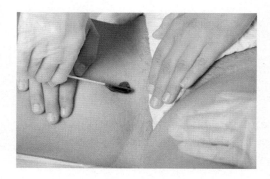

8 The next application is downward from the ridge toward the table, leaving enough space for hand placement to hold the skin taut. To facilitate this procedure, have the client bring the sole of their foot a little higher to just above the knee.

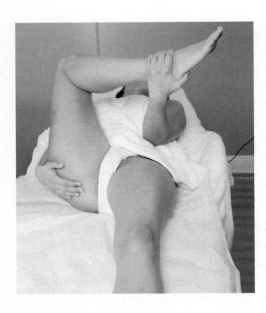

9 Next have the client lift their leg to their chest, grasping it behind the knee or drawing it across the abdomen holding it by the ankle. This should expose the last remaining third of hair that was too near the table to apply the wax. This position also ensures that the skin is nice and taut.

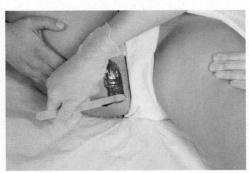

10 Apply the wax initially upwards coating the underside of the hair then back downwards over the top of the hair.

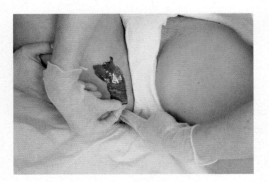

11 The removal pull for this application is upward. When the first side is completed, continue on the other side.

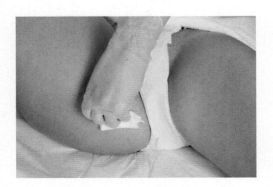

12 Apply soothing aftercare and remind the client that blood spots are normal and acceptable in this area, and a visible sign of a successful epilation.

Procedure 11-16:
Perform an American Bikini Wax with Soft Wax

Time for this service: Approximately 20 to 30 minutes, depending on the amount of hair to be removed

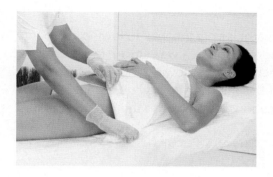

1 Complete draping by providing the client with disposable bikini bottoms or protecting the client's own undergarments with paper drapes. The client should lay face up flat or semi-reclined.

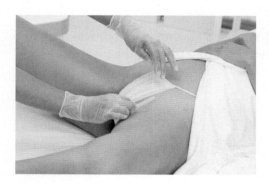

2 With an applicator select the hair to be removed, forming clean even margins on both sides and keeping hair not to be removed securely tucked away and protected from the wax.

If the hair is longer than ½ inch, it should be trimmed.

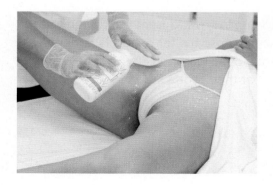

3 Cleanse and apply the pretreatment for soft wax.

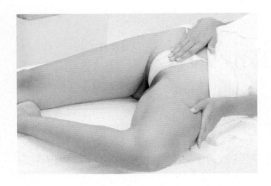

4 Starting with the side furthest away have the client place the sole of the other foot to the level of the knee on the straight leg. The client should place one hand firmly on the paper or disposable panties on the pubis, fingers straight down. The other hand is placed on the outer edge of the thigh of the bent leg to help pull the skin taut. The hands and bent leg are reversed for waxing the opposite side.

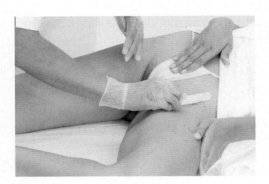

5 With a large applicator, apply the wax following the panty line up to the femoral ridge in a wax strip 2 to 3 inches wide and 4 to 6 inches long following the rules for soft wax application. If this area of hair is wide, it may take two parallel applications, so begin on the outer edge and work inward.

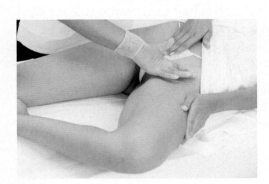

6 Remove, following the rules for soft wax removal and immediately applying pressure to the area after the removal pull.

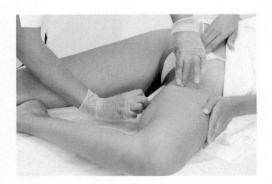

7 The next application is downward from the ridge toward the table, leaving enough space for hand placement to hold the skin taut. To facilitate the process, have the client bring the sole of their foot a little higher to just above the knee.

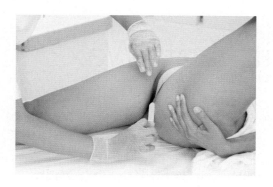

8 Next have the client lift their leg to their chest, grasping it at the ankle or behind the knee. This should expose the last remaining third of hair that was too near the table to apply the wax. This position also ensures that the skin is nice and taut. The soft wax is applied downward.

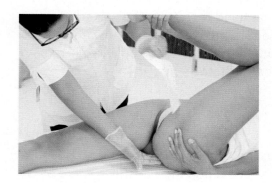

9 The removal pull for this application is upward.

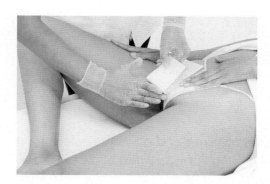

10 When the first side is completed, continue on the other side.

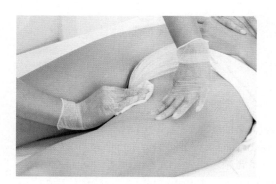

11 Apply soothing aftercare and remind the client that blood spots are normal and acceptable in this area, and a visible sign of a successful epilation.

Procedure 11-17:
Perform a Leg Waxing with Soft Wax

Time for this service: Approximately 30 minutes for half-leg treatment; approximately 45 minutes for whole leg treatment

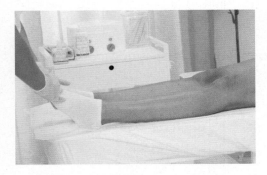

1 Complete draping with client disrobed from the waist down and fully reclined on the table with legs stretched out and flat. If the feet and toes are to be waxed along with the legs, make sure they are kept warm with socks or a towel until ready to be waxed, or the wax will remain behind and not lift off with the strip.

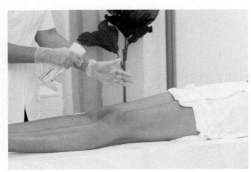

2 To pretreat the legs, mist the entire front area to be waxed with an antiseptic lotion then dust the entire area with baby powder.

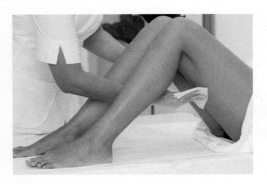

3 Have the client bend the knees and place the soles of the feet on the table. Then apply the mist and powder as far underneath as possible. For speed, prepare both legs simultaneously.

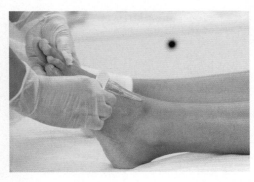

4 Begin with the leg and foot furthest away if you have to lean rather than switch sides. Give the foot a good rub with both hands until it feels warm. Apply the wax to the top of the foot, applying it downward toward the toes.

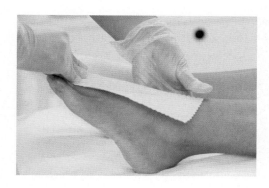

5 Apply the strip before the wax cools and pull off quickly as close to the skin as possible. Immediately apply pressure to the area.

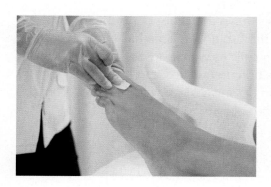

6 If there is very little hair on the toes, the wax on the strip may be sufficient to remove those hairs by pressing the wax onto the hair and quickly pulling away, making sure that the pressure is in the direction of growth, and the pull is in the opposite direction. If there is considerable hair growth, apply the wax to each toe.

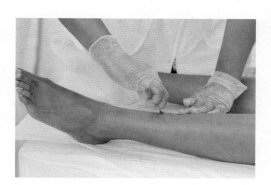

7 Rotate the foot outward. The next application is on the inside of the ankle. Apply the wax downwards toward the ankle beginning from 7 to 8 inches up the leg. Continue with the next application directly above the previous one. Proceed in the same manner until the knee is reached.

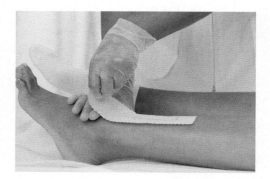

8 Rotate the foot back to the center and return. Then proceed again from the bottom, working in the same size strips, on the front of the leg up the shin bone to the knee.

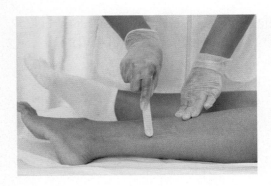

9 Rotate the foot inward. Starting again at the bottom, clear the hair in the same size strips to the outer edge of the lower leg, again working up to the knee.

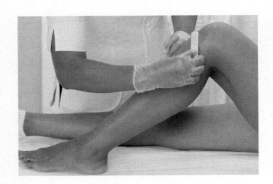

10 To wax the knees, have the client bend the leg and put the foot flat on the table. This area has coarse patches of dry, dead skin cells as well as folds of skin on some clients. This positioning ensures that the skin is tight. Apply the wax in downward, outward sections from the middle of the knee, covering the lower half.

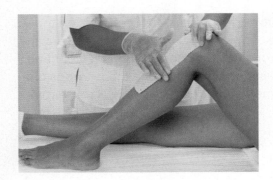

11 Apply the strip, rub firmly downward, and remove quickly upward, working your way around the knee.

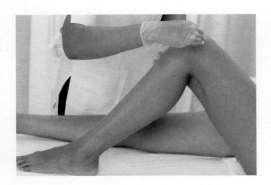

12 Next apply the wax to the top part of the knee in a downward direction over the top to the middle. Remove the wax strip.

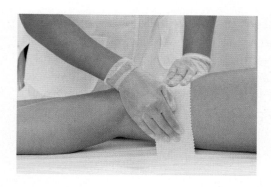

13 Next move to the upper leg. If the upper leg is not going to be waxed, you are ready to move to the other leg. The direction of hair growth on the upper leg is downward in the middle and outward on either side. Lay the leg back down and have the client rotate the foot inward for easy access. Apply the wax just above the knee to the center outward.

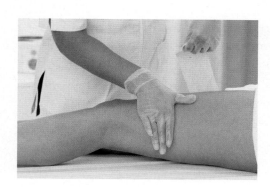

14 Continue removing the hair by applying the wax from the center outward, moving up the thigh. It is especially important to hold the skin taut for the pull on the thigh, as the skin is often looser here than on the lower leg.

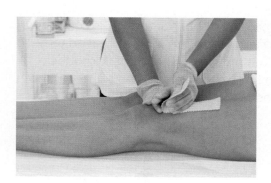

15 Rotate the leg back to the middle and apply the wax in a downward direction from 8 inches above the knee downward toward the knee.

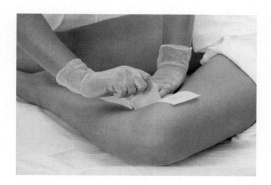

16 After the middle is cleared, to wax the inner thigh, have the client bend the leg, bringing it to the same position it would be in if getting a bikini wax with the sole of the foot resting at the level of the knee on the other leg. Begin just above the knee, applying the wax from the inside down the inner thigh, leaving enough room near the table to hold the skin taut for the removal pull. Complete the inner thigh up to the bikini area, but not including the bikini unless that is part of this service.

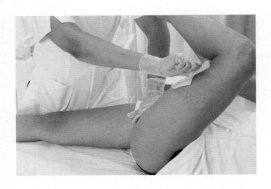

17 Next have the client grasp the ankle or under the knee, pulling the leg to the chest to expose the hairs at the back of the thigh while tightening that skin for comfort and effective removal. Be sure the skin is held as taut as possible to prevent bruising. An additional dusting of baby powder may be warranted.

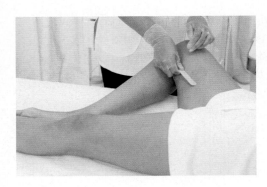

18 After completing the back of the thigh, move to the opposite leg, removing the hair in the same manner as on the first side.

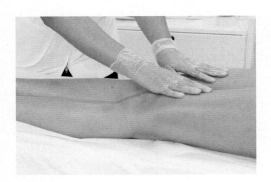

19 When the hair removal of the second leg is completed, lotion should be applied to the waxed areas to remove any residue so that the client does not stick to the paper when she turns over. This can be done with both hands simultaneously.

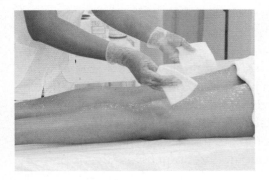

20 The client now turns over for the remaining hair removal on the back of the legs. Have the client hang her feet off the end of the table and add an additional dusting of powder if necessary.

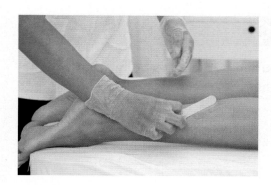

21 Begin at the bottom of the lower leg and apply wax over the calf from the outside inward, continuing up in the same manner to the back of the knee.

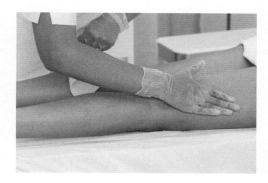

22 The hair growth pattern can vary at the back of the knee and should be determined at the time of waxing. Look for any patches of hair missed on the back of the thigh.

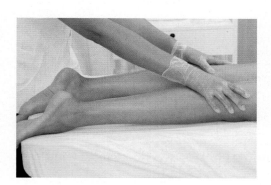

23 When all the hair has been removed from both legs, pamper the client by applying plenty of lotion and using gentle effleurage movements, massage and sooth the legs with upward movements up the middle and a little lighter stroking down the outside.

COMPETENCY PROGRESS

How are you doing with hair removal? **Check the Chapter 11 Learning Objectives below that you feel you have mastered; leave unchecked those concepts you will need to return to:**

- ☐ Explain the importance of hair removal.
- ☐ Describe the structure of hair.
- ☐ Explain the hair growth cycle.
- ☐ Identify the causes of excessive hair growth.
- ☐ Compare temporary and permanent hair removal and reduction methods.
- ☐ Explain when to use hard and soft wax methods of hair removal.
- ☐ Provide a thorough client consultation for hair removal services.
- ☐ List items needed in a wax treatment room.
- ☐ Demonstrate waxing head to toe with soft and hard waxes.

GLOSSARY

anagen AN-uh-jen	pg. 459	first stage of hair growth during which new hair is produced
axilla ag-ZIL-uh	pg. 491	the correct professional and anatomical term for the underarm; the region between the arm and the thoracic wall
blend (for electrolysis) BLEND	pg. 470	a modality of electrolysis combining alternating current (AC) and direct current (DC)
candelilla can-dih-LIH-lah	pg. 473	a hard wax used to modify the melting point and provide increased strength to hard depilatory wax
carnauba car-NOO-bah	pg. 473	a hard wax used to modify the melting point and provide increased strength to hard depilatory wax
catagen KAT-uh-jen	pg. 460	second transition stage of hair growth; in this phase, the hair shaft grows upward and detaches itself from the bulb
depilation DEP-uh-lay-shun	pg. 464	process of removing hair at the skin level
depilatory dih-PIL-uh-tohr-ee	pg. 466	substance, usually a caustic alkali preparation, used for temporarily removing superfluous hair by dissolving it at the skin level
electrolysis ee-lek-TRAHL-ih-sis	pg. 470	removal of hair by means of an electric current that destroys the hair root
epilation ep-uh-LAY-shun	pg. 464	removes hairs from the follicles; waxing or tweezing
galvanic electrolysis gal-VAN-ik ee-lek-TRAHL-ih-sis	pg. 470	direct current (DC) utilized in electrolysis
glabella glow-BELL-ah	pg. 498	the area between the eyebrows at the top of the nose

gum rosin GUM ROZ-in	pg. 469	an additive in soft wax
hair bulb HAYR BULB	pg. 457	swelling at the base of the follicle that provides the hair with nourishment; it is a thick, club-shaped structure that forms the lower part of the hair root
hair follicle HAYR FAHL-ih-kul	pg. 456	mass of epidermal cells forming a small tube, or canal; the tube-like depression or pocket in the skin or scalp that contains the hair root
hair papilla (plural: papillae) HAYR pah-PIL-uh	pg. 457	cone-shaped elevations at the base of the follicle that fit into the hair bulb; the papillae are filled with tissue that contains the blood vessels and cells necessary for hair growth and follicle nourishment
hair root HAYR ROOT	pg. 457	anchors hair to the skin cells and is part of the hair located at the bottom of the follicle below the surface of the skin; part of the hair that lies within the follicle at its base, where the hair grows
hair shaft HAYR SHAFT	pg. 457	portion of the hair that extends or projects beyond the skin, consisting of the outer layer (cuticle), inner layer (medulla), and middle layer (cortex); color changes happen in the cortex
lanugo luh-NOO-goh	pg. 458	the hair on a fetus; soft and downy hair
laser hair removal LAY-zur HAYR ree-MOOV-uhl	pg. 470	photoepilation hair reduction treatment in which a laser beam is pulsed on the skin using one wavelength at a time, impairing hair growth; an intense pulse of electromagnetic radiation
rosin ROZ-in	pg. 473	a resin used in the manufacture of soft wax
sugaring SHUH-gar-ing	pg. 467	ancient method of hair removal; the original recipe is a mixture of sugar, lemon juice, and water that is heated to form a syrup, molded into a ball, and pressed onto the skin and then quickly stripped away
syndrome SIN-drom	pg. 462	a group of symptoms that, when combined, characterize a disease or disorder
telogen TEL-uh-jen	pg. 460	also known as *resting phase*; the final phase in the hair cycle that lasts until the fully grown hair is shed
terminal hair TUR-meh-null	pg. 458	longer coarse hair that is found on the head, face and body
threading THRED-ing	pg. 466	also known as *banding*; method of hair removal; cotton thread is twisted and rolled along the surface of the skin, entwining hair in the thread and lifting it out of the follicle
trichology tri-KAHL-uh-jee	pg. 456	scientific study of hair and its diseases and care
vellus hair VEL-lus HAYR	pg. 458	also known as *lanugo hair*; short, fine, unpigmented downy hair that appears on the body, except for the palms of the hands and the soles of the feet
vermillion border ver-MILL-yun bore-dur	pg. 490	the border of the lip line

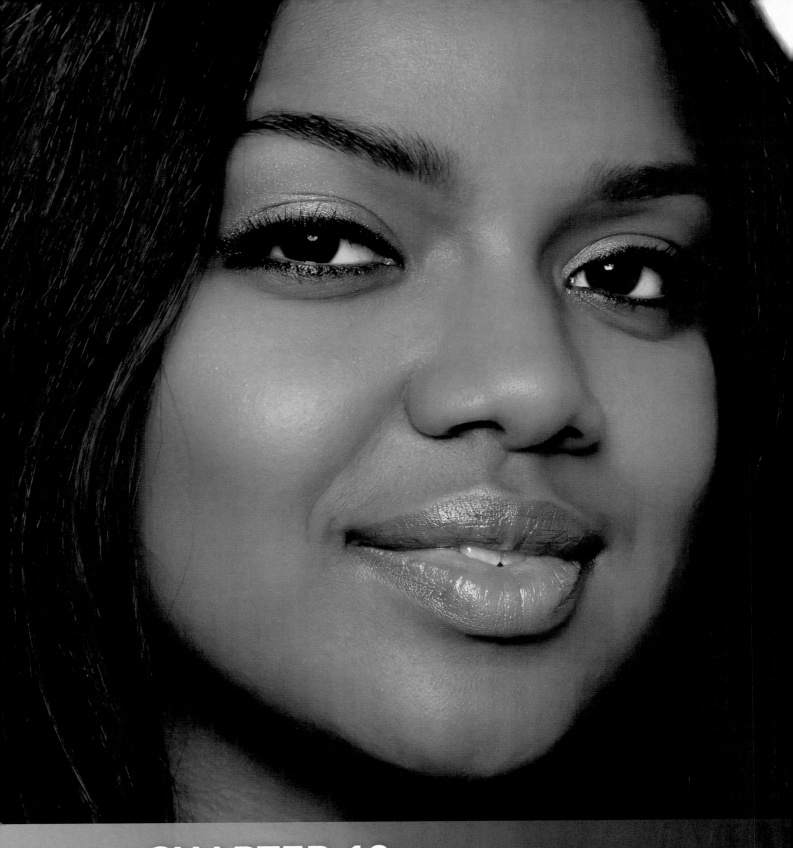

CHAPTER 12
Makeup Essentials

"Every human is an artist. The dream of your life is to make beautiful art."

–Don Miguel Ruiz

Learning Objectives

After completing this chapter, you will be able to:

1. Explain makeup essentials as it relates to an esthetician's skill set.
2. Describe the principles of cosmetic color theory.
3. Use color theory to choose and coordinate makeup color selection.
4. Identify face shapes and proportions for makeup applications.
5. Describe the different types of cosmetics and their uses.
6. Prepare the makeup station and supplies for clients.
7. Follow infection control requirements for makeup services.
8. Conduct a thorough makeup consultation with a client.
9. Perform makeup application techniques.
10. Use highlighting and contouring techniques for balance and proportion.
11. Create makeup looks for special occasions.
12. Apply makeup for the camera and special events.
13. Recognize the benefits of camouflage makeup.
14. Demonstrate the application of artificial eyelashes.
15. Describe tinting lashes and brows on a makeup client.
16. Explain the benefits of permanent makeup application.
17. Describe the benefits of a career in makeup.
18. Promote retail services as a makeup artist.

Explain Makeup Essentials as It Relates to an Esthetician's Skill Set

Whether you are interested in makeup as a stand-alone career or as a complement to your esthetics practice, having foundational knowledge of the skin is the hallmark of great makeup. The skin is the canvas the makeup artist works on; therefore, the makeup artist with training in esthetics has a distinct advantage and more opportunities available. Makeup can boost your client's confidence in their appearance which is, in itself, a rewarding experience, but it can also be a lucrative addition to an esthetician's repertoire.

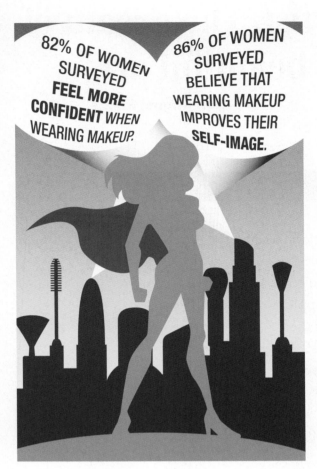

82% OF WOMEN SURVEYED **FEEL MORE CONFIDENT** WHEN WEARING MAKEUP.

86% OF WOMEN SURVEYED BELIEVE THAT WEARING MAKEUP IMPROVES THEIR SELF-IMAGE.

The cosmetics industry is a multibillion-dollar enterprise. Sales often remain steady despite the tightening of budgets at home as clients seek the latest makeup trends or to simply enhance their looks. The art of makeup can open many doors to a rewarding, diverse, and stable career.

Estheticians should have a thorough understanding of makeup because:

- Makeup knowledge and application skills add another element of expertise to enhance your reputation, grow your clientele, and increase menu services and revenues.
- Clients rely on makeup artists to design fresh makeup looks ranging from beauty and fashion to edgy and editorial.
- The makeup industry's seasonal creation of new products can offer opportunities to retail the latest color and create new looks for your clients.
- The understanding of products, color theory, makeup techniques, facial feature analysis are all part of being a successful makeup artist.
- Educated estheticians will be confident when providing consultations, product recommendations, makeup applications, and lash procedures.

Describe the Principles of Cosmetic Color Theory

The art of makeup has very few rules. Color can be used to create mood, emotion, and harmony. However, your selection of colors will depend on the rules of color theory. Color theory is the foundation of color selection, impacting every area of makeup from foundations to blush, eyeshadow, and lipsticks (**Figure 12–1**). It is important in helping clients resolve issues and create a harmonious look on every face. It will guide you as you choose proper makeup colors to enhance your clients' skin tone, dramatize their features, or completely reinvent their looks.

The Color Wheel

Understanding color theory begins with the color wheel. The color wheel is based on the three primary colors: red, yellow, and blue.

COLOR WHEEL

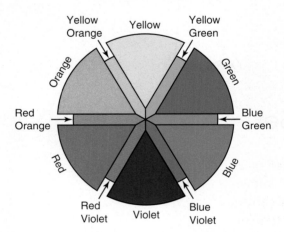

▲ **Figure 12–1** Color theory is the foundation of color selection from blush to eyeshadow and lipsticks.

The traditional color wheel is a creation of the various combinations of colors stemming from the three primary hues and resulting in 12 main divisions. The term *hue* (HYOO) refers to any color in its purest form, lacking any black (shade) or white (tint). The hue of a color represents just one dimension of a particular color. The color wheel does not change and will always serve as your core color selection guide.

PRIMARY COLORS

Primary colors (PRY-mayr-ee KUL-urz) are fundamental colors that cannot be obtained from a mixture. The primary colors are red, yellow, and blue (**Figure 12–2**). These are the main spectral colors of light seen in a prism from sunlight.

SECONDARY COLORS

Secondary colors (SEK-un-deh-ree KUL-urz) are obtained by mixing equal parts of two primary colors. The secondary colors include orange, green, and violet. Red (primary) mixed with yellow (primary) makes orange (secondary). Red (primary) mixed with blue (primary) makes violet (secondary). Yellow (primary) mixed with blue (primary) makes green (secondary) (**Figure 12–3**). Notice on the color wheel the triangular positioning of the primary colors in relation to one another and how the secondary colors fall between them.

TERTIARY COLORS

Tertiary colors (TUR-shee-ayr-ee KUL-urz) are formed by mixing equal amounts of a primary color and its neighboring secondary color on the color wheel. These colors are named by primary color first, secondary color second. For example, when we mix blue (primary) with violet (secondary), we call the resulting color blue-violet (tertiary) (**Figure 12–4**). Other examples of tertiary colors include blue-green, yellow-green (olive), orange-red (vermillion), red-violet,

PRIMARY COLORS

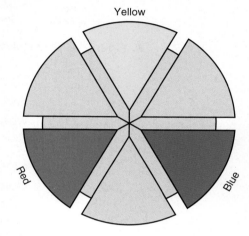

▲ **Figure 12–2** Primary colors.

SECONDARY COLORS

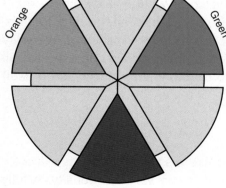

▲ **Figure 12–3** Secondary colors.

TERTIARY COLORS

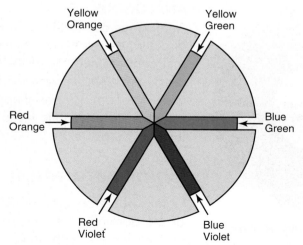

▲ **Figure 12–4** Tertiary colors.

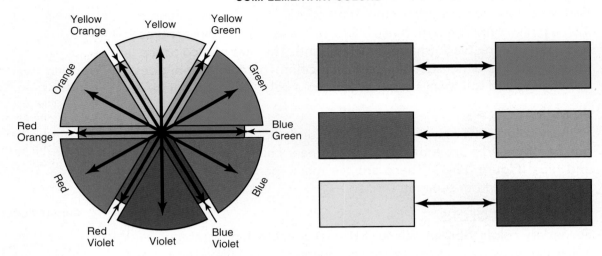

▲ Figure 12–5 Complementary colors.

and yellow-orange. These are the final six colors of the traditional color wheel. Earth tones, colors such as brown and khaki, are tertiary colors that are created by mixing three primary colors together.

COMPLEMENTARY COLORS

Complementary colors (kahm-pluh-MEN-tur-ee KUL-urz) are colors that fall directly across from each other on the color wheel. When used next to each other, they create a distinct contrast, with each intensifying the appearance of the other. This can be beneficial when you want a particular color to clearly stand out. (**Figure 12–5**). For example, if you place blue next to orange, the blue seems bluer, and the orange seems brighter. Complementary colors are frequently used when the goal of a makeup application is a vibrant, dynamic, and dramatic look, such as emphasizing eye color.

ANALOGOUS COLORS

Analogous colors (an-AL-uh-gus colorz) are colors that are located directly next to each other on the color wheel. They create minimal contrast and therefore match very well. Analogous colors are used in makeup application for soft, subtle looks, such as everyday makeup and many bridal applications; they can also be used to call attention to a specific facial feature, rather than the makeup itself (**Figure 12–6**).

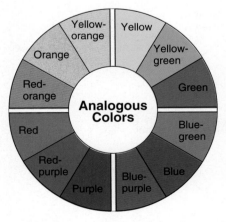

▲ Figure 12–6 Analogous colors.

Color Saturation

Color **saturation** (sach-uh-RAY-shun) refers to the pureness of a color or the dominance of hue in a color. It can vary in intensity. A fully saturated color is the truest version of that color and is extremely vibrant, strong, and intense. To use an example, the hues used for

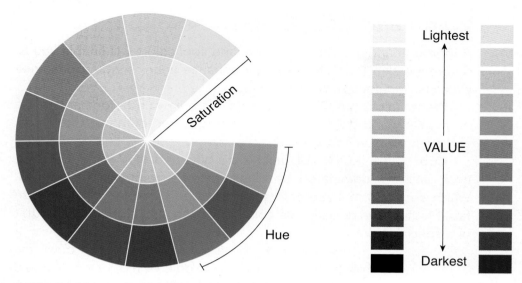

▲ Figure 12–7 Color saturation, hue, and value.

each of the 12 colors on the basic color wheel are saturated. Saturation changes as the hue moves from the outer edge of the color wheel toward the center, where it is less intense, and begins to appear gray (**Figure 12–7**).

When a color is desaturated, a large amount of pure color has been removed. Desaturated colors are colors mixed with white and located toward the inner ring of the color wheel; they contain a large amount of gray and very little remaining pure color, and they are often considered neutral. The degree of saturation is the range from the outer edge of the color wheel (fully saturated) to the center (fully desaturated), perpendicular to the value axis. The **value** (VAL-yoo) or brightness of a color is how light or dark it is. This depends on the amount of light emanating from the color. If it is lighter and closer to white, the color is brighter and higher in value.

The various degrees of saturation create tints, shades, and tones. A **tint** (TINT) occurs when white is added to a pure hue. A **shade** (SHAYD) occurs when black is added to a pure hue. A tone occurs when gray is added to a pure hue (**Figure 12–8**).

ACTIVITY

Play with Color

Using colored paper or pieces of fabric, place different colors next to each other to compare how they look. What colors are primary, complementary, and tertiary? Be sure to use the color wheel as a reference. You may also use crayons, colored pencils, or magic markers on paper to play with different color combinations. Try layering colors according to the color wheel. Which color combinations would you like to try in your next makeup look?

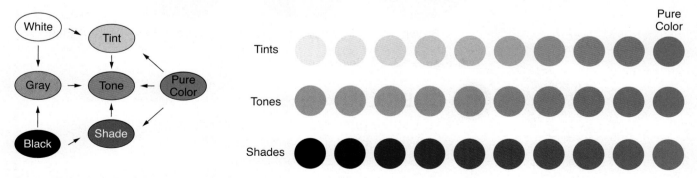

▲ Figure 12–8 Tints, tones, and shades.

Warm and Cool Colors

A thorough understanding of warm and cool colors will enable you to determine skin tone and properly enhance your client's appearance with a harmonious and flattering look.

Warm colors (WORM KUL-urz) have a yellow undertone and range from yellow and gold through the oranges, red-oranges, most reds, and even some yellow-greens.

Cool colors (KOOl KUL-urz) have a blue undertone, suggest coolness, and are dominated by blues, greens, violets, and blue-reds. Warm and cool makeup colors can be used to alter and emphasize facial features, especially eye color. They can also dramatize an outfit or a special look.

If you were to divide a color wheel in half down the middle of green and the middle of red, one half would represent warm colors and the other would represent cool colors (**Figure 12–9**). The red-yellow side of the wheel represents the warm colors, and the blue-green side represents the cool colors. The line down the center of both the green and red colors is to show that green and red can be both warm and cool. If red is orange-based, it is warm. If red is blue-based, it is cool. Green is similar. If green is yellow-based, it is warm. If green is blue-based, it is cool.

Neutral colors (NOO-trul colorz) are colors that do not complement or contrast any other color. Examples include brown and gray, along with multiple variations of each (**Figure 12–10**). They are a perfect blend of earthy tones. In makeup they represent natural, soft, flesh colors and are acceptable color choices for any skin tone. Taupe, beige and tan are widely used as neutral colors.

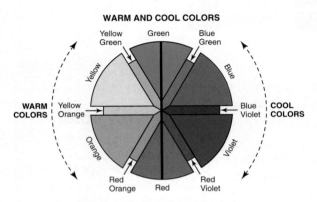

▲ Figure 12–9 Warm and Cool Colors.

Neutral Colors

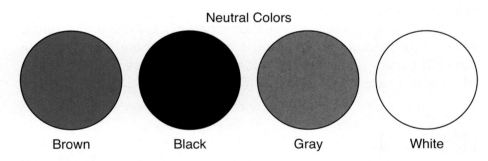

Brown   Black   Gray   White

▲ Figure 12–10 Neutral colors.

 CHECK IN

1. List the primary and secondary colors.
2. What are complementary colors?
3. Define warm and cool colors.
4. Give two examples each of warm and cool colors.

Use Color Theory to Choose and Coordinate Makeup Color Selection

Now that you understand the basics of color theory, let's look at the plethora of color palettes at your fingertips and how to choose the colors that will best suit your client. Keep in mind this is simply one way of choosing colors. The art of makeup application allows for more than one way to achieve the result you desire. Once you understand the basic rules of color selection, you can then go on to expand the ways you combine color. As you practice using these concepts and guidelines, they will become second nature and you will be increasingly confident in your color choices.

As you look at the color wheel, think of it as a tool for determining color choice. There are three main factors to consider when choosing colors for a client: skin color, eye color, and hair color.

You will also want to assess the client's face shape and features, which we will discuss shortly, during the consultation.

Color Selection at a Glance

To determine color selection, follow these steps:

1. Determine skin color:
   - Light, medium, or dark
   - Warm, cool, or neutral
2. Determine eye color:
   - Blue, green, brown, other
3. Determine hair color:
   - Warm or cool

Once you have identified these three key areas, you can begin your color selections by choosing eye makeup colors based on complementary or contrasting colors and coordinating cheek and lip colors within the same color family.

The best thing about choosing colors is the unlimited number of choices you have. Try one or all methods of choosing color. You can choose colors based on eye color and skin tone, or you might find that working with complementary colors makes you feel more comfortable.

Determine Skin Color

When determining skin color, you must first decide if the skin is fair, medium, or dark. Regardless of ethnic background, skin varies in color and tone from person to person. The **tone** [TOHN] of the skin is also known as *hue*. In terms of skin, *tone* is used to describe the warmth or coolness of a color and is generally classified as light, medium, or dark.

Then determine whether the **undertone** (UN-dur-tohn) is warm or cool. There are three general undertones:

- Cool colors (pink, red, or bluish undertones)
- Warm colors (yellow, peachy, or golden undertones)
- Neutral colors (a mix of warm and cool undertones).

To determine the client's undertone, use the neck or forearm. If the client is frequently exposed to the sun, then use the neck as the primary indicator of skin undertone. In natural light, place a white piece of paper or cloth next to clean skin and determine the color that is most apparent. Look for yellow, red (pink), green (olive), or blue (brown) undertones.

- Cool undertones will include pink and bluish hues.
- Warm undertones will range from peach to yellow and gold.

Undertone also applies to makeup products. You may have heard people refer to a color as having a lot of blue in it. This does not mean that the color is a true blue. Rather, it means that a blue pigment was mixed to create that cosmetic formula. For example, deep red lipsticks are manufactured with a blue base.

Refer to **Table 12–1** to reference skin tones and undertones. Refer to **Table 12–2** for color intensity of the skin and determining the best colors based on the tone and undertone.

TIPS ON MAKEUP APPLICATION BASED ON THE TONE AND UNDERTONE

- If skin color is light, you can use light colors for a soft, natural look. Medium to dark colors will create a more dramatic look.
- If skin color is medium, medium tones will create an understated look. Light or dark tones will provide more contrast and will appear bolder.
- If skin color is dark, dark tones will be most subtle. Medium to medium-light or bright tones will be striking and vivid.
- For a neutral skin tone, match the foundation color to the color of the skin, or use the corrective techniques discussed later in this chapter.

CONSIDERATIONS FOR ALTERING SKIN TONE

For various reasons, some clients may wish to alter their skin tone. In terms of corrective makeup, you will be dealing with two basic skin tones: ruddy and sallow.

- For **ruddy** (RHUD-ee) skin (skin that is unnaturally red, wind burned, or affected by rosacea), apply a yellow- or green-tinted foundation to affected areas, blending carefully. A yellow-based foundation will neutralize excess red in skin. A green-based foundation (an opposite color to red) will block out excess redness but may impart a flat look

▼ **TABLE 12–1** Identifying Skin Tones and Undertones

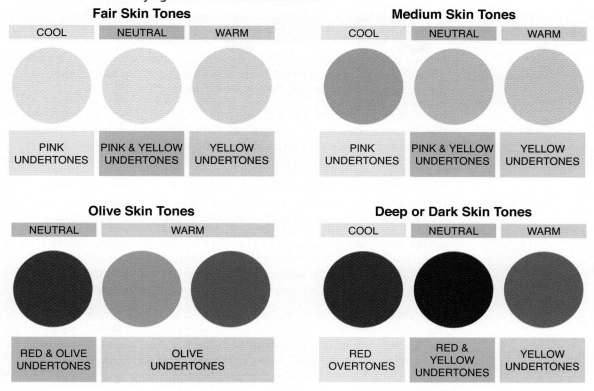

Fair Skin Tones

COOL	NEUTRAL	WARM
PINK UNDERTONES	PINK & YELLOW UNDERTONES	YELLOW UNDERTONES

Medium Skin Tones

COOL	NEUTRAL	WARM
PINK UNDERTONES	PINK & YELLOW UNDERTONES	YELLOW UNDERTONES

Olive Skin Tones

NEUTRAL	WARM	
RED & OLIVE UNDERTONES	OLIVE UNDERTONES	

Deep or Dark Skin Tones

COOL	NEUTRAL	WARM
RED OVERTONES	RED & YELLOW UNDERTONES	YELLOW UNDERTONES

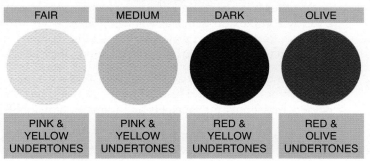

Neutral Skin Tones

FAIR	MEDIUM	DARK	OLIVE
PINK & YELLOW UNDERTONES	PINK & YELLOW UNDERTONES	RED & YELLOW UNDERTONES	RED & OLIVE UNDERTONES

to the skin overall. Choose the technique that best suits your needs. After you have applied the tinted foundation you can use a light layer of flesh tone foundation on top of the corrective color to give the skin a natural glow, setting it with translucent powder. You may not need blush at all for this application. If you do want to add blush, avoid red and pink tones. Opt instead for a nice neutral tan shade.

- For **sallow** (SAL-oh) skin (skin that has a yellowish hue), apply a pink-based foundation on the affected areas and blend carefully into the jaw and neck. Set with translucent powder. Avoid using yellow-based colors for eyes, cheeks, and lips.

Makeup Color	Color Intensity	Description
Pink	Cool/warm	Pink can be either warm or cool depending on the intensity and under-tone. Pink combines well with other shades and tints of blue, black, green, yellow, gray, purple, brown, beige, and white.
Blue	Cool	Blue is complementary to most skin tones. Lighter blues enhance darker skin, while darker blue brings out color and is complementary to lighter skin. Blue combines well with almost all other colors.
Purple	Cool/warm	Mixed with pale tints of orchid and lavender, purple is cool. Darker shades (plum) with red undertones are warm. Purple with red under-tones can bring out red in skin with rosacea or acne. Purple combines well with pink, white, gray, soft blue, beige, black, and pale yellow.
Green	Cool/warm	Green is easy on the eyes and flattering to many skin tones. Bright green can intensify red in the skin. Blue-greens are cool and generally attractive for both light and dark skin. Green combines well with other greens, blue, yellow, orange, beige, brown, white, and black.
Brown	Warm	Brown is a good basic color and can be kind to many complexion tones. Other reflecting or accent colors can be worn near the face if the skin is dark brown. Brown combines well with warm colors, green, beige, blue, pink, yellow, orange, gold, white, and black. Reddish browns may not be flattering for the same reason that purples and reds may make the skin or eyes look ruddy or tired.
Red	Warm/cool	Red is a vibrant color. Red with blue undertones is cool; with yellow undertones it is warm. Red of a specific tint or shade may not be kind to a ruddy complexion. Freckles will look darker when red is reflected onto the face. Red combines well with many other colors. Among them are black, white, beige, gray, blue, navy, green, and yellow.
Black	Neutral	Black combines well with all other colors. A black outfit can create a contrast for light skin and hair. When the skin and hair are dark, a lighter color contrast near the face acts as a frame or highlight for the face.
White	Cool/neutral	White is easy to wear, but be cautious of its undertones. Some materi-als reflect beige or yellow undertones (off-white is warm), while others appear slightly blue. White combines well with all other colors.
Gray	Neutral	A cool-based neutral gray combines well with many other colors, espe-cially cool colors.

Determine Eye Color

Just as there are many skin colors, there are many eye colors. It is easy to categorize eyes into blue, green, brown, and hazel; however, as any makeup artist knows, each of these colors has many variations. Individual eye color helps you as a makeup artist choose eyeshadow colors, depending upon whether you are trying to enhance the natural color or to make it "pop" with a contrasting color.

When selecting eye colors, neutral tones are always your safest choice. They contain elements of warm and cool, plus they complement any skin color, eye color, or hair color. Neutral colors range from taupe to brown, and from gray to white or black.

They may have a warm or cool base. For example, plum-brown, charcoal gray, and blue-gray are considered cool neutrals. An orange-brown is considered a warm neutral. Matching shadow color with eye color creates a monochromatic field with a less dramatic depth of contrast. Selecting eyeshadows in complementary colors will emphasize the eyes most. You may refer back to the color wheel for additional help in determining complementary eyeshadow colors. Remember to coordinate cheek and lip products within the same color family, adding neutrals with warm or cool colors as desired.

Complementary color choices for eye colors are summarized as follows:

- Complementary colors for blue eyes: Orange is the complementary color to blue. Because orange contains yellow and red, shadows with any of these colors in them will make eyes look bluer. Common choices include gold, warm orange-browns like peach and copper, red-browns like mauves and plums, and neutrals like taupe or camel (**Figure 12–11**).

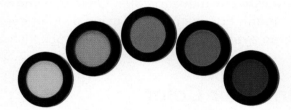

▲ **Figure 12–11** Complementary colors for blue eyes.

- Complementary colors for green eyes: Red is the complementary color to green. Because red shadows tend to make the eyes look tired or bloodshot, pure red tones are not recommended. Instead, use brown-based reds or other color options next to red on the color wheel. These include red-orange, red-violet, and violet. Popular choices are coppers, rusts, pinks, plums, mauves, and purples (**Figure 12–12**).

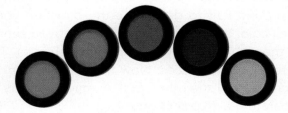

▲ **Figure 12–12** Complementary colors for green eyes.

- Complementary colors for brown eyes: Brown eyes are neutral and can wear any color. Recommended choices include contrasting colors such as greens, blues, grays, and silvers (**Figure 12–13**).

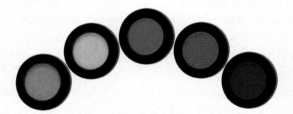

▲ **Figure 12–13** Complementary colors for brown eyes.

COORDINATE CHEEK AND LIP COLORS WITH EYE COLORS

After choosing the eye makeup, coordinate the cheek and lip makeup in the same warm or cool color family. For example, suppose your client has green eyes, and you recommended plums for her, which are cool. Now you should stay with cool colors for the cheeks and lips, so they will coordinate with the eye makeup. You could also choose neutrals because they contain both warm and cool elements and coordinate with any makeup color. Once you know color theory you can experiment. For example, try using a violet eyeshadow on a client with green eyes with an orange-red lipstick instead of a plum color.

Determine Hair Color

Use the client's hair color as a final consideration when deciding on a color palette for your makeup application. From the color combinations you've been considering based on your client's natural skin tone and eye color, take into account the client's current hair color as a final factor and look for the best palette to combine with the hair color in creating a good overall look.

Consider the hair color when choosing makeup colors, but prioritize the client's natural warm or cool skin tone. Keep in mind that the client's current hair color and natural hair color may be quite different. One could be cool and the other warm. Factor this in when trying to determine the best overall makeup colors. Try placing the color wheel next to the skin and hair to determine the direction you want to go with the overall color selection. Discussing what you see with your clients enables them to better understand your choices. They may not have considered the differences. Now they can decide whether they prefer one strategy over the other, or they may opt to try two different options in separate makeup sessions.

ACTIVITY

Use Color Theory and Coordinate!

Apply makeup to a partner using your knowledge of color theory and intensity to choose and coordinate makeup colors. Be sure to analyze your partner's skin color, eye color, and hair color to help determine your palette of choice. Have fun and experiment. If you do not like it, just wash it off and try again!

Mature and Textured Skin

Here are tips when working with mature clients or clients who have enlarged pores and textured skin due to acne scarring or excessive sun exposure:

- Products made with shimmer glitter can accentuate skin texture.
- Colors that are more matte (not shiny) can reduce the appearance of texture from fine lines and uneven skin (**Figure 12–14**).

Matte

Shimmer

iStock.com/Preto_perola

▲ **Figure 12–14** Use matte instead of shimmer to reduce the appearance of fine lines and uneven skin.

CHECK IN

5. What are the three main color selection steps used to choose makeup colors?
6. What colors are used to tone down red?

Identify Face Shapes and Proportions for Makeup Applications

Understanding face shapes is helpful for determining where to place lighter and darker tones of makeup for greater impact. You may want to use light or dark colors to accentuate or de-emphasize certain features.

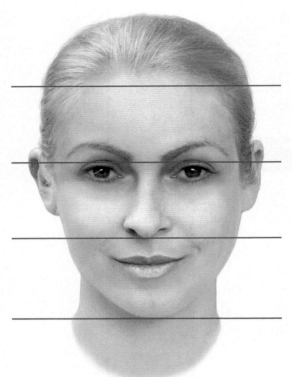

Analyzing Face Shapes

The ability to analyze face shapes is helpful in a variety of esthetic areas. The face shape can be a determining factor in hair styles, the size and shape of hats, reading or sunglasses, and jewelry. For the makeup artist, understanding how to help a client accentuate features they wish to be more prominent and de-emphasize ones they prefer to go unnoticed is a valuable skill. Please refer to the Face Shapes chart (**Table 12–3**) for a complete list of face shapes. You will refer to these standard artistic proportions when practicing highlighting and contouring makeup application techniques to be discussed later in the chapter.

OVAL-SHAPED FACE

As professionals in today's modern world, we are well aware that there is no such thing as the "perfect" face. All clients are perfect in their own way. While all face shapes are attractive in their own way, the oval face with well-proportioned features has long been considered the ideal. The face is divided into three equal horizontal sections. The first third is measured from the hairline to the tops of the eyebrows. The second third is measured from the tops of the eyebrows to the tip of the nose. The last third is measured from the tip of the nose to the bottom of the chin. The oval face is about one and a half times longer than its width across the brow (**Figure 12–15**). The ideal distance between the eyes is the width of one eye.

▲ **Figure 12–15 The oval-shaped face.**

▼ **TABLE 12–3 Face Shapes**

Face Shape	Characteristics
Oval	Widest at the temple and forehead, tapering down to a curved chin. This is considered the ideal facial shape because of its balance and overall look of symmetry.
Round	This face is widest at the cheekbone area and is usually not much longer than it is wide, having a softly rounded jawline, short chin, and rounded hairline over a rather full forehead.

Face Shape	Characteristics
Square	This face has a wide, angular jawline and forehead; the lines of this face are straight and angular.
Rectangle (oblong)	This face shape is long and narrow; the cheeks are often hollowed under prominent cheekbones. Corrective makeup can be applied to create the illusion of width across the cheekbone line, making the face appear shorter and wider.
Triangle (pear-shaped)	Like a pyramid, this face is widest at its base or jawline, tapering up to slightly narrower cheeks and reaching its apex at a narrow forehead. A jaw that is wider than the forehead characterizes the pear-shaped face. Corrective makeup can be applied to create width at the forehead, slenderize the jawline, and add length to the face.
Heart	This facial shape is wide at the temple and forehead area and tapers down to a narrow chin, forming a heart shape (inverted triangle). It is usually soft rather than angular, and has some prominence in the cheekbone area.
Diamond	Widest at the cheekbones, this face has a narrow chin and forehead. It is angular in form, and the measurements of the jaw and hairline are approximately the same.

CHECK IN

7. Why is analyzing face shapes an important skill?
8. What are the seven basic face shapes?

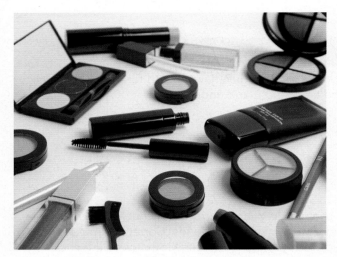

▲ **Figure 12–16** Assorted makeup products.

Describe the Different Types of Cosmetics and Their Uses

Most products come in several forms, including powders, creams, and liquids, in an assortment of containers and packages (**Figure 12–16**). Makeup formulations are evolving with a focus on maintaining healthier skin. Let's take a look at the product formulations, application techniques, and facial features of each type of product currently available.

Foundation

Foundation (fown-DAY-shun), also known as *base makeup*, is a tinted cosmetic used to even out skin tone and color, conceal imperfections, and protect the skin from the outside elements of climate, dirt, and pollution. Dark circles, blemishes, pigmentation, redness, and other concerns can be neutralized with foundation. Face makeup comes in different forms—mainly cream, liquid, powder, and mineral. Most people may need different makeup colors in the summer (darker) and winter (lighter).

- Foundations that usually contain mineral oil or other oils are referred to as **oil based** (OYL BAYST). These products are a good choice for normal to dry skin.
- Oil-free products are referred to as **water based** (WAW-tur BAYST). Water-based foundations generally give a more **matte** (MAT) (nonshiny, dull) finish and help conceal minor blemishes and discolorations. These foundations are preferred for oily skin and sensitive skin.
- **Silicone-based** (SIL-ih-kohn BAYST) products are good for occluding the skin and proving a more even surface. They can also diffuse imperfections. Silicone-based makeup is also more durable for prolonged wear and is an excellent choice for bridal makeup.
- **Alcohol-based** (AL-kuh-hawl BAYST) makeup is also available for extreme durability and is popular with special effects artists as well as for temporary tattoos. Alcohol-based makeup is not ideal for prolonged wear as it can exacerbate dry skin.

Product ingredients continue to advance. The ingredients of a foundation consist mainly of water, emollient bases, humectants, pigments, binders, fragrances, and preservatives. Sunscreen, plant extracts, vitamins, and other ingredients beneficial to the skin are also added to some face makeup (**Figures 12–17a** and **12–17b**).

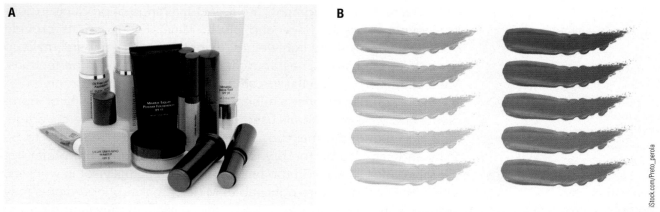

▲ **Figures 12–17a and 12–17b** Different types of foundations (a) and some examples of foundation color swatches (b).

Some **liquid foundations** (LIK-wud fown-DAY-shun) are combinations of organic and inorganic pigments in alcohol- and water-based solutions. Bentonite (a clay base) is added to help keep the products blended and absorb excess oil. The liquid formulation is generally suited for clients with oily to normal skin conditions who desire sheer to medium coverage. Other liquid foundations are oil based.

Cream (KREEM) foundations are thicker and give medium to heavier coverage. They are generally suited for dry to normal skin.

Cake makeup (KAYK MAYK-up), also known as *pancake makeup*, is a heavy cream foundation. It is normally applied to the face with a moistened cosmetic sponge, and is used for theater and film, or whenever extreme coverage is needed.

Greasepaint (GREES-paint) is a heavy cream makeup used for theatrical purposes. Certain makeup products are created for effect and work beautifully for short periods of time and for smaller areas of coverage. Most theatrical and effect makeup is made with alcohols and oils that can be comedogenic. Be sure to recommend a good skin care routine with an effective but gentle cleanser.

Powder foundations, consist of a powder base mixed with a coloring agent (pigment). Cream-to-powder foundations are moist on application but dry to a powdery finish.

Primers (PRIH-murz) are liquids or silicone-based formulas designed to go underneath foundation and other products to prepare the skin for makeup and to help keep the product on the skin. Primers provide a smooth surface for the makeup, while keeping product off the skin so that it is not broken down by the natural oils of the skin.

Mineral Makeup

Mineral makeup is composed of minerals and other ingredients and is designed to be healthy for the skin. A mineral-based foundation is considered more noncomedogenic (less likely to clog pores) and natural than liquid foundations. This makeup is not as heavy as other types

FOCUS ON
BB and CC Creams

As discussed in Chapter 6, BB creams are multitasking products for daytime use that include a moisturizing day cream, sun protection, makeup foundation coverage, age prevention, and corrective ingredients all in one easy step and can be found for all skin types.

A spinoff, CC cream (color and correct) is similar to a BB cream but provides heavier coverage, similar to a concealer. CC creams also have added lighteners and brighteners to help improve skin discolorations.

of products. Mineral pigments are found in a range of products including powders, eyeshadows, and blush. Mineral foundations provide good coverage yet are lightweight. If lightly applied, mineral makeup can refract light from lines and creases and minimize imperfections. Mineral makeup is popular as camouflage makeup after surgery.

Many companies offer a mineral makeup line. The quality of ingredients and type of minerals used in formulas will affect the coverage, look, and feel of the makeup. Some formulas have a tendency to be shiny and can also be too dry for some mature clients who prefer liquid foundation. If applied too heavily, they can actually set in wrinkles, which makes them more noticeable. Mineral makeup ingredients may include titanium dioxide, zinc oxide, mica, silica, magnesium stearate, bismuth oxychloride, iron oxides, kaolin clay, and rice powder. Synthetic preservatives, fragrances, talc, and dyes are commonly used in cosmetics, but are not recommended ingredients because they may trigger allergic reactions.

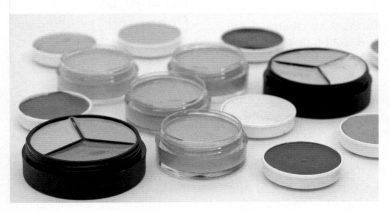

▲ Figure 12–18 Concealers in a range of colors to address a variety of issues.

Concealer

Concealers (kahn-SEEL-urs) are used to cover blemishes and discolorations and may be applied before or after foundation. They are available in pots, pencils, wands, and sticks in a range of colors to coordinate with or match skin tones (**Figure 12–18**). Concealers may contain moisturizers or control oil, depending on the formulation. The chemical composition of concealers is similar to that of cream foundation.

Face Powder

Face powder is used to add a matte, or nonshiny, finish to the face. It enhances the skin's natural color, helping to conceal minor blemishes and discolorations, and diminish excessive color and shine. Face powder is also used to set foundation.

Loose powder and pressed powder are the two most widely used forms of face powder. (**Figure 12–19**). Both types have the same basic composition. Pressed powders are compressed and held together with binders so that they will not crumble. Face powders are available in a variety of tints and shades and in different weights (sheer to heavy). Coverage depends on the weight, formulation, and application.

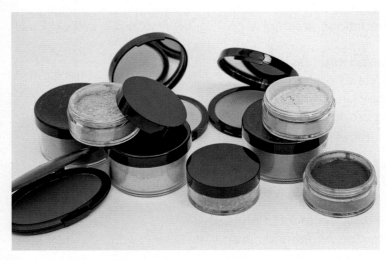

▲ Figure 12–19 Face powder.

Face powders consist of a powder base mixed with a coloring agent (pigment). Ingredients in powders may include talc, zinc oxide, titanium dioxide, dimethicone, kaolin, tocopheryl acetate, zinc stearate, and magnesium stearate.

Blush

Cheek color is available in cream, liquid, dry (pressed), and loose powder form. **Blush** (BLUSH) gives the face a natural-looking glow and helps create facial balance (**Figure 12–20**).

Powder blush is the most common cheek color and consists of ingredients similar to powders with colorants added. Cream or gel cheek colors resemble cream foundation and are generally preferred for dry and normal skin. Cream and liquid blush fall into two categories: oil based and emulsions.

Oil-based formulations are combinations of pigments in an oil or fat base. Blends of waxes (carnauba wax and ozokerite) and oily

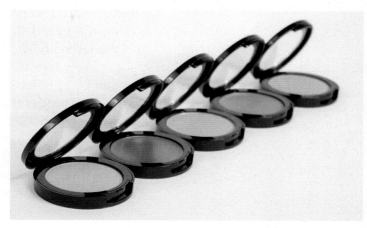

▲ **Figure 12–20** Blush.

liquids (isopropyl myristate and hexadecyl stearate) create a water-resistant product. In addition, cream cheek colors contain water, dyes, thickeners, and a variety of surfactants or detergents that enable particles to penetrate the hair follicles and cracks in the skin. Because these ingredients can potentially clog the follicles, it is important to remind clients to remove their makeup each night.

Highlighter

Highlighters are lighter than the client's skin color, and they accentuate and bring out features such as the brow bone under the eyebrow, the temples, the chin, and the cheekbones. They are typically found in liquid and powder forms.

Eyeshadow

Eyeshadows (EYE shad-ohz) accentuate and contour the eyes. Eyeshadow colors come in an endless variety—from warm to cool, neutral to bright, and light to dark. Some powder eyeshadows are designed to be used either wet or dry. They also come in a variety of finishes including matte or shimmer.

Eyeshadow is available in cream, pressed, and dry powder form (**Figure 12–21**). Stick and cream shadows are water based with oil, petrolatum, thickeners, wax, perfume, preservatives,

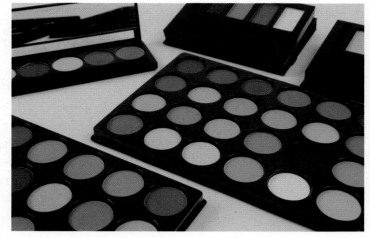

▲ **Figure 12–21** Eyeshadow.

and color added. Water-resistant shadows have a solvent base, such as mineral spirits. Pressed and dry powder eyeshadow ingredients are similar to pressed face powder, mineral makeup, and blush.

Eyeliners

Eyeliner (EYE-lyn-ur) is used to emphasize the eyes. It is available in pencil, liquid, and pressed (cake) form. With eyeliner, you can create a line on the eyelid close to the lashes to make the eyes appear larger and the lashes fuller. Pencil is the most commonly used liner. Liquid or gel eyeliners create a more dramatic look. Powder liners and eyeshadows can be applied wet or dry. When applied wet, they are more vivid and stay on longer than when applied dry.

Eyeliner pencils consist of a wax (paraffin) or hardened oil base (petrolatum) with a variety of additives to create color. Pencils are available in both soft and hard form for use on the eyebrow as well as the eye. Eyeliners contain ingredients such as alkanolamine (a fatty alcohol), cellulose ether, polyvinylpyrrolidone, methylparaben, antioxidants, perfumes, and titanium dioxide.

Eyebrow Color

Eyebrows frame the eye. The correct brow shape enhances the face and the entire makeup look. **Eyebrow pencils** (EYE-brow PEN-silz), **shadows** (SHAD-ohz), **pomades** (poh-MAYDZ), and **gel formulations** (JEL form-yoo-LAY-shunz) are used to add color and shape to the eyebrows. They can be used to darken the eyebrows, correct their shape, or fill in sparse areas. For the best results, match the natural brow color or use a close shade of brown. The chemistry of eyebrow products is often similar to that of eyeliner pencils and eyeshadows. (**Figure 12–22**).

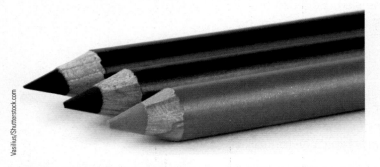

▲ **Figure 12–22** Eyebrow color.

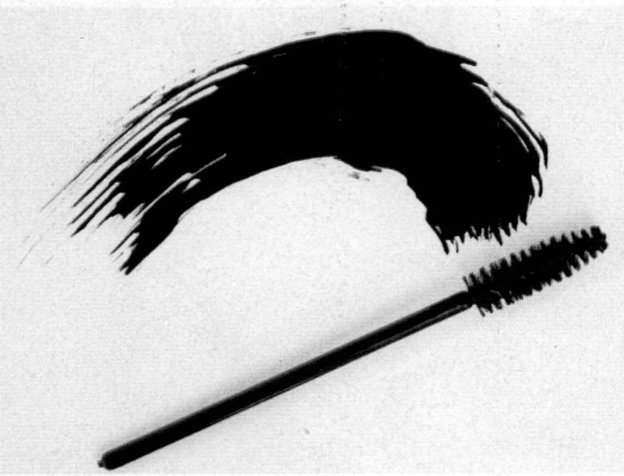

Mascara

Mascara (mas-KAIR-uh) darkens, defines, and thickens the eyelashes (**Figure 12–23**). There are two main types of mascara: regular and waterproof. Both types are available in liquid, cake, and cream form in various shades and tints. The most popular mascara is a liquid formula in black or brown. These colors enhance the natural lashes, making them appear thicker and longer.

Regular mascara (reg-YOO-lar mas-KAIR-uh) is a good daily use product that can be easily removed with regular eye makeup remover. It may not be ideal for clients with

▲ **Figure 12–23** Mascara.

seasonal allergies whose eyes water frequently, brides, or clients that may come in frequent, direct contact with wind or water.

Waterproof mascara (WAW-tur-proof mas-KAIR-uh) is designed to stay on and not smudge when it comes in contact with water. This may be ideal for clients who have watery eyes from allergies, brides, or clients who may come in frequent, direct contact with water. The waterproof mascara may require an oil-based eye makeup remover.

Mascaras are polymer products that contain water, wax, thickeners, film formers, and preservatives in their formulations. The pigments in mascara must be inert (unable to combine with other elements) and are made with carbon black, carmine, ultramarine, chromium oxide, and iron oxides. Some wand mascaras contain rayon or nylon fibers to lengthen and thicken the hair. Lash conditioners and gels are also popular products. Lash enhancers are products designed to stimulate lash growth.

Eye Makeup Removers

Makeup removers (MEYK-uhp RE-moverz) are either oil based or water based (**Figure 12-24**).

- Oil-based removers are generally mineral oil with a small amount of fragrance added. Oil-based removers are great for removing waterproof mascara, dramatic eye makeup, and artificial lashes.

- Water-based removers are a water solution to which witch hazel, boric acid, oils, lanolin or lanolin derivatives, and other solvents have been added. Water-based eye makeup remover is a good choice for removing regular mascara and light eye makeup, and is a good alternative for clients who are sensitive to oil.

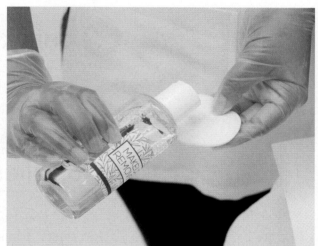

▲ Figure 12–24 Eye makeup remover.

Most products will come off with cleansers. It is not recommended to remove eye makeup while wearing contacts as this can irritate the eye.

Lip Color

Lip color (LIP KUL-ur), lipstick, and gloss give color to the face and provide a finish to your makeup design. Lip color worn alone enhances the face like no other product can. Some lip colors contain sunscreen to protect the lips from the harmful effects of the sun. Most contain moisturizers to keep lips from becoming dry or chapped.

Lip color is available in several forms: creams, glosses, pencils, and sticks (**Figure 12–25**). Formulas include oils, waxes, and dyes. Castor oil is also a common ingredient in lipsticks. Other oils used are olive, mineral, sesame, cocoa butter, petroleum, lecithin, and hydrogenated vegetable. Waxes commonly included in the ingredients are paraffin,

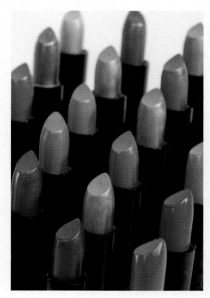

▲ Figure 12–25 Lip color.

beeswax, carnauba, and candelilla. The tinting agents D&C Red No. 27, D&C Orange No. 17 Lake, and other related tints are examples of common coloring agents. Lakes are organic pigments that are formulated to be insoluble. Iron oxides, mica, and annatto are natural colorants sometimes used in lip colors. Lip gloss, plumpers, and stains are also popular.

LIP LINER

Lip liner is a makeup product intended to fill uneven areas on the outer edges of the lips to define their shape. Lip liner is also used to outline the lips and keep lipstick inside the lip area, preventing the lip color from bleeding. Lip liner is most often found in pencil form, but consistencies vary from a firm, waxy pencil to a softer, cream pencil. Colors are available in the same broad range as lip colors, allowing you to properly match the lip liner to the chosen lip color shade.

 CHECK IN

9. List the specific categories of products used in makeup application.

Prepare the Makeup Station and Supplies for Clients

Before you begin any makeup service you will need the necessary products, tools, and supplies to prepare your makeup kit and work area for your client.

Supplies and Accessories

There are many supplies and accessories that you will find useful for your makeup applications (**Figure 12–26**; **Table 12–4**). These supplies may include:

- Sponges (SPUNJ-uz)—These are good for blending foundation, concealer, and powder. Wedge and egg-shaped sponges, known as beauty blenders, are very popular choices. Use the large, thicker end of the sponge for foundation to get more coverage and control. Use the smaller sides to blend around the eyes. Note: Sponges are porous and cannot be cleaned/disinfected and used again. They must be discarded after use.

- Spatulas (SPACH-uh-lahz)—Use spatulas to remove products such as concealer or lipstick from jars and containers. Do not put fingers into products. Use a new single-use or cleaned and disinfected spatula each time. Do not double-dip.

- Tissues (TISH-ooz)—Use tissue for blotting lipstick or powder.

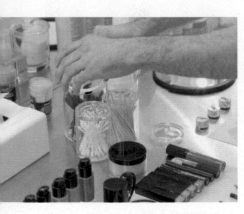
▲ **Figure 12–26 Makeup supplies.**

▼ **TABLE 12–4** Makeup Supplies Checklist

Equipment
☐ Cape and draping items
☐ EPA-registered disinfectant/cleaning supplies
☐ Tweezers
☐ Mirror
☐ Hair clip/headband
☐ Brushes
☐ Pencil sharpener
☐ Small scissors
☐ Brow comb
☐ Lash comb
☐ Lash curler
☐ Single-use items: spatulas, cotton swabs, mascara wands, mixing cups, sponges, tissues, applicators
☐ Hand towel
☐ Artist tray/palette
☐ Gloves
☐ Client chart
☐ Face charts

Skin Care Products
☐ Cleanser
☐ Toner
☐ Moisturizer
☐ Lip conditioner

Makeup Products
☐ Primer
☐ Foundation
☐ Powder
☐ Eyeshadow
☐ Eyeliner
☐ Mascara
☐ Blush
☐ Lip gloss
☐ Lip liner
☐ Lipstick
☐ Concealer
☐ Highlighter
☐ Contour color

- Wand (WOND)—Use a new, single-use wand to dip into the mascara. Do not double-dip. Roll the wand around in a circle rather than pumping it in and out because this dries out the mascara.
- **Brow comb** (BROW kohm)—A brow comb is a tool used to brush eyebrow hairs into the desired position, creating a finely groomed look. In addition to the comb itself, many brow combs have a brush on one side.
- **Lash comb** (lash KOHM)—A lash comb separates lashes so lashes look finished and are not clumpy or messy looking. They are used before applying mascara or when the mascara is still wet. Do not point combs or brushes toward the eyes or poke the skin. Point them up and away from the eye. If necessary, you can gently rest the side of your little pinky finger on the face to steady the application. If the client is sensitive around the eyes, let them apply the mascara.
- Cotton swabs (KAHT-un SWAHBZ)—These are useful for blending under the eyes and especially when cleaning up mascara or other smudges.
- Paper drapes (PAY-pur DRAYPS)—Hand-size towels made of paper that are inexpensive and easy to use to protect the client's clothing during a touch-up.
- Cleaning agents—Use brush cleaner to clean the brushes. Use hand sanitizer to clean hands (if allowed in your state) when soap and water is not available and use a disinfectant approved by the Environmental Protection Agency (EPA) on surfaces and tools. Note: A clean brush is not acceptable for use between clients, as it needs to be disinfected.
- **Brushes** (BRUSH-ez)—Use them to blend powder, blush, and eyeshadows, as they work better than sponge tips or fingers. Brushes vary in size, shape, make, use, cost, and longevity. Brushes are the artist's most essential tool, as they allow for better control and blending. They also feel nicer to the skin. Brush hair types fall into two categories: natural and synthetic. Each type of bristle has distinct features, qualities, and functions.

Disposable brushes are ideal when working with clients. If you are not using single-use brushes, then make sure you clean and disinfect synthetic brushes between clients and always have enough clean brushes on hand for multiple uses throughout the day. Art stores and brush wholesalers are good places to find a variety of brush options, and they are also cost effective.

- *Lash curler*—For straight lashes, a lash curler can be used before applying mascara.
- *Hair clips or a headband*—Use hair clips or a headband to hold the hair away from the face. Remove these items and fix the client's hair before showing them the finished look.

CAUTION!

For a brush to be able to be disinfected, it must be synthetic (not natural bristle). Most expensive brushes are natural bristle and therefore not able to be disinfected. The safest method for application is to remove a portion of the product to a palette to work from then clean/disinfect any synthetic brushes and discard disposable brushes.

- *Cape*—Use a cape or towel around the client's neck to protect their clothes. Put a tissue, clean towel, or single-use neck strip under the collar and around the neck and be sure to use a new cape with every client.

- *Tweezers*—Tweezers are used to remove individual hairs from the brow area and to remove stray hairs from above, beneath, and around the eyes and chin.

  Types of tweezers are discussed in greater detail in Chapter 11, Hair Removal.

- *Sharpeners*—Pencil sharpeners are either plastic or metal, and they are available with different-sized sharpening holes to accommodate different-sized pencils.

- *Mirror*—A high quality reflective surface for the client to view the application.

- *Mixing cups*—These can be used for blending foundation colors together or mixing foundation and moisturizer for a lighter tinted foundation. Artist's *palettes* are also great for holding products.

Use a Makeup Palette

Use a single-use spatula, or palette knife, to place a small amount of product on a palette. This will keep the main product free of pathogens such as bacteria and fungus and protect your client from infection. Palettes are either straight and flat (for mixing crèmes) or have small indentations, for working with loose products like powders. Some states require the use of a palette, so check with your state board about licensure requirements. Remember to take notes of the products you work with on the palette and add them to your client's chart.

Makeup Brushes

Makeup brushes come in a variety of shapes and sizes (**Figure 12–27**). Brushes are made of three parts: the hair (bristles), the handle, and the ferrule. By running the brush hair across the hand, you can test the hair for softness and the bristles for shedding.

- Brush hairs are either natural animal hair or synthetic. Unlike natural hair brushes, synthetic brushes can be disinfected. Sable, squirrel, mink, goat, pony, and other blends are used for brushes. Natural-hair brushes are more expensive than synthetic ones. Natural-hair brushes are more frequently used to apply dry, powder products, whereas synthetic bristles are

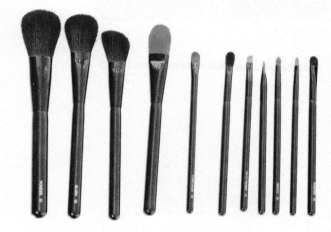

▲ Figure 12–27 Makeup brushes.

> **CAUTION!**
>
> Brushes with wooden handles should not be used on clients because wood is porous and cannot be disinfected. They may be retailed to clients for personal use.

better for moist product application. The first-cut hair is a better quality and considered cruelty free because it is sheared from the tips of the fur. Blunt cuts are less expensive and more coarse and prickly. Synthetic nylon and Taklon are stiffer bristles used for brow, concealer, and foundation brushes.

- Handle lengths vary, but 7 inches (17.5 centimeters) is the standard length for brushes. If the handle is too long, it is harder to control.
- The **ferrule** (FAIR-uhl) is the metal part that holds brushes intact. Choosing quality makeup brushes is important, so look for double-crimping of the ferrule to avoid loose handles that come apart faster.

Refer to **Table 12–5** for the most commonly used makeup brushes.

▼ **TABLE 12–5 Makeup Brushes**

Standard Brush	Type of Brush	Description and Use
Most brushes can be interchanged and used for more than one purpose.		
	Powder brush	Large, soft brush used for blending and to apply powder or blush
	Blush brush	Smaller, more tapered version of the powder brush used for applying powder blush; can be angled
	Foundation brush	Longer, flatter bristles that end in a round or oval compact shape; used for applying and blending liquid, cream, and paste foundations
	Concealer brush	Usually narrow and firm with a flat edge; used to apply concealer around the eyes, on blemishes, and other areas
	Kabuki brushes	Short brushes with dense bristles for powder or blush; mainly used in a circular motion to apply and blend powders

Standard Brush	Type of Brush	Description and Use
	Eyeshadow brushes	Available in a variety of sizes and ranging from soft to firm; the softer and larger the brush, the more blended the shadow will be; a firm brush is better for depositing dense color than for blending it; small brushes are best for dark colors
	Eyeliner brush	Fine, tapered, firm bristles; used to apply liner to the eyes
	Angle brow brush	Firm, thin bristles; angled for use on the eyebrows or for eyeliner
	Lash and brow brush	The comb side is used to remove excess mascara on lashes, and the brush side is for brows; metal lash combs are also available, but plastic is ideal because it is disposable
	Lip brush	Similar to the concealer brush, but smaller and with a more tapered, rounded edge; also used to apply concealer

CARING FOR MAKEUP BRUSHES

If you invest in high-quality makeup brushes, you will have them for years. To use them safely for years, it is best to remove makeup from the original container and use a palette for makeup applications and cleaning/disinfection after each client.

How to clean. Take good care of your brushes by cleaning them gently. A commercial cleaner can be used for quick cleaning, although spray-on instant sanitizers contain a high level of alcohol and will dry brushes over time. The alcohol does clean, but at a very high cost to the brush itself. A gentle shampoo, liquid soap, or brush solvent should be used to thoroughly clean the brushes. These products will not hurt brushes and may actually help them last longer.

The brush should always be put into running or still water with the ferrule (the metal ring that keeps the bristles and handle together) pointing downward. If the brush is pointed up, the water may remove the glue that keeps the bristles in place.

Rinse brushes thoroughly after cleaning. Avoid pulling on the brush bristles as this could loosen them. Because they will dry in the shape they are left in, reshape the wet bristles and lay the brushes flat to dry.

How to disinfect. Brushes must be cleaned and disinfected properly after each client with liquid soap and an EPA-registered disinfectant; however, natural bristles are porous and cannot be disinfected. Disposable brushes are ideal for this reason. Wooden handles are porous and cannot be disinfected. Standard brush cleaners may not be enough to disinfect brushes for clients.

DID YOU KNOW?

Do not leave the brushes in the disinfectant longer than necessary. This can cause them to wear out much faster. Always follow the manufacturer's instructions to preserve their longevity. Always ensure the disinfectant is mixed properly to reduce wear on brushes.

Rinse, dry, and then cover brushes with a towel while drying to keep them clean and put them in a clean, closed covered container or drawer when dry.

CHECK IN

10. Excluding makeup, list the supplies and accessories necessary for makeup application.
11. What are the types of makeup brushes, what is each kind used for, and how should they be cared for?

Follow Infection Control Requirements for Makeup Services

Following proper infection control is important to keep you and your clients safe. Check your local regulations for proper makeup product and brush infection control requirements. Listed here are some basic infection control rules for makeup products and services. These safety measures should be followed when applying makeup to avoid product contamination:

- Wash your hands before touching or applying makeup.
- Do not touch product contents with your fingers as this can spread bacteria from your skin, causing contamination.
- Do not touch open products with previously used applicators. This is called double dipping and can spread infection. Remove products with disposable, single-use spatulas and distribute onto clean palettes before applying.
- When using pressed powders, scrape powders with a clean spatula onto a clean palette or clean tissue before applying.
- Never apply lipstick, gloss, or eyebrow colors directly to the client from the container or tube. Use a spatula to remove the product, and then apply with a disposable applicator.
- Never apply mascara directly to the lashes from the container. Use a disposable mascara wand to remove the product then apply with a new wand.

- If the product is accidentally contaminated, follow your supervisor's directions to either throw away the product or give it to your client. Do not put it back with your clean products to reuse.

To clean multiuse applicators, pencils, and testers, follow these guidelines:

- **Applicators**—Use new or disinfected applicators, brushes, wands, and spatulas to distribute products. Disinfect multiuse tools after each use. Do not double-dip dirty spatulas, wands, or brushes back into products. Discard single-use applicators such as sponge tips, as these are porous and cannot be disinfected.

- **Pencils**—Sharpen pencils and wipe with tissue; if they cannot be sharpened, they cannot be cleaned. Pencils with autorollers or felt tips cannot be sharpened and should never be used on a client. Sharpeners must be cleaned and disinfected after each use, ensuring that all product is removed and the blade is disinfected.

- **Testers**—Keep testers clean in the retail area. To avoid contamination, assist clients who are using testers. Using fingers and double-dipping applicators will spread contaminants that can cause disease. Any contaminated makeup should be removed as a tester and discarded.

- **Palettes and supplies**—Clean and disinfect artist trays, palettes, brushes, sharpeners, and foundation mixing cups after each use.

 FOCUS ON

Safety First
Unfortunately, some facilities do not always follow proper infection control standards for makeup station testers and applications. If you see incorrect practices, bring this to the attention of the staff to help them comply with appropriate standards. A staff training session may be necessary to remind everyone of the correct procedures. Clients will appreciate knowing the testers and applicators are clean, otherwise they may be hesitant to try products or schedule any makeup services.

 CHECK IN

12. List at least five safety measures that should be followed when applying makeup to avoid product contamination.

Conduct a Thorough Makeup Consultation with a Client

The client consultation is a valuable tool for both you and the client. It allows you to spend time with your client and get to know their likes and dislikes before you begin. If possible, sit down with your client and help them fill out the client questionnaire (**Table 12–6**). This will help you to better understand your client's needs and review their information before you begin the makeup session. Your client will appreciate that you are taking the time to work through the form with them, answering any questions they may have. Some common questions to ask during a consultation are:

- What are some of your needs or expectations today?
- Will you be attending a special occasion?

Confidential Makeup Questionnaire

PLEASE PRINT Today's Date: _____

First Name: _____ Last Name: _____ Birthday _____/_____

Street _____ Apt# ___---_____ City _____ State _____ Zip _____

Phone: Home ( ) _____ Work ( ) _____ Cell ( ) _____ E-mail: _____

Referred by (circle one): Friend   Social Media   Walk-by Gift Certificate   Browser Search   Other:_____

- Have you ever had a professional makeover ☐ Yes ☐ No
- If yes, what did you like (dislike) about the session?
  _____
- What are some of your goals today?
  _____
- What special areas would you like to focus on?
  _____
- What are your favorite makeup and clothing colors?
  _____
- Describe an ideal look for your makeup.
  _____
- Do you wear contact lenses? ☐ Yes ☐ No   If yes, are they: ☐ Hard ☐ Soft
- Do you take any medications that cause your eyes to be dry or itch? ☐ Yes ☐ No
  If yes, what? _____
- Are you currently taking prescription drugs that affect your skin or have you taken any in the past? ☐ Yes ☐ No
  If yes, describe the course and length of treatment. _____
- Do you have any health condition that may cause sensitivity in your skin or eye area? ☐ Yes ☐ No
  If yes, what? _____
- Do you have any allergies? ☐ Yes ☐ No   If yes, please indicate. _____
- Do you have any allergies to skin care products? ☐ Yes ☐ No   If yes, what? _____

I fully acknowledge that I do not have any known allergies to makeup products, or contagious conditions, or have listed them above.

Signature: _____

Salon Policies

(Note: This is just an example of policies that may be used.)

1. We require a 24-hour cancellation notice.
2. Please arrive on time for appointments.
3. There is a $25 charge for a no-show appointment.
4. Health regulations do not allow us to accept returned products unless they are unopened and in their original packaging.
5. Returns are given salon credit only. No cash refunds.

I fully understand and agree to the above salon policies.

Client's Signature: _____ Date: _____

- Describe your makeup use.
- How much time do you spend applying makeup?
- What areas of concern would you like to focus on?
- What are your favorite colors?
- Do you have any makeup issues (e.g., allergies or irritations)?

Even though some of the questions listed above will be covered in the questionnaire, it is always a good idea to initiate a conversation with your client. The consultation will help to establish the parameters of work you can perform for them. Knowledge of prior illnesses, injuries, surgeries, or even whether the client wears contact lenses is useful to determine best practices for the makeup application you are planning.

Once you have completed the client consultation forms you can add client preferences such as noting colors they prefer during the makeup application on the client chart (**Table 12–7**).

▼ **TABLE 12–7 The Client Chart.**

Name: _____ Date: _____

Skin Care

Makeup remover _____

Cleanser _____

Freshener _____

Moisturizer _____

Makeup

Matte_____ Dewy_____ Shimmer/Shiny_____

Foundation: Liquid_____ Wet/dry _____ Mineral _____

Color _____

Concealer _____

Powder _____

Brow color _____

Eyeshadows _____

Orbital area _____

Crease _____

Lid _____

Eyeliner _____

Mascara _____

Lip conditioner _____

Lip pencil _____

Lipstick _____

Lip gloss _____

Other

Special Instructions

_____

_____

_____

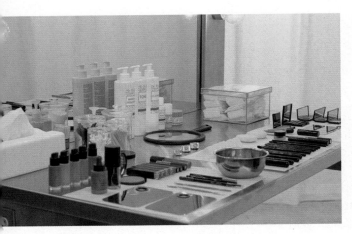

▲ Figure 12–28 Makeup station.

The Makeup Station and Consultation Area

Try to have your makeup station in a visible yet semi-private area of the salon. Make sure that your makeup kit and station are cleaned and well organized before and after each client (**Figure 12–28**). Having good visual references at hand is also suggested as you discuss makeup styles with your client. This will help to identify the desired look. Have on hand makeup examples to reference with your client for inspiration such as current magazines or digital images. Be sure to update your references on a regular basis to keep current and inspired.

LIGHTING

Adequate and flattering lighting is essential for makeup application. Indirect natural daylight from a large window can be good at the right time of day, but will be much more blue on a cloudy day than a clear day, and will shift toward orange at sunset. Because of this variability, even a space with window light will need reliably consistent artificial light.

A bright, even, frontal light source with a daylight color balance is ideal. Placing vertical strips of lights on both sides of the makeup mirror and a horizontal strip or row just above the mirror will produce consistent light. These lights can be rows of individual bulbs or fluorescent tubes. Fluorescent tubes consume very little power and radiate far less heat than conventional bulbs, but for makeup work they must be daylight color-balanced tubes. Traditional incandescent bulbs are inexpensive to purchase and are available in daylight color temperature, but they produce the most heat. LED bulbs are available in daylight color temperature and radiate much less heat than conventional bulbs. While they are more expensive to purchase than incandescent bulbs, they will save you money over time with their extremely low power consumption and long life. The lights around the makeup mirror should be the brightest light source in the room or area. If glare from overhead lights or behind the client is brighter, look for a way to turn off or block it.

Makeup Lessons versus Makeup Application

A makeup lesson includes instruction in how to duplicate the techniques you are using on the client as you work. Allow adequate time when scheduling this service so you can answer questions and let your clients practice the techniques on themselves.

In contrast, a makeup application is one where you apply the makeup, usually for an event, and the client is not given step by step instruction. Clients will usually ask questions while you do their makeup, and you should certainly do your best to provide useful perspective and commentary as time permits, but without slowing down the makeup application process. In cases where the client has a real desire to learn the techniques you're using you should invite the client back for a scheduled makeup lesson.

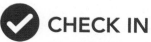 **CHECK IN**

13. List five makeup questions you should ask your client during a makeup consultation.

Perform Makeup Application Techniques

Now that you understand the many facets of selecting preferred colors for your client, let's take a look at application techniques for each product.

Foundation Application

When correctly applied, foundation creates an even canvas for the rest of the makeup application. Skin tone determines the selection of foundation color. As previously discussed, skin tones are generally classified as light, medium, and dark; undertones are warm, cool, or neutral. Warm tones have yellow undertones. Cool tones have blue undertones. Neutral skin has equal amounts of warm and cool tones.

MATCHING AND BLENDING
Foundation should always be matched as closely as possible to actual skin color. If the foundation color is too light, it will have a chalky or ghostly appearance and will "sit" on top of the skin. If the color is too dark, it will look dirty or artificial on the skin. The best way to determine the correct foundation color for your client is to apply a 1- to 2-inch (2.5- to 5-centimeter) vertical stripe of color below the cheek down onto the jawline. Blend slightly and then try other colors if necessary. The color that "disappears" and blends in is the correct one. Avoid creating a contrast between the color of the face and the color of the neck. Makeup should blend smoothly with no visible line (no line of demarcation). Different colors can be mixed together to custom-blend a color. Base makeup colors may need to be changed with the seasons and sun exposure—darker in the summer, lighter in the winter.

SUPPLIES FOR FOUNDATION APPLICATION
Foundations are applied to the face with a disposable makeup sponge or brush. Sponges are banned in some states, so be sure to consult with your local regulatory agency. The sponge can be moist or dry.

Test It Out: Foundation

Using a model (or yourself) and two different color applications, divide the face in half. Try various foundations, colors, and intensities on each side. This will give you a visual example of how different makeup will look on the same face.

DID YOU KNOW?

If you first hold a few colors of a product up next to a client's face, it will give you an idea of whether the colors would be a good potential choice. This is especially useful for foundations, eyeshadows, and blushes.

Patting (also called *stippling*), rather than rubbing, gives better coverage where it is needed. For corrective makeup applications, stippling is a technique that creates the illusion of texture on the skin where there is none. Avoid excessive rubbing and use gentle pressure while blending. Primers underneath makeup help the product go on smoother and stay on longer.

Concealer Application

In most cases, concealer should match the tone of the foundation. You can apply this under or over the foundation beneath the eyes and on other areas to conceal. Concealer is removed from the container with a spatula and may be applied with a concealer brush or a sponge. Place it sparingly over blemishes or areas of discoloration and blend. It is important to match concealer color to skin color as closely as possible.

Concealer that is noticeably lighter than the skin can appear obvious and can actually draw attention to a problem area, such as dark circles. If covering a blemish, match skin tone closely to avoid highlighting the blemish. Yellow- and green-toned concealers must be well blended and covered with foundation.

The principles that apply to choosing foundation colors also apply to concealer colors. Concealer may be worn alone, without foundation, if chosen and blended correctly. Be sure to use it sparingly and soften the edges so that the complexion looks natural.

Concealer products can also be used as a highlighter if the concealer is lighter than the skin color to accentuate and bring out features. A darker shade of concealer can be used for contouring. Light shades bring out the features, and dark shades cause them to recede.

Highlighting and Shading

Highlighters (HY-lyt-urz) are lighter than the skin color, and they accentuate and bring out features such as the brow bone under the eyebrow, the temples, the chin, and the cheekbones.

Contouring (KAHN-toor-ing) colors are darker shades used to define the cheekbones and make features appear smaller. Dark colors recede or diminish features.

These highlighting and contouring (shading) products are found in both liquid and powder forms. Depending on placement, these are applied in a variety of ways similar to shadow, blush, or concealer applications.

Face Powder Application

Face powder should match the natural skin tone and the foundation. **Translucent powder** (tranz-LOO-sent POW-dur) (colorless and sheer) blends with all foundations and will not change color when applied.

Powder sets the foundation and finishes the makeup. This is usually applied after the foundation and before the rest of the makeup. It is also applied again after the blush to help blend and set the blush. Do not use too much powder as it can make skin appear dry and draw attention to wrinkles. Make sure the client's eyes are closed to avoid getting powder in the eyes.

Apply face powder using a brush. Use a brush to blend and remove the excess powder. To apply, sweep in circular or downward motions. Depending on the client you can recommend both loose and pressed powders when suggesting products to a client.

LOOSE POWDER MAKEUP APPLICATION

Loose powder products are easy to spill. Tap jars before opening to settle the product and take out only a tiny amount (a little goes a long way) to use. A partial brushful of product is usually more than enough. Use a clean brush or new, single use, disposable spatula to remove products from the container and tap the product onto a palette to use. Replace the cap right away to avoid spillage and keep the product clean.

PRESSED POWDER MAKEUP APPLICATION

Pressed powder is compact and easy to carry for quick touch-ups during the day.

Pressed products can be turned into loose powder by loosening it up with a new, single use spatula or disinfected or new brush. This is a faster way to remove more of the pressed product out of the container.

Blush Application

Blush gives color to the face and accentuates cheekbones. Choose a color that resembles the face when blushing; in most cases that is a pink to red tone, adjusting for skin color. Apply blush just below the cheekbones, blending on top of the bones toward the top of the cheeks. When you want to get the most flattering placement of the blush to accentuate the client's cheekbones, ask the client to tilt their head back on the axis of the occipital neck point. Notice how their cheekbones become more noticeable. Then slowly turn the client's head left and right. Now you have a better idea for placement. The blush domain area is no closer to the nostrils than the center of the pupil and no lower to the jawbone than an imaginary line from the tip of the nose to the middle of the ear (**Figure 12–29**). And the blush gently kisses the temple area but does not reach the hairline in that region.

Depending on the formulation, blush is usually applied with a brush. Creams are applied with a stiff brush or sponges. Blend the color along the cheekbone so that it fades softly into the foundation. Keep blush placement away from the nose and below the temples.

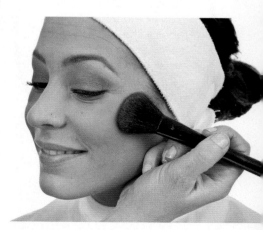

▲ **Figure 12–29 Blush application.**

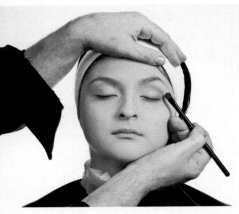

▲ Figure 12–30 Eyeshadow application.

Eyeshadow Application

Choose colors to bring out the eyes, even if the application is subtle. When applied to the lids, eyeshadow makes the eyes appear brighter and more expressive. Using color other than the eye color (i.e., a contrasting or complementary color) can enhance the eyes. Using light and dark contrasts also brings attention to the eyes.

Generally, a darker shade of eyeshadow makes the natural color of the iris appear lighter, while a lighter shade makes the iris appear deeper. The only set rules for selecting eye makeup colors are that they should enhance the client's eyes, and color choices should be flattering. Blending is the key, especially when using dark colors.

Eyeshadow colors are generally referred to as highlighters, bases, and contour/dark colors (**Figure 12–30**).

- A *highlight* color is lighter than the client's skin color. Popular choices include matte or iridescent (shiny). These colors highlight a specific area, such as the brow bone. A lighter color such as white will make an area appear larger.

- A *base* color is generally a medium tone that is close to the client's skin color. This color is used to even out the skin tone on the eye. It is often applied all over the lid and brow bone—from lash to brow, before other colors are applied—thus providing a smooth surface for the blending of other colors. If used this way, a matte finish is preferred.

- A *contour* color is deeper and darker than the client's skin color. It is applied to minimize a specific area, to create contour in a crease, or to define the eyelash line.

- Note: Eye makeup primers can be used prior to applying eye makeup to help it last longer and produce truer colors.

BRACING DURING APPLICATION

Bracing (BRAY-sing) takes practice. But it is a technique using one or both hands positioned to avoid client injury, keeping your hands steady and the client safe. For bracing around the eyes use the back side of your dominant hand on the client's face to steady yourself while using the fingers of the same hand to manipulate the applicator, brush or pencil. Around the eye area you may need only one hand. Sometimes a tissue is used under your hand. Many makeup artists use their opposite hand to hold their own wrist. For the eye, brace your hand just above the brow, not at the top of the head.

To apply eyeshadow:

- Remove the product from its container with a spatula and then use a single-use applicator or clean and disinfected brush.

- Apply the base eye color close to the lashes on the eyelid, sweeping the color slightly upward and outward.

CAUTION!

Be guided by your state on whether bracing is required for your practical exam. Some artists make small precise lines when applying any liner, eye, or lip makeup in lieu of bracing.

- End the color inside the outer edge of the brow.
- Highlighters are used under the eyebrow and on the lid. Darker colors are used in the crease. Blend to achieve the desired effect.

Eyeliner Application

Eyeliner accentuates the eyes. Eyeliner can be applied before or after eyeshadow. Some clients prefer eyeliner that is the same color as the lashes or mascara, for a more natural look. More intense colors may be preferred to match shadow colors or seasonal color trends.

As an alternative to pencils, eyeshadow used with a thin brush dipped in water works well as a wet liner. Dry shadow applied with a thin, firm brush also works. Gels and liquids are also popular. Liner is applied to the top and bottom edge of the eye on the outside of the lashes, not the inner part of the eye. Applying it on the inner mucous membrane can be unhealthy for the eye and can lead to infections.

> **CAUTION!**
>
> According to the American Medical Association, eye pencils should not be used to color the inner rim of the eyes. Doing so can lead to infection of the tear duct, causing tearing, blurring of vision, and permanent pigmentation of the mucous membrane lining the inside of the eye.

Like eyeshadow application, be cautious when applying eyeliner. You must have a steady hand and be sure that your client remains still. Brace your hand by gently resting the base of your hand on a tissue against the cheek of your client. Sharpen the eyeliner pencil and wipe with a clean tissue before and after each use, if needed. Also, remember to clean and disinfect the sharpener after each use. All product residue (wax/wood) must be removed from the sharpener. The sharpener should then be disinfected with a disinfectant approved in your state by either immersion or wipe/spray (if allowed).

Apply short, even strokes and gentle pressure. The most common placement is close to the lash line. For powder shadow liner application, scrape a small amount onto a tissue or tray and apply to the eyes with a single-use applicator or clean brush. If desired, wet the brush before dipping into the color for a more intense and lasting color.

Eyeshadow may be applied as eyeliner with an eyeliner brush to create a softer lined effect. Whether you are using shadow or pencil liner, it may be helpful to gently pull the skin taut—from right below the eyebrow and out or upward without distorting the shape of the eye—to ensure smooth application. Use a light touch when working with contact lens wearers, as they may be more sensitive to the application of product near their eyes.

Mascara Application

Dip a new single-use wand into a clean tube of mascara and apply from close to the base of the lashes out toward the tips, making sure your client is comfortable throughout the application. Bracing the hand lightly on the face allows for more control. The lower or upper lashes can be coated first. Have the client look up at the ceiling when applying mascara to the lower lashes. Let the mascara sit for a few seconds before having them look down or to the side to apply to the upper lashes.

For more coverage, use a side-to-side motion with the wand when applying it from the base to the tip of the lashes. The end of the wand can also be used to apply more mascara to the tips of the lashes. Hold the wand sideways, not pointing toward the eye. Apply mascara carefully. The most common injury with mascara application is poking the eye with the applicator. Practice applying mascara repeatedly until you feel confident enough to apply it on clients.

Dispose each wand into the lined waste receptacle. Never double-dip the same wand back into the mascara. Brush with a lash separator before the mascara dries to avoid clumps. Avoid using powder-based products after applying mascara, including face powder, as it can attach to the damp mascara and discolor the product. Save mascara application for the final step after powder.

Curl the lashes before applying the mascara. This keeps the lash curler clean and avoids getting mascara on the upper lid. You can practice curling artificial lashes while they are still in their tray or by applying them to a mannequin head. Ask your instructor to demonstrate before attempting to use an eyelash curler on a client or fellow student. Clients may prefer to curl their own lashes.

Eyebrow Color Application

Measure the brow shape and follow the shaping guidelines as closely as possible (refer to Table 12–3 on page 564). Check the brows before beginning the service to determine if any stray hairs need to be tweezed.

Usually the best starting point for the eyebrow color ranges from light brown to darker browns, and from softer to richer colors. For a client with very dark brown or black hair, choose a warm black or very dark brown. For a client with pale blonde or platinum blonde hair, choose a very soft taupe. For an older client with gray or silver-gray hair, light taupe is usually best. Additionally, for a client with red hair, taupe or dark brown works great. To determine which color is best, check the hair color using taupe for strawberry blondes and those with lighter hair colors, and dark browns for deep redheads. Using red for eyebrows can look artificial.

To color in the brows, use a sweeping motion to follow the pattern of the hair. Brace your hand just above the brow. Blend back and forth inside the brow line to achieve a natural look.

Lip Color Application

Consider your overall makeup design (evening or daytime, natural versus dramatic, etc.) as you choose a lip color. Lip products are available in numerous types (translucent/stained or opaque), colors (from light to dark), and finishes (ranging from glossy to matte).

Light colors make lips appear larger; dark colors make lips look smaller.

- **Lip gloss** (LIP GLAWS) can give a shiny, moisturized look to the lips.
- **Lip conditioner** (LIP kun-DIH-shun-ur)—Put on a lip moisturizer when starting the makeup application, so it can soak in and moisturize before starting to apply the liner. A primer, foundation, or plumper can be applied prior to the lip color.
- **Lip liners** (LIP LYN-urz) are colored pencils used to line and define the lips. Lining the lips also helps keep lip color on and keeps it from feathering. Lip liner is often used when doing corrective makeup. Lip liner comes in thin- or thick-pencil form, and the formulations are similar to eye pencils. Some lip liners can double as lipstick.

To define and shape the lips, lip liner is usually applied before the lip color. Choose a lip liner that coordinates with the natural lip color or lipstick. The liner color should not be dramatically darker or brighter than the lip shade. If a darker liner is desired, fill in most of the lip with the liner and blend the lip color and lip liner to avoid harsh lines.

To refine or correct the lip outline and help define the lines, use a small amount of foundation or powder on a small brush to erase and blend the lined area as necessary.

Sharpen the lip liner pencil and wipe with a clean tissue before each use. Also remember to clean and disinfect the sharpener before every use. All product residue (wax/wood) must be removed from the sharpener. The sharpener should then be disinfected with a disinfectant approved in the state by either immersion or wipe/spray (if allowed).

- **Lipstick**—Lip color must not be applied directly from the container unless it belongs to the client. Use a spatula to remove the lip color from the container and then take it from the spatula with a disposable lip brush. Use the tip of the brush to follow the lip line. Connect the center peaks using rounded strokes, following the natural lip line. For long-lasting color, use a liner and then a lipstick with gloss over the lipstick.

Makeup Application Tips and Guidelines

The following guidelines should be considered when applying makeup:

- Your fingernails should be short with smooth edges. Be especially cautious when working around the client's eyes!
- Although single-use tools may not be most artists' first choice, they are a clean, safe, inexpensive way to get a job done. Disposable brushes and applicators should be used to prevent the spread of infection and offer a clean application every time.
- Blending and evenness are the most important factors in a good makeup application.

FOCUS ON

Retailing

Lip colors create a good opportunity for retail sales. Suggest a few colors and finishes to your clients. Lip color is a simple way to change a look. It is an easy way for your clients to complete their look and brighten their day.

DID YOU KNOW?

Lip liner used as a base for lipstick and applied all over the lips helps color last much longer than lipstick alone. It also helps color look more natural, as it fades without leaving an obvious line around the lips.

DID YOU KNOW?

Using your wedge-style sponge, you can add a little loose powder around the outside of the lip to help prevent the color from bleeding. Dust the excess powder away with the other side of the sponge.

- Apply creams or liquids before powders. Creams over powders do not blend.

- Use a light touch. Avoid tugging on the skin or rubbing too hard, and avoid holding the client's head.

- Be cautions when lifting the skin around the eye. Lifting the skin may change the look when you let go of the skin around the eye. It is helpful to have your client open and close their eyes during application, so you can see the results of your work and make any necessary adjustments as you go.

- Be sure the client's eyes are closed when applying powder or eyeshadow.

- Apply foundation and powder downward in the direction of the hairs on the face for better blending.

- Incorporate bracing techniques to allow for a safe makeup application (**Figures 12–31a** and **12–31b**).When applying makeup to your client's eyes and lips, be sure to brace the back of your hand or fingers gently on the client's face to steady your hand during application. A tissue can be used between your bracing hand and your client's skin to avoid smudging the underlying makeup.

  - When performing a lip application, you may prefer two hands for bracing. Take your nondominant hand and place it on the edge of the chin. This offers support for your dominant working hand. You can also brace at the corner of the mouth and apply from corner to center.

  - For the eye, brace your hand just above the brow, not at the top of the head.

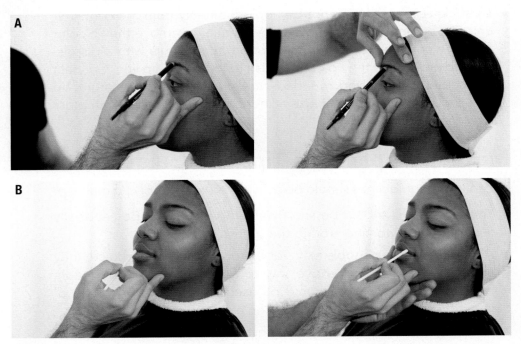

▲ **Figures 12-31a and 12-31b** Single and double bracing near the eyes (a) and single and double bracing near the lips (b).

Use Highlighting and Contouring Techniques for Balance and Proportion

Highlighting and contouring use light and dark shades of makeup to draw attention to or away from particular facial features (**Figures 12–32a** and **12–32b**). A basic rule to keep in mind for highlighting and contouring is that highlighting a feature emphasizes, and contouring or shadowing minimizes. A highlight is created when the cosmetic used is lighter than the original foundation applied. Conversely, a contour (or shading) is formed when the product used is darker than the skin or foundation color. The use of shading (using dark colors and shades) minimizes prominent features, making them appear less noticeable. Using highlighting and contouring, you can satisfy your client's desire for a more balanced appearance by enhancing or de-emphasizing facial features or shapes.

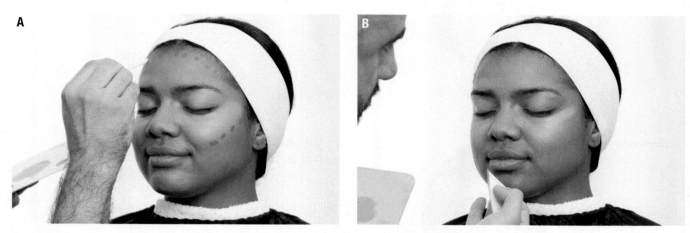

▲ **Figures 12-32a and 12-32b** Example of contour (a) and highlighting (b).

Understanding facial shapes will make it easier to balance features your clients wish to emphasize or de-emphasize. (**Table 12–8**). Products used for highlighting and contouring are foundations and powders. Experiment using lighter and darker shades to achieve the desired effect.

Jawline and Neck Area

When using highlighting and contouring on the jawline and neck the goal is to be able to blend the product so it is consistent from face to neck. From the same tonal family as your base foundation, select a color a shade lighter for highlighting and a shade darker for contouring. Be sure to use a translucent powder to help the makeup set and avoid transfer to clothing. If you wish to elongate the neck, use the lighter color all the way down the center and use the darker shades under the jaw and down both sides.

▼ **TABLE 12–8** Highlight and Contour Makeup Techniques

Facial Feature	Reshaping Techniques
Round/square face	Use two foundations, light and dark, with the darker shade blended on the outer edges of the temples, cheekbones, and jawline, and the light one from the center of the forehead down the center of the face to the tip of the chin.
Triangular face	Apply a darker foundation over the chin and neck and a lighter foundation through the cheeks and under the eyes to the temples and forehead, and then blend them together over the forehead for a smooth and natural finish.
Narrow face	Blend a light shade of foundation over the outer edges of the cheekbones to bring out the sides of the face.
Wide jaw	Apply a darker foundation below the cheekbones and along the jawline; blend into the neck.

Facial Feature	Reshaping Techniques
Double chin	To minimize a double chin, apply shading under the jawline and chin over the full area.
Long, prominent chin	To make a long or prominent chin appear less prominent, apply darker foundation over the area.
Receding chin	Highlight the chin by using a lighter foundation than the one used on the face.
Protruding forehead	Apply a darker shade of foundation over the forehead area.

Facial Feature	Reshaping Techniques
Narrow forehead	Apply a lighter foundation along the hairline and blend onto the forehead.
Wide nose	Apply foundation a shade lighter to the center of the nose. Apply darker foundation on both sides, and blend them together.
Short nose	Blend a lighter shade of foundation onto the tip of the nose and between the eyes.

For a small face and a short, thick neck use a slightly darker foundation on the side of the neck than the one used on the face. This will make the neck appear thinner.

Eye Shapes

The eyes are very important when it comes to balancing facial features. Proper application of eye colors and shadow can create the illusion of the eyes being larger or smaller and will enhance the overall look (**Table 12–9**).

Eye Shapes	Reshaping Techniques
Monolid	Shadow is used to create a desired crease and add definition to the eye area. 1. With a darker color, create a crease in the middle of the upper lid. Avoid strong colors. 2. Highlight the brow bone and hidden area. 3. Softly line upper and lower lashes using a thin line (or skip the upper liner). 4. Apply light (brown) mascara.
Small eyes	To make small eyes appear larger, extend the shadows slightly beyond the side of the eyes. 1. Place a lighter shadow over the lid, blending it out toward the temple and up to the eyebrow. 2. Apply a darker shadow to the crease and outer corners of the lower lids. 3. Blend eyeliner softly from the center to the outer corners of both eyes along the eyelashes. Another alternative is no eyeliner. 4. Apply mascara, brushing the lashes carefully.
Round eyes	Round eyes can be lengthened by extending the shadow beyond the outer corner of the eyes. 1. Apply a medium shade of shadow, blending it over the eyelid out toward the edge of the eyebrow. 2. Apply dark shadow onto the crease and blend it out toward the temple. 3. Line the eye with an eyeliner pencil. 4. Extend and blend the colors applied in steps 1 and 3 toward the outer corner of the eye. 5. Apply mascara to the lashes, heavier at the outer corners of the eyes.
Protruding eyelids	Protruding eyes can be minimized by blending a dark shadow carefully over the prominent part of the eyelid, carrying it lightly toward the eyebrow. Use a medium to deep shadow color. 1. Apply a medium shading color on the entire eyelid, and blend it toward the eyebrow. 2. Highlight the brow bone area. 3. Line the eye. 4. Apply mascara.
Deep-set eyes	For deep-set eyes, use bright, light, reflective colors. 1. Apply a light eyeshadow along the crease of the lid. 2. Blend in a medium color next to the outer corners of the eyelids. 3. Use a soft color to accentuate the eyes. 4. Clearly outline the eyes along the lashes. 5. Choose a dark shade of mascara.

Eye Shapes	Reshaping Techniques
Close-set eyes	Close-set eyes are closer together than the width of one eye. For eyes that are too close together, lightly apply darker shadow on the outer edge of the eyes and light on the inside near the nose. 1. Apply a paler shade to the lid and a darker shade to the outer corner. 2. Line the eye from the middle out to the corner, and blend the shadow outward. 3. Apply mascara in an upward and outward motion.
Wide-set eyes	For wide-set eyes, apply the darker color to the inner side of the eyelid toward the nose, and blend carefully. 1. Extend a darker shadow to the inner corner of the eye toward the nose so eyes appear closer together. 2. Blend a lighter shadow from the middle toward the outer corner. Blend the light and dark colors together in the middle, so it's not obvious. 3. Apply liner all the way to the inside edge of the eye by the nose. 4. Apply mascara with an inward motion toward the nose.
Downward sloping eyes	For drooping eyelids, shadow evenly and lightly across the lid from the edge of the eyelash line to the small crease in the eye socket. Use a light color on the lid and a medium to dark color (sparingly) above the crease. To offset the droop of the eye, which is often accompanied by a low bone structure or low lid fold, it is suggested to give the appearance of a lift to the entire eye area. 1. Tweeze the under-area of the outer portion of the brow to give a more prominent arch. 2. Lightly apply a medium-color shading shadow across the fold and smudge it up and outward. 3. Apply highlighter directly under the arch of the brow. 4. Apply eyeliner (if used) in a very thin line, and thicken it very slightly at the outside edge in a wedge-like point to give a lift to the eye.
Close-set eyes	To diminish dark circles under the eyes, apply concealer over the dark area, blending and smoothing it into the surrounding area. Set lightly with translucent powder. 1. Apply matte concealer. 2. Use a disposable sponge to very gently and lightly blend the concealer under the eye. Work from the inner corner to the outer corner until the concealer is blended. 3. Counterbalance the most prominent undertone when you choose the concealer color. 4. Apply foundation over the concealed areas. 5. Set lightly with translucent powder. Note: Powder may accentuate fine lines and dryness. Use sparingly or not at all under the eye.

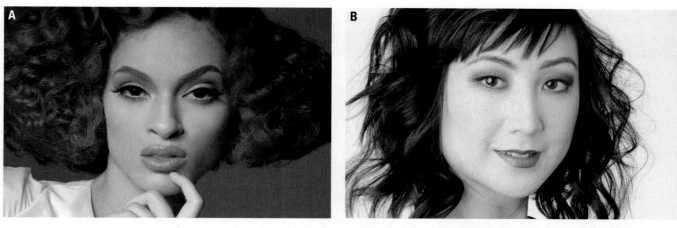

▲ **Figure 12–33a and 12–33b** Eyebrows frame the eyes (dramatic (a) and natural (b)).

Eyebrows

Reshaping and defining eyebrows can be an art unto itself. Well-groomed eyebrows are part of a complete makeup application. The eyebrow is the frame for the eye (**Figure 12–33a** and **12–33b**). Over-tweezed eyebrows may not grow back and can make the client appear older. Use caution when removing brow hairs by either tweezing or waxing. Subtle changes in the shape of the brows can make a big difference in the client's overall look. Adjustments to eyebrow shape can also be used to enhance other facial features (**Table 12–10**).

▼ **TABLE 12–10** Altering Brow Shapes

Brow Shapes	Reshaping Techniques
High arch 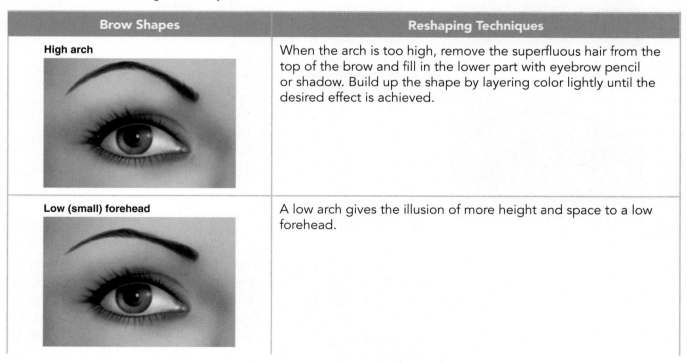	When the arch is too high, remove the superfluous hair from the top of the brow and fill in the lower part with eyebrow pencil or shadow. Build up the shape by layering color lightly until the desired effect is achieved.
Low (small) forehead	A low arch gives the illusion of more height and space to a low forehead.

Brow Shapes	Reshaping Techniques
Wide-set eyes	The eyes can be made to appear closer together by extending the eyebrow lines closer together past the inside corners of the eyes; however, care must be taken to avoid giving the client a frowning look.
Close-set eyes	To make the eyes appear farther apart, widen the distance between the eyebrows and extend them slightly outward beyond the outside of the eyes.
Round face	Arch the brows high and make them more angular to make the face appear narrower.
Long face	Making the eyebrows almost straight (less arch) can create the illusion of a shorter face. Do not extend the eyebrow lines farther than the outside corners of the eyes.
Square face	The face will appear more oval if there is a higher brow arch.

When a client wants to correct their eyebrow shape, begin by removing all unnecessary hairs and then demonstrate how to use the eyebrow pencil or shadow to fill in until the natural hairs have grown in again. When there are spaces in the eyebrow hair, they can be filled in with hair-like strokes of an eyebrow pencil or a shadow applied with an angled brush. Use an eyebrow brush or makeup sponge to soften the pencil or shadow marks.

THE IDEAL EYEBROW SHAPE

The ideal eyebrow shape can be measured by using three lines (**Figure 12–34a** and **12–34b**). The first line is vertical, measuring from the widest side of the nose and inner corner of the eye upward. This is where the eyebrow should begin. For wider nostrils, rest the applicator just above the nostril for a more accurate start point. The second line is from the outer corner of the nose to the outer corner of the eye. This is where the eyebrow should end. The third line is vertical, from the outer circle of the iris (colored part of the eye) upward to the highest point of the brow arch. The client should be looking straight ahead as you determine this line. This third line is where the highest part of the brow arch would ideally be.

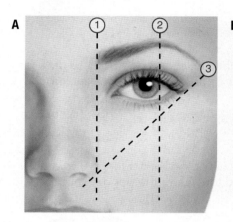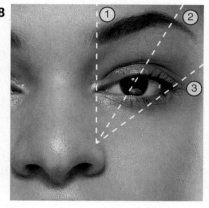

▲ **Figure 12–34** Ideal eyebrow shape.

Of course, not everyone's eyebrows fit exactly within these measurements, so use them only as guidelines. Use the thin edge of a tool such as a small ruler, brow brush, or pencil to measure these lines. If desired, use a brow pencil to draw little dots and mark the three points. This also helps mark the area for hair removal.

Lips

Lips are usually proportioned so that the curves or peaks of the upper lip fall directly in line with the center of each of the nostrils. In some cases, one side of the lips may differ from the other. Various lip colors and techniques can be used to create the illusion of better proportions, as illustrated in **Table 12–11**. It is best to follow the natural lip line as closely as possible.

ACTIVITY

Practice Brow Shapes

Draw several kinds of brow shapes on different face shapes on a piece of paper. Next, sketch in some lines and your makeup ideas showing how you would apply makeup.

─PERFORM─
Procedure 12-1
Performing a Professional Makeup Application

✓ CHECK IN

14. What is contouring or shading used for?
15. Where on the face could you apply a highlighter?
16. How do you measure the ideal eyebrow shape?

▼ **TABLE 12–11** Altering Lip Shapes

Lip Shape	Reshaping Techniques
Thin lower lip	Line just outside the lower lip to make it appear fuller. Fill in with lip color to create balance between the lower and upper lips.
Thin upper lip	Use a liner to outline the upper lip and then fill in with lip color to balance with the lower lip.
Thin upper and lower lips	Outline the upper and lower lips slightly fuller, but do not try to draw far over the natural lip line. Use a lighter color to make lips appear larger.
Cupid bow or pointed upper lip	To soften the peaks of the upper lip, use a medium-color liner to draw a softer curve inside the points. Extend the line to the desired shape. Fill in with lip color.
Large, full lips	Draw a thin line just inside the natural lip line. Use soft, flat lipstick colors that will attract less attention than shimmery or glossy lip colors.
Small mouth and lips	Outline both the upper and lower lips. Fill in lips with soft or shimmery colors to make them appear larger.
Downturned corners	Line the lips to build up the corners of the mouth. This will minimize the drooping appearance. Fill in lips with a soft color.

Lip Shape	Reshaping Techniques
Asymmetrical lips	Outline the upper and lower lips with a soft color to create the illusion of matching proportions.
Straight upper lip	Use liner to create a slight dip in the center of the upper lip, directly beneath the nostrils. Fill in with a flattering color.
Fine lines around the lips	Outline the lips with a long-lasting lip pencil, and then fill in with a product formulated to keep lip color from running into fine lines. Lighter colors work better and do not show the lines as much as dark or red colors do.

Create Makeup Looks for Special Occasions

When working with a client for a special occasion try to get as much information as possible about the event. Identifying it as an evening or outdoor event may help you create a look that will look great and last longer. If you are working with a client for an evening event, one with lower lighting that is more formal, suggest a stronger makeup look, perhaps with false eyelashes. If the event is a daytime or outdoor event, make sure you are working in similar lighting conditions to ensure the client will look great.

Events are an opportunity for clients to purchase any makeup they may want to have on hand, like the lipstick color you used, powder, or bronzer. Check with your client and see if they will need a hairstylist or other services. If you are in a salon, this is a perfect opportunity to provide all of your client's needs for the occasion. If providing this service in a spa or other esthetics treatment location, consider recommending a quality salon in your area. Helping your client with all their needs is something they will appreciate and helps to build a network of coworkers that will refer services to you. Cross-promoting is beneficial for everyone.

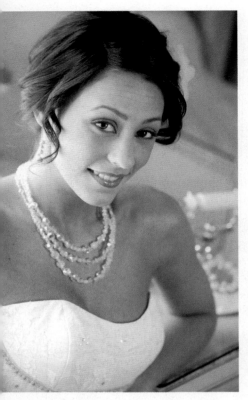

▲ Figure 12–35 Bridal makeup.

Bridal Makeup

Bridal makeup is an important part of the bride's wedding (**Figure 12–35**).

Bridal makeup is highly sought after and can be booked months in advance. A consultation or dry run is recommended to help establish both the desired look and timelines for the day of the event. This will help to ensure things go as smoothly as possible on the actual wedding day.

For the consultation, establish the bride's color preferences and the type of makeup she wants. Ask to see a photograph of the dress to determine how formal the event will be. The photo will also help in designing the right feel for the makeup. Using a scarf, practice protecting the hair and face while putting on and removing a garment. On the wedding day, many brides like to hold off starting makeup until the last possible moment, so you may have to work in tandem with the hairstylist to finish on time. It can be helpful to practice this teamwork during the consultation. Discuss the wedding day timeline at this point as well. Advocate for building in extra time to ensure you can stay on track even if there are unforeseen issues. At the consultation, be sure to suggest products the bride may want to purchase for the wedding and reception.

FOCUS ON

Special Services

Weddings and special occasions are a great opportunity for client services and retail sales. Brides and those attending special events will want to look their best. Facials, good skin care products, and waxing are an important part of preparing for a big day!

Allow plenty of time for your clients to start a beauty-maintenance program, and make sure products are effective and there are no negative skin reactions.

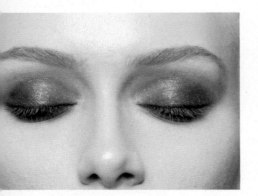

▲ Figure 12–36 Glamorous eyes.

Special-Occasion Makeup for Eyes

STRIKING CONTOUR EYES

Follow these techniques for more glamorous eyes (**Figure 12–36**):

1. Apply the base color from the lashes to the brow with a shadow brush or applicator.

2. Apply a colorful medium tone on the lid, blending from lash line to crease with the shadow brush or applicator.

3. Apply medium to deep color in the crease, blending up toward the eyebrow but ending below it. Take the color further—just outside of the eye.

4. Apply a shimmery highlight shadow under the brow bone with the shadow brush or applicator.

5. Apply eyeliner (liquid or dry) on the upper lash line from the outside corner in, tapering as you reach the inner corner. Blend with the small brush or applicator.

6. Apply shadow in the same color as the liner, directly over the liner. This will give longevity and intensity to the liner. Repeat on the bottom lash line, if desired.

7. Apply two coats of mascara with a single-use mascara wand. Do not double-dip the wand.

DRAMATIC SMOKY EYES

Follow these techniques for dramatic smoky eyes (**Figure 12–37**):

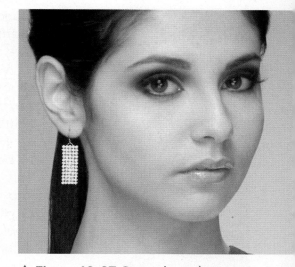

1. Use a dark gray, black, brown, or other dark color of your choice around the entire eye near the lash line on the top and bottom of the eye. Smudge with a small shadow brush or single-use applicator.

2. Apply dark shadow from the upper lash line to the crease, softening and blending as you approach the crease. The shadow should be dark from the outer to inner corner. You can choose either shimmery- or matte-finish eyeshadows. Blend out toward the edge of the brow (in a wedge shape from thickest near the eye to thin on the outside edge of color placement).

3. Apply shadow over the liner on the lower lash line, carefully blending any hard edges.

▲ **Figure 12–37** Dramatic smoky eyes.

4. If desired, add a highlight color in a shimmering or matte finish to the upper brow area with the shadow brush or applicator.

5. Apply two or three coats of mascara with a disposable wand.

6. Add individual or band lashes if desired.

 CHECK IN

17. Why is it important to get as much information as possible about the event when applying makeup for special events?

18. What are the important details to consider when planning bridal makeup?

Apply Makeup for the Camera and Special Events

In this section, we will explore makeup for photography, film, and video.

Photography and Video Applications

With the introduction of HD (high-definition) cameras, imperfections in skin (and makeup) suddenly became much more visible on screen. To counter this, some makeup artists began applying heavier foundation, but the heavier makeup was itself clearly visible, so this wasn't a good solution. Instead, today's makeup artists are meeting the high-def challenge through the use of carefully selected makeup products, strategically placed, resulting in a more natural look.

The combination of HD and bright lighting can dilute the look of makeup, but that does not mean you need to apply more makeup. Adjusting the darkness of the brows and choosing slightly more intense colors for eyes, cheeks, and lips works well without the use of heavy foundation. Airbrushing is ideal for many types of video, film, and live events. The coverage is seamless and can be used effectively on the face and body.

Whether you're working on a video shoot or a still photography shoot, ask to see the makeup on the largest available monitor so you can determine if you have enough color intensity to show up under the lighting and lens conditions in use.

High-definition makeup (HY-def-uh-nish-un MAYK-up) is designed to be invisible when using high-definition cameras (**Figures 12–38**). This makeup is formulated with super-fine microparticles that blend into the skin to provide a flawless complexion. The photochromatic pigments react with all types of lighting so skin looks natural and flawless. The optical correctors and liquid crystal pigments reflect both natural and artificial lights. High-def primers, foundations, and powders diffuse pores and smooth out the skin tone.

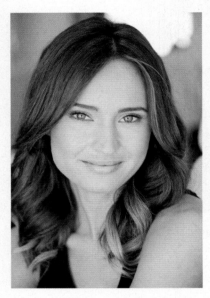

▲ **Figure 12–38** High definition makeup.

Airbrush Makeup

Airbrush makeup is used for photography, film, theater, fantasy, and bridal makeup.

Airbrush makeup is sprayed on and techniques include both freehand and stencil (**Figure 12–39**).

Airbrushing has the following benefits:

- Hygienic, long-lasting, friction- and water-resistant, yet simple to remove
- More efficient and faster to apply than traditional makeup
- Lightweight, natural, and provides a flawless look.

Airbrush makeup is used for the following applications:

- Face and body art, washable tattoos, and artificial tans
- Makeup application: foundations, shading and highlighting, use of stencils

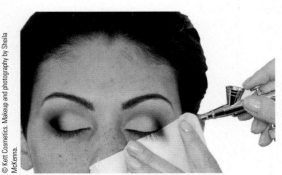

© Kett Cosmetics. Makeup and photography by Sheila McKenna.

▲ **Figure 12–39** Airbrush makeup.

- Hair- and nail-art application: hair adornments, coloration, and scalp covering
- Popular for photography, film, theater, fantasy, and bridal makeup.

 CHECK IN

19. What is high-def makeup? How is it different from ordinary makeup?
20. List the benefits of airbrushing.

Recognize the Benefits of Camouflage Makeup

Camouflage makeup is an important skill set for working with postoperative patients, persons with congenital effects or scarring, or persons experiencing illness or injury. This work is typically done in a doctor's office, hospital, or cancer center. Advanced training is required to learn specific contraindications related to working with the needs of these clients, who may have adverse reactions to certain products or methods of application. This is a rewarding career for those interested in this advanced training (**Figures 12-40a** and **12-40b**).

ACTIVITY

Tattoo Cover Up

Working on yourself or a classmate, use color theory as you work to cover a tattoo. No tattoo handy? Use a skin-safe temporary tattoo to practice covering different tattoos.

A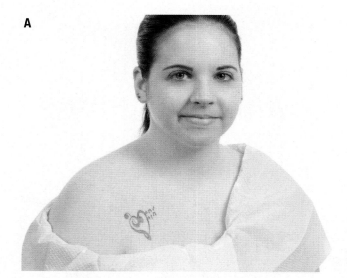

B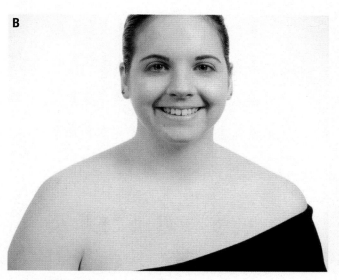

▲ Figures 12-40a and 12-40b Camouflage makeup before (a) and after (b).

 CHECK IN

21. Who can benefit from camouflage makeup?

Demonstrate the Application of Artificial Eyelashes

Artificial eyelashes are an easy way to add length, thickness, and drama to any makeup application. This service may require extra time as well as the cost of the set of lashes and thus require you to add additional charges to a client's bill.

Types of Lashes

Three types of artificial eyelashes are commonly used: band, tabs, and individual lashes.

1. **Band lashes** (BAND lash-ez), also known as *strip lashes*, are eyelash hairs on a strip that are applied with adhesive to the natural lash line (**Figure 12–41**).

2. **Tabs** (TABZ) are small clusters of three or four lashes on one point of attachment (**Figure 12–42**).

3. **Individual lashes** (in-dih-VIJ-oo-al lash-ez) are separate artificial eyelashes that are applied on top of the upper lashes one at a time. (**Figure 12–43**). These are not to be confused with the synthetic eyelash extensions that can last up to two months. Individual eyelashes attach directly to a client's own lashes at the

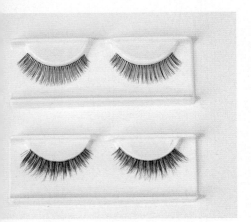

▲ **Figure 12–41** Band or strip lashes.

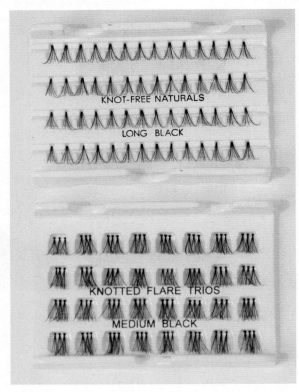

▲ **Figure 12–42** Eyelash tabs.

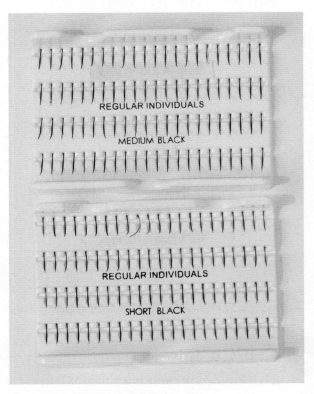

▲ **Figure 12–43** Individual lashes.

base. This process is sometimes referred to as **eye tabbing** (EYE tab-ing). Tab lashes or clusters are groupings of lashes (two to five in a group) that are applied using a technique similar to that used for individual lashes. Tab lashes create a fuller lash line in less time.

Artificial lashes are available in a variety of sizes and colors. They can be made from human hair, animal hair, or synthetic fibers. Synthetic-fiber eyelashes are made with a permanent curl and do not react to changes in weather conditions. Artificial eyelashes are available in natural colors, ranging from light to dark brown and black or auburn, as well as in bright, trendy colors. Black and dark brown are the most popular choices.

Adhesive

Eyelash adhesive is used to make artificial eyelashes adhere, or stick, to the natural lash line (**Figure 12–44**). Some clients may be allergic to adhesive. When in doubt, give the client an allergy patch test before applying the lashes.

This test may be done in one of two ways:

- Put a drop of the adhesive behind one ear. Alternatively, you can use a drop in the crook of the elbow or behind the knee.
- Attach a single individual eyelash to the base of the eyelash. Do not attach to the skin.

In either case, if there is no reaction within 24 hours, you may proceed with the application.

Contraindications

Due to the sensitivity of the eye area and the importance of healthy eyes, there are situations in which eyelash extensions should not be applied:

- Pregnancy
- Eye irritations
- Eye infections
- Eye allergies
- Blepharitis (chronic inflammation of the eyelid)
- Glaucoma (refer to Did You Know?)
- Excessive tears
- Chemotherapy*
- Thyroid problems affecting lash growth or hair loss
- Asthma (may be sensitive to the adhesive odor).

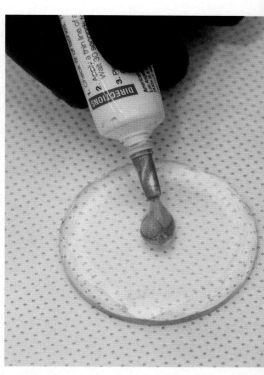

▲ **Figure 12–44** Eyelash adhesive.

ACTIVITY

Practice Makes Perfect Lashes

Apply artificial lashes to a mannequin head and practice applying mascara. This will build your skill as a gentle and steady artist.

DID YOU KNOW?

Glaucoma is a disease in which the optic nerve is damaged and can lead to progressive, irreversible loss of vision.

*Chemotherapy often causes shedding of the lashes, which act as a protective barrier to prevent dust and debris from entering the eye. Without them your client will already be having trouble with eye irritation and tearing. The fumes from the glue used to attach artificial lashes to the eyelid can worsen this irritation and watering of the eyes. Instead, show the client how to use eyeliner to create the illusion of a lash line while being careful not to allow eyeliner inside of the eyelid. A colorful lipstick can help draw attention from thinning eyelashes. The recycle growth for eyelashes is approximately 56 days.

Removing Artificial Eyelashes

To remove artificial eyelashes, use eye pads saturated with an oil-based eye makeup remover that is formulated to remove waterproof mascara. The lash base may also be softened by applying a facecloth or cotton pad saturated with warm water and a gentle facial cleanser. Hold the cloth over the eyes for a few seconds to soften the adhesive. Starting from the outer corner, remove the lashes carefully to avoid pulling out the client's own lashes. Pull strip lashes off parallel to the skin, not straight out. Use wet cotton pads or swabs to remove any makeup and adhesive remaining on the eyelid.

---PERFORM---

Procedure 12-2
Applying Artificial Lashes

 CHECK IN

22. Name and describe the two types of artificial eyelashes.

CAUTION!

Not all tints are safe or legal to use so be sure to check with local laws and regulations to determine which are allowed in your area. Use of illegal tints could result in fines and loss of your license.

- Do not use tints with aniline derivatives (coal-tar based). These are not FDA approved and can cause blindness.
- Some tints on the market may be sold by retailers, but are actually illegal in the United States.
- Vegetable dyes may be allowed in some regions but do not work as well or last as long.
- Some regions prohibit the use of any type of coloring product to tint the eyelashes and eyebrows.
- Permanent haircolor should never be used on brows.

Describe Tinting Lashes and Brows on a Makeup Client

Lash and brow tinting is used to darken lashes and brows. It is nice for clients with light hair to have some color that lasts a few weeks, rather than penciling in brows or having light eyelashes without mascara. Tint is effective for those who have enough hair to darken. If the hair is sparse, tinting may not show up enough to be effective. Tinting is a quick procedure and can be a great add-on service to facials or waxing.

The application must be precisely placed inside the brow shape. It is very important to keep the tint off of the skin unless requested for the brow area. Color takes very quickly, so any excess on the skin must be removed within seconds or it could remain there for weeks. Lashes or brows can be tinted—clients do not always want both areas tinted.

Other Eyelash Services

LASH EXTENSIONS

Lash extensions are single synthetic or natural hairs that are applied one-by-one to the client's natural lashes with a special adhesive. Fine-tipped forceps or tweezers are used to apply the lash extensions, and it can take up to two hours to apply a set. Partial applications and touch-ups take less time.

The bond will last for the life cycle of the natural lash—approximately two months. Fills, or touch-ups, are necessary as the hair grows and the extension needs to be replaced. For extensions to last, makeup application and cleansing should be gentle around the lash area. Research on the quality of the adhesive and its safety is recommended. Advanced training and practice are necessary before performing this intricate procedure on clients.

┌─────PERFORM─────┐
Procedure 12-3
Tinting Lashes
and Brows
└─────────────────┘

Lash Perming

Lash perming is the process of chemically curling the lashes. Research on the quality and safety of the perm solution is recommended. Advanced training and practice are necessary before performing this delicate procedure on clients. Always check with your regulatory agency about the legalities of performing lash services.

CHECK IN

23. What ingredient found in lash tint products should not be used?
24. How long do lash extensions last, and how best can they be applied so they will last as long as possible?

Explain the Benefits of Permanent Makeup Application

Permanent makeup requires an extensive amount of training and the intent of this section is to briefly introduce you to the topic with the understanding that many states require a special certification in addition to an esthetician's license. It is important to address the topic as it is a fast growing field and estheticians are drawn to it based on potential revenue streams.

Permanent makeup (PUR-muh-nent MAYK-up) is a cosmetic implantation technique that deposits colored pigment into the upper reticular layer of the dermis, similar to tattooing. (**Figure 12–45**). The specialized techniques used

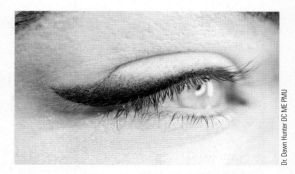

▲ **Figure 12–45** Permanent makeup application.

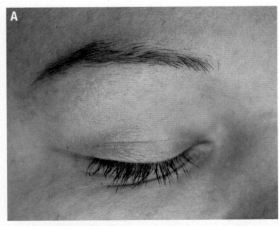

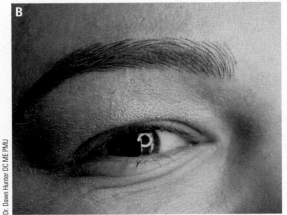

▲ Figures 12-46a and 12-46b Microblading before (a) and after (b).

Dr. Dawn Hunter DC ME PMU

for permanent cosmetics are often referred to as *micro-blading*, *micropigmentation*, *micropigment implantation*, or *dermagraphics*. Scar camouflage and body art are offered as permanent cosmetic services, although eyeliner and eyebrow tattooing are the most popular services.

One specific area growing in popularity for the eyebrows is known as *microblading*. Microblading is defined as a tattooing or semipermanent makeup technique where a small hand-held device made up of tiny needles is used to add pigment to the skin. It is considered semipermanent as the color will fade and require touch-ups. Check with your state as to the requirements to perform this technique as this is an advanced technique requiring additional training.

Permanent cosmetic procedures are performed using various methods, including traditional tattoo machines, pen or rotary machines, and the hand method (**Figure 12–46**). The process includes an initial consultation, then application of pigment, and at least one or more follow-up visits for adjusting the shape and color or density of the pigment.

Technically, permanent cosmetic procedures are considered permanent because the color is implanted into the upper reticular part of the dermal layer of the skin and cannot be washed off. As with any tattoo, however, fading can and often does occur, requiring periodic maintenance and touch-ups.

Estheticians, tattoo artists, and medical technicians perform these services. Licensing and training requirements vary from state to state. A thorough training program and hands-on experience are necessary to perform these technical services. It is recommended that clients choose a technician carefully by considering their training and experience and by looking at their portfolio. It is important to remember that the shape and proper placement of the pigment is as important as the right color. It is permanent and there is absolutely no room for error. One must have a steady hand and attention to detail to perform this service.

Considerations for Permanent Makeup

The initial procedure will generally take approximately 1 to 2.5 hours to perform. Touch-up procedures do not usually require as much time. Most clients experience some discomfort. This varies according to an

ACTIVITY

What Inspires You?

- Find five pictures of makeup looks that you like and five that you dislike. Note why you like or dislike them.
- Find one example of each look: natural, business, evening, and dramatic.
- Find a brow look you like and one you dislike.
- What is in style right now for makeup? Present an example in class.
- Find two professional articles about techniques on applying makeup.

individual's pain threshold as well as the skills of the technician performing the service. Generally, there is some swelling of the treated area. While eyebrows may show little after-effect, eyeliner and lips may show more, and the edema (inflammation) may last from 2 to 72 hours. During the procedure, there may be some bleeding and/or bruising. There is usually some tenderness for a few days. The color is much darker for the first 6 to 10 days.

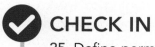 **CHECK IN**

25. Define permanent cosmetic makeup.

Describe the Benefits of a Career In Makeup

Makeup artists play an important role in the esthetics field. Many opportunities are available for makeup artists in clinical offices, film/video, theater, and fashion. These art forms give individuals a chance to be creative. A natural part of the full-service menu for spas and salons, makeup services complement other services offered by estheticians.

To thrive in this business, it is important to keep up with current styles, sell yourself, and present yourself well.

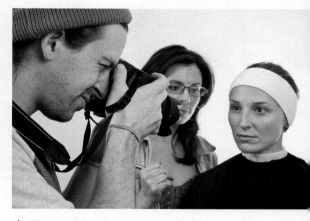
▲ **Figure 12–47** Commercial photography.

- Commercial photographers often work with freelance makeup artists. In fashion photography, a makeup artist works with models (**Figure 12–47**). Magazine and advertising layouts often require ultrafashionable hairstyles and makeup to call attention to products or clothing.

- Another exciting avenue for makeup artistry can be found in television, theater, movies, and fashion shows. In this highly competitive field, you may need a lengthy apprenticeship and acceptance into a union.

- Another option for makeup artists is a career in mortuary science. Many people believe that viewing the deceased has a comforting psychological effect on the bereaved family and friends, and the custom is widely practiced. Training includes the study of restorative art, which is the preparation of the deceased. Restoration work requires a high degree of skill and must be performed under the direction of a mortician. In this career, the esthetician or cosmetologist works only on preparing and applying cosmetics.

Freelance Makeup Artistry

Freelance makeup artists provide services outside of the salon for photography, video, and events (**Figure 12–48**). Film studios, theater productions, fashion shows, and special events all require on-location makeup artists. Men also need makeup for video, fashion, and print work (**Figure 12–49**).

Freelance makeup artistry is an exciting, fast-paced part of the makeup business. It can be challenging to work on location. You need to be flexible, quick, and organized to keep up with the crew and schedule. The work area can be limited and correct lighting is not always available, but it is rewarding to see the fruits of your labor in action. It can be an interesting and lucrative career choice to be a freelance makeup artist (**Figure 12–50**).

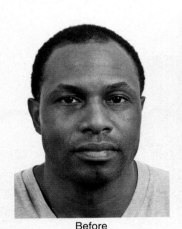

▲ **Figure 12–48** Freelance makeup artist services outside of the salon.

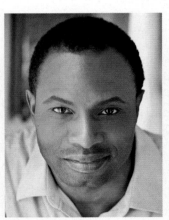

Before   After

▲ **Figure 12–49** Makeup for men.

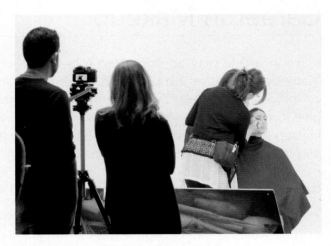

▲ **Figure 12–50** Makeup artist on set.

DID YOU KNOW?

A test, or test-shoot, is a photo-industry term describing a shoot planned to explore a new creative idea or technical solution. Typically, everyone on set, including the model, wardrobe stylist, hair stylist, and photographer, create an image or series of images without charging a fee. Typically, these images are made available to all participants for self-promotion. Contributing your time for a photography test is a great way to gain experience and create professional images for your portfolio without spending a lot of money.

A makeup artist with education and certification in esthetics has a distinct advantage. As a makeup artist you will find your clients have many questions about their skin. The skin is the canvas that makeup is applied to and therefore it is important to understand its structure and function. Knowledge of how to address your client's skin care needs will help to build their confidence in your abilities to provide other services and retail products.

MARKETING FREELANCE MAKEUP SERVICES

Create social media sites for your freelance makeup work that are separate from your personal accounts. Post before and after images of your work and post more creative images on your Instagram feed as an example. These are both effective and inexpensive ways to build a following. Be sure to get written permission from each client or model to use their image for marketing purposes. Standard model releases can be found online to use for this purpose. Additionally, tell everyone you know that you are a freelance makeup artist. Calling on photographers and production companies in your area can help you build relationships that lead to paid work.

Makeup Marketing Tips

- Promote makeup services to facial clients.
- Offer free consultations.
- Visit and hand out your business cards and brochures to photographers, bridal shops, TV studios, and ad agencies.
- Establish a relationship with physicians' offices (dermatology, cosmetic surgery).
- Create a quality portfolio to share with potential clients. It is worth having a professional photo session to create your portfolio if you are going to specialize in freelance makeup.
- Attend bridal fairs and place ads in bridal publications.
- Market yourself at event locations and venues where large functions are held.
- Think of other retail stores and locations where you could offer free consultations.
- Take advantage of all social network, media, and Internet marketing avenues.

CREATING YOUR ON-LOCATION MAKEUP KIT

Creating a makeup kit specifically for location work can be a fun experience. Each time you go out with your kit you will notice more things you can add to make working on location easier.

Start with a sturdy case with lots of compartments to keep your tools and makeup safe during air travel or bouncing down rough roads driving to location. The case should be roomy, preferably stackable, and have wheels. Alternatively, a folding hand cart can be a lifesaver, especially when moving about in big sound stages or down long hallways.

Add these essentials to your basic makeup kit (see Table 12–4):

- Foundations and powders in a range of colors to address all ethnicities
- Eyeshadows, eyeliners, brow pencils—in a variety of shades and finishes—makeup pencil sharpeners
- Regular and waterproof mascara in black and brown

ACTIVITY

Build a Makeup Kit

Put together an "on-location" makeup kit to carry with you for special-event makeup.

Think about ways you can promote your talent. Starting a blog is a great method to create a professional status and following that will help build your business. Post regularly—even every day—as it is well worth the effort and exposure. Another idea is sending your work to professional magazines, which can also give your career a boost. If featured, cut out or print the articles to showcase the work and let your new clientele see you in print.

- Cheek colors for all skin types in a variety of light as well as more intense colors and a range of finishes including matte, shimmer, and cream blush for drier skin
- Lip pencils, lip pencil sharpener, lipsticks, glosses, and a clear lip moisturizer (for men and kids as well as women)
- A professional set of makeup brushes, with extra brushes so you won't have to wait for brushes to dry between models, and brush cleaner
- A set of disposable, single-use brushes and applicators, as wells as sponges, tissues, and cotton swabs
- Hair supplies: clips, headbands, hairspray, brush, comb, hairpins
- Other supplies: tweezers, scissors, safety pins, skin oil, hand sanitizer, mirror, washcloths, drinking straws (a lipstick saver), makeup cape
- Artificial eyelashes, glue, and an eyelash curler
- Outdoors: umbrella for shade, sunscreen, water
- As needed: small portable table, chair, shower curtain and tape for privacy screen, duct tape, lights and lighting, extension cords, and multioutlet power strip
- Makeup remover wipes and eye makeup remover
- Other stylist accessories and on-location supplies: paper towels, tissues, snacks, mints, eye drops, band aids, artificial tears, antihistamine spray, an emergency eyewash kit, lined trash bin, and so on.

 CHECK IN

26. What is a test shoot?
27. Why is marketing yourself as a makeup artist important and how can you go about it?

Promote Retail Services as a Makeup Artist

Retailing cosmetics is a significant part of the business. It is also an effective way to increase your income. Most salons will pay you 5 to 10 percent of every product you retail.

As a licensed professional you will have access to both private label and commercial or consumer brands. Many national brands have programs for professional makeup artists to receive a discount off the retail price.

When considering a makeup line to retail in your salon or spa, choose a line you like working with and feel comfortable recommending to your clients. This will make retailing easier. Consider the education and support that the company may offer. Knowledge is key when working with products that you will use and retail. Choose lines that have quality assurance with a stable company that offers products in a wide assortment of foundations so you can accommodate all skin tones and ethnicities.

One of the biggest challenges clients face when purchasing cosmetics is finding the correct colors and finishes. During your makeup service, let your client know which products you are using and make them available afterward. This is an effective and convenient way for your client to shop and duplicate their look at home.

A retail section with product displays should also be accessible to your clients (**Figure 12–51**). Make testers readily available and let clients enjoy "playing" with the products. Assist them with keeping testers clean and using single-use applicators to avoid contamination.

Having an attractive display, an assortment of makeup options, and a thorough knowledge of the products you offer is a must when answering any questions your client may have and for helping to select the most beneficial items that they will enjoy using at home or for that special occasion.

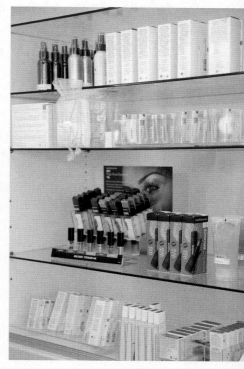

▲ **Figure 12–51** Makeup retail section.

ACTIVITY

Practice Interview Techniques

Have the students interview a professional salesperson (in any field) and ask them the top three tips they would give for sales. Discuss with the class to highlight new ways to approach retail.

The price of services and products will vary depending on the geographical location of the salon and client demographics. Lessons, makeovers, and special-occasion applications cost more than basic applications.

Web Resources

www.makeupabout.com
www.safecosmetics.org

 CHECK IN

28. List factors to keep in mind when promoting retail services.

Procedure 12-1:
Performing a Professional Makeup Application

Implements and Materials

- [ ] Skin care products
- [ ] Cleanser
- [ ] Toner
- [ ] Moisturizer (skin primer optional)
- [ ] Lip conditioner

MAKEUP
- [ ] Concealer
- [ ] Highlighter
- [ ] Contour color
- [ ] Foundation
- [ ] Powder
- [ ] Eyeshadow
- [ ] Eyeliner
- [ ] Mascara
- [ ] Blush
- [ ] Lip liner
- [ ] Lipstick
- [ ] Lip gloss
- [ ] Other: bronzers, specialty items

SUPPLIES
- [ ] Cape and draping supplies
- [ ] Client charts
- [ ] EPA-registered disinfectant
- [ ] Hair clip/headband
- [ ] Hand towel
- [ ] Lash comb
- [ ] Lash curler
- [ ] Lined waste receptacle
- [ ] Makeup brushes
- [ ] Mirror
- [ ] Pencil sharpener
- [ ] Small scissors
- [ ] Tweezers

SINGLE-USE ITEMS
- [ ] Spatulas
- [ ] Cotton (swabs and rounds)
- [ ] Mascara wands
- [ ] Sponges
- [ ] Tissues
- [ ] Applicators
- [ ] Paper towels

There are many ways to approach makeup application. The following is an example of one approach. In time, you will find a routine that works best for you and your clients. Developing your signature style will help you stand out from other artists, and make your process more efficient. Completing a makeup application includes the consultation, setup, application, and clean-up procedures (refer to Tables 12–1, 12–2, and 12–3).

Preparation

- Perform Procedure 7–1 and 8–1: Pre-Service Procedures.
- Start by setting out a few color selections: neutrals, cools, warms.
- The client's skin needs to be exfoliated and hydrated for the makeup to be applied successfully. This should happen before the procedure, but if there is extra time the client can wash and exfoliate their face at a sink. You might ask them to come in early for this.

Procedure

1 **Determine the client's needs**, choosing products and colors accordingly. Discussing skin care or waxing is appropriate with a makeup client. Go over the client questionnaire (refer to Table 12–6), making sure to ask the following questions:

- Do you wear contacts or have skin sensitivities?
- What type of look would you like to achieve?
- What makeup products do you normally wear?
- What are your typical clothing colors?
- Are you going to a special occasion or event?

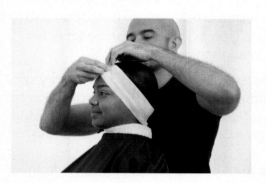

2 **Wash your hands.**

3 **Drape the client** and use a headband or hair clip to keep their hair out of their face.

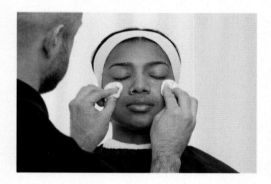

4 **Cleanser**—After washing your hands, cleanse the face if the client is wearing makeup or if the skin is oily.

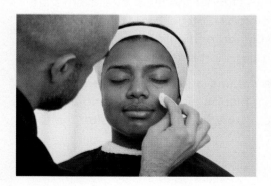

5 **Toner**—Use a cotton pad to apply toner to help remove any traces of makeup and restore the pH balance of the skin.

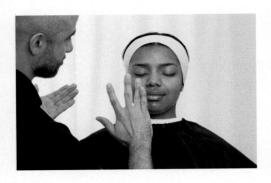

6 **Moisturizer**—Apply a small amount of moisturizer to prepare the skin for makeup. Apply a primer if applicable.

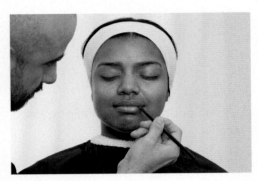

7 **Lip conditioner**—Use a new, single-use spatula to remove the product from the container. Apply with a disposable or disinfected brush. To give it more time to soak in and moisturize, put on the lip conditioner when starting the makeup application.

Note: If lips are chapped, have clients rub off the dry skin with a wet washcloth, esthetic wipes, or a lip scrub before starting the service. Tissue or paper towels are drying and leave lint on the lips so are not recommended for this.

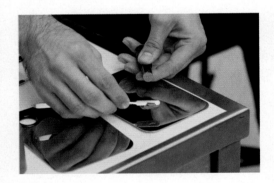

8 **Concealer**—Use a spatula to remove the product from the container. Choose a color similar to the foundation and the same color as the skin.

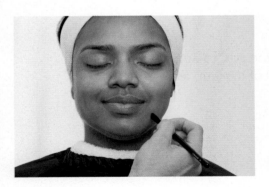

9 Match the surrounding skin closely in areas where you wish to cover darkness (under the eyes, over blemishes, over red or dark-colored splotches). You can use a concealer a shade lighter for highlighting. Apply with a brush or sponge, using short strokes.

Note: Always use creams and liquids before applying powders for ease of blending. If you are using a powder concealer or contour powder, apply these after the foundation.

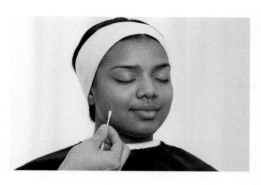

10 **Foundation**—Select a few colors you wish to work with to blend and match the skin. Use a spatula to retrieve the product from the container, placing the product on a palette or directly on a disposable sponge. Apply to the jawline to check for a match with the skin.

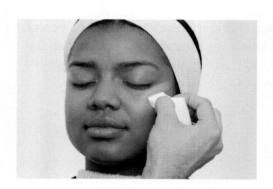

11 Cover the skin with a thin layer of product using even strokes. Blend along the jaw and edges of the face. Blend downward in the direction of the growth of facial hair and downward as well around the hairline. Pat gently around the eyes.

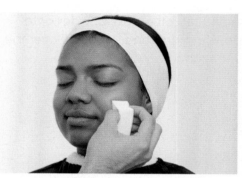

12 **Highlighter**—Use a spatula to remove the product from the container. Apply a lighter color than the client's skin tone to accentuate and bring out features along the brow bone, temples, chin, or above the cheekbones. Blend well with a brush or sponge.

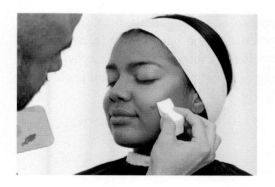

13 **Contouring**—Use a spatula to get the product out of the container. Using a small amount, apply a darker shade under the cheekbones and to other features you want to appear smaller. Blend well.

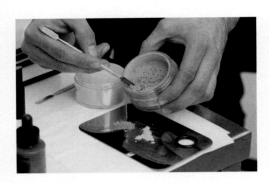

14 **Powder**—Pour a little powder on a clean palette or tissue to avoid cross-contamination.

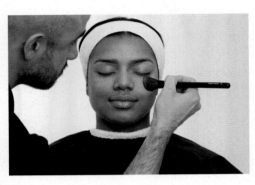

15 Apply to the brush and tap off excess powder onto the tissue. Use a powder brush and sweep all over the face to set the foundation.

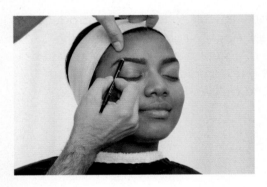

16 **Eyebrows**—Use a shade that is close to the hair color, or a shade the client likes. Brace your hand just above the brow and apply color by using short strokes with a pencil or eyeshadow with a brush.

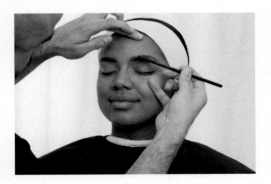

17 Smudge with a brush or a makeup sponge, going in the direction opposite to the hair growth to blend. Then smooth brows back into place with a brow brush.

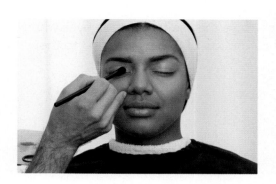

18 **Eyeshadow**
Light—Choose a light base color and apply all over the eyelid, from the lash line up to the brow. Stop color at the outside corner of the eye up to the outside corner of the brow. To steady your hand and avoid eye injury, gently rest the base of your hand against the cheek of your client. Sometimes a tissue is used under your hand. For the eye, brace your hand just above the brow.

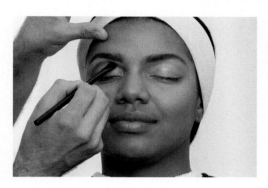

19 *Dark*—Apply a darker shade to the crease: partially on top of the crease and partially underneath the crease. First tap the excess powder off the brush. Never blow on brushes. Apply the most color from the outside corner of the eye into the crease area above the inside of the iris.

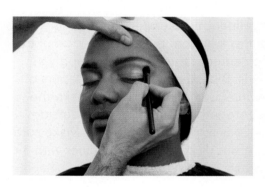

20 This dark color covers three-quarters of the way above the outside part of the eye. Blend the color.
Optional: Apply the eyeliner before applying the dark shadow color.

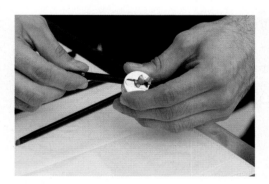

21 **Choose an eyeliner**—Sharpen the liner before and after use. Shadow as wet liner can also be used for liner and applied with a single-use or clean brush. Eyeshadow can be applied as liner with a thin brush dipped in water. Dry shadow can also be applied with a thin, firm brush for a more natural look. Make sure the liner is not too rough or so dry that it drags on the eye. Liquid liners require applicators that are disposable or that can be disinfected. Each dip into the liquid will require a new applicator.

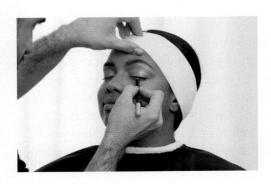

22 **Apply eyeliner**—Have the client shut their eyes when you apply the liner on top of the eyelids next to the lashes.

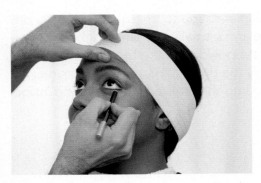

23 Have the client look up and away as you apply the lower liner under the eyes. Apply the liner underneath the lower lashes.

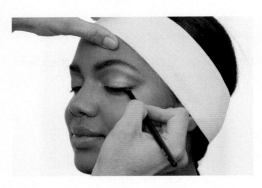

24 **Complete the eyeliner and blend**—Bring the liner three-quarters of the way from the outside edge of the eye in toward the center of the eye, ending softly at the inside of the iris. Blend so that the color tapers off. Bringing the liner in closer to the nose can make the eyes appear closer together. Lining only the outside corner makes the eyes appear farther apart. Make sure the line does not abruptly stop. Blend the liner with a firm, small liner brush.

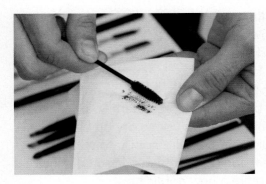

25 **Mascara**—Dip the disposable wand then wipe off excess product.

Note: Some artists prefer to do the lower lashes first to avoid mascara touching the tops of the eye area when the client looks up for the lower application.

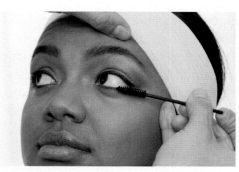

26 **Apply to lower lashes**—Have the client put their chin down while looking up at the ceiling with their eyes to apply mascara to the bottom lashes. Be sure to brace the hand lightly on the face for more control. Comb and separate before the mascara dries.

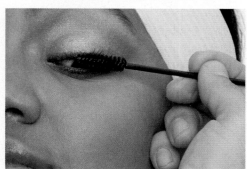

27 **Apply to upper lashes**—Wipe excess product off the wand. Have the client look down and focus on a fixed point to apply mascara to the upper lashes, brushing from the base to the tip. Be sure to brace the hand lightly on the face for more control. Use a lash comb before the product dries and before the client looks in a different direction to avoid smudging.

Note: Use a cotton-tipped swab or small stiff brush with a little foundation or powder on it to fix or erase smudges.

Optional: Curl the lashes before applying mascara. Hold the curler on the base of the lashes without pulling and release the curler before moving it away from the lashes.

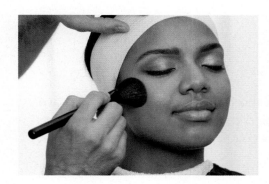

28 **Blush**—The order in which you apply blush is a personal choice. (Note: If you are using a cream blush, apply this before applying powders.) Tap off the excess powder from the brush. Apply blush just below the cheekbones, blending back and forth along the cheekbone. For optimum results, the color should stop below the temple and should not go lower than the nose. The blush domain area is no closer to the nostrils than the center of the pupil and no closer to the jawbone than an imaginary line from the tip of the nose to the middle of the ear. And blush should blend to the hairline, but not into it. A more horizontal application of blush will tend to widen the face, whereas a more vertical application will make it look narrower. Following the cheekbones usually works best.

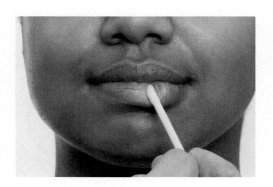

29 **Optional: lip conditioner**—This step applies if lips are dry or you did not already apply lip moisturizer. Use a spatula to get the product out of the container. Use a disposable brush to apply. Put on a lip moisturizer so it can soak in and moisturize before you start applying the liner.

Note: Some artists use a primer or foundation on the lips under the lip color to help keep it on.

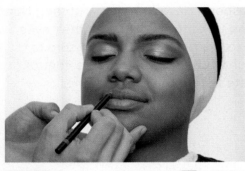

30 **Lip liner**—Sharpen the liner. Have the client smile and stretch their lips. Brace at the corner of the mouth. With the lips pulled tight, the liner and lipstick brush glide on more smoothly. Line the outer edges of the lips first with small firm strokes; then fill in and use the liner as a lipstick. This keeps the lipstick and color on longer.

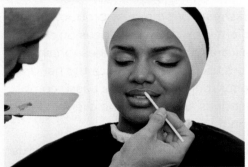

31 **Lipstick**—Use a spatula to get the product out of the container. Have the client select a color from among two or three choices. Apply the lipstick evenly with a lip brush. Rest your ring finger near the client's chin to steady your hand. Ask the client to relax their lips and part them slightly. Brush on the lip color. Then ask the client to smile slightly so that you can smooth the lip color into any small crevices.

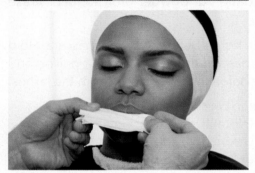

32 **Blot the lips with tissue** to remove excess product and set the lip color. Finish with gloss if desired.

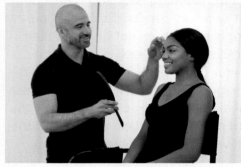

33 **Show the client the finished application**—Remove the cape and hair clips so they can see the finished look. Discuss the colors and any product needs they may have.

FINISHED LOOK

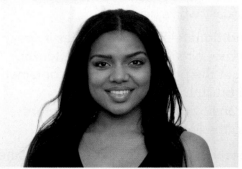

POST-SERVICE

- Complete Procedures 7–2 and 8–9: Post-Service Procedures.

Procedure 12-2:
Applying Artificial Lashes

Note: This procedure is intended for strip lashes and individual lashes.

Implements and Materials

SUPPLIES
- ☐ Disinfectant
- ☐ Headband or hair clip
- ☐ Tweezers
- ☐ Eyelash comb/brush
- ☐ Eyelash curler
- ☐ Hand mirror
- ☐ Small (manicure) scissors
- ☐ Adjustable light
- ☐ Adhesive tray or foil to put adhesive on
- ☐ Disinfected dappen dish or small palette to hold the lashes before application
- ☐ Makeup cape
- ☐ Hand sanitizer
- ☐ Lined waste container

PRODUCTS
- ☐ Artificial eyelashes
- ☐ Eyelid and eyelash cleanser
- ☐ Lash adhesive
- ☐ Eyelash adhesive remover
- ☐ Eye makeup remover

SINGLE-USE ITEMS
- ☐ Cotton swabs
- ☐ Cotton pads
- ☐ Toothpick or hairpin
- ☐ Mascara wand
- ☐ Paper towels

Preparation

- Perform Procedures 7–1 and 8–1: Pre-Service Procedures.
- Discuss with the client the desired length of the lashes and the effect they hope to achieve.
- Wash your hands and put on gloves.
- Place the client in the makeup chair with their head at a comfortable working height. The client's face should be well and evenly lit; avoid shining the light directly into the eyes. Work from behind or to the side of the client. Avoid working directly in front of the client whenever possible.
- If the client wears contact lenses, she must remove them before starting the procedure.
- If the client is only having artificial lashes applied and you have not already done so, remove mascara so that the lash adhesive will adhere properly. Work carefully and gently. Follow the manufacturer's instructions carefully.

Note: If the artificial lash application is in conjunction with a makeup application, complete the makeup without applying mascara to the lashes, finish with the false lashes, and then add mascara, which is usually needed only on the lower lashes.

Procedure

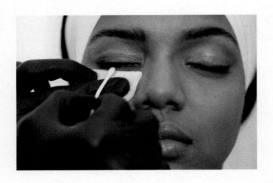

1 Brush the client's eyelashes to make sure they are clean and free of foreign matter, such as mascara particles.

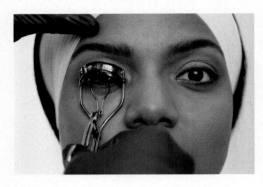

2 If the client's lashes are straight, they can be curled with an eyelash curler before you apply the artificial lashes.

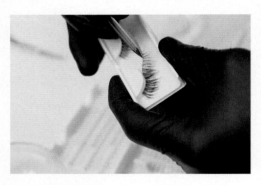

3 Carefully remove the eyelash band from the package. Tweezers work well for this.

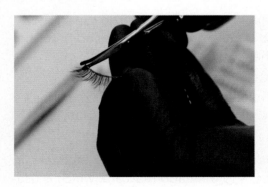

4 Start with the upper lash. Hold this up to the eye to measure the length. Use your fingers to bend the lash into a horseshoe shape to make it more flexible so it fits the contour of the eyelid. If the band lash is too long to fit the curve of the upper eyelid, trim the outside edge.

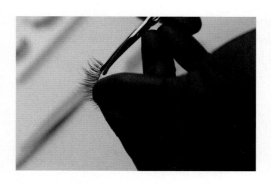

5 Feather straight band lashes to make uneven lengths on the end ("w" shapes) by nipping into them with the points of your scissors if desired. This creates a more natural look.

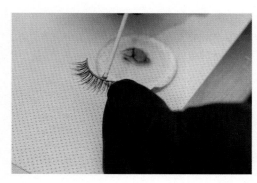

6 Using a disposable brush or rounded end of a toothpick, apply a thin strip of lash adhesive to the base of the false lashes and allow a few seconds for it to set.

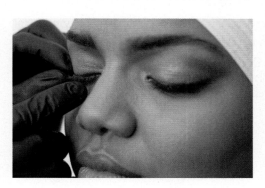

7 **Apply the lashes**

For strip lashes—Apply the lashes by holding the ends with the fingers or tweezers. Start with the shorter part of the lash and place it on the natural lashes at the inner corner of the eye, toward the nose.

Note: You may wish to apply eyeliner before the lash is applied if it will not affect the false lash adhesion.

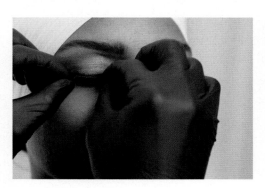

8 Position the rest of the artificial lash as close to the client's own lash as possible, not on the skin. Make sure there is not an excess of glue and that the client can open their eyes once applied. Remove any excess glue and reposition the lashes as necessary.

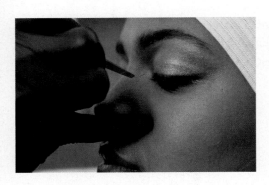

9 **For individual lashes**—Using tweezers, apply one at a time until you have five or six lashes that are evenly spaced across the lash line.

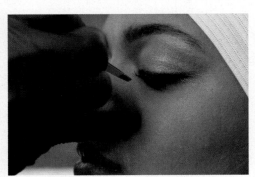

10 Use longer lashes on the outer edges of the eye, medium length in the middle, and short on the inside by the nose. Cut lash lengths as needed.

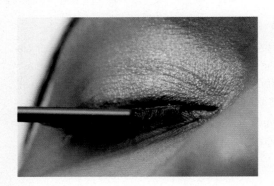

11 Use the rounded end of a lash liner brush, or tweezers, to press the lash on without adhering the brush or tweezers to the glue. Be very careful and gentle when applying the lashes. Remove any excess glue and rebrush or reposition lashes as necessary.

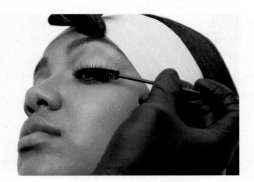

12 An additional liquid liner may be used to finish the look if it does not affect the false lash adhesion. Adding a coat of mascara can help false lashes adhere to natural lashes.

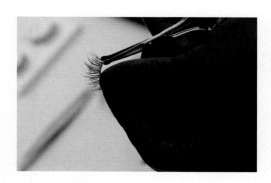

13 Optional: Apply the lower lash, if desired. Trim the lash as necessary. Scissors should not be used near the client's eyelashes as you might accidentally cut their natural lashes. Always cut the lashes away from the client. Once cut, place the lashes near the eye to check the size. If additional cutting is required, bring them down away from the client's eyes. When ready, apply adhesive in the same way you did for the upper lash. Place the lash on top of or beneath the client's lower lash. Place the shorter lash toward the center of the eye and the longer lash toward the outer part.

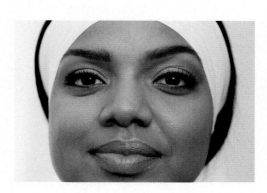

14 Check the finished application and make sure the client is comfortable with the lashes. Remind the client to take special care with artificial lashes when swimming, bathing, and cleansing the face. Water, oil, or cleansing products will loosen artificial lashes. Band lash applications last one day and are meant to be removed nightly.

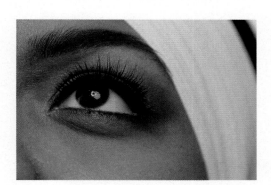

FINISHED LOOK

POST-SERVICE

- Complete Procedures 7–2 and 8–9: Post-Service Procedures.

Procedure 12-3:
Tinting Lashes and Brows

Implements and Materials

SUPPLIES
- EPA-registered disinfectant
- Headband
- Hand towels
- Plastic mixing cup
- Distilled water
- Small bowl of water
- Timer
- Brow comb or mascara wand
- Eyeliner brush
- Small scissors
- Lined waste container
- Emergency eyewash kit

PRODUCTS
- Cleanser or eye makeup remover
- Witch-hazel
- Petroleum jelly/occlusive cream
- Lash tint kits: colors may include black for lashes and brown for brows unless client requests otherwise

SINGLE-USE ITEMS
- Cotton swabs
- Round cotton pads
- Protective paper sheaths

Preparation

- Perform Procedures 7–1 and 8–1: Pre-Service Procedures.

Procedure

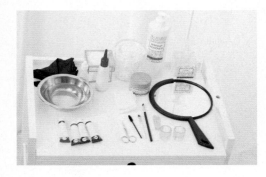

1 Wash hands and put on gloves.

2 Gather and set out supplies.

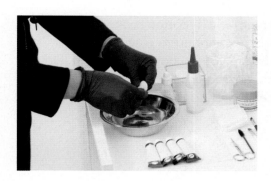

3 Wet cotton pads and cotton swabs.

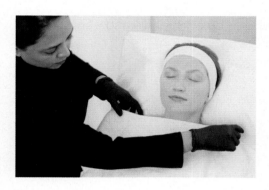

4 Conduct the client consultation, and have the client sign the release form. Drape the client with a headband and towel around the neck.

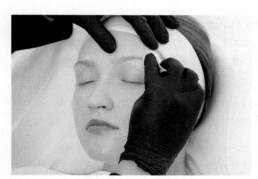

5 Cleanse the brow and/or lash area. All makeup must be removed and the area clean and dry before applying tint.

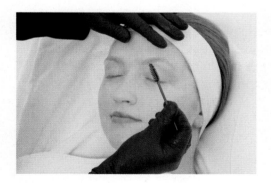

6 Brush brows into place.

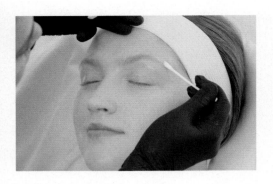

7 Apply protective cream with a cotton swab directly next to the area where you are tinting to protect the skin, covering the area where you do not want the tint. Do not touch the hairs with cream because this interferes with the color. Apply cream around the brow area.

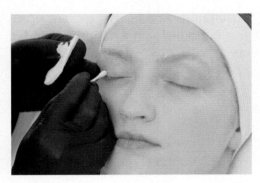

8 Apply cream on the skin below the eye and above the lashes, just next to the lash line.

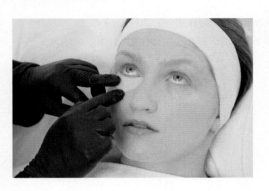

9 **Apply pads for lash tinting**—Apply pads under the eyes and over the cream to keep tint from bleeding onto the skin. Use the paper sheaths in the tint kit.

You may have to cut or adjust pad shapes to fit under the eyes. Pads should be under the lashes as close to the eye as possible without holding or interfering with the lower lashes.

To make cotton pads—Wet the pads and squeeze out excess water, tearing them so they are half as thick. Then fold in half to make half-moon-shaped pads.

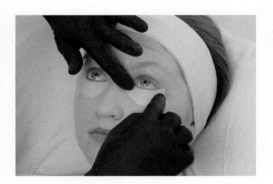

10 Adjust the pads—Have the client close their eyes, and adjust the pad so it sits next to the eye, not bunched up too close to the eye. If the pad is too close or too wet, tint may wick into the eye and onto the skin.

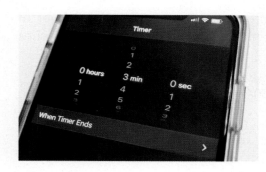

11 Prepare your timer according to the manufacturer's directions and have wet pads and cotton swabs ready to use for rinsing. *Note:* You can start with the lashes and do the brows while the lash tint is processing. Generally, tint can sit on the lashes longer than the brows if you are going for a natural brow look.

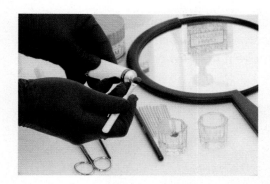

12 **Prepare the tint**— Place the amount of product you need into a cup-shaped palette. The brow tint can be diluted with water in a 1:1 ratio in a mixing cup to lighten the color.

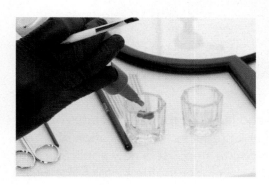

13 Some tint kits have only one bottle and combine the tint and developer into one application. If your kit requires the addition of developer to the tint be sure to add it at this time and mix well.

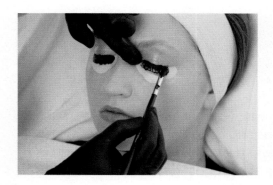

14 **Apply the lash tint**—For the lashes, brush the product from the base of the lashes to the ends. Do not double-dip—use a new applicator each time to reapply.

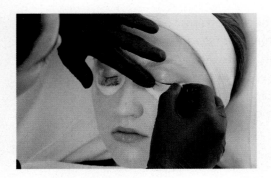

Note: Some manufacturers may suggest a second layer of protective sheaths that may be fitted over the tinted lashes at this time.

15 **Apply the brow tint**—For the brows, apply the color from the inside to the outside edge. Do not double-dip—use a new applicator each time to reapply and work across the brows. **Caution:** Brows can absorb color quickly, so be ready to remove it right away to avoid excess color.

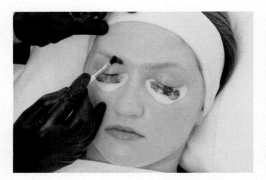 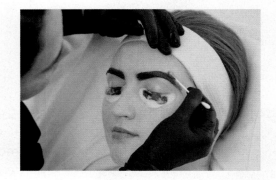

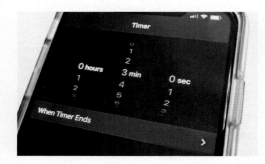

16 Begin the timer and leave on for three minutes or as directed. If your kit requires the application of developer in a separate step, use a new applicator to carefully apply the developer (bottle #2 for some kits) for one minute or as directed.

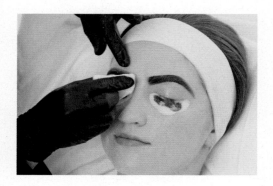

17 Rinse each area with water at least three times with wet cotton swabs and cotton pads without dripping water into the eyes. Have an emergency eyewash kit available in case any product gets into the client's eye.

Tip: Before rinsing, you can replace the under-eye shields if necessary (if color is bleeding through the pads to the skin). Make sure the tint does not touch the skin.

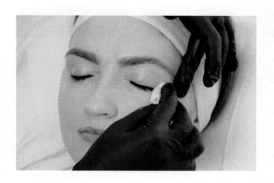

18 Remove the protective pads and continue to rinse the area thoroughly.

> # CAUTION!
> To avoid eye damage, do not let tint or water drip into the client's eyes. Have the client keep their eyes closed throughout the treatment.

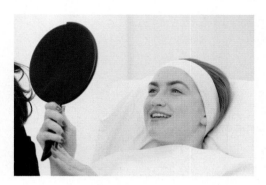

19 Ask the client if they feel any discomfort and have them flush the eyes with water at the sink if necessary. It is common for the eyes to feel a little grainy after tinting, so rinsing is a good idea. Show the application to the client.

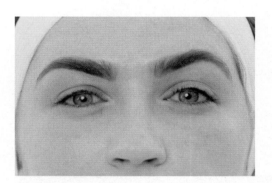

FINISHED LOOK

POST-SERVICE

- Complete Procedures 7–2 and 8–9: Post-Service Procedures.

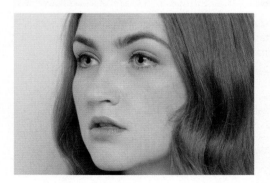

COMPETENCY 👁 PROGRESS

How are you doing with makeup essentials? **Check the Chapter 12 Learning Objectives below that you feel you have mastered; leave unchecked those concepts you will need to return to.**

- ☐ Explain makeup essentials as it relates to an esthetician's skill set.
- ☐ Describe the principles of cosmetic color theory.
- ☐ Use color theory to choose and coordinate makeup color selection.
- ☐ Identify face shapes and proportions for makeup applications.
- ☐ Describe the different types of cosmetics and their uses.
- ☐ Prepare the makeup station and supplies for clients.
- ☐ Follow infection control requirements for makeup services.
- ☐ Conduct a thorough makeup consultation with a client.
- ☐ Perform makeup application techniques.
- ☐ Use highlighting and contouring techniques for balance and proportion.
- ☐ Create makeup looks for special occasions.
- ☐ Apply makeup for the camera and special events.
- ☐ Recognize the benefits of camouflage makeup.
- ☐ Demonstrate the application of artificial lashes.
- ☐ Describe tinting lashes and brows on a makeup client.
- ☐ Explain the benefits of permanent makeup application.
- ☐ Describe the benefits of a career in makeup.
- ☐ Promote retail services as a makeup artist.

GLOSSARY

alcohol based AL-kuh-hawl BAYST	pg. 566	refers to makeup with extreme durability that is popular with special effects artists as well as for temporary tattoos; alcohol-based makeup is not ideal for prolonged wear as it can exacerbate dry skin
analogous colors an-AL-uh-gus colorz	pg. 554	colors that are located directly next to each other on the color wheel
band lashes BAND lash-ez	pg. 606	also known as *strip lashes*; eyelash hairs on a strip that are applied with adhesive to the natural lash line
blush BLUSH	pg. 569	makeup that gives the face a natural-looking glow and helps create facial balance
bracing BRAY-sing	pg. 586	technique using one or both hands positioned to avoid client injury, keeping your hands steady and the client safe
brow comb BROW kohm	pg. 574	a tool used to brush eyebrow hairs into the desired position, creating a finely groomed look; in addition to the comb itself, many brow combs have a brush on one side

brushes (makeup) BRUSH-ez	pg. 574	Used for applying and blending powder, blush, and eyeshadows, as they work better than sponge tips or fingers; brushes vary in size, shape, make, use, cost, and longevity; brushes are the artist's most essential tool, as they allow for better control and blending
cake makeup KAYK MAYK-up	pg. 567	also known as *pancake makeup*; a heavy-coverage makeup pressed into a compact and applied to the face with a moistened cosmetic sponge
complementary colors kahm-pluh-MEN-tur-ee KUL-urz	pg. 554	primary and secondary colors opposite one another on the color wheel
concealers kahn-SEEL-urs	pg. 568	cosmetics used to cover blemishes and discolorations; may be applied before or after foundation
cool colors KOOl KUL-urz	pg. 556	colors with a blue undertone that suggest coolness and are dominated by blues, greens, violets, and blue-reds
contouring KAHN-toor-ing	pg. 584	refers to makeup colors that are darker shades used to define the cheekbones and make features appear smaller
eyebrow gel formulations EYE-brow JEL form-yoo-LAY-shunz	pg. 570	makeup used to add color and shape to the eyebrows
eyebrow pencils EYE-brow PEN-silz	pg. 570	makeup used to add color and shape to the eyebrows
eyebrow pomades EYE-brow poh-MAYDZ	pg. 570	makeup used to add color and shape to the eyebrows
eyebrow shadows EYE-brow SHAD-ohz	pg. 570	makeup used to add color and shape to the eyebrows
eyeliner EYE-lyn-ur	pg. 570	makeup used to emphasize the eyes; it is available in pencil, liquid, and pressed (cake) form
eyeshadows EYE shad-ohz	pg. 569	makeup used to accentuate and contour the eyes
eye tabbing EYE tab-ing	pg. 607	procedure in which individual synthetic eyelashes are attached directly to a client's own lashes at their base
ferrule FAIR-uhl	pg. 576	the metal part that holds makeup brushes intact
foundation fown-DAY-shun	pg. 566	also known as *base makeup*; a tinted cosmetic used to cover or even out skin tone and coloring of the skin
greasepaint GREES-paint	pg. 567	heavy makeup used for theatrical purposes
high-definition makeup HY-def-uh-nish-un MAYK-up	pg. 604	designed to be invisible when using high-definition cameras; formulated with super-fine microparticles that blend into the skin to provide a flawless complexion
highlighters HY-lyt-urz	pg. 584	makeup that is lighter than the skin color; accentuate and bring out features such as the brow bone under the eyebrow, the temples, the chin, and the cheekbones
hue HYOO	pg. 553	any color in its purest form, lacking any black (shade) or white (tint); the hue of a color represents just one dimension of a particular color
individual lashes in-dih-VIJ-oo-al lash-ez	pg. 606	separate artificial eyelashes that are applied on top of the lashes one at a time
lash comb lash KOHM	pg. 574	separates lashes so they look finished and are not clumpy or messy looking; used before applying mascara or when the mascara is still wet

lip color LIP KUL-ur	pg. 571	makeup that gives color to the face and provides a finish to your makeup design
lip conditioner LIP kun-DIH-shun-ur	pg. 589	an application such as a lip moisturizer that is put on when starting the makeup application, so it can soak in and moisturize before starting to apply the liner; a primer, foundation, or plumper can be applied prior to the lip color
lip gloss LIP GLAWS	pg. 589	can give a shiny, moisturized look to the lips
lip liners LIP LYN-urz	pg. 589	colored pencils used to line and define the lips
liquid foundation LIK-wud fown-DAY-shun	pg. 567	type of foundation made of suspension of organic and inorganic pigments in alcohol- and water-based solutions; bentonite (a clay base) is added to help keep the products blended and absorb excess oil; the liquid formulation is generally suited for clients with oily to normal skin conditions who desire sheer to medium coverage
makeup removers MEYK-uhp RE-moverz	pg. 571	either oil-based or water-based formulations to remove various types of makeup
mascara mas-KAIR-uh	pg. 570	makeup that darkens, defines, and thickens the eyelashes
matte MAT	pg. 566	nonshiny; dull
neutral colors NOO-trul colorz	pg. 556	colors that do not complement or contrast any other color; examples include brown and gray, along with multiple variations of each
oil based OYL BAYST	pg. 566	refers to foundations that contain mineral oil or other oils
permanent makeup PUR-muh-nent MAYK-up	pg. 609	cosmetic implantation technique that deposits colored pigment into the upper reticular layer of the dermis, similar to tattooing
primary colors PRY-mayr-ee KUL-urz	pg. 553	yellow, red, and blue; fundamental colors that cannot be obtained from a mixture
primers PRIH-murz	pg. 567	liquids or silicone-based formulas designed to go underneath foundation and other products to prepare the skin for makeup and to help keep the product on the skin; primers provide a smooth surface for the makeup, while keeping product off the skin so that it is not broken down by the natural oils of the skin
regular mascara reg-YOO-lar mas-KAIR-uh	pg. 570	makeup that darkens, defines, and thickens the eyelashes; a good daily use product that can be easily removed with regular eye makeup remover
ruddy RHUD-ee	pg. 558	refers to skin that is red, wind burned, or affected by rosacea
sallow SAL-oh	pg. 559	refers to skin that has a yellowish hue
saturation sach-uh-RAY-shun	pg. 554	refers to the pureness of a color or the dominance of hue in a color
secondary colors SEK-un-deh-ree KUL-urz	pg. 553	colors obtained by mixing equal parts of two primary colors
shade SHAYD	pg. 555	refers to degree of saturation; occurs when black is added to a pure hue
silicone based SIL-ih-kohn BAYST	pg. 566	refers to products that are good for occluding the skin and proving a more even surface; they can also diffuse imperfections

tabs TABZ	pg. 606	small clusters of three or four artificial eyelashes on one point of attachment
tertiary colors TUR-shee-ayr-ee KUL-urz	pg. 553	intermediate colors achieved by mixing a secondary color and its neighboring primary color on the color wheel in equal amounts
tint TINT	pg. 555	refers to degree of saturation; occurs when white is added to a pure hue
tone (skin) TOHN	pg. 557	also known as *hue*; in terms of skin, this is a term used to describe the warmth or coolness of a color; generally classified as light, medium, or dark
translucent powder tranz-LOO-sent POW-dur	pg. 584	colorless and sheer makeup that blends with all foundations and will not change color when applied
undertone (skin) UN-dur-tohn	pg. 558	also known as *contributing pigment*; a subdued shade of a color; a color on which another color has been imposed and which can be seen through the other color; the underlying color that emerges during the lifting process of melanin that contributes to the end result
value VAL-yoo	pg. 555	also known as *brightness of a color*; how light or dark it is, which depends on the amount of light emanating from the color
warm colors WORM KUL-urz	pg. 556	the range of colors with yellow undertones; from yellow and gold through oranges, red-oranges, most reds, and even some yellow-greens
water based WAW-tur BAYST	pg. 566	refers to oil-free products; water-based foundations generally give a more matte finish and help conceal minor blemishes and discolorations
waterproof mascara WAW-tur-proof mas-KAIR-uh	pg. 571	makeup that darkens, defines, and thickens the eyelashes; is designed to stay on and not smudge when it comes in contact with water

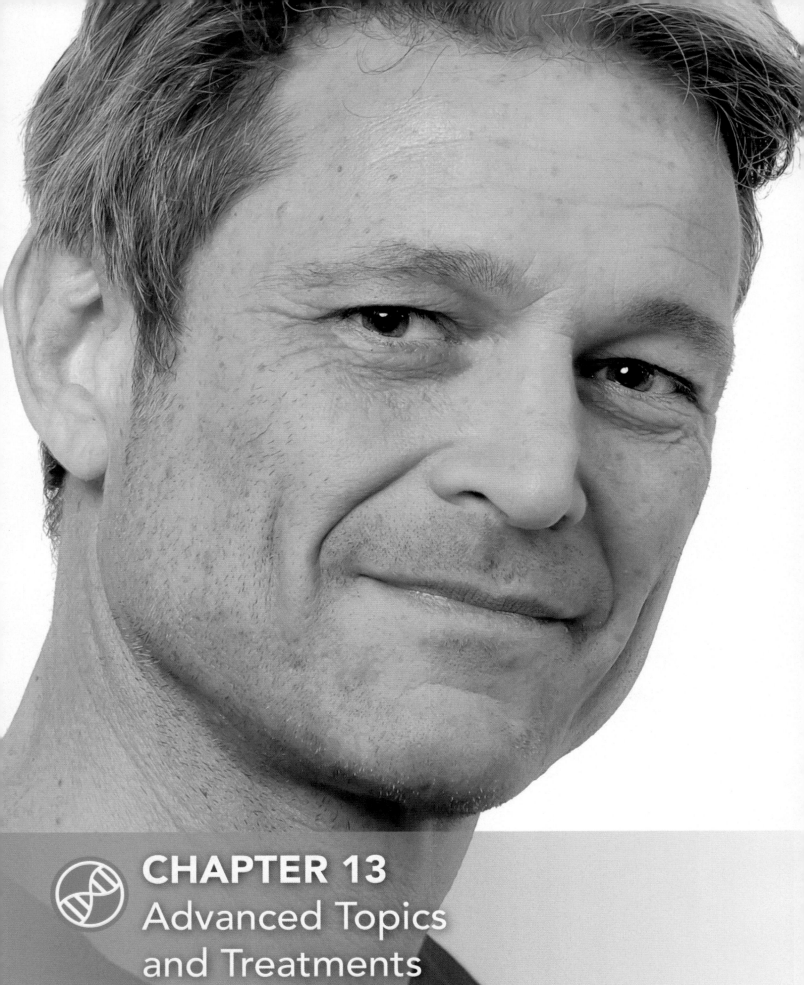

CHAPTER 13
Advanced Topics
and Treatments

"Love what you do and care to be different."

−Joel Gerson

Learning Objectives

After completing this chapter, you will be able to:

1. Explain advanced skin care topics and treatments for licensed, trained estheticians.
2. Describe chemical exfoliation and peels.
3. Identify how to safely and effectively use chemical exfoliation and peels.
4. Discuss the benefits of microdermabrasion by type of device.
5. Explain the benefits of laser technology.
6. Explain the benefits and types of light therapy.
7. Discuss microcurrent treatments.
8. Discuss ultrasound.
9. Discuss microneedling and nano infusion.
10. Describe spa body treatments.
11. Discuss common treatments used to address cellulite.
12. Explain the benefits of manual lymphatic drainage.
13. Describe the field of medical esthetics.

Explain Advanced Skin Care Topics and Treatments for Licensed, Trained Estheticians

Understanding the foundations of the equipment, indications, and contraindications will enable you to employ combination therapies that will yield greater results and client satisfaction. Advanced treatments have expanded the esthetician's repertoire to include more results-driven treatments such as chemical exfoliation and microdermabrasion, microcurrent, ultrasound, and light emitting diode (LED) (**Figure 13–1**).

Estheticians should study and have a thorough understanding of advanced topics and treatments because:

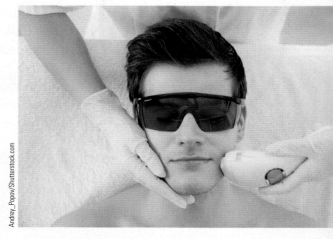

▲ **Figure 13–1** With new technologies being developed, the world of esthetics continues to grow.

- Advanced machine technology is always being developed and improved upon, and some of these technologies are expansions from the original formats.
- Offering advanced treatments will keep technicians competitive in the marketplace.
- The esthetician's professional expertise in analyzing the skin and recommending the best program helps make these procedures safe and effective.

Describe Chemical Exfoliation and Peels

What is chemical exfoliation? In the field of skin care, we define the process of removing excess accumulations of dead skin cells from the corneum layers of the epidermis as *superficial peeling*, *exfoliation*, *keratolysis*, and *desquamation*. These are interchangeable terms. This process can be accomplished mechanically (microdermabrasion), manually (scrubs), or chemically by the use of specific products (enzymes, alpha hydroxy acid (AHA), beta hydroxy acid (BHA), light Jessner's, and light trichloroacetic acid (TCA) peels) formulated to achieve this result. Advanced training and certification are necessary to perform exfoliating treatments and peels. Peels and chemical exfoliation services are efficient and take less time than the more relaxing, in-depth facials. Peels and chemical exfoliation services yield more significant results, help produce a clinical change in the skin, and are commonly used to address photoaging, acne, and hyperpigmentation, in addition to other conditions.

Chemical exfoliation and chemical peels come in many different formulations and strengths. Your regulatory agency will determine the guidelines regarding the strength and pH of the products you can use. You will determine the treatment protocol, including the type of acid, the procedure time, the strength, the application process, and the assisting ingredients. Protocols vary depending on the product line, but the basic process consists of applying the product, neutralizing, and removing it within a few minutes. Some peels do not require neutralizing, as they are self-neutralizing.

Acid, Alkaline, and pH Relationships

To understand the strengths of peels and the different formulations, it is important to understand acid, alkaline, and pH relationships. pH is an especially important consideration in peel products.

- Acids have a pH of 0 to 6; neutral is 7.
- Alkalines range from 8 to 14.

CAUTION!

Each regulatory agency is different, so check your local laws to see what is acceptable related to performing exfoliation services under your esthetics license.

The average pH of skin is 5.0 (typically between 4.5 to 5.5). Acids penetrate the skin and can be a cause of irritation because of their small molecular size. A pH of less than 3 is not recommended for salon peels, and most states do not allow use of a lower pH. *Buffering agents* are ingredients added to products to help make them less irritating. Products with a higher acid percentage and a lower pH are more irritating. The acid needs to have a pH lower than the skin's pH to be effective (**Figure 13–2**).

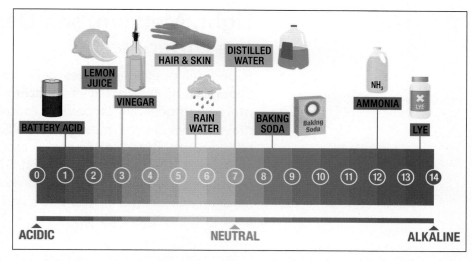

▲ **Figure 13–2** Potential hydrogen (pH) scale is used to measure the acidity and alkalinity of substances.

Putting it into perspective:

- A spa level of 30 percent concentration of glycolic acid is usually formulated to have a pH of 3 if it is buffered properly.
- Physician peels have a higher percentage concentration and lower pH.
- Over-the-counter (OTC) AHA home care product formulations contain from 2 to 15 percent acid.
- AHA home care product formulations sold by spas range from 5 to 10 percent acid.
- Physicians carry home care products with higher percentages of acid.

Peels are sometimes used to restore a skin's natural glow, which can be inhibited in hyperkeratinized skin and skin that is not functioning optimally at the physiological level. The **cell renewal factor (CRF)** (sell re-new-uhl fack-tor), or *cell turnover rate,* is the rate of cell mitosis and migration from the dermis to the top of the epidermis. This process slows down with age. The average rate of cell turnover rate for babies is 14 days; for teenagers, 21 to 28 days; for adults, 28 to 42 days; for those 50 and older, 42 to 84 days. Keeping cell mitosis going is one of the goals of skin preservation.

Factors influencing the CRF include genetics, the natural environment, and one's medical history, lifestyle, personal care, and exfoliation methods. The keratinized corneum layer is composed of approximately 15 to 20 layers and varies in thickness in different body areas. While exfoliating is great for the skin, a hydrolipidic balance must be maintained, especially for alipidic (dry) skin. Overpeeling is detrimental to the skin, and monitoring the client during a treatment plan is imperative.

Light, Medium, and Deep Peels—What Is the Difference?

Superficial peeling removes cells from only the stratum corneum. Superficial or light peels (chemical exfoliators) are esthetician administered and generally (according to state-mandated license scope and practice) include enzymes, glycolic acid (30 percent or less), lactic acid (30 percent or less), and in some cases Jessner's solution and low percentage TCA (one to three layers). The term *chemical exfoliation* is sometimes used in place of the word *peel* to differentiate between the medium and deeper clinical *peels* and the lighter chemical exfoliation used in spas (**Figure 13–3**).

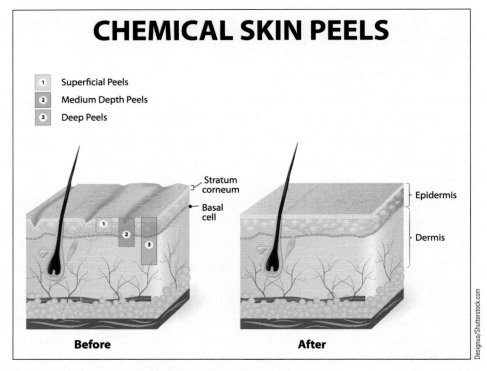

▲ **Figure 13–3** Before and after chemical skin peels.

Physicians use high strength peel formulations that are designed to penetrate deeper into the skin (the dermal layer). These peels are commonly referred to as *medium* or *deep peels*. Peels administered by physicians make use of the following chemicals:

- Resorcinol
- Phenol (carbolic acid, also called *Baker's peel*)
- Trichloroacetic acid (TCA)
- Glycolic acid (50 percent or more)
- **Jessner's peel** (JEZZ-nuhrz PEEL); 4 to 10 layers, which contains lactic acid, salicylic acid, and resorcinol in an ethanol solvent

- TCA, a medium-depth peel that removes the epidermis down to the dermis
- Phenol, a highly acidic deep peel that peels down into the dermis. This peel is not commonly used, but is still important to be aware of.

Medium-depth peels are performed primarily with stronger TCA concentrations by physicians to remove the entire epidermis and part of the papillary dermis. Although not used often, deep peels are performed primarily with a phenol solution by physicians to peel deep within the dermis. There has been a movement toward the use of ablative lasers (erbium and fractional CO_2) versus deep peeling solutions due to the ability to control the depth of the procedure with the former method. With lasers, you can limit the number of passes but peel solutions may penetrate beyond the desired depth.

General Effects of Chemical Exfoliation and Peels

Peels and chemical exfoliation result in:

- Improved texture of the skin, barrier function, and moisture retention
- Increased cell renewal factor (CRF), hydration, and intercellular lipids
- Reduced fine lines, wrinkles, and surface pigmentation
- Skin that looks and feels smoother and softer
- Improved skin conditions such as acne, hyperpigmentation, clogged pores, and dry skin
- Potential stimulation of elastin and collagen production.

Keep in mind the more intense the peel, the better the results, but you must also use caution to avoid complications. The client should also be made aware of the differences in "downtime" as it pertains to peel intensity.

General Contraindications to and Precautions for Chemical Exfoliation and Peels

Exfoliated skin needs to be protected from sun exposure and tanning to avoid hyperpigmentation and damage to the skin. Sunscreen must be used daily when using AHAs or other strong exfoliating products or treatments.

Chemical exfoliation and peels can result in burns that may require medical attention and can scar a client. It is important to obtain as much training as possible in working with chemicals. Consult with the client before applying a chemical exfoliant, follow the manufacturer's instructions, and whenever possible perform a patch test (inner arm, inner wrist, inside crease of elbow, or behind the ear) 24 to 48 hours before giving a treatment to watch for adverse reactions to the product.

Chemical exfoliation contraindications include the following:

- Recent cosmetic surgeries, laser resurfacing, chemical peels, or dermabrasion
- Recent injectables, fillers, or Botox® (*Note:* Depends on how recent and the depth of the peel, so ask your physician or specialist that administered the treatment.)
- Use of Retin-A® or other medications that exfoliate or thin the skin (For example, client must be off Accutane six months prior to the service.)
- Allergies or sensitivities to products or ingredients
- Pregnancy
- Active herpes simplex
- Hyperpigmentation tendencies
- Inflamed rosacea or acne
- Infectious diseases
- Open sores or suspicious lesions
- Sunburn or irritated skin
- Photosensitizing medications (make skin very sensitive to sun)
- Other contraindicated drugs or medication.

To prevent skin damage, warn your clients to avoid sun exposure, scrubs, rubbing, pulling dead skin, depilatories, waxing, benzoyl peroxide, and exfoliating or glycolic acid products for at least 24 to 48 hours before or after any chemical exfoliation procedure. Recommend a longer period of time if the client's condition warrants it.

> ## CAUTION!
>
> As you learn more about facials and related treatments, you will become more familiar with the term *contraindication*. A contraindication is a predetermined condition that exists in your client that excludes them from using certain ingredients or products and/or from having certain treatments.

✓ CHECK IN

1. What are the benefits of chemical exfoliation?
2. What are general contraindications for chemical exfoliation?

Identify How to Safely and Effectively Use Chemical Exfoliation and Peels

It is important to identify the types of chemical exfoliation and peels available in the market today, and to understand the benefits and contraindications for each.

What Is an Enzyme Peel?

Enzyme treatments are often referred to as enzyme peels or an enzyme mask. Whereas physical exfoliants work to slough off dead cells sitting on the surface of the skin, enzymes are proteolytic in nature and work to digest the keratin (protein) in dead skin cells on the surface of the skin. Enzyme treatments, depending on their composition and your client's skin, can be gentle enough to repeat once a week. You will find that most clinical facials include the use of an enzyme mask for enhanced exfoliation and to assist in preparing the skin for easier extractions. Enzymes can also be combined with microdermabrasion (may be referred to as microdermabrasion peel combination), LED, and many other advanced treatments to prepare the skin to yield greater results and/or enhance exfoliation.

You will find that enzyme treatments come in a couple of different forms such as ready to use masks or a powder with a liquid activator that you need to mix just prior to application.

Ingredients found in enzymes include:

- Bromelain, which is derived from pineapples
- Papain, which is derived from the papaya fruit
- Pancreatin and trypsin, which are derived from meat by-products.

Always follow the manufacturer's directions for mixing, applying, and removing any enzyme treatment.

WHEN TO USE ENZYMES

When determining whether a treatment is appropriate for a client, consider the following factors: skin type, sebaceous gland activity, skin conditions, the client's philosophy of sun exposure, their cosmetic and product use, and whether they are using Retin-A, other acids/AHAs, and/or acne drugs such as Tetracycline or Doxycycline.

Enzyme peels can be applied once every one to two weeks but are usually used in conjunction with a clinical facial or to prepare for an advanced treatment such as microdermabrasion ultrasound or LED. Enzymes are not typically used prior to a chemical peel.

EFFECTS OF AN ENZYME PEEL

The results are very superficial, temporary, and provide a refreshed dewy complexion but none of the in-depth clinical changes such as those as seen with AHA, BHA, Jessner's, or TCA peels.

- Because most solutions will be in the form of a mask, you may be unable to see the skin's response and you will rely on information obtained from the client to determine if the mask is processing according to expectations. (There should be no reaction beyond very light tingling or the absence of any tingling.)
- If you are applying a mask you can see the skin through it, it is expected to initially see the skin experience a very light erythema or even turn pink. The client may experience minimal or no tingling while the solution is actively processing. You are looking for pinkness, not redness, as this is an enzyme peel.

CONTRAINDICATIONS AND BEST PRACTICES FOR ENZYME PEELS

- Remember to always consult the manufacturer's instructions.
- Eyewear is always recommended to protect the client and technician. OSHA requires that anytime a corrosive agent is used, the technician must wear protective eyewear with side shields. An OSHA-approved emergency eyewash station is also required. Not all enzymes are categorized as corrosive, so you must consult the SDS sheet provided by the manufacturer for full information.
- The manufacturer will provide instructions on the application and removal processes. The general application process for a basic enzyme peel involves cleansing, toning, applying the enzyme peel, processing according to the manufacturer's instructions, rinsing, and applying moisturizer and a product with SPF.
- Some areas of the face may process sooner than others and you may need to perform spot removal on those areas. Some clients' entire face may process sooner than the manufacturer's recommended minimal processing time, in which case you will need to remove the entire peel immediately.
- The best rule of thumb as a newer esthetician, who may not yet have mastered efficient application and removal processes, is to be prepared to remove the peel just prior to reaching the endpoint to ensure you can complete neutralization and removal before the client becomes overprocessed. It is also recommended to have a closed container of extra 4" × 4" moistened esthetic wipes available for use if needed, as you will need them readily accessible.

┌─── PERFORM ───┐
Procedure 13-1
Enzyme Mask
└───────────────┘

┌─── PERFORM ───┐
Procedure 13-2
Back Facial with Enzyme Mask
└───────────────┘

What Is an AHA or a BHA Peel?

Alpha hydroxy acids (AHAs) are mild acids that come in different percentages and pH levels and help to dissolve the desmosomes between cells to keep skin cells exfoliated. AHAs penetrate the corneum via the intercellular matrix and loosen the bonds between the cells. The intercellular matrix between the skin cells consists of ceramides, lipids, glycoproteins, and active enzymes. AHAs also stimulate the production of intercellular lipids. *Glycolic acid*, a commonly used AHA, can penetrate the epidermis more effectively because it has the smallest molecular size of the AHAs. Follow the light glycolic peel procedure as described in Procedure 13–3 (**Figure 13–4**).

Most AHA peels you will use will not be at a level that will yield any peeling or flaking.

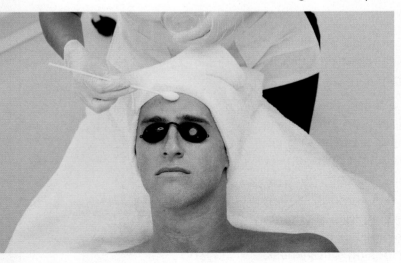

▲ **Figure 13–4 A glycolic acid exfoliation treatment.**

AHAs include:

- Glycolic acid is derived from sugar cane and is the strongest AHA.
- Lactic acid is derived from milk.
- Tartaric acid is derived from grapes.
- Malic acid is derived from apples.
- Citric acid is derived from citrus fruit (citric acid is now considered an AHA, rather than a BHA).
- Mandelic acid is derived from bitter almond.

BHAs work under the same premise as AHAs but are better suited to dissolve oil and are primarily used for oily skin and acne. You will find that BHA peels are usually stronger than AHA peels, but this will depend on the chemical formulations. You may encounter some slight flaking or mild peeling, depending on the strength of the BHA peel.

BHAs include salicylic acid, which is derived from sweet birch, willow bark, and wintergreen and has antiseptic and anti-inflammatory properties.

WHEN TO USE AHA PEELS

- When determining whether an AHA peel treatment is appropriate for a client, consider the following factors: skin type, sebaceous gland activity, skin conditions, the client's philosophy of sun exposure, their cosmetic and other product use, and whether they are using Retin-A, and/or other acids/AHAs, or acne drugs such as Tetracycline or Doxycycline.

- It is preferred (but not required) that clients begin a home care regimen to prepare the skin for peels, but not every client is willing to commit in this way. Pretreating assists in providing optimal outcomes because you are beginning the plan with a more acclimated and prepared skin surface. A home care plan should include at least a cleanser, retinol and/or AHA cream, vitamin C, and a product with sunscreen. Other products should be added according to the issues that you are targeting such as skin lightening products for pigmentation issues.

- Home care plans that work in tandem with the in-office clinical treatment plan are very important. The best way to convey their importance to a client is by emphasizing that you are providing the peel to assist in restoring the skin to optimal functioning capacity, but you are not performing any home maintenance; neglecting the home maintenance is like taking two steps forward and one step back. The home care plan is similar to the pretreatment plan mentioned earlier in this discussion.

- Treatment plans begin with a series of treatments to jump-start progress. A series can consist of six to eight peels administered once a week over six to eight weeks. During the series and at the end of the series, monitor the client's progress and determine if the goals have

—PERFORM—
Procedure 13-3
Light Glycolic Peel

CAUTION!
When employing BHA peels, keep in mind that aspirin is derived from salicylates, so clients who are allergic to aspirin may be allergic to salicylic ingredients. Clients must be directed to follow all home care regimens to ensure optimal outcomes and to minimize complications.

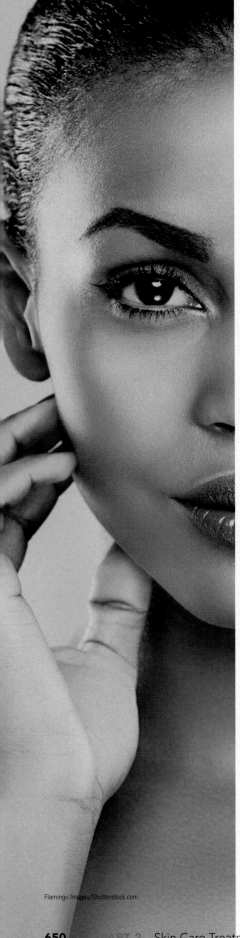

been met or if you need to administer another series (your assessment determines the number of sessions and the length of the series), move up to a stronger peel, or move to the maintenance phase.

- In the maintenance phase, you maintain the results by administering a monthly maintenance peel. You may also boost progress throughout the year by adding a series when desired. An example would be to schedule a series every fall to address any summer photodamage.

- Some technicians' treatment plans work on a graduated peeling system where you start with the mildest level peel, such as a 2 percent lactic acid, for the first couple of peels in the series and then move up to a low-dose glycolic acid, working up to a 20 percent glycolic acid and then ending with a 30 percent glycolic acid.

- Stronger superficial peel treatment plans are administered to clients whose skin is cleared for this level of peeling and to those who want to achieve faster results or have conditions that are better addressed with a stronger superficial peel such as severe sun damage, more in-depth age-related skin issues, or hyperpigmentation. An example is a series of 5 percent TCA peels once every three to four weeks or 10 percent TCA once every four weeks. When working at this advanced level, the technician needs to be very diligent in monitoring progress to ensure they are administering the next peel only well after the skin has recovered from the previous peel. Client input is paramount.

- Photo documentation before and after peels and during the series is advantageous because it is good business practice for your personal records and it is also beneficial documentation of the client's progress. Important reminder: Peel schedules depend on the product's strength and the client's tolerance of the procedure.

WHEN TO USE BHA PEELS

- Pretreatment and home care guidelines are the same as for AHAs, but you may add in products specifically for clients with oilier skin and with acne, for example, an acne and blemish serum.

- BHAs are used primarily on clients with oilier skin and with acne. You will find these peels usually come in strengths of 20 to 30 percent and are much stronger than AHAs, so you will most likely administer the peels only once every two or more weeks. Clients will notice flaking and peeling, so it is important to mention this in the consultation.

- It is advisable to start with a lower strength and work up once you have a baseline for the client's reaction to the procedure.

- A series can be implemented according to your client's goals and the outcomes achieved.

- The maintenance phase begins once the goals have been met and you want to maintain the results.

CONTRAINDICATIONS AND BEST PRACTICES OF AHA AND BHA PEELS

You generally follow the same course of action during and after both AHA and BHA peels, including the following:

- Before a chemical exfoliation service, discuss potential issues and contraindications during the client consultation. Explain the procedures, expected outcomes, and realistic goals.

- In a diagnostic facial or skin analysis before scheduling treatments, note on the client intake form the condition of the skin, including dehydration, hyperpigmentation, open lesions, and any other skin conditions. Also choose the type of exfoliant based on the condition of the client's skin and the desired results.

- Always keep in mind the manufacturer's instructions throughout the process and while performing the peel consultation.

- Eyewear is always recommended to protect the client and technician. OSHA requires that any time a corrosive agent is used, the technician must wear protective eyewear with side shields. An OSHA-approved emergency eyewash station is also required.

- Other precautions may be taken such as applying occlusive barriers to the corners of the eyes, the mouth, and around the nostril area.

- Because the sun is stronger during the summer and outdoor exposure is more frequent, chemical exfoliation and other exfoliation procedures (e.g., microdermabrasion) should be used with extreme caution during those months and should be avoided in some cases where the client is not willing to take precautions to avoid inadvertent exposure during their daily activities.

- The manufacturer will provide instructions on the application and removal process. General application for basic peel involves cleansing, toning, applying the peel, processing according to the manufacturer's instructions, neutralizing if directed by the manufacturer, rinsing, and applying moisturizer and a product with SPF.

- During the application there will be slight stinging and tingling and you may want to provide clients a fan to cool the face during the application.

- During the neutralizing or rinsing step, the peel may temporarily reactivate for a few seconds due to the water rehydrating the peel, and the client may experience an increased tingling or stinging sensation.

- Immediately after application the client will have a rosy glow and even mild erythema of the skin.

- With a BHA peel, there may be salicylic crystal residue present, which should not be confused with frosting from a Jessner's or TCA peel. In some cases when a 30 percent BHA is used the client may experience frosting around thinned skin such as under the eyes, at the corners of the eyes and mouth, or even around blemishes (which is why some manufacturers recommend using an occlusive barrier in some areas).

- Sometimes a Wood's lamp is used with BHA applications to view the accuracy and evenness of the peel application, as the peel can be illuminated by the lamp.

What Is a Jessner's or a TCA Peel?

A Jessner's peel is categorized as a stronger superficial peel and utilizes a Jessner's solution, which is a mixture of salicylic acid, resorcinol, lactic acid, and ethanol. You may find some of these formulas contain 2 percent phenol. Trichloracetic acid peels are also known as TCA peels. Some states allow estheticians to perform superficial peeling with a Jessner's or a TCA. These peels are achieved at a superficial level by applying low percentages and fewer layers than are found with the medium-level peelings performed by physicians, which remove the entire epidermis and part of the papillary dermis.

Both Jessner's and TCA peels work on the premise of protein coagulation; therefore, there will be flaking and peeling. How much peeling will depend on the intensity of the peel and the client. These peels are not neutralized and sometimes may remain on the face, with the client rinsing the residue off several hours later. Clients must be directed to follow all home care regimens to ensure optimal outcomes and to minimize complications.

WHEN TO USE JESSNER'S AND TCA PEELS

- When determining whether a specific treatment is appropriate for a client, consider the following factors: skin type, sebaceous gland activity, skin conditions, the client's philosophy of sun exposure, their cosmetic and product use, and whether they are using Retin-A, other acids/AHAs, or acne drugs such as Tetracycline or Doxycycline.

- Pretreatment and home care guidelines are the same as those for AHAs, but you may add in products specifically to address aging or sun-damage such as antioxidants or skin lightening agents. For those who have oilier and acneic skin you may add in products such as an acne and blemish serum.

- Jessner's peels are primarily used on clients with oilier skin and acne but are also used to address sun damage. The Jessner's solution is usually applied in several layers, according to the manufacturer's directions. You will find these peels are much stronger than AHAs, so you will most likely administer the peels only once every three to four or more weeks. Clients will notice flaking and peeling, so it is important to mention this in the consultation.

- TCA peels are used primarily for clients experiencing aging and sun damage. The TCA solution is usually applied in several layers, according to the manufacturer's directions. You will find these peels are much stronger than AHAs, so you will most likely administer the peels only once every three to four or more weeks. Clients will notice flaking and peeling, so it is important to mention this in the consultation.

- It is advisable to start with a lower strength and work up once you have a baseline for the client's reaction to the procedure.

- Series can be implemented according to your client's goals and the outcomes achieved. An example of a series is four TCA peels administered once every three to four weeks, then moving to maintenance with lower-dose peels such as a 30 percent AHA once a month.

- The maintenance phase begins once the goals have been met and you and the client want to maintain the results. Always remember that if you are using a more advanced peel before the maintenance phase, a lower-dose peel will not fully maintain the results, and a refresher peel (or series) needs to be administered periodically.

CONTRAINDICATIONS AND BEST PRACTICES FOR JESSNER'S AND TCA PEELS

The same course of action is generally followed during and following both Jessner's and TCA peels, including the following specifics:

- During the client consultation before a chemical exfoliation service, discuss the issues the client would like to address along with contraindications. Explain the procedures, the expected outcome, and realistic goals. In a diagnostic facial or skin analysis before scheduling treatments, note on the client intake form the condition of the skin, including dehydration, hyperpigmentation, open lesions, and any other skin conditions. Also choose the type of exfoliant based on the client's skin condition and the results desired.

- Remember to always consult the manufacturer's instructions throughout the process and while performing the prepeel consultation.

- Eyewear is always recommended to protect the client and technician. OSHA requires that anytime a corrosive agent is used, the technician must wear protective eyewear with side shields. An OSHA-approved emergency eyewash station is also required.

- Other precautions may be taken such as applying occlusive barriers to the corners of the eyes, mouth, and around the nostril area.

- Because sun is stronger during the summer and outdoor exposure is more frequent, chemical exfoliation and other exfoliation procedures (e.g., microdermabrasion) should be used with extreme caution during those months and should be avoided in some cases in which the client is not willing to take precautions to avoid inadvertent exposure during their daily activities.

- The manufacturer will provide instructions on the application and removal processes. The general application process for Jessner's and TCA peels involves cleansing, toning, applying the peel, processing according to the manufacturer's instructions, rinsing if directed by the manufacturer, and applying moisturizer and a product with SPF protection.

- During the application process there will be more stinging and tingling than is experienced with AHA and BHA peels, and you may

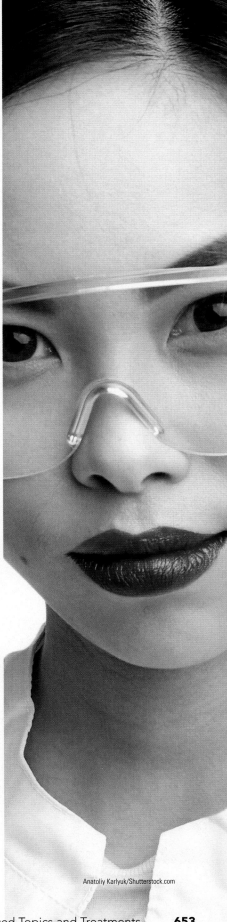

Anatoliy Karlyuk/Shutterstock.com

want to provide clients with a fan to cool the face during the application. Sometimes a Wood's lamp is used with BHA applications to view the accuracy and evenness of the peel application, as the peel can be illuminated with the lamp.

- Immediately after application the client will have mild erythema, pink or reddening of the skin, and there may be areas of frosting of the skin or an overall light frost (depending on depth of the peel) due to protein coagulation. With more superficial Jessner's or TCA peels, the frost will present as a whitish opaque haze but you will still see the pink or redness below. With medium or deeper peels, when more layers have been added, the frost will become more pronounced.

- A few hours later and especially the next day, the skin will become bronzed and will tighten over the next few days.

- Flaking or peeling will begin over the areas of the face that move the most, then all other areas will experience the same. The intensity of flaking or peeling will depend on the peel type and level of peel. It is important for clients to be instructed not to pick or peel off loose skin as this may cause a wound that could result in postinflammatory hyperpigmentation or scarring.

- Once the peel process has been completed and the skin has normalized, clients can return to their normal skin care products.

What Is a Designer Peel?

To yield more targeted results, additional ingredients may be added to formulas, including pigment lighteners, acne ingredients, and moisturizers or hydrators (Table 13–1).

▼ TABLE 13–1 Beneficial Ingredients to Combine with Chemical Exfoliation

Skin Condition	Beneficial Ingredients
Mature and/or sensitive skin	Glycolic acid, lactic acid, ceramides, hyaluronic acid, phospholipids, linoleic acid, aloe vera, allantoin, kojic acid, licorice root, peptides
Hyperpigmentation	Glycolic acid, kojic acid, licorice root, mulberry extract, bearberry extract, azelaic acid, ascorbic acid
Acne	Glycolic acid, lactic acid, salicylic acid, azelaic acid, citric acid

 CHECK IN

3. How do alpha hydroxy acids exfoliate the skin?
4. What are enzyme peels and typical results?
5. What type of skin conditions benefit most from BHA peels?
6. What is a Jessner's peel?

Discuss the Benefits of Microdermabrasion by Type of Device

Microdermabrasion (MI-kroh-DERMA-bray-shun) is a machine-based exfoliation treatment that uses a crystal spray or diamond tips to gently polish dead skin cells from the skin's surface. Today, many microdermabrasion models are available for use by estheticians and physicians. Physician-grade machines typically consist of stronger vacuum settings and more abrasive diamond tips (**Figure 13–5**).

Crystal Microdermabrasion

The crystal microdermabrasion procedure is achieved by spraying high-grade microcrystals, composed of corundum (kah-RUN-dum) powder, aluminum oxide, or a similar abrasive material across the skin's surface through a hand piece.

The crystal microdermabrasion technique is similar to running the vacuum/suction machine across the face. Crystals are first sprayed on the skin through the hand piece, and then are vacuumed off simultaneously. Because not all crystals are removed by the vacuum this treatment is considered messy and requires additional clean-up for the esthetician, and the crystal dust can pose a respiratory hazard for the esthetician. The used crystals are collected in a collection tube and must be disposed of according to the biohazard clean-up process recommended by the machine manufacturer. Crystals can also be used manually without the machine—this process is considered gentler on the skin and is called manual microdermabrasion.

DID YOU KNOW?

Estheticians should wear a mask during crystal microdermabrasion treatments, but there is still concern over lingering crystal residue on surfaces as the crystal dust can pose a respiratory hazard for the esthetician.

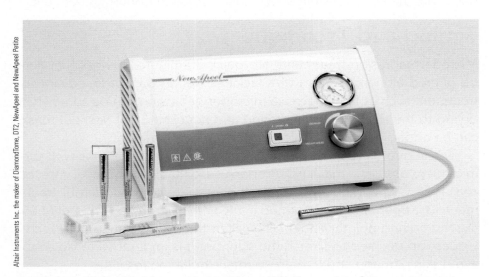

Altair Instruments Inc. the maker of DiamondTome, DT2, NewApeel and NewApeel Petite

▲ **Figure 13–5** Physician-grade machines typically consist of stronger vacuum settings and more abrasive diamond tips.

Crystal-Free Microdermabrasion

The crystal-free microdermabrasion technique consists of a diamond-tip applicator that gently polishes away the upper layers of the skin without the use of messy crystals and has gained popularity over the crystal option as it yields the same results without the clean-up or expense of crystals (**Figure 13–6**). Follow the steps described in Procedure 13–4: Crystal-Free Microdermabrasion (Diamond Tip).

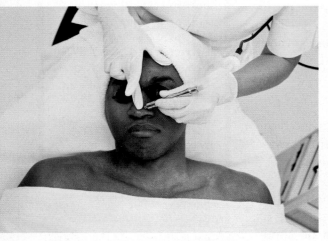

▲ **Figure 13–6** Microdermabrasion machines exfoliate the skin.

Hydradermabrasion (Wet Microdermabrasion)

A procedure similar to microdermabrasion, that is called *hydradermabrasion* or *wet microdermabrasion*, is gaining popularity. This noninvasive and nonirritating procedure combines mechanical and liquid exfoliation with serum penetration and hydration via a machine similar to the closed loop system as found with a crystal microdermabrasion machine. Serum is expelled through a hand piece that has interchangeable tips. In the initial stages of the treatment, the hand piece is used with an abrasive tip that comes into contact with the skin to provide a deep cleansing, extraction, and exfoliation action. The hand piece then uptakes the used serum and deposits it in a collection jar to be discarded after the treatment. The tip is then changed out to focus on deposition and penetration of specific target serums such as growth factors and brightening as well as serums to sooth and hydrate the skin. This treatment can also be combined with LED or microcurrent for additional antiaging benefits. The benefit of this technology is that it provides reliable exfoliation without the drying after-effects of microdermabrasion or the harshness of some chemical peels with the added benefit of extended hydration following treatment.

Timing and Technique

Microdermabrasion treatments are quick 30-minute services that can be offered alone or as part of a facial as well as part of an advanced treatment such as LED. Because microdermabrasion can be somewhat drying to the skin, a quick hydrating and nourishing gel or sheet mask can be added as part of a microdermabrasion treatment.

Technique plays a vital role in creating optimal outcomes with the microdermabrasion machine. Proper use of the hand piece, rate of crystal flow, and vacuum setting all contribute to a successful treatment. The treatment is performed in the area of stretched skin between the thumb and pointer finger, also called the action zone. Other techniques can be used to stretch the skin, but it is imperative to do so to avoid skin damage and to gain optimal exfoliation results.

The number of passes used during the treatment will be determined by the client's skin type and condition, the presence of erythema, and how the client tolerates the treatment. Typically passes consist of horizontal, vertical, and diagonal directional applications (**Figure 13-7**). The cross-hatching method involves using only two passes, can be used to complete the treatment quicker, and is one of the more popular approaches. On sensitive types you may find you use only one pass. More sensitive areas such as the neck may also require fewer passes, and one to two passes are commonly used. Higher vacuum settings, time in contact with the skin, and more passes yield more aggressive treatments. The endpoint for a microdermabrasion treatment is the presence of erythema.

Reading a manual does not provide instant experience in using this machine. Training and certification are mandatory. Microdermabrasion machines should be used by licensed, trained skin care professionals only.

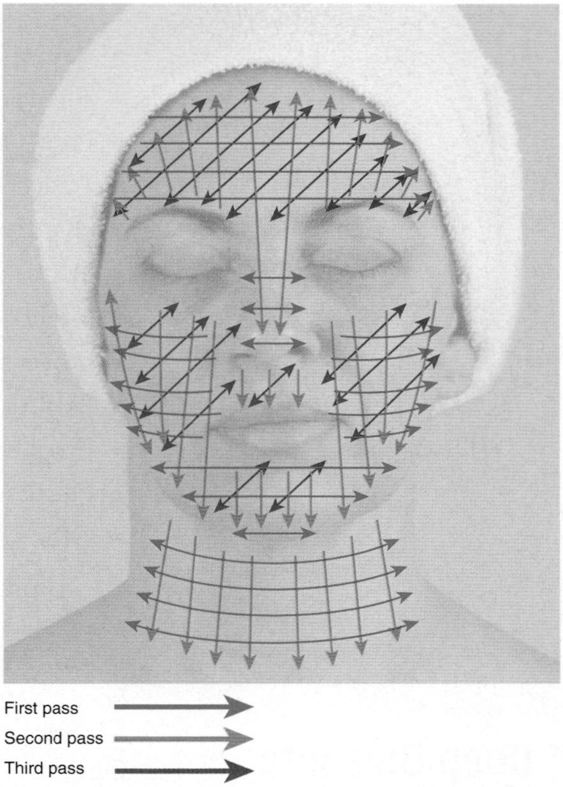

WHEN TO USE MICRODERMABRASION

Those who cannot tolerate acids may be candidates for microdermabrasion.

The difference between AHAs and microdermabrasion is that AHAs are chemical in nature and penetrate the epidermis, whereas microdermabrasion is a surface-level mechanical method of exfoliation. While microdermabrasion does exfoliate the epidermis effectively as well as stimulate cell metabolism and circulation, the benefits of the acids penetrating the skin and stimulating cell mitosis and cell turnover rate are not achieved with microdermabrasion. Generally, you can think of microdermabrasion as a more effective tool for surface exfoliation and AHAs as more effective below the surface. Using both peels and microdermabrasion in a treatment series is a common practice.

First pass
Second pass
Third pass

▲ **Figure 13-7** Systematically work your way around the face in horizontal, vertical and diagonal directional applications.

EFFECTS OF MICRODERMABRASION

Microdermabrasion can be used to diminish the following conditions:

- Sun damage
- Pigmentation
- Open and closed comedones
- Fine lines and wrinkles
- Enlarged pores and coarsely textured skin.

In addition to the typical exfoliation benefits, the vacuum mechanism stimulates cell metabolism and blood flow.

CONTRAINDICATIONS AND PRECAUTIONS FOR MICRODERMABRASION

Microdermabrasion contraindications include the following:

- Recent cosmetic surgeries, laser resurfacing, chemical peels, or dermabrasion

- Recent injectables, fillers, or Botox®
- Use of Retin-A, or other medications that exfoliate or thin the skin
- Allergies or sensitivities to products or ingredients
- Pregnancy (some healthcare providers may clear client for service)
- Active herpes simplex
- Hyperpigmentation tendencies
- Inflamed rosacea or acne
- Infectious diseases
- Open sores or suspicious lesions
- Sunburn or irritated skin
- Fragile skin, couperose skin
- Photosensitizing medications (makes skin very sensitive to sun)
- Other contraindicated drugs or medications.

To prevent skin damage, warn your clients to avoid sun exposure, excessive sweating, scrubs, rubbing, depilatories, waxing, benzoyl peroxide, and exfoliating or glycolic acid products for at least 24 to 48 hours before or after any chemical exfoliation procedure. Recommend a longer period of time if the client's condition warrants it. Other considerations:

- Do not use microdermabrasion so aggressively that the client is uncomfortable.
- Once the skin shows erythema or redness, this is considered the endpoint for the procedure.
- To avoid eye damage or breathing in crystals during microdermabrasion, technicians need to wear protective eyewear and protective masks.
- Clients must use protective eyewear and must keep eyes closed at all times.
- Avoid getting crystals in the client's mouth, nose, or ears.
- Improper use of microdermabrasion can cause hypopigmentation and hyperpigmentation. It can also lead to sensitivity and other problems. Any strong exfoliation procedure requires sun abstinence and daily sunscreen.

BEST PRACTICES AND SAFETY CONSIDERATIONS FOR MICRODERMABRASION

- Before a microdermabrasion service, discuss the issues and contraindications during the client consultation. Explain the procedures, the expected outcome, and realistic goals.
- In a diagnostic facial or skin analysis before scheduling treatments, note on the client intake form the condition of the skin, including dehydration, hyperpigmentation, open lesions, and any

ACTIVITY

Deep Dive into Microdermabrasion and Exfoliation

Research microdermabrasion machines and chemical exfoliation products. See what is offered in spas. Which product and/or manufacturer do you like? Why do you think one is better than the others? What services would you choose to offer? How much would you charge per treatment?

other skin conditions. Also choose the level of exfoliation with the microdermabrasion treatment based on the client's skin condition and the results desired.

- Remember to always consult the manufacturer's instructions throughout the process and while performing the microdermabrasion consultation.

- Eyewear is always recommended to protect the client and technician. A mask for the technician is also required.

- Microdermabrasion exfoliation procedures should be used with extreme caution during outdoor exposure and should be avoided in some cases where the client is not willing to take precautions to avoid inadvertent exposure during their daily activities.

- The manufacturer will provide instructions on the application and treatment process. General application steps for microdermabrasion involves cleansing, toning, proceeding with microdermabrasion treatment, rinsing or additional cleansing, and applying moisturizer and a product with SPF.

- It is preferred (but not required) that clients begin on a home care regimen to prepare the skin for microdermabrasion, but not every client is willing to commit. Pretreating assists in providing optimal outcomes because you are beginning the plan with a more acclimated and prepared skin surface. A home care plan should include, at minimum, a cleanser, retinol and/or AHA cream, vitamin C, and a product with SPF. Other products can be added in according to the issues that you are targeting such as skin lightening products in the case of pigmentation issues.

- Home care plans that work in tandem with the in-office clinical treatment plan are very important. The best way to convey this to a client is to communicate that you are providing the microdermabrasion treatment to assist in restoring the skin to optimal functioning capacity, and not performing any home maintenance will be similar to taking two steps forward and one step back. The home care plan should be like the pretreatment plan mentioned earlier in this discussion.

- Treatment plans begin with a series of treatments to jump-start progress. A series can consist of six to eight microdermabrasion treatments administered once a week over six to eight weeks. During the series and at the end of the series, monitor the client's progress and determine if the goals have been met or if you need to administer another series (the number of treatments and length of the series will be determined by your assessment) or move to the maintenance phase.

- During the maintenance phase, you maintain the results by administering a monthly maintenance microdermabrasion treatment. You may also boost progress throughout the year by adding a series when desired. An example would be to schedule a series every fall to address any summer photodamage.

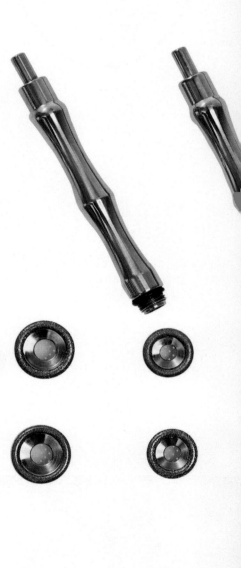

- Photo documentation before and after treatments and during the series is advantageous, as it is good business practice for your personal records and it also is beneficial documentation of the client's progress.

- Important reminder: The treatment schedule will depend on the client's tolerance to the procedure.

SAFETY AND MAINTENANCE OF MICRODERMABRASION MACHINES

- Daily care and proper use prevents unnecessary machine repairs.

- Microdermabrasion machines consist of internal motors, hoses, filters, and hand pieces. Hoses and hand pieces must be dry so that the crystals will flow properly.

- Use only the crystals recommended by the manufacturer. It is not necessary to overuse crystals to obtain good results. A constant, even flow of crystals will give a smooth and effective treatment. Crystals should flow onto the skin's surface only.

- Avoid breathing the crystals or getting them in the eyes or the nose.

- Carefully clean up crystals while wearing rubber gloves and a mask. Machines that have separate crystal containers for clean and used crystals are preferred. This way the used crystals stay contained and do not come into contact with the technician. These sealed containers are safer to dispose of properly. Follow the manufacturer's directions for disposal and maintenance.

- The treatment room and linens also need to be cleaned and checked for crystal residue and contamination.

✓ **CHECK IN**

7. What benefits does microdermabrasion have on the skin?

▲ **Figure 13–8** Client undergoing laser hair treatment in the axilla.

Leon Prete LMT and Barbara Prete, CE SafeLase for Cosmetic Laser Training

Explain the Benefits of Laser Technology

Lasers (LAY-zurs) are medical devices used for hair removal and skin treatments (**Figure 13–8**). Laser is an acronym that stands for *light amplification stimulation emission of radiation*. Lasers are high-powered devices that use intense pulses of electromagnetic radiation and a single wavelength at one time. One of the many differences between lasers and other light therapies is that, depending upon the skin condition you are treating, lasers are designed to focus all of the light-power with the same color, traveling to a specific depth, in one direction. In contrast, other light therapies, such as intense pulsed light (IPL), have multiple colors, depths, and wavelengths and the light may be scattered. The most important point to know about light therapy is that the equipment you use is selected based on the skin type and condition you are treating. Different wavelengths affect different components of the skin. Lasers work by means of a medium (solid, liquid or gas, or semiconductor) that emits light when excited by a power source. The medium is placed in a specifically designed chamber with mirrors located at both ends of the inside. The chamber is stimulated by an energy source such as electrical current, which in turn excites the particles. The reflective surfaces create light that becomes trapped and goes back and forth through the medium, gaining energy with each pass. The medium determines the wavelength of the laser and thus its use (**Figure 13–9**).

Lasers and IPL are strong machines that are rated as Class IV medical devices by the U.S. Food and Drug Administration (FDA). LED is rated as a safer Class I or II device and is regulated less strictly. Not all states allow estheticians to use lasers or IPL, and some states will not even allow the use of LED unless you are under a doctor's supervision.

When to Use and Effects of Laser Technology

All lasers and light therapy methods use selective *photothermolysis*. Remember that *thermolysis* means heat effect. Lasers emit light waves of the same wavelength, while nonlaser photo devices, such as IPL, use a spectrum of different wavelengths. For skin rejuvenation, heating and damaging the dermal tissue stimulates fibroblasts to repair and rebuild tissue such as collagen. The laser is a precise tool used for surgical procedures. In laser skin resurfacing, pulsed lasers are so precise that they can be directed to "burn" off the surface of the skin without ever touching the lower dermis.

These different treatments can stimulate collagen production, reduce spider veins, reduce hair growth, or peel the skin (**Figure 13–10**). Some

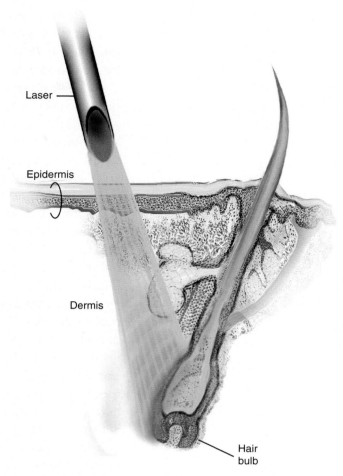

▲ **Figure 13–9** Lasers are designed to focus all of the light-power with the same color, traveling to a specific depth, in one direction.

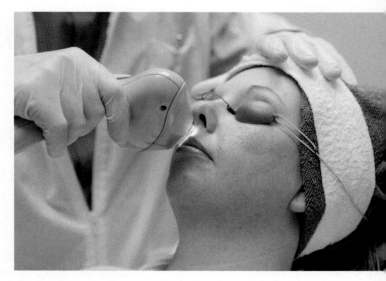

▲ **Figure 13–10** Laser treatment in progress.

lasers target specific substances—such as melanin, dark hair, blood vessels, skin growths, and pigmentation—that absorb the energy from the laser. A 755 Alexandrite Laser is known as the gold standard laser for hair reduction in lower Fitzpatrick clients.

A laser produces colored light. Wavelengths are selected to treat a range of skin conditions. For instance, one laser is designed to produce yellow light. Yellow light will selectively absorb into the color red. Laser light passes harmlessly through the skin and targets only the hemoglobin of the red blood cells. The laser energy then heats and destroys the cells, leaving the normal skin cells completely intact.

Lasers are now more commonly used for noninvasive procedures. Types of lasers include the alexandrite, diode, and Nd:YAG. Another treatment is referred to as *photodynamic* therapy and is best for primarily treating actinic keratoses. Many manufacturers have different names for their devices and specific treatments, which can be confusing. New devices are constantly coming on the market.

Lasers combined with radio frequencies are considered to be even more effective. This combined energy technology targets and heats connective tissue to stimulate collagen production and produce a firming effect. Radio waves of a certain frequency penetrate and are absorbed by the tissues. The strong damaging heat effect is what promotes skin healing and tightening. It is also effective for hair removal and used for cellulite reduction. Using radio waves in the skin is a similar process to how a microwave cooks food. Medical devices that use this technology are very strong, while those sold for home use are much weaker.

Lasers and light therapy are advanced topics. It is not necessary at this stage to learn all of the details concerning these devices. They are mentioned to familiarize you with the technology, which continues to evolve. See Chapter 11, Hair Removal, for additional information on lasers used for hair removal.

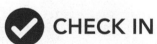 CHECK IN

8. What types of skin conditions do lasers treat?

Explain the Benefits and Types of Light Therapy

Light therapy is the application of light rays to the skin for the treatment of wrinkles, capillaries, pigmentation, or unwanted hair. Light therapy uses different types of devices: lasers, intense pulsed light (IPL), and light-emitting diode (LED) technologies. The power and effectiveness of the machines vary and depend on such factors as the wavelength, heat, and penetration power. The range of wavelengths used in light therapy are visible, infrared, and far infrared (Figure 13–11).

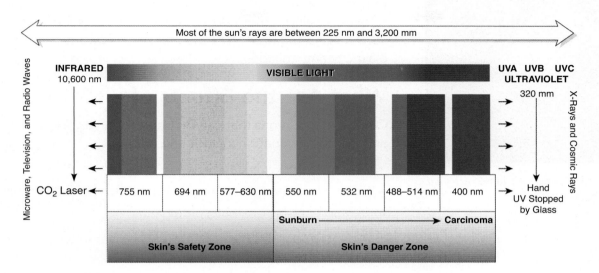

| Most of the sun's rays are between 225 nm and 3,200 mm |

INFRARED 10,600 nm   VISIBLE LIGHT   UVA UVB UVC ULTRAVIOLET

Microware, Television, and Radio Waves

320 mm

X-Rays and Cosmic Rays

CO_2 Laser ←

| 755 nm | 694 nm | 577–630 nm | 550 nm | 532 nm | 488–514 nm | 400 nm |

→ Hand UV Stopped by Glass

Sunburn ————————→ Carcinoma

Skin's Safety Zone   Skin's Danger Zone

▲ Figure 13–11 Wavelengths used in light therapy.

What Is Infrared Light and When Do You Use It?

Light therapy with the use of infrared heat has been used for years to treat physical conditions such as pain and to promote healing. Infrared lamps have been used in salons for heating conditioners and chemicals in hair treatments. They are also used in spas and saunas for relaxation and warming up muscles, detoxifying the body, and reducing pain. There are uses of near infrared light for signs of aging (such as for wrinkles), wound healing, and increasing circulation as it has the longest wavelength of all of the light therapies and thus can penetrate the deepest into the skin.

Therapeutic lamps are also used for light therapy. Color therapy uses different colors of light for various psychological effects: Red is considered stimulating, while green is calming (Figure 13–12).

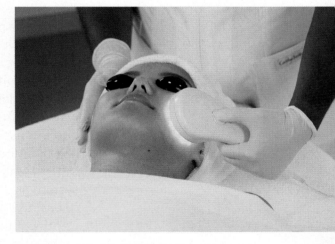

▲ Figure 13–12 LED Light Therapy has many benefits for your client.

What Is IPL and When Do You Use It?

Intense pulse light (in-TENS PULSE LYHT) devices are similar to lasers. IPL devices use pulses of multiple wavelengths (versus single in lasers) to reduce pigmentation, remove surface capillaries, and rejuvenate the skin. Intense pulse light emits light absorbed by hemoglobin (vascular), melanin (pigmented lesions), and hair follicles (hair removal).

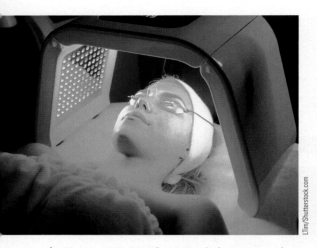

▲ **Figure 13–13** Therapeutic lamps are also used for light therapy.

Photorejuvenation (FO-toh-rih-joo-vin-A-shun) is another term used for the growing technology that utilizes light therapy to enhance the skin (**Figure 13–13**). It is the nonablative (not causing injury to the skin) treatment of extrinsic and intrinsic signs of aging such as superficial vascular and pigmented irregularities, along with a loss of elasticity and collagen.

What Are the Effects of IPL?

Common conditions that can be treated with an IPL device and photorejuvenation include the following:

- Fine lines and wrinkles
- Skin texture changes including roughness and coarseness
- Telangiectasias or small spider veins
- Pigmented lesions or dyschromia
- Poikiloderma of Civatte
- Rosacea symptoms: erythema or redness, flushing, and papules.

What LED Is and When to Use It

LED is the acronym for **light-emitting diode** (LYT EE-mitt-ing DYE-ode), a device used to reduce acne, increase skin circulation, and improve the collagen content in the skin. LED technology is nonthermal, meaning it does not use heat. LED technology works on the premise of nonthermal, nonablative cellular stimulation called photomodulation. This action triggers a photobiochemical response versus relying on thermal injury (as with lasers).

Estheticians use LED light for skin rejuvenation. LED individual wavelengths are used at low intensity and are not as strong as the laser and intense pulse light modalities. LED uses visible light such as blue, red or amber, and infrared (invisible). Different colors of light produce different effects on the skin. LED has been shown to help the lymph system and increase ATP energy production in the cells. LED works by releasing light onto the skin to stimulate specific responses, at precise depths of the skin. Each color of light corresponds to a different depth in the skin (**Table 13–2**). The LED color of light is also seeking color in the skin known as a chromophore. The term *chromophore* is derived from the Greek term *chroma* meaning "color." A **chromophore** (krohma-for) is a color component within the skin such as blood or melanin. When the colored light reaches a specific depth in the skin, it triggers a reaction such as stimulating circulation or reducing the amount of bacteria.

Hand-held devices are increasingly popular. The use of machines, light therapy, and medical esthetics continues to develop. Scientific discoveries and advances are changing the face of the antiaging industry.

Effects of an LED Treatment

Depending on the type of equipment, the LED can be blue, red, yellow, or green (Table 13–2).

▼ **TABLE 13–2** Effects of LED (Light-Emitting Diode) Therapy

Effects of LED (Light-Emitting Diode) Therapy	
Color (nm [nanometers])	**Beneficial Effects**
Red light (RED LYT) 640–660 nm	Increases cellular processes Boosts collagen and elastin production Stimulates wound healing
Yellow light (YEL-oh LYT) 575–595 nm	Reduces inflammation Improves lymphatic flow Detoxifies and increases circulation
Green light (GREEN lyte) 500–525 nm	Lessens hyperpigmentation Reduces redness Calms and soothes
Blue light (BLOO LYT) 410–450 nm	Improves acne Reduces bacteria *Used with medications for precancerous lesions

*Medical procedure only

Contraindications and Best Practices for LED

The following conditions are contraindicated for LED treatments:

- Pregnancy
- Open or unidentified skin lesions
- Seizure disorders
- Autoimmune disorders
- Clients taking photosensitizing medications
- As with all light therapies, it is important to make certain that you have viewed the client consultation form for any contraindications.
- Light therapy should not be performed on anyone who has light sensitivities (photosensitivities), has phototoxic reactions, is taking antibiotics, has cancer or epilepsy, is pregnant, or is under a physician's care. If you are unsure whether you should apply a treatment, always refer the client to their healthcare provider.
- LEDs are used in facials for approximately 15 minutes. Protective eyewear are used to protect both the technician's and client's eyes. The thyroid area should also be covered. The thyroid can be

stimulated by the LED device as demonstrated by the off-label use of red light LED in the treatment of hypothyroidism by physicians.

Safety and Maintenance for LED Machines

LED machines should be maintained in accordance with the manufacturer's instructions. The machines and protective eyewear should be disinfected after each use.

CHECK IN

9. What is light therapy?
10. What is light therapy used for?
11. What are LEDs used for?

Discuss Microcurrent Treatments

Microcurrent (mi-kroh-CUR-ent), or wave therapy, devices mimic the way the brain relays messages to the muscles. Therefore, microcurrent is used by the medical field to treat many conditions, such as Bell's palsy and stroke paralysis. The growing uses of microampere electrical neuromuscular stimulation include healing muscles and wounds, controlling pain, and even fusing bones. There is even greater potential for this type of therapy. In the esthetics realm, microcurrent is used to relax muscles, and strengthen and tone the muscles by stimulating motor nerves and contractions of the muscles.

The standard technique utilizes two hand-held probes placed on facial muscle groups (**Figures 13–14**). A specific movement technique is used on all of the designated facial points. An ampoule may be applied under the conducting gel or a conducting gel alone may be placed on the skin before beginning the treatment. The electrical current is regulated according to the skin's resistance. For visible results, treatments are given once a week for at least 10 sessions. Treatments must be given every four weeks to maintain the benefits and results.

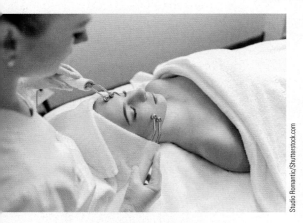

▲ **Figure 13–14** Ionizing with microcurrent.

When to Use Microcurrent

Many biological processes are associated with electrical impulses. Facial skin tone and muscles are all related to this system. As we age, impulses slow down, causing the skin to sag. Muscles may not completely contract after use, such as in the case of sagging jowls (jaw muscles). The same effect can be seen on the rest of the body as well. That is why exercise and stretching are extremely important as one ages.

- Microcurrent is thought to aid in the healing and repair of tissues and to influence metabolism.

- It works gently and helps speed up the natural regenerative processes of the body when the correct intensity of current and frequency are used.

- Firmer and healthier skin are expected treatment results.

Microcurrent devices are designed to work in harmony with the natural bioelectrical currents found in the body.

Some models of hand-held devices are combined with ultrasound technology (**Figure 13–15**) for additional penetration and added exfoliation effects.

Microcurrent combined with light therapy can be even more effective. When using any electrical device, you should obtain a complete client health history and conduct a consultation before treatment. Contraindications are the same as those described for other electrical devices.

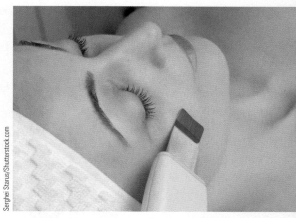

▲ **Figure 13–15** Ultrasound technology

Effects of Microcurrent

In esthetics, microcurrent is used primarily to tone and stimulate facial muscles. Considered a passive form of exercise, this therapeutic technique helps stimulate motor nerves until a contraction of the muscles can be seen. Microcurrent has the ability to firm muscles and boost cellular activity. It improves blood and lymph circulation and can also assist with product absorption. In the past, faradic current has been used to stimulate motor nerves.

Contraindications and Precautions for Microcurrent

As with all electrical current devices, microcurrent should not be used on clients with the following health conditions:

- Open wounds, muscular diseases, advanced diabetes, pacemakers, epilepsy, cancer, pregnancy, hemophilia, phlebitis, thrombosis; anyone currently under a healthcare provider's care for a condition that may be contraindicated

- Typical recommended use of microcurrent treatments with injectables: wait two weeks after the injection procedure.

Best Practices and Safety Considerations for Microcurrent

As microcurrent movements are complex, potentially lengthy, and specific to the manufacturer's recommendations and because the treatment depends on proper positioning, it is important to review

CAUTION!

As with all electrical current devices, microcurrent should not be used on clients with the following health conditions: pacemakers, epilepsy, cancer, pregnancy, phlebitis, or thrombosis. Microcurrent should also not be used on anyone currently under a healthcare provider's care for a condition that may be contraindicated. If you are unsure about treating a client, refer them back to their healthcare provider to obtain consent.

DID YOU KNOW?

Most high-tech devices such as LED and microcurrent require multiple sessions to achieve desired results.

muscle location, origin, and insertion. Improper placement could result in no improvement. Always follow the instructions and recommendations provided by the manufacturer of your device.

Safety and Maintenance of Microcurrent

Microcurrent machines should be maintained in accordance with the manufacturer's instructions. The machines and protective eyewear should be disinfected after each use.

 CHECK IN
12. What is microcurrent and what does it do for the skin?

Discuss Ultrasound

Ultrasound and *ultrasonic* are synonymous terms referring to a frequency that is above the range of sound audible to the human ear. This equipment uses noninvasive sound waves to create results-oriented treatments. **Ultrasonic** (ULL-trah-son-ik) equipment is based on high-frequency mechanical oscillations produced by a metal spatula-like tool.

When to Use and Effects of Ultrasound Technology

Ultrasound (ULL-trah-sow-nd) technology in esthetics can be used for product penetration and for cellulite reduction. The vibrations, created through a water medium, help cleanse and exfoliate the skin by removing dead skin cells. Ultrasound penetrates deeply—it stimulates tissue, increases blood flow, and promotes oxygenation. Keep in mind that the lower the frequency, the greater the penetration; conversely, a higher frequency has less penetration. Cellulite is affected through the heat manipulation of the tissue and lymphatic movements performed with the device. Heat is created, and the vibration in the cells stimulates circulation, metabolism, and lymph drainage. The heat damage from ultrasound and other modalities (such as lasers) is what stimulates collagen production.

Ultrasound also sends waves through the skin to assist in product penetration. This process is called *sonophoresis* (SAHN-oh-for-EE-sus), which is similar to iontophoresis (iontophoresis uses electrically charged ions, so an electrical charge is needed from electrodes). Some esthetic ultrasound equipment is rated as an FDA Class II device and may not be within an esthetician's scope of practice outside of a medical facility. Advanced training and technical research on equipment claims are necessary before using any advanced esthetic machine. Different

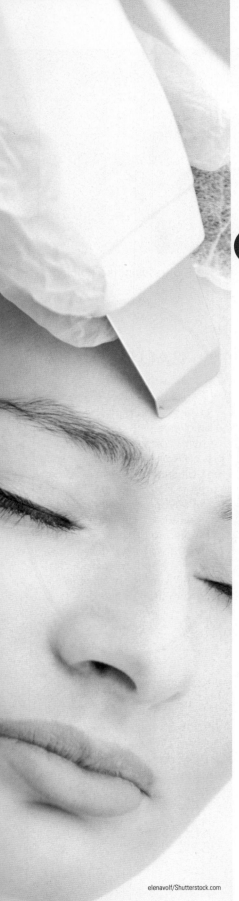
elenavolf/Shutterstock.com

frequencies of ultrasound are also used for medical imaging, physical therapy, and pain management. Lower-frequency ultrasonic devices are used for toothbrushes and jewelry cleaners.

Hand-held devices for a consumer's personal skin care that are used at home are milder but should be used in moderation to avoid damaging the skin.

Because of its gentle, nonabrasive nature, this treatment can be a viable choice for clients with sensitive skin conditions or rosacea versus other exfoliating services. As gentle as ultrasonic therapy is, some clients are still not good candidates.

Contraindications and Precautions for Ultrasound Technology

Ultrasound contraindications include open or unidentified skin lesions, heart conditions, pacemakers or electrical implants, epilepsy, pregnancy, advanced diabetes, and cancerous lesions; or on anyone currently under a doctor's care for a condition that may be contraindicated. Like all machines, overuse can be damaging.

Best Practices and Safety Considerations for Ultrasound Technology

To avoid excessive heat buildup and unstable cavitation, it is important to maintain constant movement of the handpiece on moist skin. Caution should be exercised with fragile skin and in thin, delicate areas such as near the eye.

Safety and Maintenance for Ultrasound Machines

Ultrasound machines should be maintained in accordance with the manufacturer's instructions. The machine should be disinfected after each use.

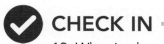 **CHECK IN**

13. What is ultrasound and what is it used for in esthetics?

Discuss Microneedling and Nano Infusion

It should be noted that not all states allow estheticians to perform microneedling or dermal rolling and categorize it as a medical procedure, requiring physician supervision.

Microneedling or Dermal Rolling

Cosmetic and medical rolling, also called **microneedling** (MI-kroh-NEED-ling) or *dermal rolling*, is a form of collagen induction therapy (CIT). This procedure causes tiny needle pricks across the skin from rollers or electronic handpieces that induce collagen formation during the wound healing process (**Figure 13–16**).

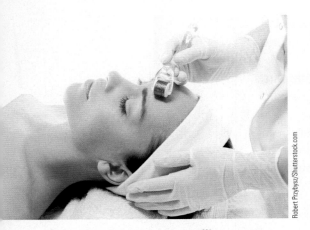

▲ **Figure 13–16** Microneedling causes tiny needle pricks across the skin from rollers or electronic handpieces that induce collagen formation from the wound healing process.

Nano Infusion

Nano Infusion is a popular technology used by estheticians in states that do not allow microneedling in an esthetician's scope of practice. Nano Infusion technology includes the use of a microneedling handpiece but with needle-free Nano Tips versus the standard microneedling tip that has needles that puncture the skin and can penetrate to the epidermal or dermal level, depending on how aggressive you are with the microneedling handpiece settings. The Nano Infusion tip is a popular alternative treatment because it is not invasive. It uses a single use sterile cartridge, made of silicone or surgical steel pyramid-like modules that are microscopic. The pyramid modules are smaller than one single strand of human hair, and almost invisible to the naked eye. This specialized design, allows for a safe treatment with no downtime as the Nano Tips do not penetrate into the dermis. The science behind this treatment is to create thousands of micro-channels per minute on top of the skin while the vibratory action of the microneedling handpiece assists in penetrating in the topical product of choice.

CHECK IN

14. What is microneedling?
15. What is Nano Infusion?

CAUTION!

Instruct your clients to drink lots of water to flush the system and rehydrate the body after detoxifying body treatments. If they do not replenish the water in the body, clients may feel tired or sick. Additionally, detoxifying treatments are not as effective when the body is not flushed and rehydrated with water.

Describe Spa Body Treatments

Spa treatments provide a wonderful, relaxing experience. Body treatments have a therapeutic effect and treat the skin of the whole body. They include wraps, scrubs, and masks. Be mindful of contraindications and allergies to ingredients (e.g., seaweed, nuts) before working on clients.

When to Use and Effects of Spa Body Treatments

- **Body wraps** (BAHD-ee RAPs) are treatments where product is applied on the body and then covered or wrapped up. Wraps are used for various reasons and can remineralize, hydrate, stimulate, detoxify, or promote relaxation. The product used will determine the effects and results. Aloe, gels, lotions, oils, seaweed, herbs, clay, or mud products can all be used for wraps. Linens or plastic can be used to wrap clients and to promote product penetration. Blankets or sheets are the cocoon of the "wraps." Inch-loss wraps, another type of wrap, are designed to flush toxins out of the body and promote inch loss. Inch-loss wraps have a diuretic effect and are controversial in their effectiveness. If done properly, detoxifying the body may aid in weight reduction (**Figure 13–17**).

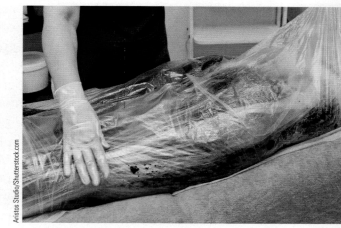

▲ **Figure 13–17** Aloe, gels, lotions, oils, seaweed, herbs, clay, or mud products can all be used for wraps.

- **Body scrubs** (BAHD-ee scrubz) use friction to exfoliate and hydrate, increase circulation, and nourish skin using a combination of ingredients such as ground nuts, apricot kernels, cornmeal, jojoba beads, honey, salt, or sugar combined with oil or lotion. Exfoliation treatments are also called *polishes* and *glows* (**Figure 13–18**). Exfoliation prepares the skin to receive additional products or treatments. Dry brushing is also beneficial and is used to exfoliate and stimulate the skin.

- **Body masks** (BAHD-ee masks) remineralize and detoxify the body using primarily clay, mud, or seaweed mixtures. Certain body masks are used to treat cellulite. Clients are usually wrapped up after the mask application, and thus masks are similar to wraps. The ingredients and procedure used in the treatment determine whether the process is called a *mask* or a *wrap* (**Figure 13–19**).

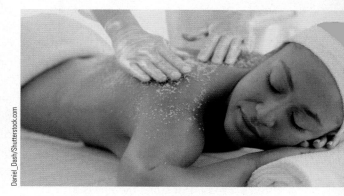

▲ **Figure 13–18** A salt exfoliation treatment.

- **Hydrotherapy** (hy-druh-THAIR-uh-pee) is another spa treatment that uses water in its three forms (ice, steam, and liquid). Hydrotherapy tubs, Scotch hoses, Vichy (VIH-shee) showers (**Figure 13–20**), Watsu®

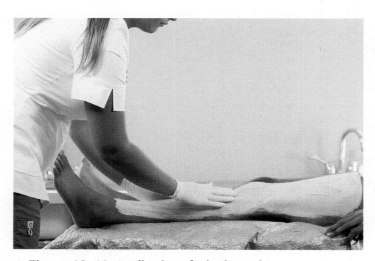

▲ **Figure 13–19** Application of a body mask.

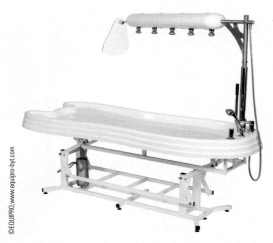

▲ **Figure 13–20** The Vichy shower is used in hydrotherapy treatments.

massages, hot tubs, steam rooms, saunas, cold-plunge pools, foot soaks, and whirlpool baths are all different forms of hydrotherapy found in spas.

All spa treatments, especially intensive hydrotherapy treatments, can be powerful, so proper training is important before offering these services.

- **Balneotherapy** (bal-nee-oh-THAYR-uh-pee) is the treatment of physical ailments using therapeutic water baths (**Figure 13–21**). Mineral, mud or fango, Dead Sea salt, seaweed, enzymes, or peat are used in the baths (*balneum* is Latin for bath).

- **Stone massage** (STON mass-aje) is the technique of using hot stones and cold stones in massage or other treatments (**Figure 13–22**). Facial stone massage can be incorporated into regular facials.

- **Foot reflexology** (FOOT reflex-OL-oo-jee) is the technique of applying pressure to the feet based on a system of zones and areas on the feet that directly correspond to the anatomy of the body (**Figure 13–23**). Reflexology is performed on the feet, hands, and ears as these are the areas that correspond to the body zones. It causes relaxation, increased circulation, and balance to the entire body. Estheticians are not usually trained in reflexology, so be aware of your scope of practice and licensing regulations. Reflexology is generally performed by licensed massage therapists. Massage can be dangerous if performed incorrectly.

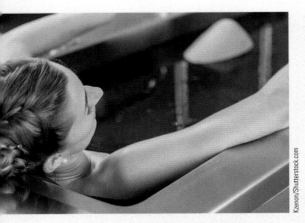

▲ **Figure 13–21** Balneotherapy is another type of hydrotherapy

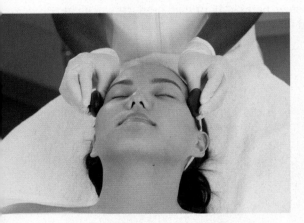

▲ **Figure 13–22** Hot stone therapy is a relaxing option for your client.

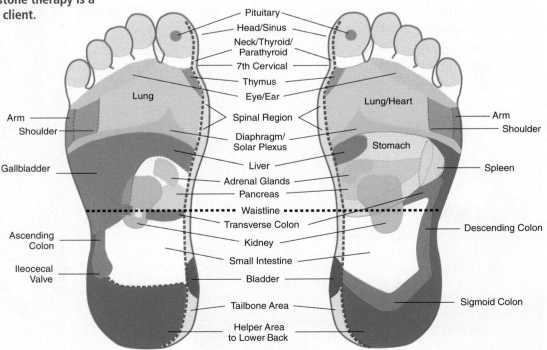

▲ **Figure 13–23** Foot reflexology chart.

- **Ayurvedic** (ah-yur-VAY-dic) concepts are based on three *doshas*, or mind and body types. Treatments include *Shirodhara* (**Figure 13–24**), massage, and facials using ancient Indian concepts and ingredients suited to the three body/mind types: *pitta*, *kapha*, and *vatta*. Ayurveda originated over 5,000 years ago in India. It is a philosophy of medicine and balancing life and the body through various methods ranging from massage to eating habits. *Ayur* means "life, vital power"; *veda* means "knowledge." *Ayurveda* translates from Sanskrit as "science of health or wellness." Shirodhara is an ayurvedic treatment that consists of running warm oil on the third-eye area of the forehead for 30 minutes. This relaxing, meditative process releases stress and calms the mind.

- *Sunless tanning* product application is a service offered as an alternative to tanning (**Figure 13–25**). It is sprayed on or applied manually.

- **Endermology** (ENDER-mol-oh-gee) is a treatment for cellulite. It helps stimulate the reduction of adipose tissue by a vacuum massage that combines a vigorous massage along with suction. Machines and other endermology methods are used in spas and in medical facilities.

- **Reiki** (RAY-KEE) is a Japanese technique for stress reduction and relaxation that also promotes healing. It is administered by "laying on hands" and is based on the idea that an unseen "life-force energy" flows through us and is what causes us to be alive.

- Other energy practices include energy balancing and chakras. According to ancient Hindu philosophy, our bodies have seven major vortexes through which we process our life force energy (sometimes known as *ki*, or *chi*). A block in any of these power centers can create unbalance, disease, or an overwhelming sense of tiredness and feeling "stuck." The focus of the chakra balancing is to identify any blocks in the chakras, open them up, and reconnect your energy body.

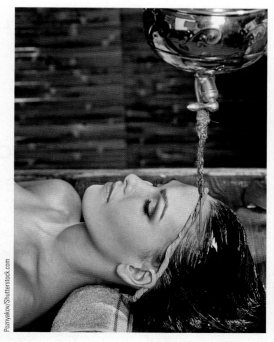

▲ Figure 13–24 Shirodhara is an ayurvedic treatment that consists of running warm oil on the third-eye area of the forehead.

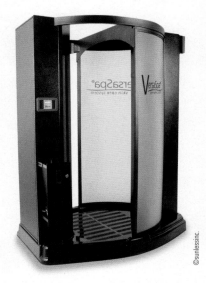

▲ Figure 13–25 Sunless tanning options are a safe alternative for your clients to get golden skin

ACTIVITY

Learn More About Spa Treatments

To learn more about spa treatments, here is a research idea: Check out the spa menus and brochures in your area or on Internet sites. Professional trade journals and spa suppliers offer excellent information on a variety of treatment procedures. Many spa magazines are also good resources to gain insight into the industry. What body treatment services are you most interested in learning about? A nice way to learn is to experience the treatment yourself. Book an appointment to have a spa research day!

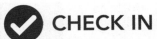
Discuss Common Treatments Used to Address Cellulite

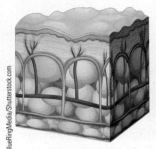 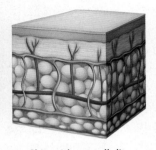

Skin with cellulite   Skin without cellulite

▲ **Figure 13–26** Cellulite skin versus smooth skin.

BlueRingMedia/Shutterstock.com

Cellulite (SEL-yoo-lyt) appears as dimpled or bumpy skin caused primarily by female hormones and genetics. Cellulite consists of fat cells. Dermal fat cells do swell, but that is not the only cause of cellulite. Cellulite is visible when dermal fat cells are closer to the surface of the skin (**Figure 13–26**). This occurs from damage to the dermis. If water is lost and the tissue is weakened, then dermal fat begins to push into the dermis.

Additionally, if the epidermis is weakened or dehydrated, cellulite is more visible.

Keeping collagen and elastin healthy helps reduce cellulite. To repair cellulite, cells and connective tissue need to be strengthened and hydrated through nutrients and water intake. Drinking water is not enough—our cells have to be able to hold onto the water. Wasted water in the body builds up and leads to water retention and puffiness. Blood flow and the circulation of nutrients through blood vessels up to the skin also affect cellulite. Repairing cell damage, connective tissue damage, and stratum corneum damage is important in treating cellulite.

The following recommended nutrients and ingredients may be beneficial for cellulite reduction:

- Lecithin and lipids for cell walls
- Glycosaminoglycans (GAGs) for moisturizing and firming
- Glucosamine to build GAGs and connective tissue
- B vitamins to retain moisture and provide nutrients
- Amino acids for building collagen and elastin
- Essential fatty acids to attract water for the connective tissue
- Antioxidants
- Anti-inflammatories
- Aloe vera, an anti-inflammatory that improves hydration and contains enzymes and minerals
- AHAs
- Alpha lipoic acid.

The effectiveness of some endermology treatments is controversial. Detox diets, liposuction, and muscle-stimulating systems do not minimize cellulite. Some body wraps result in only a temporary water loss. Electronic devices with vacuums may reduce cellulite temporarily.

Manual lymph drainage, mesotherapy (microinjection to the dermis to melt fat), dermal fillers, lasers, chemical peels, and microdermabrasion have all been tried to help reduce cellulite. Most of these techniques are considered to provide temporary results, and their effectiveness varies. Increasing blood flow, stimulating collagen and elastin, attracting water to cells, and repairing cell membranes are recommended to reduce cellulite. Additionally, reducing wasted water, preventing free radical damage, and reducing inflammation is part of a healthy approach to treating cellulite and the skin. Exercise, along with a healthy low-fat diet with a reduced intake of processed foods, is thought to help reduce cellulite.

Professional cellulite treatments must be performed consistently in continuous sessions. A common spa treatment consists of exfoliation with a scrub or dry brushing followed by a detoxifying mask and wrap. These stimulate the metabolism and circulation. To finish the service, a cellulite treatment cream is applied.

Exfoliation and skin brushing are also good for blood vessels and circulation. Another popular treatment is *thalassotherapy* (thuh-LA-soh-THAIR-uh-pee). Thalassotherapy is the use of seawater as a form of therapy. Therapeutic benefits from sea and seawater products include many minerals and nutrients. Massage can also help soften hardened cellulite. Cellulite is a common condition for most women, and improving the health of the skin is a continual process.

Explain the Benefits of Manual Lymph Drainage

Manual lymph drainage (MLD) (MAN-yoo-ul LIMF DRAY-nij) stimulates lymph fluid to flow through the lymphatic vessels.

When to Use Manual Lymph Drainage and Effects of This Modality

This technique helps to cleanse and detoxify the body. Congestion, water, and waste in the lymphatic vessels create edema in the tissue. Moving this fluid out of the body with light massage movements will decrease the swelling from excess fluid (**Figure 13–27**). MLD is a great addition to a facial or other treatments. It is also used both before and after surgery because it expedites healing and enhances cell metabolism. Mechanical lymph drainage is a very beneficial service performed with machines. Advanced training courses in MLD are available for both

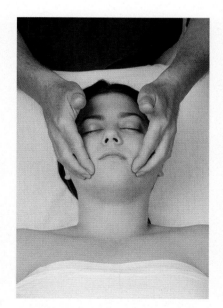

▲ **Figure 13–27** Manual lymph drainage can cleanse and detoxify the body.

estheticians and massage therapists; however, some states require an advanced license before an esthetician can perform this service.

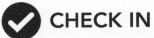

CHECK IN

18. Explain the benefits of manual lymphatic drainage.

Describe the Field of Medical Esthetics

Medical esthetics is a multibillion-dollar industry. The industry is constantly developing new products and services for our youth-oriented society. Plastic surgery, laser treatments, and injectables focus on maintaining a youthful appearance. Medical esthetics integrates surgical and nonsurgical procedures with esthetic treatments. Estheticians also perform services such as peels, microdermabrasion, and light therapy. Some assist with medical procedures and monitor patient recovery.

Additionally, home care products recommended by the esthetician help patients heal faster and maintain their skin's health. Because medical esthetics is evolving, the esthetician's role can be shaped to fit the facility's needs. Each setting varies, so it is important to define the responsibilities included in the esthetician's job description.

Clinical estheticians are well trained, experienced, and in some cases certified; however, not all estheticians must be certified to work in medical esthetics. Most clinical procedures must be done in a medical office under a healthcare provider's supervision. Medi-spas are medical clinics and spas combined in one location and offer both esthetic and medical services.

The most popular medical spa services are chemical peels, microdermabrasion, Botox®, fillers, laser hair removal, and light therapy/photorejuvenation. Estheticians are not qualified to perform certain procedures, but it is important to be familiar with all of them because many clients will be asking questions and utilizing these procedures. Society is now flooded with information on medical esthetics. It is part of modern society's continued quest for instant gratification and maintenance of physical beauty. Medical spas are a fast-growing segment in the beauty industry.

Pre- and Postoperative Care

Estheticians perform pre- and postoperative treatments and provide patient education before cosmetic surgery. These are important for faster patient recovery time. Estheticians also provide facials, light peels, extractions, and microdermabrasion prior to surgery. Camouflage makeup, retail sales, and patient home care counseling are other responsibilities in medical esthetics.

Preoperative care focuses on preparing the skin for the procedure. Getting the skin in its optimum state and as healthy as possible makes the surgery less traumatic on the tissue and shortens recovery time. Increasing the skin's metabolism and reducing cellular debris on the surface are part of conditioning the skin. Plan and schedule for pre- and postop care are outlined by the medical staff before a patient's surgery.

Postop care includes providing skin care for rapid wound healing and the avoidance of infection. Decreasing inflammation, soothing and moisturizing, and providing for sun protection are the goals. Massage, hydration, protection, and camouflage makeup are often part of postop care. Home care instructions for long-term maintenance are also important. Permanent makeup, sometimes referred to as *micropigmentation*, is another technique utilized in clinical esthetics.

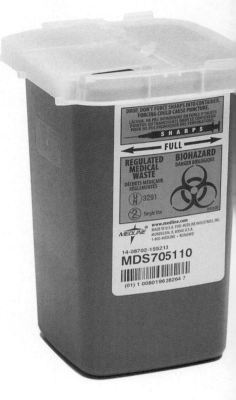

Microdermabrasion and Chemical Peels

Glycolic (gly-KAHL-ik) treatments can be performed to precondition the skin before laser resurfacing or surgery. These "lunchtime peels" can enhance the strength and barrier function of the epidermis. Microdermabrasion benefits to the epidermis are similar to those provided by AHA treatments, although the effects are more superficial.

Documentation

A patient's chart is a record of what the patient conveys, what the esthetician observes, assessment and analysis, and a plan of action for treatment. Protocols from clinical procedures are followed. Patient informed consent forms and treatment records are required and are part of the standard charting procedure.

Other Clinical Procedures

Numerous opportunities for estheticians are found in specialized clinical settings. Laser and medical centers offer hair reduction, spider vein removal, nonablative wrinkle treatments, and other types of laser procedures. Nonablative (non-uh-BLAY-tiv) procedures do not remove tissue. Nonablative wrinkle treatments use intense pulsed light (IPL) to bypass the epidermis and stimulate collagen in the dermis to promote wrinkle reduction. Estheticians can assist healthcare providers in these procedures if the technician is properly trained and certified.

Other common procedures performed by healthcare providers include injectables of dermal fillers and Botox®.

INJECTABLES
Botox® and dermal fillers are injectables that are a large part of the industry. Injectables have become the fastest-growing product in the

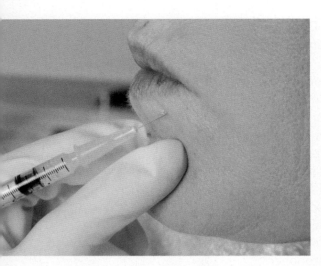

▲ **Figure 13–28** Botox® is a treatment some client's desire.

medical spa industry. **Injectable fillers** (in-JEK-tuh-bul FIL-urz) are substances used in nonsurgical procedures to fill in or plump up areas of the skin. FDA-approved fillers are non-toxic, durable, biocompatible, and easy to use—these are the necessary attributes of a safe filler.

BOTOX®

Botox® injection is a popular nonsurgical clinical service. **Botox®** (Bow-tocks) is a neuromuscular-blocking serum (botulinum toxin) that paralyzes nerve cells on the muscle when this serum is injected into it. Botox® is injected into the muscles to cause paralysis or diminished movement by blocking neurotransmitters. This relaxes tissues and diminishes lines. The **glabella** (gluh-BEL-uh) is the area between the eyebrows where muscles cause creasing from squinting or frowning. The glabella has strong muscles and is the most common site for Botox® injections (**Figure 13–28**). Millions of Botox® injections are performed annually in the United States.

DERMAL FILLERS

Dermal fillers (DUR-mul FILL-erz) are used to fill lines, wrinkles, and other facial imperfections. As we age, dermal collagen, hyaluronic acid, and fat are lost and skin loses its shape. The first fillers were from animal sources, specifically bovine collagen. Today, collagen treatments use a filler, usually a bovine (cow) derivative, to fill in wrinkles or to make lips larger. Dermal fillers last longer when used in conjunction with Botox®.

Today's fillers are obtained from a variety of sources. Many are combined substances and materials. Collagen may be derived from human or animal sources. Synthetic sources are silicone and hyaluronic acids (HAs). The newest trend is to use both nonanimal (Restylane®) and animal-based (Hylaform®) hyaluronic acid fillers. Juvéderm® is one of the many cross-linked HA fillers. Hyaluronic acid is a polysaccharide found in the body and connective tissues. A component of the skin's natural moisturizing function, it holds up to 1,000 times its weight in water. Cross-linking is a process in which ingredients are combined to increase a product's stability and durability.

Another type of filler is aqueous calcium (Radiesse® FN), which is calcium based. Another injectable that is not a filler, but a dermal stimulator, is called poly-L-lactic acid (PLLA). This product (marketed as Sculptra®) increases fibroblast activity and collagen production. New products are coming on the market regularly.

Surgical Procedures

There are two types of surgery: reconstructive and cosmetic.

- **Reconstructive surgery** (REE-con-struct-if SIR-JUR-ee) is defined as that which restores a bodily function. This type of surgery is necessary for accident survivors and those with congenital disfigurements or other diseases.

- Cosmetic surgery (kahz-MET-ik SUR-juh-ree), also known as *esthetic surgery*, is elective surgery for improving and altering the appearance.

COSMETIC SURGICAL PROCEDURES

Common cosmetic surgery procedures are facelifts, forehead lifts, eye lifts, nose reconstruction, laser resurfacing, and deep peels.

- A rhytidectomy (rit-ih-DEK-tuh-mee) is a facelift. This procedure removes excess fat at the jawline; tightens loose, atrophic muscles; and removes sagging skin (**Figure 13–29a** and **Figure 13–29b**).

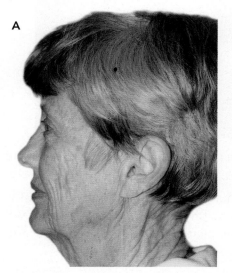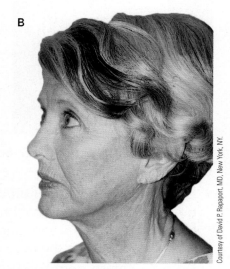

▲ **Figures 13–29a and 13–29b** Before (a) and after (b) a facelift.

- A forehead lift, also called a *brow lift*, can be performed separately or in combination with an eye lift.
- A blepharoplasty (BLEF-uh-roh-plas-tee) is an eye lift. It removes fat and skin from the upper and lower lids, making them less baggy and crinkled-looking (**Figure 13–30a** and **Figure 13–30b**). When sagging eyelids impede a patient's ability to see, it is a medical condition that may be covered by insurance.

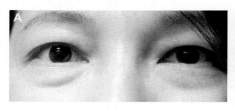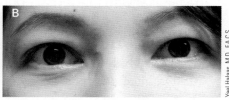

▲ **Figures 13–30a and 13–30b** Before (a) and after (b) an eye lift.

- A transconjunctival blepharoplasty (trans-kon-junk-TIE-vul BLEF-uh-roh-plas-tee) is performed inside the lower eyelid to remove bulging fat pads, which are often congenital.

- **Rhinoplasty** (RY-noh-plas-tee) is nose surgery that makes a nose smaller or changes the appearance in some other way. Sometimes rhinoplasty is necessary for health reasons and to improve the patient's ability to breathe.

- **Laser resurfacing** (LAY-zur re-SUR-fas-ing) is used to smooth wrinkles or lighten acne scars. Collagen remodeling stimulates the growth of new collagen in the dermis (**Figure 13–31a** and **Figure 13–31b**). This type of laser treatment removes the epidermal layer and requires a recovery period.

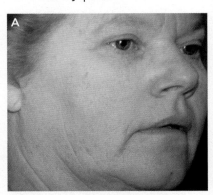 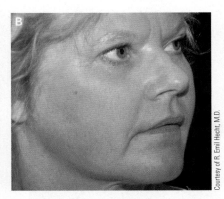

▲ **Figures 13–31a and 13–31b** Before (a) and after (b) a laser resurfacing treatment.

- **Dermabrasion** (dur-muh-BRAY-zhun) is a strong exfoliation method that uses a mechanical brush to physically remove tissue down to the dermis. It is a very deep exfoliation used primarily on scars. Lasers are replacing the use of this medical procedure.

  Do not confuse dermabrasion with microdermabrasion. Microdermabrasion is a mild, superficial mechanical exfoliation method.

- **Trichloroacetic acid (TCA) peels** (TRY-klor-oh-AH-seed-ick ASUD PEELZ) are deep peels used to address sun damage and wrinkles.

- **Phenol** (FEE-nohl) peels are the strongest peels and can be toxic. They are still used and are less expensive, but they require a longer recovery period than TCA peels or laser resurfacing.

BODY PROCEDURES

Many individuals are having elective surgeries. It is therefore important to be familiar with these procedures, especially if you are offering body treatments.

- *Sclerotherapy* (sklair-oh-THAIR-uh-pee) minimizes varicose veins (dilated blood vessels) and other varicosities by injecting chemical agents into the affected areas. Lasers are a secondary method of vein therapy. Over 50 percent of women and 40 percent of men have varicose veins and smaller spider veins (telangiectasia) on their legs.[1] Potential causes are heredity, race, gender, posture, hormones, and pregnancy. Trauma

[1] Office on Women's Health in the U.S. Department of Health and Human Services. "Varicose veins and spider veins." https://www.womenshealth.gov/a-z-topics/varicose-veins-and-spider-veins. Accessed February 22, 2018.

and injury causes inflammation to vessels. Phlebitis (fluh-BY-tus) is the inflammation of a vein. To take pressure off veins keep the legs elevated, wear compression stockings, avoid crossing the legs, exercise, and avoid being in stationary positions for extended periods of time.

- **Mammoplasty** (MAYM-oh-plas-tee) is breast surgery that enlarges the breasts or reconstructs them. This procedure is also referred to as breast augmentation, or implants. Breast reduction reduces or repositions the breasts. This is sometimes performed for health reasons, primarily to alleviate back pain.

- **Liposuction** (ly-POH-suk-shun) is the procedure that surgically removes pockets of fat.

- An **abdominoplasty** (ab-DOM-un-oh-plas-tee) removes excessive fat deposits and loose skin from the abdomen to tuck and tighten the area.

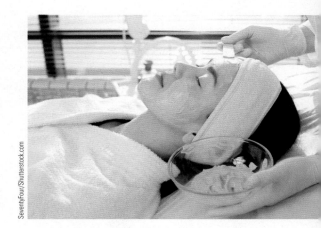

Web Resources

Here are some great websites for more information:
American Society of Plastic Surgeons: www.plasticsurgery.org
eMedicine: www.emedicine.com
Mayo Clinic: www.mayoclinic.com
The medical journal for skin care professionals: www.pcijournal.com

The Clinical Esthetician

Working as a clinical esthetician in medical esthetics can be enriching (**Figure 13–32**). This specialty requires compassion and patience because you will work with people who are in pain or who are experiencing physical trauma. Many patients feel more comfortable with the esthetician than they do with a physician, who may not have time for more personal and empathetic discussions. Remember to stay focused on the treatment goals and maintain a professional role at all times. The role of an esthetician can be invaluable in a medical setting in providing pre- and postoperative care and other patient services and education.

A career in esthetics is always exciting and fascinating. Advanced areas of study range from medical esthetics to exotic body treatments. Light therapy and AHAs for skin care are two of the most effective tools available today to estheticians. Opportunities for advanced training are limitless.

There are many services one can specialize in. As the industry continues to grow, keep up with modern technology and changes, even if they are not on your service menu. After basic esthetic techniques are mastered, it is a natural progression to add advanced treatments to the services currently offered. This is the beauty of esthetics: the increased ability to improve the health of the skin as the industry evolves. Educated and skilled technicians will always be in demand.

▲ **Figure 13–32** The role of an esthetician can be invaluable in a medical setting in providing pre- and postoperative care and other patient services and education.

 CHECK IN

19. What services do medical estheticians provide?
20. What are injectable fillers used for?
21. What are the medical terms for facelift, eye lift, and nose surgery?

Procedure 13-1:
Perform An Enzyme Mask Service

Regulatory Alert: Not all states allow estheticians to perform peels. Check with your regulatory agency prior to performing advanced procedures. As with all peels and procedures, make certain to obtain and maintain the highest level of training, certification, and licensure available within your scope of practice.

Materials, Implements, and Equipment

- ☐ 2" × 2" Esthetic wipes or cotton rounds
- ☐ 4" × 4" Moistened esthetic wipes (or single-use sponges, cotton compresses, or facial cloths to be used with water in a bowl)
- ☐ Cleanser
- ☐ Disposable spatula or fan brush

- ☐ Enzyme mask
- ☐ Gloves
- ☐ Goggles/protective eyewear
- ☐ Hand sanitizer
- ☐ Magnifying lamp
- ☐ Makeup remover
- ☐ Moisturizer
- ☐ Post-Service supplies (disinfection solution, paper towels, etc.)

- ☐ Protective eyewear
- ☐ Standard treatment table setup with linens
- ☐ Sun protection
- ☐ Toner (appropriate for client's skin)

Procedure

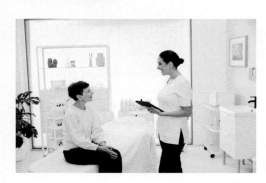

1 Complete Procedure 7–1: Pre-Service including proper draping. Ensure the client is cleared for this service prior to proceeding. Discuss the expected outcome of this treatment with the client so they have realistic expectations of what the treatment can and cannot accomplish.

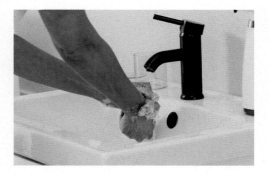

2 Wash your hands and put on gloves.

CAUTION!
As a new esthetician, until you are familiar with your client's reaction to this treatment, it is better to be more conservative than to encounter an adverse reaction.

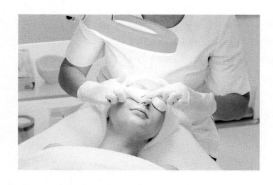

3 Perform a visual analysis of the skin to ensure the skin is intact and to ensure the treatment is not contraindicated. Complete Procedure 5–1: Skin Analysis.

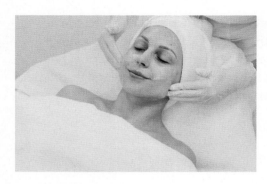

4 Apply a cleanser suitable to remove makeup with your gloved hands. Massage the cleanser to loosen makeup. Remove the cleanser.

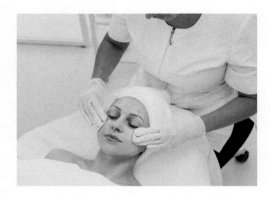

5 Using 2″ × 2″ gauze pads or cotton rounds moistened with toner, remove any residue.

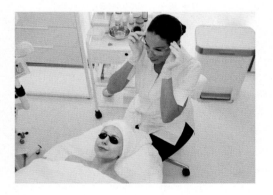

6 Apply goggles to your client and yourself to protect the eyes from any irritants.

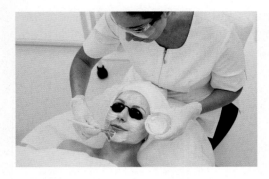

7 Using a disposable spatula or fan brush, apply the enzyme mask beginning at the forehead and moving to the temples, then to the right and left cheeks, chin, upper lip, and nose.

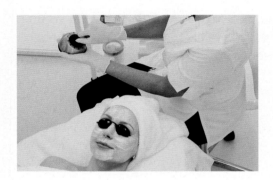

8 Set a timer and process the mask according to the manufacturer's instructions. NOTE: Remove sooner if client cannot tolerate the treatment or if the peel has processed prior to the recommended minimal end time. **Endpoint goal: very light erythema.**

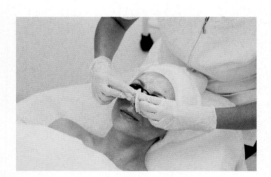

9 Remove the mask using 4" × 4" moistened esthetics wipes or chosen material.

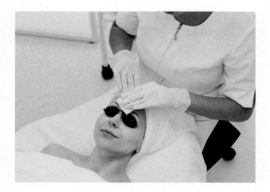

10 Apply toner to the skin to remove residue.

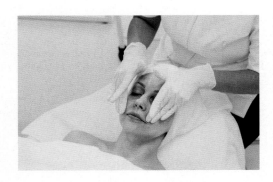

11 Apply moisturizer and sun protection.

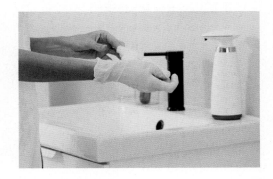

12 Remove your gloves and wash your hands.

13 Discuss your observations and any recommendations with the client.

14 Perform Procedure 7–2 and 8-9: Post-Service.

Expected response to enzyme peel mask:

There should be no reaction beyond very light tingling or the absence of any tingling. If you are applying a mask you can see the skin through, it is expected to initially see the skin experience a very light erythema or even turn pink. The client may experience minimal or no tingling while the solution is actively processing. You are looking for pinkness, not redness, as this is an enzyme peel.

Procedure 13-2:
Perform a Back Facial with Enzyme Mask

Materials, Implements, and Equipment

- ☐ 2" × 2" Esthetic wipes or cotton rounds
- ☐ 4" × 4" Esthetic wipes pads (or single-use sponges, cotton compresses, or facial cloths to be used with water in a bowl)
- ☐ Cleanser to remove makeup
- ☐ Disposable applicator or brush

- ☐ Enzyme mask
- ☐ Gloves
- ☐ Goggles/protective eyewear
- ☐ Hand sanitizer
- ☐ Magnifying lamp
- ☐ Moisturizer
- ☐ Post-Service supplies (disinfectant solution, paper towels, etc.)

- ☐ Standard treatment table setup with linens
- ☐ Steamer (optional)
- ☐ Sun protection
- ☐ Toner (appropriate for client skin)
- ☐ Warm towels in hot towel cabinet

Procedure

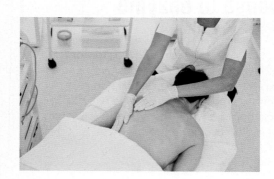

1 Complete Procedure 7–1: Pre-Service. Ensure the client is cleared for this service prior to proceeding.

2 Cleanse and analyze the skin. Apply a cleanser suitable for the client's skin type with your gloved hands. Massage the cleanser in circular motions. Remove the cleanser using 4" × 4" moistened gauze pads or chosen material. Complete Procedure 5–1: Skin Analysis.

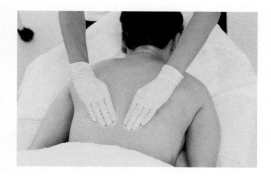

3 Using 2" × 2" esthetic wipes or cotton rounds moistened with toner, remove any residue.

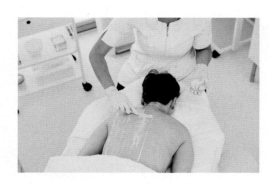

4 Using a disposable spatula or brush apply the enzyme mask to the back area.

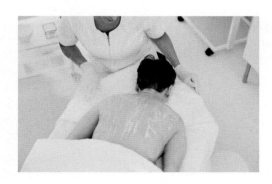

5 Process the mask according to the manufacturer's instructions. (Remove sooner if client cannot tolerate the treatment or if the peel has processed prior to the recommended minimal end time.)

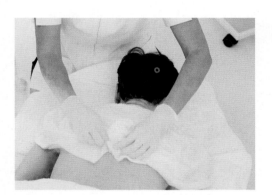

6 Remove the mask using warm towels, 4" × 4" moistened esthetic wipes, or chosen material.

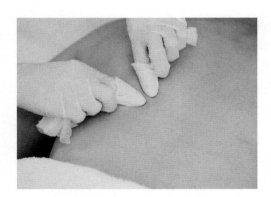

7 Option: Perform extractions.

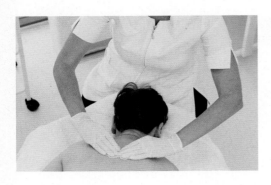

8 Using 2″ × 2″ esthetic wipes or cotton rounds moistened with toner, remove any residue.

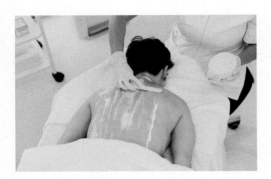

9 Using a disposable spatula or brush apply a mask suitable for the client's skin type to the back area.

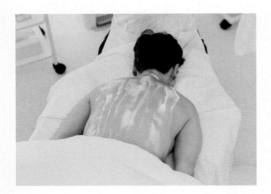

10 Process the mask.

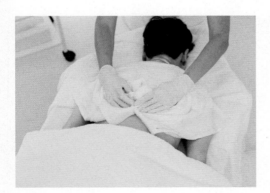

11 Remove the mask using warm towels, 4″ × 4″ moistened esthetic wipes or chosen material.

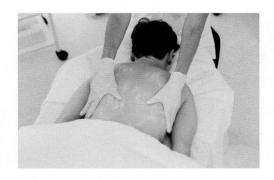

12 Apply moisturizer in circular motions and then sun protection.

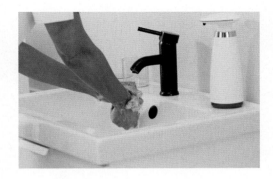

13 Remove your gloves and wash your hands.

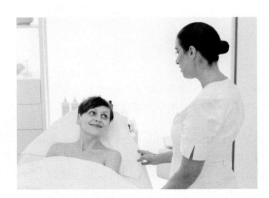

14 Discuss your observations and any recommendations with the client.

15 Perform Procedure 7–2 and 8-9: Post-Service.

Procedure 13-3:
Perform a Light Glycolic Peel

Regulatory alert: Not all states allow estheticians to perform peels. Check with your regulatory agency prior to performing advanced procedures.

Materials, Implements, and Equipment

- ☐ 2" × 2" Esthetic wipes or cotton rounds
- ☐ 4" × 4" Moistened esthetic wipes (or single-use sponges, cotton compresses, or facial cloths to be used with water in a bowl)
- ☐ Cleanser
- ☐ Gloves
- ☐ Goggles/protective eyewear

- ☐ Hand sanitizer
- ☐ Large tipped cotton applicators
- ☐ Light glycolic peel
- ☐ Magnifying lamp
- ☐ Moisturizer
- ☐ Peel neutralizer
- ☐ Post-Service supplies (disinfectant solution, paper towels, etc.)

- ☐ Protective ointment
- ☐ Standard treatment table setup with linens
- ☐ Sun protection
- ☐ Toner (appropriate for client skin)

Procedure

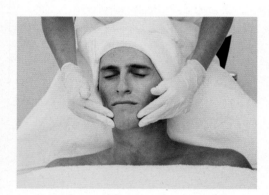

1 Complete Procedure 7–1: Pre-Service. Ensure the client is cleared for this service prior to proceeding.

2 Cleanse and analyze the skin. Apply a cleanser suitable for the client's skin type with your gloved hands. Massage the cleanser in circular motions. Remove the cleanser using 4" × 4" moistened gauze pads or chosen material. Complete Procedure 5–1: Skin Analysis.

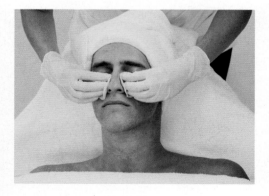

3 Using 2" × 2" esthetic wipes or cotton rounds moistened with toner, remove any residue.

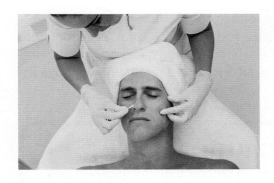

4 Apply a protective ointment around the eyes, corners or the nose and on the lips.

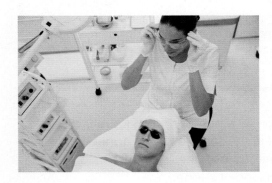

5 Apply protective eyewear to your client and then to yourself.

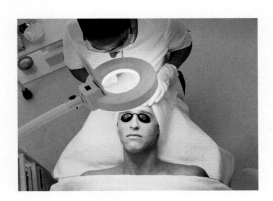

6 Carefully analyze the client's skin with the magnifying lamp.

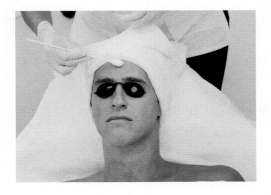

7 Using a large tipped cotton swab, apply the peel beginning at the forehead and moving to the temples, then to the right and left cheeks, chin, upper lip, and nose.

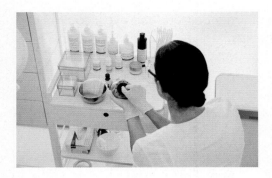

8 Process the peel according to the manufacturer's instructions (neutralize and remove sooner if client cannot tolerate the treatment or if the peel has processed prior to the recommended minimal end time). **Endpoint goal: mild erythema**.

> # CAUTION!
> Some areas of the face may process sooner than others, and you may need to perform spot neutralization and removal on those areas. Sometimes a client's entire face may process sooner than the manufacturer's recommended minimal processing time and you may need to neutralize and remove the peel immediately.

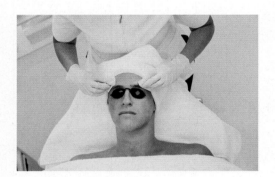

9 Using 2" × 2" esthetic wipes or chosen material, neutralize the peel in the same order as applied unless you need to spot neutralize other areas first due to the peel reaching its endpoint sooner.

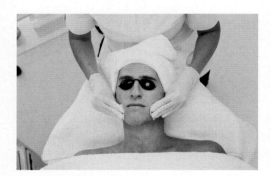

10 Remove the peel using damp 4" × 4" esthetic wipes or chosen material.

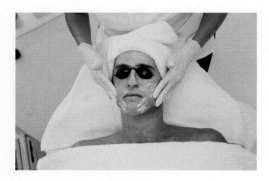

11 Apply moisturizer and sun protection liberally.

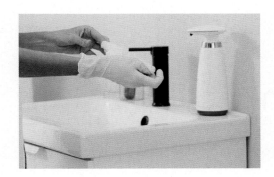

12 Remove your gloves and wash your hands.

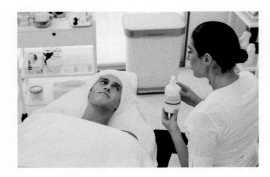

13 Discuss your observations and any recommendations with the client.

14 Perform Procedure 7–2 and 8-9: Post-Service.

> ## Expected response to light glycolic peel solution:
> It is expected to initially see slight or mild erythema, which may be expressed in an uneven or a spotty appearance. The client may experience tingling or itchiness while the solution is actively processing. You are looking for slight or mild erythema as this is a light glycolic peel.

Procedure 13-4:
Perform Crystal-Free Microdermabrasion (Diamond Tip)

Regulatory alert: Not all states allow estheticians to perform microdermabrasion. Check with your regulatory agency prior to performing advanced procedures.

Materials, Implements, and Equipment

- ☐ 2" × 2" Gauze pads or cotton rounds
- ☐ 4" × 4" Moistened gauze pads (or single-use sponges, cotton compresses, or facial cloths to be used with water in a bowl)
- ☐ Cleanser to remove makeup

- ☐ Crystal-free microdermabrasion machine (diamond tip) and handpiece
- ☐ Gloves
- ☐ Goggles/protective eyewear
- ☐ Hand sanitizer
- ☐ Magnifying lamp
- ☐ Moisturizer

- ☐ Post-Service supplies (disinfectant solution, paper towels, etc.)
- ☐ Standard treatment table setup with linens
- ☐ Sun protection
- ☐ Toner (appropriate for client skin)

Procedure

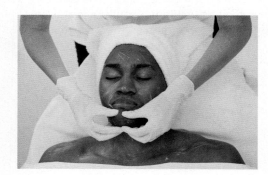

1 Complete Procedure 7–1: Pre-Service. Ensure the client is cleared for this service prior to proceeding.

2 Cleanse and analyze the skin. Apply a cleanser suitable for the client's skin type with your gloved hands. Massage the cleanser in circular motions. Remove the cleanser using 4" × 4" moistened gauze pads or chosen material. Complete Procedure 5–1: Skin Analysis.

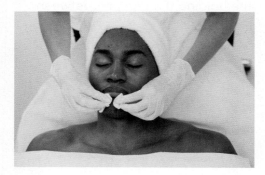

3 Using 2" × 2" esthetic wipes or cotton rounds moistened with toner, remove any residue.

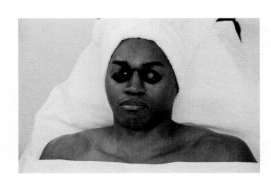

4 Apply goggles to protect the eye area.

5 Engage the crystal-free handpiece with the hose of the microdermabrasion machine. Test the intensity of the suction over your gloved hand and adjust accordingly.

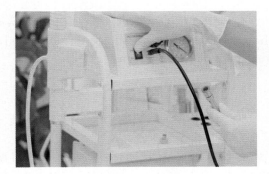

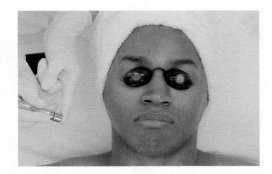

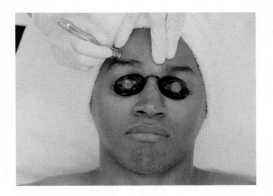

6 Begin at the forehead, then move to the temples, to the right and left cheeks, chin, upper lip, and nose.

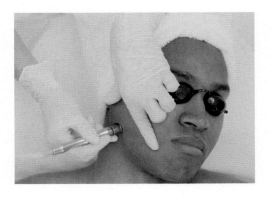

7 Use light, even pressure holding the skin taut between the thumb and the forefinger as you move from one section to the next.

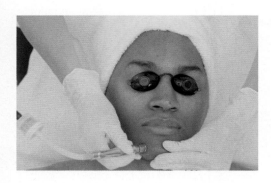

8 The number of passes should range between one and three depending on the thickness and sensitivity of the client's skin, the machine settings and, the point the erythema occurs. More sensitive clients and areas receive fewer passes.

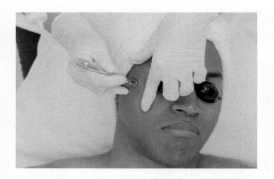

9 Passes typically proceed as follows: horizontal, vertical, then diagonal. Passes can be performed independently over the entire face and then proceed to the next direction until the treatment is completed. However, cross-hatching with two passes consisting of a horizontal then vertical action is used most frequently.

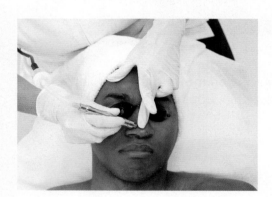

10 For smaller areas, such as the upper lip and nose, change the diamond tip size that best fits the area being treated.

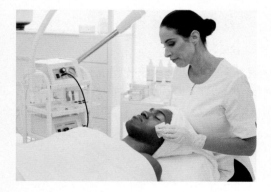

11 Using 2" × 2" esthetic wipes or cotton rounds moistened with toner, remove any residue.

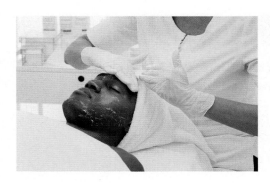

12 Apply moisturizer and sun protection.

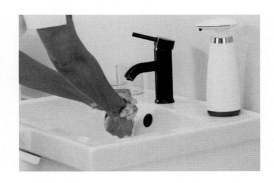

13 Remove your gloves and wash your hands.

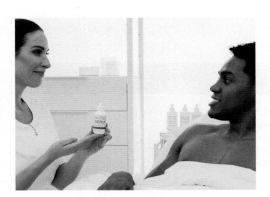

14 Discuss your observations and any recommendations with the client.

15 Perform Procedure 7–2 and 8-9: Post-Service.

Expected response to microdermabrasion:

It is expected to initially see slight or mild erythema. The client may experience pressure and a slight abrasive sensation associated with the handpiece. You are looking for slight erythema, not redness, as this is an esthetic-level microdermabrasion. Endpoint goal: mild erythema.

COMPETENCY ⊘ PROGRESS

How are you doing with advanced topics and treatments? **Check the Chapter 13 Learning Objectives below that you feel you have mastered; leave unchecked those objectives you will need to return to:**

- ☐ Explain advanced skin care topics and treatments for licensed, trained estheticians.
- ☐ Identify how to safely and effectively use chemical exfoliation and peels.
- ☐ Discuss the benefits of microdermabrasion by type of device.
- ☐ Explain the benefits of laser technology.
- ☐ Explain the benefits and types of light therapy.
- ☐ Discuss microcurrent treatments.
- ☐ Discuss ultrasound.
- ☐ Discuss microneedling and nano infusion.
- ☐ Describe spa body treatments.
- ☐ Discuss common treatments used to address cellulite.
- ☐ Explain the benefits of manual lymphatic drainage.
- ☐ Describe the field of medical esthetics.

GLOSSARY

abdominoplasty ab-DOM-un-oh-plas-tee	pg. 681	procedure that removes excessive fat deposits and loose skin from the abdomen to tuck and tighten the area
ayurvedic ah-yur-VAY-dic	pg. 673	one of the world's oldest holistic healing systems; it originated in India and is thought to be as much as 5,000 years old; *Ayurveda* translates from Sanskrit as "science of health or wellness"
balneotherapy bal-nee-oh-THAYR-uh-pee	pg. 672	body treatments that use mud or fango, Dead Sea salt, seaweed, enzymes, or peat baths
blepharoplasty BLEF-uh-roh-plas-tee	pg. 679	a plastic surgery procedure that removes excess skin and/or fat in the upper or lower eyelids
blue light BLOO LYT	pg. 665	a light-emitting diode for use on clients to improve acne and reduce bacteria
body masks BAHD-ee masks	pg. 671	a body treatment involving the application of an exfoliating, hydrating, purification, or detoxification mask to the entire body; masks may include clay, cream, gel, or seaweed bases
body scrubs BAHD-ee scrubz	pg. 671	use of friction and products to exfoliate, hydrate, increase circulation, and nourish the skin
body wraps BAHD-ee RAPs	pg. 670	wraps that remineralize, hydrate, stimulate, or promote relaxation by using aloe, gels, lotions, oils, seaweed, herbs, clay, or mud

Botox® Bow-tocks	pg. 678	neuromuscular-blocking serum (botulinum toxin) that paralyzes nerve cells on the muscle when this serum is injected into it
cell renewal factor sell re-new-uhl fack-tor	pg. 643	abbreviated CRF; also known as *cell turnover rate*; the rate of cell mitosis and migration from the dermis to the top of the epidermis
cellulite SEL-yoo-lyt	pg. 674	dimpling of the skin caused by protrusion of subcutaneous fat; due to an irregularity in distribution of fat in the area, usually found on the thighs, hips, buttocks, and abdomen
chromophore krohma-for	pg. 664	the colored cells or target in the epidermis or dermis that absorbs a laser beam's thermal energy, causing the desired injury or destruction of material
cosmetic surgery kahz-MET-ik SUR-juh-ree	pg. 679	also known as *esthetic surgery*; elective surgery for improving and altering the appearance
dermabrasion dur-muh-BRAY-zhun	pg. 680	medical procedure; strong exfoliation method using a mechanical brush to physically remove tissue down to the dermis
dermal fillers DUR-mul FILL-erz	pg. 678	products used to fill lines, wrinkles, and other facial imperfections
endermology ENDER-mol-oh-gee	pg. 673	treatment for cellulite; helps stimulate the reduction of adipose tissue by a vacuum massage that combines a vigorous massage along with suction
foot reflexology FOOT reflex-OL-oo-jee	pg. 672	technique of applying pressure to the feet based on a system of zones and areas on the feet that directly correspond to the anatomy of the body; reflexology is also performed on the hands and ears
green light GREEN lyte	pg. 665	a light-emitting diode for use on clients with hyperpigmentation or for detoxifying the skin
hydrotherapy hy-druh-THAIR-uh-pee	pg. 671	spa treatments that use water
injectable fillers in-JEK-tuh-bul FIL-urz	pg. 678	substances used in nonsurgical procedures to fill in or plump up areas of the skin; Botox® and dermal fillers are injectables
intense pulse light in-TENS PULSE LYHT	pg. 663	abbreviated IPL; a medical device that uses multiple colors and wavelengths (broad spectrum) of focused light to treat spider veins, hyperpigmentation, rosacea and redness, wrinkles, enlarged hair follicles and pores, and excessive hair
Jessner's peel JEZZ-nuhrz PEEL	pg. 644	light to medium peel of lactic acid, salicylic acid, and resorcinol in an ethanol solvent
lasers LAY-zurs	pg. 660	acronym for *light amplification stimulation emission of radiation*; a medical device that uses electromagnetic radiation for hair removal and skin treatments
laser resurfacing LAY-zur re-SUR-fas-ing	pg. 680	a laser procedure utilizing a CO_2 or an erbium laser that involves vaporization of the epidermis and/or dermis for facial rejuvenation; used to smooth wrinkles or lighten acne scars and stimulate growth of new collagen
light-emitting diode LYT EE-mitt-ing DYE-ode	pg. 664	abbreviated LED; a device used to reduce acne, increase skin circulation, and improve the collagen content in the skin
liposuction ly-POH-suk-shun	pg. 681	a surgical procedure used to remove stubborn areas of fat

mammoplasty MAYM-oh-plas-tee	pg. 681	surgery to alter the shape or contours of the breast
microcurrent mi-kroh-CUR-ent	pg. 666	used in a device that mimics the body's natural electrical energy to re-educate and tone facial muscles; improves circulation and increases collagen and elastin production
microdermabrasion MI-kroh-DERMA-bray-shun	pg. 655	form of mechanical exfoliation
microneedling MI-kroh-NEED-ling	pg. 670	the use of a dermal roller or an electronic handpiece to induce puncture wounds to the skin that induce collagen formation during the wound healing process
nonablative non-uh-BLAY-tiv	pg. 677	procedure that does not remove tissue; wrinkle treatments that bypass the epidermis to stimulate collagen in the dermis for wrinkle reduction are nonablative
phenol FEE-nohl	pg. 680	carbolic acid; a caustic poison; used for peels and to disinfect metallic implements
reconstructive surgery REE-con-struct-if SIR-JUR-ee	pg. 678	defined as *restoring a bodily function*; necessary surgery for accident survivors and those with congenital disfigurements or other diseases
red light RED LYT	pg. 665	a light-emitting diode for use on clients in the stimulation of circulation and collagen and elastin production
Reiki RAY-KEE	pg. 673	universal life-force energy transmitted through the palms of the hands that helps lift the spirits and provide balance to the whole self: body, mind, and spirit
rhinoplasty RY-noh-plas-tee	pg. 680	plastic or reconstructive surgery performed on the nose to change or correct its appearance
rhytidectomy rit-ih-DEK-tuh-mee	pg. 679	a facelift procedure that removes excess fat at the jawline; tightens loose, atrophic muscles; and removes sagging skin
stone massage STON mass-aje	pg. 672	use of hot and cold stones in massage or other treatments
transconjunctival blepharoplasty trans-kon-junk-TIE-vul BLEF-uh-roh-plas-tee	pg. 679	procedure performed inside the lower eyelid to remove bulging fat pads, which are often congenital
trichloroacetic acid (TCA) peels TRY-klor-oh-AH-seed-ick ASUD PEELZ	pg. 680	a strong peel used to diminish sun damage and wrinkles
ultrasonic ULL-trah-son-ik	pg. 668	frequency above the range of sound audible to the human ear; vibrations, created through a water medium, help cleanse and exfoliate the skin by removing dead skin cells; contraindications include epilepsy, pregnancy, and cancerous lesions; synonymous with ultrasound

ultrasound ULL-trah-sow-nd	pg. 668	frequency above the range of sound audible to the human ear; vibrations, created through a water medium, help cleanse and exfoliate the skin by removing dead skin cells; also used for product penetration; cellulite reduction; stimulating tissue, increasing blood flow, and promoting oxygenation
yellow light YEL-oh LYT	pg. 665	a light-emitting diode that aids in reducing inflammation and swelling

Appendix A: Resources

Alberts, B., and Johnson, A. D. (2015). *Molecular Biology of the Cell*, 6th ed. New York: Garland Science.

Baker, J. T. (2016). *Secrets of Successful Spa Owners*. Self-published.

Bialosky, Joel E. *et al.* (2008). "The mechanisms of manual therapy in the treatment of musculoskeletal pain: a comprehensive model." *Manual Therapy* 14(5): 531–538. Available at https://www.ncbi.nlm.nih.gov/pmc/articles/PMC2775050/

Crane J. D. *et al.* (2012). "Massage therapy attenuates inflammatory signaling after exercise-induced muscle damage." *Science Translational Medicine*. doi: 10.1126/scitranslmed.3002882. Available at https://www.medpagetoday.com/neurology/painmanagement/30996

Culp, J., and Campbell, T. (2013). *Esthetician's Guide to Client Safety & Wellness*. New York: Cengage Learning.

Deitz, S. (2013). *Skin Care Practices and Clinical Protocols*. New York: Cengage Learning.

Goldberg, D. J., and Alexander, L. B. (2018). *Disorders of Fat and Cellulite*. New York: Informa Healthcare.

James, W. D., Elston, D. M., and McMahon, P. J. (2018). *Andrews' Diseases of the Skin Clinical Atlas*. New York: Elsevier.

Kolster, B. C., and Waskowiak, A. (2018). *The Reflexology Atlas*. New York: Simon & Schuster.

Lees, M. (2014). *Clearing Concepts: A Guide to Acne Treatment*. New York: Cengage Learning.

Lees, M. (2012). *Skin Care Beyond the Basics*, 4th ed. New York: Cengage Learning.

Lees, M. (2011). *The Skin Care Answer Book*. New York: Cengage Learning.

Martini, F. H., Tallitsch, R. B., and Nath, J. L. (2017). *Human Anatomy*, 9th ed. New York: Pearson.

Michalun, M. V., and DiNardo, J. C. (2014). *Skin Care and Cosmetic Ingredients Dictionary*, 4th ed. New York: Cengage Learning.

Pierce, A. (2013). *Milady's Aesthetician Series: Treating Diverse Pigmentation*. New York: Cengage Learning.

Pugliese, M. Q., and Hancock, S. (2018). *The Esthetician's Guide to Outstanding Esthetics*. Self-published.

Schmaling, S. (2012). *Milady's Aesthetician Series: Aging Skin*. New York: Cengage Learning.

Shapiro, B. (2018). *Skin Deep: Women on Skin Care, Makeup, and Looking Their Best*. New York: New York Times.

Simon, S. (2018). "How to Spot Skin Cancer." American Cancer Society. Available at https://www.cancer.org/latest-news/how-to-spot-skin-cancer.html [Accessed February 1, 2019].

Touch Research Institute. (2012). University of Miami, Miller School of Medicine. Available at http://www6.miami.edu/touch-research/

Weis-Bohlen, S. (2018). *Ayurveda Beginner's Guide*. San Antonio, TX: Althea Press.

Wolff, K., and Johnson, R. A. (2017). *Fitzpatrick's Color Atlas & Synopsis of Clinical Dermatology*, 8th ed. New York: McGraw-Hill.

Worwood, V. A. (2016). *The Complete Book of Essential Oils and Aromatherapy*. San Rafael, CA: New World Library.

Appendix B: Conversions

U.S. Measurement-Metric Conversion Tables

The following tables show standard conversions for commonly used measurements in Milady Standard Esthetics: Fundamentals, 12th Edition.

Conversion Formula for Inches to Centimeters: (number of) inches x 2.54 = centimeters

LENGTH	
Inches	**Centimeters**
⅛ inch (.125 inches)	0.317 centimeters
¼ inch (.25 inches)	0.635 centimeters
½ inch (.50 inches)	1.27 centimeters
¾ inch (.75 inches)	1.9 centimeters
1 inch	2.54 centimeters
2 inches	5.1 centimeters
3 inches	7.6 centimeters
6 inches	15.2 centimeters
12 inches	30.5 centimeters

Conversion Formula for U.S. Fluid Ounces to Milliliters:
(amount of) U.S. fluid ounce (fl. oz.) x 29.573 milliliters (ml)

Conversion Formula for U.S. Fluid Ounces to Liters:
(amount of) U.S. fluid ounce (fl. oz.) x .029573 liters (l)

VOLUME (liquid)	
U.S. Fluid Onces	**Milliliters/liters**
1 fluid ounce (⅛ cup)	29. 57 milliliters/.02957 liters
2 fluid ounces (¼ cup)	59.14 milliliters/.05914 liters
4 fluid ounces (½ cup)	118.29 milliliters/.11829 liters
6 fluid ounces (¾ cup)	177.43 milliliters/.17743 liters
8 fluid ounces (1 cup)	236.58 milliliters/.23658 liters
16 fluid ounces (1 pint)	473.16 milliliters/.47316 liters
32 fluid ounces (1 quart)	946.33 milliliters/.94633 liters
33.81 fluid ounces (1 liter)	1,000 milliliters/1 liter
64 fluid ounces (½ gallon)	1,892.67 milliliters/1.8926 liters
128 fluid ounces (1 gallon)	3,785.34 milliliters/3.78534 liters

Conversion Formula for Degrees Fahrenheit (°F) to Degrees Celsius (°C): $°C = (°F-32) \times (5/9)$ *

TEMPERATURE	
Degrees Fahrenheit (°F)	**Degrees Celsius (°C)**
32°	0°
40°	4.444°
50°	10°
60°	15.556°
70°	21.111°
80°	26.667°
98.6°	37°
200°	93.333°
300°	148.889°
400°	204.444°

*** If you have a Fahrenheit temperature of 40 degrees and you want to convert it into degrees on the Celsius scale: Using the conversion formula, first subtract 32 from the Fahrenheit temperature of 40 degrees to get 8 as a result. Then multiply 8 by five and divide by nine (8 x 5)/9 to get the converted value of 4.444 degrees Celsius.

Glossary/Index

A

Abdominoplasty, procedure that removes excessive fat deposits and loose skin from the abdomen to tuck and tighten the area, *681, 698*

Abduction, muscles that draw a body part, such as a finger, arm, or toe, away from the midline of the body or of an extremity. In the hand, abduction separates the fingers, *46, 70*

Absorption, the transport of fully digested food into the circulatory system to feed the tissues and cells, *68, 70*

Acai berry, berry rich in antioxidants, vitamins A, B, C, and E; protects, replenishes; helps heal damaged skin, *228, 254*

Accessory nerve, also known as *eleventh cranial nerve;* a type of motor nerve that controls the motion of the neck and shoulder muscles, *50, 51, 53, 70*

Accutane®. *See* Isotretinoin

Acids,
  in chemical exfoliation, 642–643

Acne, chronic inflammatory skin disorder of the sebaceous glands that is characterized by comedones and blemishes; commonly known as acne simplex or acne vulgaris, *131, 156*
  benzyl peroxide for, 229
  facial masks for, 242
  facial treatments, 335–344
    extraction techniques, 338–340
    home care, 337–338
    procedure, 340–344
    suggestions for clients with, 337
  grades of, 134
  laser resurfacing for acne scars, 680
  laser resurfacing for scars of, 680
  LED for, 664
  light therapy for, 662–666
  medications for, 137–138
  skin, 236
  sulfur in acne products, 234
  triggers, 134–137
  types, 131–138

Actinic keratosis, pink or flesh-colored precancerous lesions that feel sharp or rough; resulting from sun damage, *129, 156*

Acupressure, *391*

Adapalene (Differin®), *137*

Adduction, muscles that draw a body part, such as a finger, arm, or toe, inward toward the median axis of the body or of an extremity. In the hand, adduction draw the fingers together, *46, 70*

Adenosine triphosphate (ATP), transports chemical energy within cells for metabolism, *29, 70*

Adhesive, *607*

Adipose tissue, specialized connective tissue considered fat, which gives smoothness and contour to the body and cushions and insulates the body, *31, 70, 86, 91*

Adrenal glands, glands that are located at the top of the kidneys assisting in the regulation of metabolism, stress response and blood pressure, and support of immune system health through the generation of specific hormones, *64, 70*

Advanced topics and treatments. *See also* Chemical exfoliation; Exfoliation; Laser; Light therapy
  cellulite, 674–675
  laser technology, 660–662
  for licensed and trained estheticians, 641–642
  light therapy, 662–666
  manual lymph drainage, 392, 675–676
  medical aesthetics, 681
  microcurrent treatments, 666–668
  microdermabrasion, 655–660
  microneedling and nano infusion, 669–670
  procedures
    back facial with enzyme mask, 686–689
    crystal-free microdermabrasion (diamond tip), 694–697
    enzyme mask service, 682–685
    light glycolic peel, 690–693
  spa body treatments, 670–675
  ultrasound and ultrasonic technology, 668–669

Aesthetics, 6

Africa, *19*

Age of Extravagance, *19*

Aging
  facial treatments for, 325–330
  factors causing, 174–175
  lifestyle choices and, 110–112
  physiology of, 113
  skin, 237
  UVA and UVB radiation, 107–108

Blush, makeup that gives the face a natural-looking glow and helps create facial balance, *569, 585, 636*

Body dysmorphic disorder, psychological disorder in which the client has a preoccupation with their appearance; they tend to fixate on minor appearance imperfections and see them as disfiguring, *152–153, 156*

Body masks, a body treatment involving the application of an exfoliating, hydrating, purification, or detoxification mask to the entire body. Masks may include clay, cream, gel, or seaweed bases, *671, 698*

Body scrubs, use of friction and products to exfoliate, hydrate, increase circulation, and nourish the skin, *671, 698*

Body systems, also known as *systems,* groups of body organs acting together to perform one or more functions. The human body is composed of 11 major systems, *32, 71*

Body wraps, wraps remineralize, hydrate, stimulate, or promote relaxation by using aloe, gels, lotions, oils, seaweed, herbs, clay, or mud, *670–671, 698*

Boil. *See* Furuncle

Botanicals, ingredients derived from plants, *216, 254*

Botox®, neuromuscular-blocking serum (botulinum toxin) that paralyzes nerve cells on the muscle when this serum is injected into it, *678, 699*

Bracing, technique using one or both hands positioned to avoid client injury, keeping your hands steady and the client safe, *586, 636*

Brain, part of the central nervous system contained in the cranium; largest and most complex nerve tissue; controls sensation, muscles, glandular activity, and the power to think and feel, *49, 71. See also* Cranium
endocrine system and, *63*
and spinal cord, *49*

Brain stem, structure that connects the spinal cord to the brain, *49, 71*

Brazilian waxing, *494*

Breastbone, *39*

Brighteners, *219*

Bromhidrosis, foul-smelling perspiration, usually in the armpits or on the feet, *154, 157*

Brow comb, a tool used to brush eyebrow hairs into the desired position, creating a finely groomed look; in addition to the comb itself, many brow combs have a brush on one side, *574, 636*

Brows. *See* Eyebrows

Brushes (makeup), Used for applying and blending powder, blush, and eyeshadows, as they work better than sponge tips or fingers; brushes vary in size, shape, make, use, cost, and longevity; brushes are the artist's most essential tool, as they allow for better control and blending, *574, 575–578, 637*

Buccal nerve, nerve that affects the muscles of the mouth, *51, 52, 71*

Buccinator, thin, flat muscle of the cheek between the upper and lower jaw that compresses the cheeks and expels air between the lips, *43, 71*

Bulla (plural: bullae), large blister containing watery fluid; similar to a vesicle, but larger, *124, 157*

C

Cake makeup (pancake makeup), a heavy-coverage makeup pressed into a compact and applied to the face with a moistened cosmetic sponge, *567, 637*

Calendula, anti-inflammatory plant extract, *229, 254*

Calming influence, *673*
aromatherapy, *392*
facial masks, *241*
shirodhara, *673*

Camouflage, makeup, *605*

Candelilla, a hard wax used to modify the melting point and provide increased strength to hard depilatory wax, *473, 548*

Capillaries, tiny, thin-walled blood vessels that connect the smaller arteries to the veins. Capillaries bring nutrients to the cells and carry away waste materials, *56, 71*

Carbomers, ingredients used to thicken creams; frequently used in gel products, *215, 254*

Carbuncle, cluster of boils; large inflammation of the subcutaneous tissue caused by staphylococci bacterium; similar to a furuncle (boil) but larger, *154, 157*

Cardiovascular system, body system consisting of the heart, arteries, veins, and capillaries for the distribution of blood throughout the body, *54, 71*

Career planning, licensure, *389*

Career(s)
brow specialists, *7–9*
day spa esthetician, *6–7*
in education, *13*
esthetics writer, *11*
in makeup, *611–614*
makeup artist, *9*
mortuary science, *9*
oncology-trained esthetician, *15–16*
waxing specialists, *7–9*

Carnauba, a hard wax used to modify the melting point and provide increased strength to hard depilatory wax, *473, 548*

Carpus (wrist), a flexible joint composed of eight small, irregular bones (carpals) held together by ligaments, *40, 71*

Catagen, second transition stage of hair growth; in the catagen stage, the hair shaft grows upward and detaches itself from the bulb, *460, 548*

Cataphoresis, process of forcing an acidic (positive) product into deeper tissues using galvanic current from the positive pole toward the negative pole; tightens and calms the skin, *428, 452*

Cell membrane, part of the cell that encloses the protoplasm and permits soluble substances to enter and leave the cell, *29, 72*
basic structure of, *29*
reproduction and division, *29–30*

Cell renewal factor (CRF), cell turnover rate, *643, 699*

Cells, basic unit of all living things; minute mass of protoplasm capable of performing all the fundamental functions of life, *28, 72*
metabolism, *30*
skin, *85–86*

Cellulite, dimpling of the skin caused by protrusion of subcutaneous fat; is due to an irregularity in distribution of fat in the area, usually found on the thighs, hips, buttocks, and abdomen, *674–675, 699*

Central nervous system (CNS), cerebrospinal nervous system; consists of the brain, spinal cord, spinal nerves, and cranial nerves, *48, 72*

Ceramides, glycolipid materials that are a natural part of skin's intercellular matrix and barrier function, *107, 116*

Certificate or license, esthetician's, scope of practice, *388–389*

Certified colors, inorganic color agents also known as *metal salts;* listed on ingredient labels as D&C (drug and cosmetic), *214, 254*

Certified nursing assistants (CNAs), *7*

Cervical cutaneous nerve, nerve located at the side of the neck that affects the front and sides of the neck as far down as the breastbone, *51, 53, 72*

Cervical nerves, nerves that originate at the spinal cord, whose branches supply the muscles and scalp at the back of the head and neck; affect the side of the neck and the platysma muscle, *51, 52*

Cervical vertebrae, the seven bones of the top part of the vertebral column, located in the neck region, *38, 72*

Chamomile, plant extract with calming and soothing properties, *229, 254*

Cheekbones, *37*

Chelating agents, a chemical added to cosmetics to improve the efficiency of the preservative, *212–213, 255*

Chemical exfoliants, chemical agent that dissolves dead skin cells and the intercellular matrix, or "glue," that holds them together (desmosomes), *240, 255*

Chemical exfoliation, *314, 642–654*
acid, alkaline, and pH relationships, *642–643*
AHA and BHA, *648–652*
cell renewal factor and, *643*
contraindications for, *645–646*
designer peel, *654*
general effects of, *645*
light, medium, and deep peels compared, *644–645*
safely and effectively using, *646–654*

Chemistry, cosmetic, *13–14, 198*
ingredients in, *204–205*
pH, *642–643*

Chest
bones, *38–39*
waxing, *492–493*

Chewing muscles, *44*

Chicken pox. *See* Herpes zoster

Chin, waxing, *490, 509*

China, *18*

Circulatory system (cardiovascular system, vascular system), system that controls the steady circulation of the blood through the body by means of the heart and blood vessels, *32, 54–59, 72*

Clavicle (collarbone), bone joining the sternum and scapula, *39, 72*

Clay masks, oil-absorbing cleansing masks that draw impurities to the surface of the skin as they dry and tighten, *242, 255*

Clean-up, end-of-the-day, *284*

Cleansers, soap or detergent that cleans the skin, *199, 238–239, 255*
client home-care instruction sheet, *250*

Client
Client Assessment Form (waxing procedures), *478, 479*
Client Chart (makeup), *581*
Client Consent Form (skin analysis), *183*
Client Intake Form and Medical History (skin analysis), *180–183*
Client Intake Form, *307–309*
Client Questionnaire (makeup), *580*
consultation for hair removal, *478–483*
consulting on home care, *319–320*
draping and hand washing, *310–311*
home-care instruction sheet for skin products, *250*
indications and contraindications, *481, 482*
meeting and greeting, *302–303*
on schedule, *302*

Client (*Continued*)
  preparing for facial treatment, 303–304
  Service Record (skin analysis), 184–185
  wax intake form, 479
  Wax Release Form (waxing procedures), 478–480
Client consultation, *579–581*
  for hair removal, 478–483
  questions during, 186–188
  skin analysis, 179–188
Client home-care instruction sheet, *250*
Clindamycin, *137*
Clinical aesthetician, *681*
Clinical esthetics, previously known as *medical esthetics;* **the integration of surgical procedures and esthetic treatments,** *7, 24*
  career in, 7
Clogged follicles
  causes of, 131–132
  types of, 132–133
Clothing, gloves, *190*
CNS. *See* Central nervous system
Coconut oil, derived from coconut, one of the fattiest and heaviest oils used as an emollient, *207, 255*
Coenzyme Q10, powerful antioxidant that protects and revitalizes skin cells, *230, 255*
Cold receptors, *87*
Cold sores. *See* Herpes simplex virus 1
Collagen, fibrous, connective tissue made from protein; found in the reticular layer of the dermis; gives skin its firmness. Topically, a large, long-chain molecular protein that lies on the top of the skin and binds water; derived from the placentas of cows or other sources, *92, 116*
  aging and, 113
Collagenase, *93*
Collarbone, *39*
Color(s)
  analogous, 554
  complementary, 554
  cool, 556
  eye, 560–562
  eyebrow, 588
  foundation (base makeup), 566–567
  hair, 562
  intense pulsed light, 663–664
  intensity, 560
  lip, 588–589
  primary, 553
  saturation, 554–555
  secondary, 553
  selection, 557–563
  skin, 87
  tertiary, 553–554

  warm, 556
  wheel, 552–554
Color agents, substances such as vegetable, pigment, or mineral dyes that give products color, *214, 255*
  types of, 214
Color theory
  makeup color selection, 557–563
  principles of, 552–556
Color therapy, *665*
Combination skin, treating, *235*
Comedo (plural: comedones), mass of hardened sebum and skin cells in a hair follicle; an open comedo or blackhead when open and exposed to oxygen. Closed comedos are whiteheads that are blocked and do not have a follicular opening, *132, 157*
Comedogenic, tendency for an ingredient to clog follicles and cause a buildup of dead skin cells, resulting in comedones (blackheads), *136, 157, 203*
Common carotid arteries, arteries that supply blood to the face, head, and neck, located on either side of the neck, having an internal and external branch, *58, 72*
Communicable disease. *See* Contagious disease
Communication. *See also* Client consultation
  esthetician, 299
  importance of, prior to bikini waxing, 494
  pheromones and, 104
Complementary colors, primary and secondary colors opposite one another on the color wheel, *554, 637*
Concealers, cosmetics used to cover blemishes and discolorations; may be applied before or after foundation, *568, 584, 637*
Concentrate
  aromatherapy essential oils, 392
  mask (pack, masque) products, 241–243
  serums, 243–244, 317
Conjunctivitis (pinkeye), very contagious infection of the mucous membranes around the eye; chemical, bacterial, or viral causes, *149, 157*
Connective tissue, fibrous tissue that binds together, protects, and supports the various parts of the body such as bone, cartilage, and tendons. Examples of connective tissue are bone, cartilage, ligaments, tendons, blood, lymph, and fat, *31, 72*
Consent Form, a customary written agreement between the esthetician (salon/spa) and the client for applying a treatment, whether routine or preoperative, *186, 194*
  using, 186
Contact dermatitis, inflammatory skin condition caused by contact with a substance or chemical. Occupational disorders from ingredients in cosmetics and chemical solutions can cause contact dermatitis (a.k.a. dermatitis venenata). Allergic

contact dermatitis is from exposure to allergens; irritant contact dermatitis is from exposure to irritants, *145, 157*
   allergic, *145–146*
   irritant, *146–147*
Contagious disease, *149–152. See also* Virus
Contouring, refers to makeup colors that are darker shades used to define the cheekbones and make features appear smaller, *584, 637*
Contraindications, factor that prohibits a treatment due to a condition; treatments could cause harmful or negative side effects to those who have specific medical or skin conditions, *177, 194*
   AHA and BHA peels, *651–652*
   artificial eyelashes, *607–608*
   for chemical exfoliation, *645–646*
   for electric mitts and boots, *437*
   for electrotherapy, *413*
   for enzyme peels, *648*
   epilepsy, *433*
   facial massage, *388–389*
   for galvanic machine, *429*
   for hair removal services, *481*
   high blood pressure, *433*
   high-frequency machines, *433*
   Jessner's and TCA peels, *653–654*
   for LED, *665–666*
   for magnifying lamp, *416–417*
   for microcurrent, *667*
   for microdermabrasion, *657–658*
   for paraffin wax, *436*
   pregnancy, *433*
   for rotary brush, *420*
   for skin analysis, *177–178*
   for skin treatment, *178–179*
   for spray machine, *435*
   for steamer, *422–423*
   ultrasonic and ultrasound, *669*
   for vacuum machine, *425*
   for warm towels from a hot towel cabinet, *414–415*
   for waxing procedure, *481, 482*
   for, Wood's lamp, *418*
Cool colors, colors with a blue undertone that suggest coolness and are dominated by blues, greens, violets, and blue-reds, *556, 637*
Corium, *92*
Corneocytes, another name for a stratum corneum cell; hardened, waterproof, protective keratinocytes; these "dead" protein cells are dried out and lack nuclei, *97, 116*
Corrugator muscle, facial muscle that draws eyebrows down and wrinkles the forehead vertically, *43, 72*
Cosmeceutical, term used to describe high-quality products or ingredients intended to improve the skin's health and appearance, *199, 255*

Cosmetic chemists, *13–14*
Cosmetic ingredient
   main types, in cosmetic chemistry, *204–227*
   natural *vs.* synthetic, *201–202*
   sources *vs.* product names, *201–204*
Cosmetic surgery (esthetic surgery), elective surgery for improving and altering the appearance, *679*
   clinical esthetician for, *681, 699*
   procedures, *678–681*
Cosmetics, as defined by the U.S. Food And Drug Administration (FDA): articles that are intended to be rubbed, poured, sprinkled, or otherwise applied to the human body or any part thereof for cleansing, beautifying, promoting attractiveness, or altering the appearance, *198, 255. See also* Skin care products
   as acne trigger, *136*
   buyer of, *11*
   chart for comparing product lines, *252*
   FDA regulations for, *198–199*
   FD&C Act defining, *198–199*
   ingredient sources *vs.* product names, *201–204*
Couperose, redness; capillaries that have been damaged and are now larger, or distended, blood vessels; commonly seen with telangiectasia, *114, 116, 172*
Cranium, oval, bony case that protects the brain, *36, 72*
Cream, *567*
CRF. *See* Cell renewal factor
Cruelty-free, term used to describe products that are not tested on animals at any stage of the production process; nor are any of its ingredients tested on animals, *203, 255*
Crust, dead cells form over a wound or blemish while it is healing, resulting in an accumulation of sebum and pus, sometimes mixed with epidermal material; an example is the scab on a sore, *126, 157. See also* Desincrustation
Crystal microdermabrasion, *655*
Crystal-free microdermabrasion, *656*
Cuticle, nail, *102*
Cutis, *92*
Cyst, closed, abnormally developed sac containing fluid, infection, or other matter above or below the skin, *131, 157*

D

Day spa esthetician, *6–7*
Décolleté, also referred to as *décolletage* (dek-UH-luh-taj); pertaining to a woman's lower neck and chest, *171, 194*
Defecation, elimination of feces from the body, *68, 72*

Dehydrated skin, *235*

Dehydration, lack of water, *172, 194*

Delivery systems, systems that deliver ingredients to specific tissues of the epidermis, *210–211, 255*

Deltoid, large, triangular muscle covering the shoulder joint that allows the arm to extend outward and to the side of the body, *45, 72*

Deoxyribonucleic acid (DNA), the blueprint material of genetic information; contains all the information that controls the function of every living cell, *29, 72*
personal appearance and, 31

Department of Agriculture, U. S., *202*

Depilation, process of removing hair at skin level, *464, 548*

Depilatory, substance, usually a caustic alkali preparation, used for temporarily removing superfluous hair by dissolving it at the skin level, *466, 548*

Depressor anguli oris (triangularis muscle), muscle extending alongside the chin that pulls down the corner of the mouth, *43, 72*

Dermal fillers, products used to fill lines, wrinkles, and other facial imperfections, *679, 699*

Dermal papillae, membranes of ridges and grooves that attach to the epidermis; contains nerve endings and supplies nourishment through capillaries to skin and follicles, *86, 92, 116*

Dermatillomania, a form of obsessive-compulsive disorder in which the person picks at their skin to the point of injury, infection, or scarring; a person with dermatillomania finds the picking stress relieving and not painful; it can often be socially isolating because severe dermatillomania can be disfiguring, *152, 157*

Dermatitis, any inflammatory condition of the skin; various forms of lesions, such as eczema, vesicles, or papules; the three main categories are atopic, contact, and seborrheic dermatitis, *145, 157*
types of, 145–148

Dermatologist, physician who specializes in diseases and disorders of the skin, hair, and nails, *122, 157*

Dermatology, medical branch of science that deals with the study of skin and its nature, structure, functions, diseases, and treatment, *122, 157*

Dermis, also known as the *derma, corium, cutis,* or *true skin;* support layer of connective tissue, collagen, and elastin below the epidermis, *92, 100, 116*

Desincrustation, process used to soften and emulsify sebum and blackheads in the follicles, *314, 383, 427, 452*

Desmosomes, the structures that assist in holding cells together; intercellular connections made of proteins, *96, 116*

Desquamation, *97, 326, 342, 642*

Detergents, type of surfactant used as cleansers in skin-cleansing products, *209, 255*
types of, 211

Diaphoresis, excessive perspiration due to a medical condition, *155, 157*

Diaphragm, muscular wall that separates the thorax from the abdominal region and helps control breathing, *66, 72*

Diet, as acne trigger, *136–137*

Differin®. *See* Adapalene

Digestion, breakdown of food by mechanical and chemical means, *68, 72*

Digestive enzymes, chemicals that change certain kinds of food into a form that can be used by the body, *67, 72*

Digestive system (gastrointestinal system), responsible for breaking down foods into nutrients and wastes; consists of the mouth, stomach, intestines, salivary and gastric glands and other organs, *33, 67–68, 73*

Digital image board, *578*

Digital nerve, sensory-motor nerve that, with its branches, supplies impulses to the fingers, *54, 73*

Digits, also known as *phalanges;* the bones in the fingers, three in each finger and two in each thumb, totaling 14 bones, *40, 73*

Disinfectants, *145*
EPA-registration number on label, 190
log, example of, 283

Dispensary, room or area used for mixing products and storing supplies, *276, 295*

Disposables. *See* Single-use items

DNA. *See* Deoxyribonucleic acid

Drug
FD&C Act defining, 199
product as cosmetic and, 199

Dry skin, *235*

Duct glands, *103–104*

Ductless glands, also known as *endocrine glands;* glands that release secretions called hormones directly into the bloodstream, *63, 73*

E

Ears
greater auricular nerve, 53
muscles, 44
reflexology applied to, 672

Eccrine glands, sweat glands found all over the body with openings on the skin's surface through pores; not attached to hair follicles, secretions do not produce an offensive odor, *104, 116*

Echinacea, derivative of the purple coneflower; prevents infection and has healing properties; used internally to support the immune system, *230, 255*

ECM. *See* Extracellular matrix

Eczema, inflammatory, painful itching disease of the skin, acute or chronic in nature, with dry or moist lesions. This condition should be referred to a physician. Seborrheic dermatitis, mainly affecting oily areas, is a common form of eczema, *146, 157*

Edema, swelling caused by a fluid imbalance in cells or a response to injury or infection, *154, 157*

Education, career in, *13*

Educator, *13*

Effleurage, light, continuous stroking movement applied with the fingers (digital) or the palms (palmar) in a slow, rhythmic manner, *389, 409*

EGF. *See* Epidermal growth factor

Egypt, ancient, *18*

Elastase, *93*

Elastin, protein fiber found in the dermis; gives skin its elasticity and firmness, *92, 116*

Electric mitts and boots, *436–437*

Electricity,
electrotherapy, *412–413, 431*

Electrode, *412–413, 430–434*

Electrolysis, removal of hair by means of an electric current that destroys the hair root, *470–471, 548*

Electronic tweezing, *464–465*

Electrotherapy, the use of electrical devices to treat the skin and provide therapeutic benefits, *412, 431*

Eleventh cranial nerve (accessory nerve), a motor nerve that controls the motion of the neck and shoulder muscles, *51, 53, 73*

Emollients, oil or fatty ingredients that lubricate, moisturize, and prevent water loss, *206, 255*
types of, *207–208*

Emulsifiers, surfactants that cause oil and water to mix and form an emulsion; an ingredient that brings two normally incompatible materials together and binds them into a uniform and fairly stable blend, *209–210, 255*

Endermology, treatment for cellulite; helps stimulate the reduction of adipose tissue by a vacuum massage that combines a vigorous massage along with suction, *673, 699*

Endocrine glands, Also known as *ductless glands;* ductless glands that release hormonal secretions directly into the bloodstream. They are a group of specialized glands that affect the growth, development, sexual activities, and health of the entire body, *33, 63, 73*

Endocrine system, group of specialized glands that affect the growth, development, sexual activities, and health of the entire body, *63, 73*

End-of-day clean-up, *284*

Endothelium, *114*

Environment
as acne trigger, *135–136*
skin health and, *110*

Environmental Protection Agency (EPA), disinfectant registration with, *190*

Enzyme peels, *646–648*
contraindications, *648*
defined, *646–647*
effects of, *647*
using, *647*

Enzymes, a group of complex proteins produced by living cells that act as catalysts in specific chemical reactions in the body, such as digestion, *68, 73*
collagenase and elastase, *93*

Enzymes (for exfoliation), provide gentle exfoliation and dissolve keratin proteins within dead skin cells on the surface, *217, 255*

EPA. *See* Environmental Protection Agency

Ephelids, also known as *freckles*, are tiny round or oval pigmented areas of skin on areas exposed to the sun (FIGURE 4–11). Also referred to as *macules*, they are small flat colored spots on the skin, *143, 157*

Epicranius (occipitofrontalis), the broad muscle that covers the top of the skull and consists of the occipitalis and frontalis, *42, 73*

Epidermal growth factor, abbreviated EGF; stimulates cells to reproduce and heal, *88, 116*

Epidermis, outermost layer of skin; a thin protective layer with many cells, mechanisms, and nerve endings; is made up of five layers: stratum germinativum, stratum spinosum, stratum granulosum, stratum lucidum, and stratum corneum, *86, 94–95, 99, 100, 116*

Epilation, removes hairs from the follicles; waxing or tweezing, *464, 548*

Epilepsy, treatments contraindicated for, *433*

Epithelial tissue, protective covering on body surfaces, such as the skin, mucous membranes, and lining of the heart; digestive and respiratory organs; and glands, *31, 73*

Equipment. *See also* Furniture
makeup station and supplies, *572–578*
purchasing facial machines, *438*

Ergonomics in treatment room, *273*

Erythema, redness caused by inflammation; a red lesion is erythemic, *154, 157*

Essential oils, oils derived from herbs; have many different properties and effects on the skin and psyche, *213, 255*

Ester of vitamin C, *222*

Esthetician, also known as *aesthetician;* a specialist in the cleansing, beautification, and preservation of the health of skin on the entire body, including the face and neck, *6, 24. See also* Careers; Professional image
business options for, 17
certificate or license to practice, 389
cranial nerves of concern to, 51–52
oncology-trained, 15–16
professional appearance, elements of, 264–265
professional image checklist, 265
scope of practice, 388–389
skin care products and ingredients and, 197–198
types of massage movements used by, 389–392

Esthetic surgery. *See* Cosmetic surgery

Esthetics, also known as *aesthetics;* from the Greek word *aesthetikos* (meaning "perceptible to the senses"); a branch of anatomical science that deals with the overall health and well-being of the skin, the largest organ of the human body, *6, 24*
future of, 20–24
oncology, 130
types of, 16–20
writer, 11

Ethanol. *See* Alcohol

Ethmoid bone, light, spongy bone between the eye sockets that forms part of the nasal cavities, *36, 37, 73*

Eumelanin, a type of melanin that is dark brown to black in color; people with dark-colored skin produce mostly eumelanin; there are two types of melanin; the other type is pheomelanin, *98, 116*

Excoriation, skin sore or abrasion produced by scratching or scraping, *126, 158*

Excretory system, group of organs-including the kidneys, liver, skin, large intestine, and lungs-that purify the body by elimination of waste matter, *33, 68–69, 73, 89*
secretory nerve regulation of, 103

Exercise
skin aging from deficient, 176
for strengthening hands and wrists, 274

Exfoliants, mechanical and chemical products or processes used to exfoliate the skin, *239–241, 255*

Exfoliation, peeling or sloughing of the outer layer of skin, *216, 255. See also* Chemical exfoliation
types of chemical ingredients for, 217–218, 314–315

Exhalation, breathing outward; expelling carbon dioxide from the lungs, *67, 73*

Exocrine glands, also known as *duct glands;* produce a substance that travels through small, tubelike ducts, sweat and oil glands of the skin belong to this group, *34, 73*

Express facial, a professional service designed to improve the appearance of the skin that takes less than 30 minutes, *321–322, 383*

Extension, when muscles straighten. when the wrist, hand, and fingers form a straight line, for example, *47, 73*

External jugular vein, vein located on the side of the neck that carries blood returning to the heart from the head, face, and neck, *58, 73*

Extracellular matrix (ECM), 94

Extraction, manual removal of impurities and comedones, *316, 383*

Extrinsic factors, primarily environmental factors that contribute to aging and the appearance of aging, *176, 194*

Eye color, 560–562

Eye shapes, makeup for, 594–597

Eye tabbing, procedure in which individual synthetic eyelashes are attached directly to a client's own lashes at their base, *607, 637*

Eye treatments, *317*

Eyebrow gel formulations, makeup used to add color and shape to the eyebrows, *570, 637*

Eyebrow pencils, makeup used to add color and shape to the eyebrows, *570, 637*

Eyebrow pomades, makeup used to add color and shape to the eyebrows, *570, 637*

Eyebrow shadows, makeup used to add color and shape to the eyebrows, *570, 637*

Eyebrows
color, 570, 588
makeup for, 597–599
muscles around, 42–43
specialists, 7–9
tinting of, 608–609
tweezing, 496–498
waxing, 488–489
with hard wax procedure, 499–501
with soft wax procedure, 502–504

Eyelash adhesive, *607*

Eyeliner, makeup used to emphasize the eyes; it is available in pencil, liquid, and pressed (cake) form, *570, 587, 637*

Eyes
applying artificial eyelashes, 625–629
artificial eyelashes, 606–608
lash and brow tinting, 608–609, 630–635

Eyeshadows, makeup used to accentuate and contour the eyes, *569–570, 586*

F

Friction, invigorating rubbing technique requiring pressure on the skin with the fingers or palm while moving them under an underlying structure, *390, 409*

Frontal bone, bone forming the forehead, *36, 37, 74*

Frontalis, front (anterior) portion of the epicranius; muscle of the scalp that raises the eyebrows, draws the scalp forward, and causes wrinkles across the forehead, *42, 74*

Functional ingredients, ingredients in cosmetic products that allow the products to spread, give them body and texture, and give them a specific form such as a lotion, cream, or gel. Preservatives are also functional ingredients, *204, 256*

Furniture
   checklist of, *269–272*
   treatment room, *269–272, 274, 284*

Furuncle, also known as *boil*; a subcutaneous abscess filled with pus; furuncles are caused by bacteria in the glands or hair follicles, *154, 158*

G

Galvanic current, *426–430*
   contraindications for, *429*
   effects of using, *427–429*
   iontophoresis, *428–429*
   safety and maintenance, *430*
   when to use, *426–427*

Galvanic electrolysis, direct current (DC) utilized in electrolysis, *470, 548*

Gastrointestinal system, responsible for changing food into nutrients and waste, also called the digestive system, *67, 74*

Genital herpes. *See* Herpes simplex virus 2

Genetic and hereditary factors
   personal appearance and, *31*
   skin aging, *175–176*
   skin color, *87*

Genetic, related to heredity and ancestry of origin, *164, 194*

Glabella, the corregator and procerus muscles; considered an area or region between the eyebrows at the top of the nose, and or on the frontal bone. Not specifically a muscle or a bone, *43, 74, 498, 548, 678*

Glands, specialized organs that remove certain elements from the blood to convert them into new compounds, *62, 74, 103–104*

Glossopharyngeal nerve, *50*

Gloves, *190, 414*

Gluten-free, *203*

Glycation, caused by an elevation in blood sugar, glycation is the binding of a protein molecule to a glucose molecule resulting in the formation of damaged, nonfunctioning structures, known as Advanced Glycation End products (a.k.a. AGES). Glycation alters protein structures and decreases biological activity, *112–113, 117, 176*
   skin aging from, *176*

Glycerin, formed by a decomposition of oils or fats; excellent skin softener and humectant; very strong water binder; sweet, colorless, oily substance used as a solvent and as a moisturizer in skin and body creams, *230, 256*

Glycoproteins, skin-conditioning agents derived from carbohydrates and proteins that enhance cellular metabolism and wound healing, *226, 256*

Glycosaminoglycans, a water-binding substance such as a polysaccharide (protein and complex sugar) found between the fibers of the dermis, *93, 113, 117*

Gommage (roll-off masks), exfoliating creams that are rubbed off the skin, *241, 256*

Goosebumps, *103*

Granger, Mary, *10*

Greasepaint, heavy makeup used for theatrical purposes, *567, 637*

Greater auricular nerve, nerve at the sides of the neck affecting the face, ears, neck, and parotid gland, *53, 74*

Greater occipital nerve, nerve located in the back of the head, affects the scalp as far up as the top of the head, *53, 74*

Greece, ancient, *18*

Green light, a light-emitting diode for use on clients with hyperpigmentation or for detoxifying the skin, *665, 699*

Green tea, powerful antioxidant and soothing agent; antibacterial, anti-inflammatory, and a stimulant, *231, 256*

Gum rosin, an additive in soft wax, *469, 549*

H

Hair
   excessive growth, *460–463*
   follicle, *100–101*
   growth cycle, *458–460*
   types of, *458*

Hair bulb, swelling at the base of the follicle that provides the hair with nourishment; it is a thick, club-shaped structure that forms the lower part of the hair root, *457, 549*

Hair color, *562*

Hair follicle, mass of epidermal cells forming a small tube, or canal; the tube-like depression or pocket in the skin or scalp that contains the hair root, *456, 549*

Hair papilla (plural: papillae), cone-shaped elevations at the base of the follicle that fit into the hair bulb. The papillae are filled with tissue that contains the blood vessels and cells necessary for hair growth and follicle nourishment, *92, 117, 457, 549*

Hair removal
    client consultations, *478–483*
    diseases, disorders and syndromes affecting hair growth, *462–463*
    hair growth cycle, *458–460*
    hard *vs.* soft, *477*
    hard wax, *473–475*
        dos and don'ts, *474–475*
        posttreatment, *474*
        pretreatment for, *473–474*
        technique, *474*
    importance of, *455–456*
    medicines affecting hair growth, *463*
    methods of, *463–472*
    permanent, *470–472*
    procedures
        axilla waxing with hard wax, *510–512*
        axilla waxing with soft wax, *513–515*
        bikini waxing with hard wax, *536–538*
        bikini waxing with soft wax, *538–541*
        chin waxing with hard wax, *509*
        eyebrow tweezing, *496–498*
        eyebrow waxing with hard wax, *499–501*
        eyebrow waxing with soft wax, *502–504*
        leg waxing with soft wax, *542–547*
        lip waxing with hard wax, *505–506*
        lip waxing with soft wax, *507–508*
        men's back waxing with hard wax, *528–531*
        men's back waxing with soft wax, *532–535*
        men's chest waxing with hard wax, *524–525*
        men's chest waxing with soft wax, *526–527*
    soft wax
        blending, *476*
        dos and don'ts, *476*
        posttreatment, *476*
        pretreatment for, *475*
        speed waxing, *476*
        technique for, *475*
    structure of hair, *456–458*
    temporary, *464–470*
    types of hair, *458*
    wax treatment room, *483–487*

Hair root, anchors hair to the skin cells and is part of the hair located at the bottom of the follicle below the surface of the skin; part of the hair that lies within the follicle at its base, where the hair grows, *457, 549*

Hair shaft, portion of the hair that extends or projects beyond the skin, consisting of the outer layer (cuticle), inner layer (medulla), and middle layer (cortex). Color changes happen in the cortex, *91, 457, 549*

Hand-applied sugaring method, *467–468*

Hands
    bones, *39–40*
    chapped, *126*
    electric mitts for, *437*
    waxing, *492*
        with hard wax procedure, *516–519*
        with soft wax procedure, *520–523*

Head. *See also* Face
    arteries and veins, *58–59*
    bones, *36*
    cervical nerves, *53, 391*
    muscles, *42–43*
    nerves, *50–53*

Headband, *190*

Healing botanicals, substances from plants such as chamomile, aloe, plant stem cells, and botanical oils that help to heal the skin, *224, 256*

Heart, muscular cone-shaped organ that keeps the blood moving within the circulatory system, *55–56, 74*

Heat, skin receptors for, *87*

Hemp seed oil, derived from hemp seeds, very light botanical oil used as an emollient, *207, 256*

Henna, a dye obtained from the powdered leaves and shoots of the mignonette tree; used as a reddish hair dye and in temporary design tattooing, *18, 25*

Herbs, hundreds of different herbs that contain phytohormones are used in skin care products and cosmetics; they heal, stimulate, soothe, and moisturize, *213, 256*

Herpes simplex virus 1, strain of the herpes virus that causes fever blisters or cold sores; it is a recurring, contagious viral infection consisting of a vesicle or group of vesicles on a red, swollen base. The blisters usually appear on the lips or nostrils, *150, 158*

Herpes simplex virus 2, strain of the herpes virus that infects the genitals, *150, 158*

Herpes zoster (shingles), a painful viral infection skin condition from the chickenpox virus; characterized by groups of blisters that form a rash in a ring or line, *150, 158*

High-definition makeup, designed to be invisible when using high-definition cameras; formulated with super-fine microparticles that blend into the skin to provide a flawless complexion, *604, 637*

High-energy visible light, abbreviated as *HEV;* light emitting from electronic devices, reported to penetrate the skin more deeply than UV rays; damages collagen, hyaluronic acid, and elastin, *108, 117*

Highlighters, makeup that is lighter than the skin color; accentuate and bring out features such as the brow bone under the eyebrow, the temples, the chin, and the cheekbones, *569, 584, 637*

Highlighting and contouring techniques, *591–601*
  eye shapes, 594–597
  eyebrows, 597–599
  jawline and neck area, 591–594
  lips, 599–601

Hirsutism, condition pertaining to an excessive growth or cover of hair, *173, 194, 461–462*

Histology, also known as *microscopic anatomy;* the study of the structure and composition of tissue, *28, 74*
  reasons to study physiology and, 83–85

Hives. *See* Urticaria

Holistically, a system of evaluating the entire individual in an interdisciplinary style, recognizing that body systems work synergistically, *166, 194*

Home care
  for acne, 337–338
  skin care instruction sheet, 250
  skin care products, 248–250

Hormone replacement therapy (HRT), *115*

Hormones, secretions produced by one of the endocrine glands and carried by the bloodstream or body fluid to another part of the body, or a body organ, to stimulate functional activity or secretion, such as insulin, adrenaline, and estrogen, *63, 74*
  as acne trigger, 135
  aging and, 113
  pheromones, 104
  skin aging from, 176
  skin functions controlled by, 85
  telangiectasia and, 114

Hot towel cabinet, *413–415*

HRT. *See* Hormone replacement therapy

Hue, any color in its purest form, lacking any black (shade) or white (tint); the hue of a color represents just one dimension of a particular color, *553, 637*

Humectants, ingredients that attract water; humectants draw moisture to the skin and soften its surface, diminishing lines caused by dehydration, *220, 256*

Humerus, uppermost and largest bone in the arm, extending from the elbow to the shoulder, *40, 74*

Hyaluronic acid, hydrating fluids found in the skin; hydrophilic agent with water-binding properties, *93, 117*

Hydradermabrasion, *656*

Hydration
  facial masks for, 241
  See also Water

Hydrators, ingredients that attract water to the skin's surface, *220, 244–245, 256*

Hydrolipidic, hydrolipidic film is an oil-water balance that protects the skin's surface, *87, 116*

Hydrophilic agents, ingredients that attract water to the skin's surface, *220, 256*

Hydrotherapy, spa treatments that use water, *671–672, 699*

Hyoid bone, u-shaped bone at the base of the tongue that supports the tongue and its muscle, *38, 74*

Hyperhidrosis, excessive perspiration caused by heat, genetics, medications, or medical conditions; also called diaphoresis, *154, 158*

Hyperkeratosis, thickening of the skin caused by a mass of keratinized cells (keratinocytes), *148, 158*

Hyperpigmentation, over-production of pigment, *142, 158, 236–237*

Hypertrichosis, condition of abnormal growth of hair, characterized by the growth of terminal hair in areas of the body that normally grow only vellus hair, *173, 194, 461*

Hypertrophy, abnormal growth of the skin; many are benign, or harmless, *148, 158*

Hypoallergenic, refers to ingredients or products that may be less likely to cause allergic reactions, *203, 256*

Hypodermis, *99*

Hypoglossal nerve, *50*

Hypopigmentation, absence of pigment, resulting in light or white splotches, *142, 158*

I

Impetigo, contagious bacterial infection often occurring in children; characterized by clusters of small blisters or crusty lesions, *150, 158*

Implements, tools used by technicians to perform services. Implements can be reusable or disposable, *276, 295*
  refresher on cleaning and disinfecting, 282–283

INCI. *See* International Nomenclature Cosmetic Ingredient

India, Ayurvedic healing system from, *673*

Individual lashes, separate artificial eyelashes that are applied on top of the lashes one at a time, *606, 637*

Infection control,
  makeup, 578–579

Lamellar granules, epidermal cells composed of keratin, lipids, and other proteins, *96, 117*

Langerhans immune cells, guard cells of the immune system that sense unrecognized foreign invaders, such as bacteria, and then process these antigens for removal through the lymph system, *93, 96, 117*

Lanolin, emollient with moisturizing properties; also, an emulsifier with high water-absorption capabilities, *203, 256*

Lanugo, the hair on a fetus; soft and downy hair, *458, 549*

Laser (light amplification stimulation emission of radiation), a medical device that uses electromagnetic radiation for hair removal and skin treatments, *660, 699*
FDA on, *471*
hair removal, *471–472*
resurfacing, *680*
technology and procedures, *660–662*

Laser hair removal, photoepilation hair reduction treatment in which a laser beam is pulsed on the skin using one wavelength at a time, impairing hair growth; an intense pulse of electromagnetic radiation, *470, 549*

Laser resurfacing, a laser procedure utilizing the CO_2 or erbium laser that involves vaporization of the epidermis and/or dermis for facial rejuvenation; used to smooth wrinkles or lighten acne scars and stimulate growth of new collagen, *680, 699*

Lash comb, separates lashes so they look finished and are not clumpy or messy looking; used before applying mascara or when the mascara is still wet, *574, 637*

Lash extensions, *609*

Lash perming, *609*

Latissimus dorsi, large, flat, triangular muscle covering the lower back, *44, 75*

Lavender, antiallergenic, anti-inflammatory, antiseptic, antibacterial, balancing, energizing, soothing, and healing, *204, 256*

Lecithin, *674*

LED. *See* Light-emitting diode
contraindications for, *665–666*
effects of, *665*
safety and maintenance for, *666*

Leeder, Alex, *8*

Leg(s)
hirsutism, *461*
waxing, *494, 542–547*

Lentigo, freckles; small yellow-brown colored spots; lentigenes that result from sunlight exposure are actinic, or solar; lentigo patches are referred to as *large macules, 142, 158*

Lesion flashcard, *128*

Lesions, mark, wound, or abnormality; structural changes in tissues caused by damage or injury, *123, 158*
primary, *123–125*
secondary, *126–127*

Lesser occipital nerve, also known as *smaller occipital nerve;* located at the base of the skull, affects the scalp and muscles behind the ear, *53, 75*

Leukocytes, white blood cells that have enzymes to digest and kill bacteria and parasites. These white blood cells also respond to allergies, *94, 105, 117*

Leukoderma, skin disorder characterized by light, abnormal patches; causes are congenital, acquired, postinflammation, or other causes that destroy pigment-producing cells; vitiligo and albinism are leukodermas, *144, 159*

Levator anguli oris (caninus), is a muscle that raises the angle of the mouth and draws it inward, *43, 75*

Levator labii superioris (quadratus labii superioris), is a muscle that elevates the lip and dilates the nostrils, as in expressing distaste, *43, 75*

Levator palpebrae superioris muscle, thin muscle that controls the eyelid and can be easily damaged during makeup application, *43, 75*

LGFB. *See* Look Good Feel Better

License, esthetician. *See* Certificate or license, esthetician's

Licensed massage therapist (LMT), *388*

Licensed practical nurses (LPNs), *7*

Licorice, anti-irritant used for sensitive skin; helps lighten pigmentation, *231, 256*

Lifestyle
as acne trigger, *136*
skin health and, *110–112*

Light-emitting diode, abbreviated LED; a device used to reduce acne, increase skin circulation, and improve the collagen content in the skin, *664–666, 699*

contraindications for, *665–666*

effects of, *665*

safety and maintenance for, *666*

Lighteners, *219*

Lighting, *582*

Lip color, makeup that gives color to the face and provides a finish to your makeup design, *571–572, 588–589, 638*

Lip conditioner, an application such as a lip moisturizer that is put on when starting the makeup application, so it can soak in and moisturize before starting to apply the liner; a primer, foundation, or plumper can be applied prior to the lip color, *589, 638*

Lip gloss, can give a shiny, moisturized look to the lips, *589, 638*

Lip liners, colored pencils used to line and define the lips, *572, 589, 638*

Lip treatments, *317*

Lipids, fats or fat-like substances; lipids help repair and protect the barrier function of the skin, *206, 257*

Liposomes, closed-lipid bilayer spheres that encapsulate ingredients, target their delivery to specific tissues of the skin, and control their release, *211, 257*

Liposuction, a surgical procedure used to remove stubborn areas of fat, *681, 699*

Lips
    chapped, *126*
    herpes simplex virus 1, *150*
    makeup for, *599–601*
    waxing, *489–490*
        with hard wax, *505–506*
        with soft wax, *507–508*

Liquid foundations, type of foundation made of suspension of organic and inorganic pigments in alcohol- and water-based solutions; bentonite (a clay base) is added to help keep the products blended and absorb excess oil; the liquid formulation is generally suited for clients with oily to normal skin conditions who desire sheer to medium coverage, *567, 638*

Liquid paraffin, emollient ingredient derived from petroleum sources, *207, 257*

Liver, a gland in the abdominal cavity that secretes enzymes necessary for digestion, synthesizes proteins, and detoxifies the blood. It regulates sugar levels in the blood and helps with decomposition of red blood cells and produces hormones necessary for body functions, *60, 75*

LMT. *See* Licensed massage therapist

Look Good Feel Better (LGFB), *16*

Loupe. *See* Magnifying lamp

Lubricant, coats the skin and reduces friction; mineral oil is a lubricant, *208, 257*

Lungs, spongy tissues composed of microscopic cells in which inhaled air is exchanged for carbon dioxide during one respiratory cycle, *66, 75*

Lymph, clear, yellowish fluid that circulates in the lymph spaces (lymphatic) of the body; carries waste and impurities away from the cells, *60, 75*

Lymph nodes, gland-like structures found inside lymphatic vessels; filter the lymphatic vessels and help fight infection, *60, 75*

Lymph vessels, located in the dermis, these supply nourishment within the skin and remove waste, *93, 117. See* Manual lymph drainage

Lymphatic/immune system, a vital factor to the circulatory and to the immune system made up of lymph, lymph nodes, the thymus gland, the spleen, and lymph vessels that act as an aid to the blood system; the lymphatic and immune system are closely connected in that they protect the body from disease by developing immunities and destroying disease-causing microorganisms, *60–62, 75*

Lymphocyte, *93*

M

Macule (plural: maculae), flat spot or discoloration on the skin, such as a freckle. Macules are neither raised nor sunken, *124, 159*

Magnifying lamp (loupe), *416–417*

Makeup
    application techniques
        blush, *585*
        concealer, *584*
        eye shadow, *586–587*
        eyebrow color, *588*
        eyeliner, *587*
        face powder, *584–585*
        foundation, *583–584*
        highlighting and shading, *584*
        lip color, *588–589*
        mascara, *587–588*
        tips and guidelines, *589–590*
    applications, *558, 563–565*
    artificial eyelashes, *606–608*
        adhesive, *607*
        contraindications, *607–608*
        removing, *608*
        types of lashes, *606–607*
    brushes, *575–578*
    for camera and special events
        airbrush makeup, *604–605*
        photography and video applications, *604*
    camouflage, *605*
    career as makeup artist, *9*
    career in, *611–614*
    client consultations, *579–581*
        Client Chart, *581*
        Client Questionnaire, *580*
    color selection, *557–563*
    cosmetic color theory, *552–556*
    esthetician's skill set relates to, *551–552*
    freelance makeup artistry, *612–613*
    highlighting and contouring techniques, *591–601*
        eye shapes, *594–597*

Melanosomes, pigment carrying granules that produce melanin, a complex protein, *88, 96, 98–99, 118*

Melasma, a form of hyperpigmentation that is characterized by bilateral patches of brown pigmentation on the cheeks, jawline, forehead, and upper lip due to hormonal imbalances such as pregnancy, birth control pills, or hormone replacement therapy, *173, 195*

Melasma, also referred to as *pregnancy mask;* skin condition that is triggered by hormones that cause darker pigmentation in areas such as on the upper lip and around the eyes and cheeks, *65, 76, 142*

Men
    back waxing
        with hard wax procedure, 528–531
        with soft wax procedure, 532–535
    chest waxing
        with hard wax procedure, 524–525
        with soft wax procedure, 526–527
    facial treatments for, 344–348
    hirsutism, 461
    waxing
        back, 493
        eyebrow, with soft wax, 489
        lower body, 493–494
        upper body, 492

Mental nerve, nerve that affects the skin of the lower lip and chin, *51, 52, 76*

Mentalis, muscle that elevates the lower lip and raises and wrinkles the skin of the chin, *43, 76*

Metabolism, (1) a chemical process taking place in living organisms whereby the cells are nourished and carry out their activities; (2) the process of changing food into forms the body can use as energy. Metabolism consists of two parts: anabolism and catabolism, *30, 76*

Metacarpus (palm), consists of five long, slender bones called metacarpal bones, *40, 76*

Methylparaben, one of the most frequently used preservatives because of its very low sensitizing potential; combats bacteria and molds; non-comedogenic, *212, 257*

Microcirculation, *113–114*

Microcurrent (device), used in a device that mimics the body's natural electrical energy to reeducate and tone facial muscles; improves circulation and increases collagen and elastin production, *666–668, 700*
    contraindications for, 667
    effects of, 667
    maintenance of, 668
    safety considerations for, 667–668
    using, 666–667

Microdermabrasion, form of mechanical exfoliation, *655–660, 700. See also* Dermabrasion
    crystal, 655
    crystal-free, 656
    timing and technique, 656–660
    wet, 656

Microneedling, the use of a dermal roller or an electronic handpiece to induce puncture wounds to the skin that induce collagen formation during the wound healing process, *670, 700*

Microscopic anatomy, *28*

MicroSpa, *8*

Middle ages, *19*

Milia, epidermal cysts; small, firm papules with no visible opening; whitish, pearl-like masses of sebum and dead cells under the skin. Milia are more common in dry skin types and may form after skin trauma, such as a laser resurfacing, *132–133, 159*

Miliaria rubra (prickly heat), acute inflammatory disorder of the sweat glands resulting in the eruption of red vesicles and burning, itching skin from excessive heat exposure, *155, 159*

Mineral makeup, *567–568*

Mineral oil, lubricant derived from petroleum, *232, 257*

Minerals, *223*

Mitochondria, cell structure that takes in nutrients, breaks them down, and creates energy for the cell, called ATP, adenosine triphosphate, *29, 76*

Mitosis, cells dividing into two new cells (daughter cells); the usual process of cell reproduction of human tissues, *29, 76, 95*

MLD. *See* Manual lymph drainage

Modelage masks (thermal masks), thermal heat masks; facial masks containing special crystals of gypsum, a plaster-like ingredient, *242, 257*

Moisturizers, products formulated to add moisture to the skin, *199, 244–245, 257, 317*
    client home-care instruction sheet, 250

Mole, pigmented nevus; a brownish spot ranging in color from tan to bluish black. Some are flat, resembling freckles; others are raised and darker, *148–149, 159*

Moles, *130*

Mortuary science, *9*

Motor nerves, also known as *efferent nerves;* carry impulses from the brain to the muscles or glands. These transmitted impulses produce movement, *50, 103, 391*

Mouth. *See also* Lips
    cold sores, 150
    herpes simplex virus 1, 150
    muscles, 43

Muscle tissue, tissue that contracts and moves various parts of the body, *31, 76*

Muscular system, body system that covers, shapes, and supports the skeleton tissue; contracts and moves various parts of the body, *32, 40–47, 76*

N

Nail, an appendage of skin, *102*

Nape, back of the neck, *36, 76*

Nasal bones, bones that form the bridge of the nose, *37, 76*

Nasal nerve, nerve that affects the point and lower sides of the nose, *51, 52, 76*

Nasalis muscle, two-part muscle which covers the nose, *43, 76*

Natural, all natural, terms often used in marketing for skin care products and ingredients derived from natural sources, *202, 257*

Neck
  arteries and veins, *58–59*
  bones, *38*
  makeup for, *591–594*
  motor nerve points, *391*
  muscles, *44, 53, 391*
  nerves, *50–53, 391*
  treatment option for, *171*

Nerve tissue, tissue that controls and coordinates all body functions, *31, 76*

Nerves, whitish cords made up of bundles of nerve fibers held together by connective tissue, through which impulses are transmitted, *49, 77, 103*
  types of, *49–50*

Nervous system, body system composed of the brain, spinal cord, and nerves; controls and coordinates all other systems and makes them work harmoniously and efficiently, *32, 48–54, 77*
  divisions of, *48–49*

Neurology, the scientific study of the structure, function, and pathology of the nervous system, *48, 77*

Neurons, also known as *nerve cell*; cells that make up the nerves, brain, and spinal cord and transmit nerve impulses, *29, 77*

Nevus, also known as *birthmark*; malformation of the skin due to abnormal pigmentation or dilated capillaries, *143, 159*

Nodules, these are often referred to as tumors, but these are smaller bumps caused by conditions such as scar tissue, fatty deposits, or infections, *124, 159*

Nonablative, procedure that does not remove tissue; wrinkle treatments that bypass the epidermis to stimulate collagen in the dermis for wrinkle reduction are nonablativ, *677, 700*

Noncertified colors, colors that are organic, meaning they come from animal or plant extracts; they can also be natural mineral pigments, *214, 257*

Nose muscles, *43*

NSAIDs, nonsteroidal anti-inflammatory drugs; over-the-counter medication used to reduce inflammation, such as ibuprofen, *179, 195*

Nucleoplasm, fluid within the nucleus of the cell that contains proteins and DNA; determines our genetic makeup, *29, 77*

Nucleus, the central part, core. 1) In histology the dense, active protoplasm found in the center of a eukaryotic cell that acts as the genetic control center; it plays an important role in cell reproduction and metabolism. 2) In chemistry, the center of the atom, where protons and neutrons are located, *29, 77*

Nutrition
  diet as acne trigger, *136–137*
  skin aging from deficient, *176*
  skin and poor, *111*

O

Occipital bone, hindmost bone of the skull, below the parietal bones; forms the back of the skull above the nape, *36, 77*

Occipitalis, back of the epicranius; muscle that draws the scalp backward, *42, 77*

Occipitofrontalis, *42*

Occupational Safety and Health Association (OSHA), *267*

Oculomotor nerve, *50*

Oil based makeup, refers to foundations that contain mineral oil or other oils, *566, 638*

Oil glands, *89*

Oil soluble, compatible with oil, *218, 257*

Oily skin, *235–236*

Olfactory nerve, *50*

Olfactory nerves, "smell" receptors in the nose that communicate with parts of the brain that serve as storehouses for emotions and memories, *214, 257*

Oncology, the study and treatment of cancer and tumors, *15, 25*
  esthetics, *130*
  -trained esthetician, *15–16*

Onychomycosis, a fungal infection that produces symptoms of thick, brittle, discolored nails; the fungus lives off the keratin in the nails, *150, 159*

Ophthalmic nerve, branch of the fifth cranial nerve that supplies the skin of the forehead, upper eyelids, and interior portion of the scalp, orbit, eyeball, and nasal passage, *51, 52, 77*

Optic nerve, *50*

Orbicularis oculi, ring muscle of the eye socket; closes the eyelid, *43, 77*

Orbicularis oris, flat band around the upper and lower lips that compresses, contracts, puckers, and wrinkles the lips, *43, 77*

Organelle, small structures or miniature organs within a cell that have their own function, *29, 77*

Organic, term used to describe natural-sourced ingredients that are grown without the use of pesticides or chemicals, *202, 257*

Organs, structures composed of specialized tissues designed to perform specific functions in plants and animals, *32, 77*

Origin, part of the muscle that does not move; it is attached to the skeleton and is usually part of a skeletal muscle, *41, 77*

OSHA. *See* Occupational Safety and Health Association

Oval-shaped face, *564–565*

Ovaries, function in sexual reproduction as well as determining male and female sexual characteristics, *64, 77*
    endocrine glands and, *63*

Oxygen, smoking and reduced, *111–112*

P

Pacinian corpuscle, *91*

Pain
    massage to relieve, *385*
    nerve endings to register, *86–87*

Palm oil, derived from the oil palm tree; one of the fattiest and heaviest oils used as an emollient, *207, 257*

Palpation, manual manipulation of tissue by touching to make an assessment of its condition, *164, 195*

Pancreas, secretes enzyme-producing cells that are responsible for digesting carbohydrates, proteins, and fats. The islet of Langerhans cells within the pancreas control insulin and glucagon production, *64, 77*

Papaya, natural enzyme used for exfoliation and in enzyme peels, *240, 257*

Papillary layer, top layer of the dermis next to the epidermis, *86, 92, 100, 118*

Papule, pimple; small elevation on the skin that contains no fluid but may develop pus, *125, 131, 159*

Parabens, one of the most commonly used groups of preservatives in the cosmetic, pharmaceutical, and food industries; provide bacteriostatic and fungistatic activity against diverse organisms, *212, 257*

Paraffin wax, *435–436*

Paraffin wax masks, mask used to warm the skin and promote penetration of ingredients through the heat trapped under the surface of the paraffin, *242, 257*

Parathyroid glands, regulate blood calcium and phosphorus levels so that the nervous and muscular systems can function properly, *63, 64, 77*

Parietal bones, bones that form the sides and top of the cranium, *36, 77*

Patch test, *200*

PCOS. *See* Polycystic ovarian syndrome

Pectoralis major and minor, muscles of the chest that assist the swinging movements of the arm, *44, 77*

Peptides, chains of amino acids that stimulate fibroblasts, cell metabolism, collagen, and improve skin's firmness. Larger chains are called polypeptides, *223, 257*

Percussion. *See* Tapotement

Performance ingredients, ingredients in cosmetic products that cause the actual changes in the appearance of the skin, *204, 257*

Perioral dermatitis, acne-like condition around the mouth. These are mainly small clusters of papules that could be caused by toothpaste or products used on the face, *147, 159*

Peripheral nervous system, abbreviated PNS; system of nerves and ganglia that connects the peripheral parts of the body to the central nervous system; has both sensory and motor nerves, *48, 77*

Peristalsis, moving food along the digestive tract, *68, 78*

Permanent makeup, cosmetic implantation technique that deposits colored pigment into the upper reticular layer of the dermis, similar to tattooing, *609–611, 638*

Pétrissage, kneading movement that stimulates the underlying tissues; performed by lifting, squeezing, and pressing the tissue with a light, firm pressure, *390, 409*

Petrolatum, emollient ingredient derived from petroleum sources, *233, 258*
    pH, in chemical exfoliation, *642–643*

pH adjusters, acids or alkalis (bases) used to adjust the pH of products, *215, 258*

Phalanges (digits), the bones in the fingers, three in each finger and two in each thumb, totaling 14 bones, *40, 78*

Phenol, carbolic acid; a caustic poison; used for peels and to sanitize metallic implements, *680, 700*

Pheomelanin, a type of melanin that is red and yellow in color; people with light-colored skin produce mostly pheomelanin; two types of melanin; the other is eumelanin, *98, 118*

Pheromones, *104*

Photography, makeup application for, *604*

Photorejuvenation, *664*

Photosensitivity, high sensitivity of the skin to UV light, usually following exposure or ingestion of certain medications, or chemicals that result in accelerated response of the skin to UV radiation, *176, 195*

Phthalates, plasticizers used in skin care formulas to moisturize and soften skin, and to dissolve or blend ingredients, *219, 258*

Physiology, study of the functions or activities performed by the body's structures, *28, 78*
   reasons to study histology and, *83–85*

Pigmentation, *418, 587, 649, 662. See also* Melanin
   abnormal, *143*
   disorders, *142–144, 333–334, 472*
   of melasma, *142*
   microdermabrasion and, *657, 659*
   tan, *143*

PIH. *See* Post inflammatory hyperpigmentation

Pilosebaceous unit, the hair unit that contains the hair follicle and appendages: the hair root, bulb, dermal papilla, sebaceous appendage, and arrector pili muscle, *132, 159*

Pineal gland, a gland located in the brain. Plays a major role in sexual development, sleep, and metabolism, *63, 64, 78*

Pinkeye. *See* Conjunctivitis

Pituitary gland, a gland found in the center of the head. The most complex organ of the endocrine system. It affects almost every physiologic process of the body: growth, blood pressure, contractions during childbirth, breastmilk production, sexual organ functions in both women and men, thyroid gland function, and the conversion of food into energy (metabolism), *63, 64, 78*

Plant stem cells, derived from plants to protect or stimulate our own skin stem cells; health and anti-aging benefits, *225, 258*

Plasma, fluid part of the blood and lymph that carries food and secretions to the cells and carbon dioxide from the cells, *57, 78*

Platelets (thrombocytes), much smaller than red blood cells; contribute to the blood-clotting process, which stops bleeding, *57, 78*

Platysma, broad muscle extending from the chest and shoulder muscles to the side of the chin; responsible for depressing the lower jaw and lip, *44, 78*

PNS. *See* Peripheral nervous system

Poikiloderma of Civatte, a skin condition caused by actinic bronzing (chronic sun exposure) to the sides of the face and neck. The skin turns a reddish-brown hue with a distinct white patch under the chin. Poikiloderma is benign, meaning it is not cancerous, *143, 159, 174*

Poison ivy, *148*

Polycystic ovarian syndrome (PCOS), Often shortened and pronounced "peecos," is a hormonal condition that impacts women in child bearing years believed to have a genetic component. PCOS symptoms include acne, thinning hair in a male hair growth pattern of baldness as in sparse hair density at the front and top of the scalp. It also causes abnormal hair growth on the face, arms, thighs, neck, and breasts. *139–140, 173*

Polyglucans, ingredients derived from yeast cells that help strengthen the immune system and stimulate metabolism; hydrophilic and help preserve and protect collagen and elastin, *226, 258*

Polymers, chemical compounds formed by combining a number of small molecules (monomers) into long chain-like structures; advanced vehicles that release substances onto the skin's surface at a microscopically controlled rate, *211, 258*

Pores, tube-like opening for sweat glands on the epidermis, *86, 89, 118*

Posterior auricular nerve, nerve that affects the muscles behind the ear at the base of the skull, *51, 52, 78*

Postinflammatory hyperpigmentation, abbreviated as *PIH*; darkened pigmentation due to an injury to the skin or the residual healing after an acne lesion has resolved; often deep red, purple, or brown in appearance, *143, 159*

Preservatives, chemical agents that inhibit the growth of microorganisms in cosmetic formulations; they kill bacteria and prevent products from spoiling, *211, 258*
   types of, *212–213*

Primary colors, yellow, red, and blue; fundamental colors that cannot be obtained from a mixture, *553, 638*

Primary lesions, primary lesions are characterized by flat, nonpalpable changes in skin color such as macules or patches, or an elevation formed by fluid in a cavity, such as vesicles, bullae, or pustules, *123–125, 159*

Primers, liquids or silicone-based formulas designed to go underneath foundation and other products to prepare the skin for makeup and to help keep the product on the skin; primers provide a smooth surface for the makeup, while keeping product off the skin so that it is not broken down by the natural oils of the skin, *567, 638*

Procerus, muscle that covers the bridge of the nose, depresses the eyebrows, and causes wrinkles across the bridge of the nose, *43, 78*

Pronate, when muscles turn inward. for example, when the palm faces downward, *47, 78*

Protoplasm, colorless, jellylike substance in cells; contains food elements such as protein, fats, carbohydrates, mineral salts, and water, *29, 78*

Pruritus, persistent itching, *154, 160*

Pseudofolliculitis (razor bumps), resembles folliculitis without the pus or infection, *154, 160, 348, 383*

Psoriasis, skin disease characterized by red patches covered with white-silver scales. It is caused by an overproliferation of skin cells that replicate too fast. Immune dysfunction could be the cause. Psoriasis is usually found in patches on the scalp, *149, 150*

Pulmonary circulation, sends the blood from the heart to the lungs to be purified, then back to the heart again, *56, 78*

Pustule, raised, inflamed papule with a white or yellow center containing pus in the top of the lesion referred to as the head of the pimple, *125, 131, 160*

Q

Quadratus labii inferioris muscle, a muscle associated with lifting the wings of the nose and upper lip. It is sometimes called the levator labii superioris, *43, 78*

Quaternium-15, all-purpose preservative active against bacteria, mold, and yeast. Probably the greatest formaldehyde-releaser among cosmetic preservatives; may cause dermatitis and allergies, *212, 258*

R

Radial nerve, a sensory-motor nerve that, with its branches, supplies the thumb side of the arm and back of the hand, *54, 78*

Radius, smaller bone in the forearm on the same side as the thumb, *39, 40, 78*

Razor bumps. *See* Pseudofolliculitis

Reactive skin, *236*

Receptors, sensory nerve endings located close to the surface of the skin, *49, 78*

Reconstructive surgery, defined as: restoring a bodily function; necessary surgery for accident survivors and those with congenital disfigurements or other diseases, *678–679, 700*

Red blood cells, also known as *red corpuscles* or *erythrocytes;* produced in the red bone marrow; blood cells that carry oxygen from the cells back to the lungs, *57, 78*

Red light, a light-emitting diode for use on clients in the stimulation of circulation and collagen and elastin production, *665, 700*

Reflex, automatic reaction to a stimulus that involves the movement of an impulse from a sensory receptor along the sensory nerve to the spinal cord. A responsive impulse is sent along a motor neuron to a muscle, causing a reaction (for example, the quick removal of the hand from a hot object). Reflexes do not have to be learned; they are automatic, *50, 79*

Registered nurse (RN), *7*

Regular mascara, makeup that darkens, defines, and thickens the eyelashes; a good daily use product that can be easily removed with regular eye makeup remover, *570–571, 638*

Reiki, universal life-force energy transmitted through the palms of the hands that helps lift the spirits and provide balance to the whole self: body, mind, and spirit, *673, 700*

Relaxation
aromatherapy, 392
shirodhara, 673

RN. *See* Registered nurse

Renaissance era, *19*

Reproductive system, body system that includes the ovaries, uterine tubes, uterus, and vagina in the female and the testes, prostate gland, penis, and urethra in the male. This system performs the function of producing offspring and passing on the genetic code from one generation to another, *33, 64–65, 79*
herpes simplex virus 2, 150

Respiration, process of inhaling and exhaling; the act of breathing; the exchange of carbon dioxide and oxygen in the lungs and within each cell, *33, 66, 79*

Respiratory system, body system consisting of the lungs and air passages; enables breathing, which supplies the body with oxygen and eliminates carbon dioxide as a waste product, *33, 66, 79*

Retailing, makeup, *615*

Retention hyperkeratosis, hereditary factor in which dead skin cells build up and do not shed from the follicles as they do on normal skin, *133, 160*

Reticular layer, deeper layer of the dermis that supplies the skin with oxygen and nutrients; contains fat cells, blood vessels, sudoriferous (sweat) glands, hair follicles, lymph vessels, arrector pili muscles, sebaceous (oil) glands, and nerve endings, *86, 92, 100, 118*

Retin-A®. *See* Retinoic acid; Tretinoin

Retinoic acid (Retin-A®), vitamin A derivative that has demonstrated an ability to alter collagen synthesis and is used to treat acne and visible signs of aging; side effects are irritation, photosensitivity, skin dryness, redness, and peeling, *137, 221*

Retinol, natural form of vitamin A; stimulates cell repair and helps to normalize skin cells by generating new cells, *218, 221, 258*

Rhinoplasty, plastic or reconstructive surgery performed on the nose to change or correct its appearance, *680, 700*

Rhytidectomy, a face-lift procedure that removes excess fat at the jawline; tightens loose, atrophic muscles; and removes sagging skin, *679, 700*

Rhytids, wrinkles, *172, 195*

Ribs, twelve pairs of bones forming the wall of the thorax, *38, 79*

Ringworm. *See* Tinea corporis

Risorius, muscle of the mouth that draws the corner of the mouth out and back, as in grinning, *43, 79*

Roll-off masks. *See* Gommage

Rome, *ancient, 18*

Rosacea, chronic condition that appears primarily on the cheeks and nose and is characterized by flushing (redness), telangiectasis (distended or dilated surface blood vessels), and, in some cases, the formation of papules and pustules, *114, 118, 140–141, 331–333*

Rosin, a resin used in the manufacture of soft wax, *140–141, 473, 549*

Rotary brush, machine used to lightly exfoliate and stimulate the skin; also helps soften excess oil, dirt, and cell buildup, *419–421, 453*

Ruddy, refers to skin that is red, wind burned, or affected by rosacea, *558, 638*

S

Safety
of electric mitts and boots, 437
for galvanic machine, 430
high-frequency machines, 434
of hot towel cabinet, 415
of iontophoresis, 428–429
of LED, 666
of magnifying lamp, 417
of microcurrent, 667–668
of microdermabrasion, 658–660
of paraffin wax, 436
product, 200–201
of rotary brush, 420
of spray machine, 435
of steamer, 423–424
ultrasonic and ultrasound, 669
of vacuum machine, 425
of Wood's lamp, 419

Safety data sheets (SDSs), *273*

Sales manager, career as, *10*

Salesperson, *10*

Salicylic acid, beta hydroxy acid with exfoliating and antiseptic properties; natural sources include sweet birch, willow bark, and wintergreen, *218, 258*

Sallow, refers to skin that has a yellowish hue, *559, 638*

Salon or spa
adverse chemical reactions in, 145
professional image of, 268–269

Saponification, chemical reaction during desincrustation where the current transforms the sebum into soap, *427, 453*

Saturation, refers to the pureness of a color or the dominance of hue in a color, *554, 638*

Scale, flaky skin cells; any thin plate of epidermal flakes, dry or oily. An example is abnormal or excessive dandruff, *127, 160*

Scapula (shoulder blade), one of a pair of large, flat triangular bones of the shoulder, *38, 79*

Scar, light-colored, slightly raised mark on the skin formed after an injury or lesion of the skin has healed up. The tissue hardens to heal the injury. Elevated scars are hypertrophic; a keloid is a hypertrophic (abnormal) scar, *127, 160*

SCM. *See* Sternocleidomastoid

SDSs. *See* Safety data sheets

Seaweed, seaweed derivatives such as algae have many nourishing properties; known for its humectant and moisturizing properties, vitamin content, metabolism stimulation and detoxification, and aiding skin firmness, *228, 258*

Sebaceous filaments, similar to open comedones, these are mainly solidified impactions of oil without the cell matter, *132, 160*

Sebaceous glands (oil glands), protect the surface of the skin. Sebaceous glands are appendages connected to follicles, *86, 89, 91, 118, 457*

Sebaceous hyperplasia, benign lesions frequently seen in oilier areas of the face. An overgrowth of the sebaceous gland, they appear similar to open comedones; often doughnut-shaped, with sebaceous material in the center, *133, 160*

Seborrhea, severe oiliness of the skin; an abnormal secretion from the sebaceous glands, *133, 160*

Seborrheic dermatitis, common form of eczema; mainly affects oily areas; characterized by inflammation, scaling, and/or itching, *147, 160*

Sebum, oil that provides protection for the epidermis from external factors and lubricates both the skin and hair, *89, 103, 118, 131*

Secondary colors, colors obtained by mixing equal parts of two primary colors, *553, 638*

Secondary skin lesions, skin damage, developed in the later stages of disease, that changes the structure of tissues or organs, *126–127, 160*

Secretion, *89*

Secretory nerves, *103*

Self-tanning products, *248*

Sensitive skin, *236*

Sensitization, the development of hypersensitivity due to repeated exposure to an allergen that can take months or years to develop due to the allergen and intensity of exposure, *145, 160*

Sensory nerves (afferent nerves), carry impulses or messages from the sense organs to the brain, where sensations such as touch, cold, heat, sight, hearing, taste, smell, pain, and pressure are experienced; sensory nerve endings called receptors are located close to the surface of the skin, *49, 79, 87, 103*

Serums, concentrated liquid ingredients for the skin designed to penetrate and treat various skin conditions, *243, 258, 317*

Seventh cranial nerve (facial nerve), the chief motor nerve of the face. It emerges near the lower part of the ear and extends to the muscles of the neck, *51, 52, 79*

Shade, refers to degree of saturation; occurs when black is added to a pure hue, *555, 638*

Shadows, *570*

Shaving, *465*

Shiatsu, *391–392*

Shingles. *See* Herpes zoster

Shirodhara, *673*

Shoulder
   bones, 38
   muscles, 45–47

Silicone-based makeup, refers to products that are good for occluding the skin and proving a more even surface; they can also diffuse imperfections, *566, 638*

Single-use items
   handling of, 283–284
   treatment room, 277–278, 280

Sinusoidal current, a smooth, repetitive alternating current; the most commonly used alternating current waveform, used in the high frequency machine and can produce heat, *430, 453*

Skeletal system, physical foundation of the body, composed of the bones and movable and immovable joints, *32, 34, 39–40, 79*
   number of bones and composition, 35
   primary functions of, 35

Skin analysis
   Client Consent Form, 183
   client consultation, 179–188
   Client Intake Form and Medical History, 180–183
   contraindications for service, 177–179
   Fitzpatrick Scale for, 167–168
   Fitzpatrick skin types, 170–171
   genetic skin types, 164–167
   healthy habits for skin, 177
   performing, 188–193
   process of, 163–164
   sensitive skin, 169
   Service Record, 184–185
   skin conditions, causes of, 172–174
   skin conditions vs. skin types, 172–174

Spa. *See also* Salon or spa
  body treatments, 670–675
  career as spa esthetician, 6–7
Spatula-applied sugaring method, *468–469*
Special occasion, *601–603*
  airbrush makeup, 604–605
  bridal, 602
  for eyes, 602–603
  photography and video applications, 604
  for special events, 603–605
SPF. *See* Sun protection factor
Sphenoid bone, forms the sides of the eye socket, *36, 37, 79*
Spinal cord, portion of the central nervous system that originates in the brain, extends down to the lower extremity of the trunk, and is protected by the spinal column, *49, 79*
Spray machine, spray misting device, *434–435, 453*
Springer, Pamela, *21*
Squalane, derived from olives; desensitizes and nourishes; an emollient, *233, 258*
Squamous cell carcinoma, type of skin cancer more serious than basal cell carcinoma; characterized by scaly, red or pink papules or nodules; also appear as open sores or crusty areas; can grow and spread in the body, *129, 160*
Stasis dermatitis, chronic inflammatory state in the legs due to poor circulation; the legs may sometimes have ulcerations, along with scaly skin, itching, and hyperpigmentation, *147, 160*
State board member, *14–15*
State licensing inspector, *14*
Steamer, *421–424*
Steatoma, sebaceous cyst or subcutaneous tumor filled with sebum; ranges in size from a pea to an orange. It usually appears on the scalp, neck, and back; also called a *wen, 154, 160*
Sternocleidomastoid (SCM), muscle of the neck that depresses and rotates the head, *44, 79*
Sternum (breastbone), the flat bone that forms the ventral support of the ribs, *39, 79*
Stone massage, use of hot stones and cold stones in massage or in other treatments, *672, 700*
Stratum corneum (horny layer), outermost layer of the epidermis, composed of corneocytes, *86, 91, 97–98, 100, 118*
Stratum germinativum, also known as *basal cell layer*; active layer of the epidermis above the papillary layer of the dermis; cell mitosis takes place here to produce new epidermal skin cells (responsible for growth), *95–96, 100, 118*
Stratum granulosum (granular layer), layer of the epidermis composed of cells filled with keratin that resemble granules; replace cells shed from the stratum corneum, *86, 91, 100, 118*
Stratum lucidum, clear, transparent layer of the epidermis under the stratum corneum; thickest on the palms of hands and soles of feet, *86, 91, 97, 100, 118*
Stratum spinosum (spiny layer), layer of the epidermis above the stratum germinativum layer containing desmosomes, the intercellular connections made of proteins, *86, 91, 96–97, 100, 118*
Stress, skin aging from, *175*
Striae, dermal scars due to rapid expansion or stretching of connective tissue leaving deep red, pink, or purple linear marks on the skin that gradually fade to light pink or silver over time. they often occur during growth phases in puberty, pregnancy, and weight gain, *174, 195*
Subcutaneous layer (hypodermis), subcutaneous adipose (fat) tissue located beneath the dermis; a protective cushion and energy storage for the body, *86, 91, 99, 118*
Subcutis tissue, also known as adipose tissue; fatty tissue found below the dermis that gives smoothness and contour to the body, contains fat for use as energy, and also acts as a protective cushion for the outer skin, *91, 118*
Suction machine. *See* Vacuum machine
Sudoriferous glands (sweat glands), excrete perspiration, regulate body temperature, and detoxify the body by excreting excess salt and unwanted chemicals, *89, 104, 118*
  disorders of, 154–155
Sugaring, ancient method of hair removal. The original recipe is a mixture of sugar, lemon juice, and water that is heated to form syrup, molded into a ball, and pressed onto the skin and then quickly stripped away, *467–469, 549*
Sulfur, reduces the activity of oil glands and dissolves the skin's surface layer of dry, dead cells; commonly used in acne products, *234, 258*
Sun exposure, *128*
Sun protection factor, abbreviated SPF; indicates the ability of a product to delay sun-induced erythema, the visible sign of sun damage; the SPF rating is based only on UVB protection, not UVA exposure, *246, 258*
  rating, 246–247
  types of, 247
Sun protection product, *318*
Sunscreen ingredients, *226–227*
Supinate, when muscles rotate, for example, in the forearm, the radius turns outward and the palm upward, *47, 80*

Supraorbital nerve, nerve that affects the skin of the forehead, scalp, eyebrow, and upper eyelid, *51, 52, 80*

Supratrochlear nerve, nerve that affects the skin between the eyes and upper side of the nose, *51, 52, 80*

Surfactants, *208*
  types, *209–210*

Sweat glands. *See* Sudoriferous glands

Sweat pore, *91*

Syndrome, a group of symptoms that, when combined, characterize a disease or disorder

Systemic circulation, circulation of blood from the heart throughout the body and back again to the heart, *56, 80*

T

Tabs, small clusters of three or four artificial eyelashes on one point of attachment, *606, 639*

Tan, increase in pigmentation due to the melanin production that results from exposure to UV radiation; visible skin damage. Melanin is designed to help protect the skin from the sun's UV radiation, *143, 160*

Tapotement (percussion), movements consisting of short, quick tapping, slapping, and hacking movements, *390, 409*

Tazarotene (Tazorac®), *137*

TCA peels. *See* Trichloroacetic acid peels

T-cells, identify molecules that have foreign peptides and also help regulate immune response, *105, 118*

Tea tree oil, soothing and antiseptic; antifungal properties, *234, 258*

"Tech neck," rhytids that develop due to the repeated movement of looking down at a cell phone or other electronic device, *171, 195*

Telangiectasia, capillaries that have been damaged and are now larger, or distended blood vessels; commonly called *couperose skin, 114, 118, 141, 169, 195*

Telogen, also known as *resting phase;* the final phase in the hair cycle that lasts until the fully grown hair is shed, *460, 549*

Temporal bones, bones forming the sides of the head in the ear region, *36, 80*

Temporal nerve, nerve affecting the muscles of the temple, side of the forehead, eyebrow, eyelid, and upper part of the cheek, *51, 53, 80*

Temporalis muscle, temporal muscle; one of the muscles involved in mastication (chewing), *44, 80*

Terminal hair, longer coarse hair that is found on the head, face and body, *458, 549*

Tertiary colors, intermediate color achieved by mixing a secondary color and its neighboring

primary color on the color wheel in equal amounts, *553–554, 639*

Testes, male organs which produce the male hormone testosterone, *64, 80*

Tetrahexyldecyl ascorbate, *222*

TEWL. *See* Transepidermal water loss

Textured skin, *563*

Thermal masks. *See* Modelage masks

Thermolysis, heat effect; used for permanent hair removal, *431, 453, 661, 700*

Thermolysis, heat effect; a modality of electrolysis utilizing alternating current (AC); used for permanent hair removal, *431, 453, 470, 549, 661, 700*

Thickeners, *215*

Thorax, also known as *chest* or *pulmonary trunk;* consists of the sternum, ribs, and thoracic vertebrae; elastic, bony cage that serves as a protective framework for the heart, lungs, and other internal organs, *38, 80*

Threading, also known as *banding;* method of hair removal; cotton thread is twisted and rolled along the surface of the skin, entwining hair in the thread and lifting it out of the follicle, *466–467, 549*

Thymus gland, *63*

Thyroid gland, a gland located in the neck; controls how quickly the body burns energy (metabolism), makes proteins, and how sensitive the body should be to other hormones, *64, 80*

Tinea, a contagious condition caused by fungal infection and not a parasite; characterized by itching, scales, and, sometimes, painful lesions, *151, 161*

Tinea corporis (ringworm), a contagious infection that forms a ringed, red pattern with elevated edges, *151, 161*

Tinea versicolor, also known as *sun spots;* a noncontagious fungal infection which is characterized by white or varicolored patches on the skin and is often found on arms and legs, *144, 161*

Tint, refers to degree of saturation; occurs when white is added to a pure hue, *555, 639*

Tissue, collection of similar cells that perform a particular function, *31, 80*

Titanium dioxide, inorganic physical sunscreen that reflects UV radiation, *227, 258*

Tone (skin), also known as *hue;* in terms of skin, this is a term used to describe the warmth or coolness of a color; generally classified as light, medium, or dark, *557, 639*

Toners, also known as *fresheners* or *astringents;* liquids designed to tone and tighten the skin's surface, *239, 258, 317*
  client home-care instruction sheet, *250*

Touch, *skin receptors, 86–87*

Urea, properties include enhancing the penetrative abilities of other substances; antiinflammatory, antiseptic, and deodorizing action that protects the skin's surface and helps maintain healthy skin, *205, 258*

Urticaria, also known as *hives*; caused by an allergic reaction from the body's histamine production, *127, 161*

USDA. *See* Department of Agriculture, U. S.

UVA radiation (aging rays), longer wavelengths ranging between 320 to 400 nanometers that penetrate deeper into the skin than UVB; cause genetic damage and cell death. UVA contribute up to 95 percent of the sun's ultraviolet radiation, *107–108, 119*

UVB radiation (burning rays), these wavelengths range between 290 to 320 nanometers. UVB rays have shorter, burning wavelengths that are stronger and more damaging than UVA rays. UVB cause burning of the skin as well as tanning, skin aging, and cancer, *108, 119*

V

Vacuum machine (suction machine), device that vacuums/suctions the skin to remove impurities and stimulate circulation, *424–426, 453*

Vagus nerve, located in the abdominal cavity, a nerve of the autonomic nervous system, *54, 80*

Value, also known as *brightness of a color*; how light or dark it is, which depends on the amount of light emanating from the color, *555, 639*

Varicella-zoster virus. *See* Herpes zoster

Varicose veins, vascular lesions; dilated and twisted veins, most commonly in the legs, *141, 161*

Vasoconstricting, refers to something that causes vascular constriction of capillaries and reduced blood flow, *333, 383*

Vasodilation, vascular dilation of the blood vessels, *140, 161*

Vegan, a product that is labeled vegan should not contain any animal ingredients or animal by-products, *203, 259*

Vehicles, spreading agents and ingredients that carry or deliver other ingredients into the skin and make them more effective, *211, 259*

Veins, thin-walled blood vessels that are less elastic than arteries; they contain cuplike valves to prevent backflow and carry impure blood from the various capillaries back to the heart and lungs, *56, 80*
of head, face, and neck, *58–59*
layers of skin and, *86*

Vellus hair, also known as *lanugo hair*; short, fine, unpigmented downy hair that appears on the body, with the exception of the palms of the hands and the soles of the feet, *458, 549*

Venules, small vessels that connect the capillaries to the veins. They collect blood from the capillaries and drain it into veins, *56, 81*

Vermillion border, the border of the lip line, *490, 549*

Verruca (wart), hypertrophy of the papillae and epidermis caused by a virus. It is infectious and contagious, *152, 161*

Vertebral column, *38*

Vesicle, small blister or sac containing clear fluid. Poison ivy and poison oak produce vesicles, *125, 161*

Vestibulocochlear nerve, *50*

Vibration, in massage, the rapid shaking movement in which the technician uses the body and shoulders, not just the fingertips, to create the movement, *390–391, 409*

Vichy shower, *671*

Victoria (queen), *19*

Victorian Age, *19*

Video makeup, *604*

Vitamin A, *221, 223, 234, 336*

Vitamin B. *See* B vitamins

Vitamin B3, *223*

Vitamin B5, *222*

Vitamin C, *222*

Vitamin C phosphate, *222*

Vitamin E, *222*

Vitamin K, *223*

Vitamins, *221–223*
skin aging from deficient, *176*

Vitiligo, pigmentation disease characterized by white patches on the skin from lack of pigment cells; made worse by sunlight, *144, 161*

W

Warm colors, the range of colors with yellow undertones; from yellow and gold through oranges, red-oranges, most reds, and even some yellow-greens, *556, 639*

Wart. *See* Verruca

Water based makeup, refers to oil-free products; water-based foundations generally give a more matte finish and help conceal minor blemishes and discolorations, *566, 639*

Water, *204–205. See also* Balneotherapy
hydrolipidic film, *87*

Water soluble, mixable with water, *217, 259*

Waterproof mascara, makeup that darkens, defines, and thickens the eyelashes; is designed to stay on and not smudge when it comes in contact with water, *571, 639*

Wax, postwax instructions and precautions, *481*

Wax equipment, *483–487*
    consumables, 484
    contaminated waste items, disposal of, 486
    disposable items, 484
    draping and disposable protection, 485–486
    gloves, 486
    hand washing and infection control measures, 486
    hygiene and infection control, 485
    mastering clean-up, 486
    table and chair protection, 485

Wax release form, *478–480*

Wax treatment
    essentials, 484
    room, 483–487

Waxing, *469–470*
    arm and hand, 492, 516–523
    back, 493
    bikini, 493–494, 536–541
    chest, 492–493
    chin, 490
    eyebrows, 488–489, 499–504
    facial, during facial, 477–478
    general, dos and don'ts, 487–488
    leg, 494, 542–547
    lip, 489–490, 505–508
    lower body, 493–494
    men's back, 528–535
    men's chest, 524–527
    sides of face, 490
    underarm (axilla), 491, 510–515
    upper arm, 492
    upper body on women and men, 492

Waxing specialists, *7–9*

Wet microdermabrasion, *656*

Wheal, itchy, swollen lesion caused by a blow, insect bite, skin allergy reaction, or stings. Hives and mosquito bites are wheals. Hives (urticaria) can be caused by exposure to allergens used in products, *125, 161*

White blood cells (white corpuscles, leukocytes), perform the function of destroying disease causing germs, *57, 81, 94*

Witch hazel, extracted from the bark of the hamanelis shrub; can be a soothing agent or, in higher concentrations, an astringent, *234, 259*

Women
    waxing, 488–494
        face, 488–489
        lower body, 493–494
        upper body, 492

Wood's Lamp, filtered black light that is used to illuminate skin disorders, fungi, bacterial disorders, and pigmentation, *188, 195, 417–419, 453*

Wrinkle treatments, *678*

Wrist. *See* Carpus

Y

Yellow light, light-emitting diode that aids in reducing inflammation and swelling, *665, 701*

Z

Zinc oxide, mineral physical sunscreen ingredient that reflects UVA and UVB rays; also used to protect, soothe, and heal the skin; is somewhat astringent, antiseptic, and antimicrobial, *205, 259*

Zygomatic bones (malar bones, cheekbones), bones that form the prominence of the cheeks; the cheekbones, *37, 81*

Zygomatic nerve, nerve that affects the skin of the temple, side of the forehead, and upper part of the cheek, *51, 52, 81*

Zygomaticus, consists of major and minor muscles extending from the zygomatic bone to the angle of the mouth that elevates the lip, as in laughing, *43, 81*